ORAL MICROBIOLOGY AND IMMUNOLOGY

ORAL MICROBIOLOGY AND IMMUNOLOGY

EDITED BY

Richard J. Lamont
Department of Oral Biology
University of Florida College of Dentistry
Gainesville, Florida

Robert A. Burne
Department of Oral Biology
University of Florida College of Dentistry
Gainesville, Florida

Marilyn S. Lantz
School of Dentistry
University of Michigan
Ann Arbor, Michigan

Donald J. LeBlanc
Global Research and Development
Pfizer, Inc.
Ann Arbor, Michigan

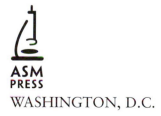

ASM
PRESS

WASHINGTON, D.C.

Address editorial correspondence to ASM Press, 1752 N St. NW, Washington, DC 20036-2904, USA

Send orders to ASM Press, P.O. Box 605, Herndon, VA 20172, USA
Phone: (800) 546-2416 or (703) 661-1593
Fax: (703) 661-1501
E-mail: books@asmusa.org
Online: estore.asm.org

Library of Congress Cataloging-in-Publication Data

Oral microbiology and immunology / edited by Richard J. Lamont ... [et al.].
p. ; cm.
Includes bibliographical references and index.
ISBN-13: 978-1-55581-262-1 (pbk.)
ISBN-10: 1-55581-262-7 (pbk.)
1. Mouth—Microbiology. 2. Mouth—Immunology. I. Lamont, Richard J., 1961–
[DNLM: 1. Mouth Diseases—microbiology. 2. Mouth—microbiology. 3. Tooth Diseases—microbiology. WU 140 O627 2006]

QR47.O73 2006
617.5′22—dc22

2006009411

10 9 8 7 6 5 4 3 2 1

Cover and interior design: Susan Brown Schmidler

Cover photo: Porphyromonas gingivalis invasion of gingival epithelial cells. The host cell nuclei (blue) and actin cytoskeleton (red) are also stained. Courtesy of Ozlem Yilmaz, University of Florida College of Dentistry.

Contents

4   Isolation, Classification, and Identification of Oral Microorganisms   73

EUGENE J. LEYS, ANN L. GRIFFEN, PURNIMA S. KUMAR, AND MARK F. MAIDEN

12 Periodontal Diseases   253

Susan Kinder Haake, Diane Hutchins Meyer, Paula M. Fives-Taylor, and Harvey Schenkein

15 Endodontic Microbiology   349

Burton Rosan and Louis Rossman

16 Systemic Disease and the Oral Microbiota   361

Susan Camp, Yu Lei, Massimo Costalonga, Yongshu Zhang, Alexandre Zaia, Reka Vajna, Karen F. Ross, and Mark C. Herzberg

18 Infection Control in Dentistry   423

J. Christopher Fenno, Wilson A. Coulter, and Dennis E. Lopatin

Contributors

Robert A. Burne
Department of Oral Biology, University of Florida College of Dentistry, Gainesville, FL 32610

Susan Camp
Department of Oral Sciences, School of Dentistry, University of Minnesota, Minneapolis, MN 55455

Richard D. Cannon
Department of Oral Sciences and Orthodontics, University of Otago, P.O. Box 647, Dunedin, New Zealand

Michael F. Cole
Department of Microbiology and Immunology, Georgetown University School of Medicine, 3900 Reservoir Rd. NW, Washington, DC 20007

Massimo Costalonga
Department of Oral Sciences, School of Dentistry, University of Minnesota, Minneapolis, MN 55455

Wilson A. Coulter
School of Dentistry, Queen's University, Grosvenor Rd., Belfast BT12 6BP, United Kingdom

J. Christopher Fenno
Department of Biologic and Materials Sciences, University of Michigan, 1011 N. University Ave., Ann Arbor, MI 48109-1078

Norman A. Firth
Department of Stomatology, University of Otago, P.O. Box 647, Dunedin, New Zealand

Paula M. Fives-Taylor
Department of Microbiology and Molecular Genetics, 116 Stafford Hall, University of Vermont, 95 Carrigan Dr., Burlington, VT 05405

Hansel M. Fletcher
Department of Microbiology and Molecular Genetics, School of Medicine, Loma Linda University, Loma Linda, CA 92350

Thomas R. Flynn
Department of Oral and Maxillofacial Surgery, Harvard School of Dental Medicine, 188 Longwood Ave., Boston, MA 02115

Ann L. Griffen
Department of Pediatric Dentistry, The Ohio State University, 305 W. Twelfth Ave., Columbus, OH 43210

Susan Kinder Haake
Section on Periodontics, UCLA School of Dentistry, Los Angeles, CA 90095

Mark C. Herzberg
Department of Oral Sciences, School of Dentistry, University of Minnesota, Minneapolis, MN 55455

Jeffrey D. Hillman
Department of Oral Biology, University of Florida College of Dentistry, Gainesville, FL 32610

Howard F. Jenkinson
Department of Oral and Dental Science, Dental Hospital and School, University of Bristol, Lower Maudlin St., Bristol BS1 2LY, United Kingdom

Mogens Kilian
Institute of Medical Microbiology and Immunology, Faculty of Health Sciences, Bartholin Building, University of Aarhus, DK-8000 Aarhus C, Denmark

Purnima S. Kumar
Department of Oral Biology, The Ohio State University, 305 W. Twelfth Ave., Columbus, OH 43210

Richard J. Lamont
Department of Oral Biology, College of Dentistry, University of Florida, Gainesville, FL 32610-0424

Marilyn S. Lantz
Department of Periodontics, Prevention, and Geriatrics, School of Dentistry, University of Michigan, Ann Arbor, MI 48109-1078

Donald J. LeBlanc
Antibacterial Molecular Sciences, Global Research and Development, Ann Arbor Laboratories, Pfizer, Inc., Ann Arbor, MI 48105

Yu Lei
Department of Oral Sciences, School of Dentistry, University of Minnesota, Minneapolis, MN 55455

Eugene J. Leys
Department of Oral Biology, 3185 Postle, The Ohio State University, 305 W. Twelfth Ave., Columbus, OH 43210

Dennis E. Lopatin
University of Michigan School of Dentistry, 1011 N. University Ave., Campus Box 1078, Ann Arbor, MI 48109-1078

Peter M. Lydyard
Department of Immunology and Molecular Pathology, Windeyer Institute for Medical Sciences, Royal Free and University College Medical School, 46 Cleveland St., London W1T 4JF, United Kingdom

Mark F. Maiden
Department of Molecular Genetics, The Forsyth Institute, 140 Fenway, Boston, MA 02115

Robert E. Marquis
Department of Microbiology and Immunology and Center for Oral Biology, University of Rochester Medical Center, Rochester, NY 14642-8672

Diane Hutchins Meyer
Department of Microbiology and Molecular Genetics, 116 Stafford Hall, University of Vermont, 95 Carrigan Dr., Burlington, VT 05405

Ann Progulske-Fox
Department of Oral Biology, University of Florida College of Dentistry, Gainesville, FL 32610

Robert G. Quivey, Jr.
Center for Oral Biology, Department of Microbiology and Immunology, University of Rochester School of Medicine and Dentistry, Rochester, NY 14642

Burton Rosan
School of Dental Medicine, University of Pennsylvania, 4010 Locust St., Philadelphia, PA 19104-6002

Karen F. Ross
Department of Oral Sciences, School of Dentistry, University of Minnesota, Minneapolis, MN 55455

Louis Rossman
Department of Endodontics, School of Dental Medicine, University of Pennsylvania, 4010 Locust St., Philadelphia, PA 19104-6002

Matti Sällberg
Division of Clinical Virology, F68, Karolinska Institutet at Huddinge University Hospital, S-141 86 Huddinge, Sweden

Frank A. Scannapieco
Department of Oral Biology, School of Dental Medicine, University at Buffalo, The State University of New York, Buffalo, NY 14214

Harvey Schenkein
Department of Periodontics, School of Dentistry, Virginia Commonwealth University, Richmond, VA 23298

Constantine Simos
Oral Surgery Group, 109 Livingston Ave., New Brunswick, NJ 08901-2410

Reka Vajna
Department of Oral Sciences, School of Dentistry, University of Minnesota, Minneapolis, MN 55455

Alexandre Zaia
Department of Oral Sciences, School of Dentistry, University of Minnesota, Minneapolis, MN 55455

Yongshu Zhang
Department of Oral Sciences, School of Dentistry, University of Minnesota, Minneapolis, MN 55455

Preface

The oral cavity represents the entry portal for both the respiratory tract and the gastrointestinal tract, and as such it is subject to unique ecological constraints. The microbial inhabitants of this ecosystem therefore differ from those found anywhere else in the body or, indeed, anywhere else in the world. Mostly harmless by nature, these microorganisms can cause disease when opportunity presents. In fact, microbial diseases of the oral cavity, such as caries (tooth decay) and periodontal (gum) disease, are among the most common infectious diseases of humans. Despite their importance, most microbiology textbooks pay scant attention to oral microorganisms. This book seeks to redress the balance. The first two chapters provide an orientation to general microbiology and immunology; then the heart and soul of the text is devoted to oral microorganisms, the diseases they cause, the host responses they engender, and the means for their control and destruction. If you are a dental student, a dental practitioner, or involved in any health-related discipline, this book will provide you with a complete resource on oral microbiology and oral immunology.

In a multiauthored endeavor such as this, it is the contributors of the individual chapters who deserve all the credit. Our gratitude is also extended to numerous colleagues, too many to mention, who reviewed and critiqued the manuscript. Finally, we thank the staff at ASM Press for their infinite patience and support.

About the Editors

Richard J. Lamont received a bachelor of science degree from the University of Edinburgh and a doctorate from the University of Aberdeen. After a postdoctoral fellowship at the University of Pennsylvania, he accepted a faculty position at the University of Washington, later moving to the University of Florida. His primary research interests are in the molecular basis of the formation and development of the dental plaque biofilm and in the cellular interactions between oral bacteria and the host epithelium. He has been teaching microbiology and immunology to dental students and residents since 1988.

Robert A. Burne received his bachelor of science degree in microbiology from the Pennsylvania State University. He completed his Ph.D. training in 1987 at the University of Rochester School of Medicine and Dentistry, where he initiated molecular genetic studies of polysaccharide metabolism by *Streptococcus mutans*. He pursued postdoctoral training at Rochester, focusing on pH homeostasis in oral streptococci, and assumed a faculty position there in the School of Medicine and Dentistry in 1990. In 2001, he moved to the University of Florida, where he continues his studies on the molecular genetics, physiology, and pathogenesis of oral biofilm bacteria.

Marilyn S. Lantz received her bachelor's degree in chemistry from Queens College of the City University of New York and her Ph.D. in biochemistry from the City University of New York. She received her D.M.D. from Southern Illinois University and her certificate in periodontology and M.S.D. degree from the University of Connecticut. She has held faculty positions at the Southern Illinois University School of Dental Medicine, the University of Connecticut School of Dental Medicine, the University of Alabama School of Dentistry, the University of Pittsburgh School of Dental Medicine (where she served as chair of the Department of Periodontics), and Indiana University School of Dentistry (where she served as chair of the Department of Oral Biology). Her research interests have centered on mechanisms of bacterial pathogenesis in periodontitis,

xxiv About the Editors

and she has taught microbiology and periodontics to dental students and residents since 1984. Since 2000, she has held the positions of professor of periodontics and oral medicine and associate dean for academic affairs at the University of Michigan School of Dentistry.

Donald J. LeBlanc received his bachelor's and master's degrees in biology from St. Michael's College in Winooski, Vt., and Fordham University in Bronx, N.Y., respectively. He obtained a Ph.D. in microbiology from the University of Massachusetts at Amherst, where he conducted his dissertation research on the evolution of bacterial carbohydrate catabolic pathways. Don obtained postdoctoral training in bacterial genetics at Georgetown University in Washington, D.C., and in molecular biology at the National Cancer Institute in Bethesda, Md. He spent the first 6 years of his independent research career as a research microbiologist at the National Institute for Dental Research in Bethesda, followed by 7 years as chief of the Bacterial Virulence Section at the National Institute for Allergy and Infectious Diseases at Fort Detrick, Frederick, Md. He moved on to an academic career, accepting the position of professor in the Department of Microbiology at the University of Texas Health Science Center in San Antonio. After 8 years in San Antonio, he moved to Indianapolis, Ind., to serve for 3 years as director of the Graduate Program in Oral Biology at the Indiana University School of Dentistry. Most of Don's National Institutes of Health and academic research involved studies on the physiology and genetics of streptococci, enterococci, and lactococci, as well as oral bacterial species, and on the genetic basis of antibiotic resistance. The final 7 years of Don's professional career involved the pursuit of antibiotic discovery research in the pharmaceutical industry, from which he retired in October 2005.

SECTION 1 GENERAL PRINCIPLES OF ORAL MICROBIOLOGY

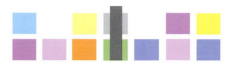

General Microbiology

Robert A. Burne

INTRODUCTION

Antony van Leeuwenhoek was a Dutch scientist who, in many respects, started the discipline of microbiology. Using simple microscopes that he had fashioned in his workshop, van Leeuwenhoek made the first observations of bacteria and microorganisms, which he called "animalcules." In 1683, van Leeuwenhoek scraped material from his own teeth, describing "a little white matter, which is as thick as if 'twere batter." He continued, "I then most always saw. . .that in the said matter there were many very little living animalcules." When observing a sample from an old man who had not cleaned his teeth, van Leeuwenhoek found "an unbelievably great company of living animalcules, a-swimming more nimbly than any I had ever seen up to this time. Moreover, the other animalcules were in such enormous numbers, that all the water. . . seemed to be alive." These observations of the oral microbiota were among the first recorded sightings of live bacteria. Today, we know that the human oral cavity is a highly dynamic ecosystem that supports the growth of a tremendous number of very diverse organisms. In fact, there are roughly a million microorganisms per milliliter of saliva. The organisms present in saliva, mostly bacteria and a few fungi, are there because they are shed from the hard and soft tissues of the oral cavity and nasopharynx and they multiply in retained pools of saliva. The use of microbiological techniques, coupled with sophisticated and sensitive technologies in molecular biology, has helped us begin to gain an appreciation for the diversity of the oral microbiota. Recent estimates place the number of different species of bacteria in the oral cavity at somewhere near 600. Research into the genetics, physiology, and biochemistry of the oral microbiota has shown that the normal colonizers are a critical component in oral health and has led to an understanding of the importance of oral ecology in the development of diseases.

To fully understand how oral microorganisms persist and, under certain circumstances, cause disease, it is necessary to have an understanding of the structure, function, and biological activities of the oral microbiota. Why? Knowledge of the structural components of a microorganism is important because determinants on the cell surface dictate which tissues

3

the organisms can colonize. Likewise, many components that contribute to the ability of the organisms to cause disease and damage host tissues are located on the cell surface. It is also important to have an appreciation for the wide variety of biological and biochemical activities that oral microorganisms possess. The metabolic capabilities of the cells—their ability to degrade the substances secreted in saliva and ingested in the diet—are of major importance in oral health and disease. How effectively organisms utilize the available nutrients determines whether an organism will establish and compete effectively at particular sites in the mouth. Moreover, the end products produced from metabolism of these nutrients, such as organic acids, have harmful effects on the tissues of the mouth. The following sections of this chapter highlight key features of the classification, structure, and functions of bacteria with the goal of providing a foundation for the more detailed descriptions of oral microbes, oral microbial ecology, growth of the oral microbiota, and the virulence mechanisms used by oral pathogens that are presented in the remainder of this text.

CLASSIFICATION SCHEMES FOR BACTERIA

The system that is commonly used for classification of life on Earth is derived from that developed by Carl Linnaeus in the 18th century. This classification scheme, originally used for systematics of plants and animals, has been useful in accommodating new forms of life as they were discovered through the centuries. Today, life on Earth is divided into three primary domains: *Eukarya*, which are eukaryotes, and *Bacteria* and *Archaea*, which are prokaryotes, the oldest and most diverse forms of life on the planet (Table 1). Archaea, which are sometimes referred to as archaebacteria, differ genetically and metabolically from true bacteria. In fact, archaea are considered to bridge a major gap in evolution between prokaryotes and eukaryotes. The prokaryotes are distinguished from eukaryotes, members of the domain *Eukarya*, most notably by the lack of a nuclear membrane, which separates the chromosomal DNA of the

TABLE I General differences between prokaryotes and eukaryotes

Property	Domain		
	Eukarya	**Bacteria**	**Archaea**
Nuclear membrane	+	−	−
Chromosomes	>1	1	1
Chromosome organization	Linear	Circular	Circular
Murein in cell wall	−	+	−
Cell membrane lipids	Ester-linked glycerides; unbranched, polyunsaturated	Ester-linked glycerides; unbranched; saturated or monounsaturated	Ether-linked; branched; saturated
Cell membrane sterols	Present	Absent	Absent
Organelles	Present	Absent	Absent
Ribosome size	80S	70S	70S
Transcription/translation coupling	No	Yes	Yes

organisms from the cytoplasmic contents. Eukaryotes also possess a variety of organelles and subcellular structures—like mitochondria, the Golgi apparatus, and the endoplasmic reticulum—that are lacking in prokaryotes. There are a variety of other fundamental differences between these two general classes of life, some of which are summarized in Table 1. Among the more notable differences, the transcription of DNA to mRNA and the translation of RNA to protein occur in separate compartments in eukaryotes, but not in prokaryotes.

Members of each of the domains can be found in the oral cavity, although the vast majority of the oral microbiota is composed of bacteria. Through highly sensitive techniques, archaea have been detected in the oral cavity, but, at least from what is currently known, they appear to represent a small minority of the total organisms present on oral soft or hard tissues. Fungi, which are eukaryotic microorganisms, can also be present in the mouth, but generally are there in low numbers and flourish only when there is a restriction of access to saliva or a reduction in immunological competence (see chapter 14). Because bacteria comprise the overwhelming majority of oral microorganisms, most of this introductory chapter focuses on bacteria.

BACTERIAL CLASSIFICATION

Most bacteria can be lumped into two categories, gram-positive and gram-negative, based on a differential staining technique developed by a Danish bacteriologist, Christian Gram. The Gram stain reveals a major structural difference between the two major groups of bacteria based on the thickness and degree of cross-linking of the cell wall. Detailed molecular studies have revealed that this relatively simple staining reaction also discloses a major evolutionary split between two major classes of bacteria. Among the bacteria, there are also organisms that cannot appropriately be classified on the basis of Gram staining, such as the agent of tuberculosis, *Mycobacterium tuberculosis*, which has a cell envelope made of mycolic acids and waxes, making it substantially different from most bacteria. Instead of Gram staining, mycobacteria can be stained by the Ziehl-Neelsen staining technique, which is also called acid-fast staining. In contrast, *Mycoplasma* species and closely related organisms are completely devoid of a cell wall, and thus, these organisms are negative in the Gram reaction—even though genetically they are more closely related to gram-positive bacteria. Gram staining and similar techniques remain useful for bacterial identification, but the phylogenetic relationships, i.e., the evolutionary relationships of bacteria, are now based almost exclusively on comparisons of nucleotide and protein sequences of organisms. Chapters 4 and 9 explain in detail many of the techniques and rationale used to speciate bacteria and outline the current phylogenetic relationships of the oral microbiota.

One of the most fascinating aspects of studying microorganisms is the tremendous diversity in microbial structure, metabolic capacities, and environments in which these organisms can thrive. In nature, there are bacteria that grow optimally at pH values around 2 (acidophiles), whereas others will only grow well at pH values near 10 (alkalophiles). Some prokaryotes grow very poorly at temperatures above 15°C (psychrophiles), whereas some thrive at 100°C in hydrothermal vents miles below the surface of the ocean (thermophiles). Some microorganisms can grow with jet fuel or kerosene as the primary carbon and energy source; some create tiny magnets inside and use them for directed movement; some emit light; and others detoxify mercury in the environment. A variety of bacteria can corrode metals and many synthesize products of significant economic importance, such as antibiotics or complex polysaccharides that are used in foods or pharmaceuticals.

Bacteria in and on the human body outnumber the cells composing the body by about 10 to 1, but the list of bacteria that colonize humans is fairly small compared to the total number of known bacteria, and the number that routinely cause disease is substantially smaller still. Interestingly, the oral microbial community is among the most diverse group of organisms colonizing the various environments of a human host. To begin to become familiar with the organisms that comprise the oral microbiota in health and diseases, some of the more abundant and significant oral microorganisms are listed in Table 2.

TABLE 2 Microorganisms of importance in the oral cavity

Gram-positive bacteria	Gram-negative bacteria
Streptococcus mutans	Fusobacterium nucleatum
S. sanguis	F. periodonticum
S. oralis	
S. mitis	Haemophilus parainfluenzae
S. sanguis	
S. parasanguis	Porphyromonas gingivalis
S. salivarius	P. endodontalis
S. anginosus	
	Prevotella intermedia
Rothia dentocariosa	P. loescheii
	P. denticola
Actinomyces naeslundii	P. melanogenica
A. gerensceriae	P. nigrescens
A. odontolyticus	P. oralis
Lactobacillus casei	Bacteroides odontolyticus
L. salivarius	B. ureolyticum
L. fermentum	
L. plantarum	Tannerella forsythensis
Eubacterium nodatum	Neisseria subflava
Peptostreptococcus micros	Veillonella parvula
P. anaerobius	
	Actinobacillus actinomycetemcomitans
Propionibacterium acnes	
	Capnocytophaga ochracea
	C. gingivalis
	Treponema denticola
	T. socranskii
	T. pertinovorum

BACTERIAL ARCHITECTURE

Most bacteria are about 1 to 5 μm across the largest dimension of the cell, although there are some interesting exceptions, including a few unusual marine bacteria that are as large as 100 μm in diameter. A bacterial colony that is roughly 3 mm in diameter that forms on an agar plate can contain upward of 100 million organisms. Bacteria also come in a wide variety of shapes: coccoid or spherical, bacillary or rod-shaped, fusiform or long thin rods that taper at the ends, helical or corkscrew-shaped, curved, irregular, or a combination of shapes. In addition, many bacteria can form complex, multicellular structures or can differentiate into alternative shapes with clearly distinct functions and metabolic potential.

Membranes

As with all living cells, biological membranes separate the contents of the cell from the surroundings. The cytoplasmic membrane of the bacteria separates an amazingly concentrated collection of proteins, nucleic acids, lipids, and other constituents from its surroundings. The protein concentration of a typical bacterial cell is estimated at 350 mg of protein per ml, compared, for instance, with plasma that contains only tens of milligrams per milliliter. Gram-positive bacteria possess a single plasma membrane, or cytoplasmic membrane. Gram-negative bacteria are characterized by the presence of two membranes, a cytoplasmic membrane and an outer membrane (Fig. 1). The space between the inner and outer membranes of gram-negative bacteria is known as the periplasm or periplasmic space. The membranes of bacteria are not radically different from those of mammalian or plant cells in the sense that they consist of a phospholipid bilayer. However, unlike eukaryotic membranes, the membranes of bacteria lack sterols, such as cholesterol, and are composed primarily of saturated or monounsaturated fatty acids, rather than polyunsaturated fatty acids. Membranes of archaea also are composed of a phospholipid bilayer, but the membrane lipids are attached to the glycerol moiety by ether linkages, rather than the ester linkages typical of bacteria and

FIGURE 1 Schematic diagram illustrating the differences between the surface of gram-positive and gram-negative bacteria. See text for details.

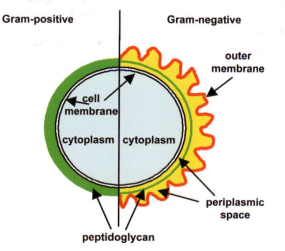

eukaryotes. The actual composition of membranes of a given bacterial species, i.e., the number of carbons in the lipids and whether the lipids are monounsaturated or completely unsaturated, can change depending on growth conditions. However, the lipid composition of a given species remains fairly consistent when the bacteria are grown under similar conditions. On the other hand, the membrane lipid composition of different species of bacteria can vary quite a bit. Consequently, it has been possible to distinguish between even fairly closely related bacteria by comparing the composition of the lipids in the membranes of isolated bacteria grown under defined conditions.

Many biologically important proteins and enzymes are embedded in the membranes of bacteria. The cytoplasmic membrane of bacteria houses the machinery for respiration, for sensing environmental signals, and for transporting compounds and macromolecules into and out of the cell. Many membrane proteins also contribute to the virulence of the organisms. For example, membrane proteins can mediate adherence to the host or can have a biochemical activity that is detrimental to host tissues, such as degradation of host proteins. The association of proteins with membranes occurs by three principal mechanisms. First, a protein can contain multiple hydrophobic domains and can weave its way in and out of the membrane, with hydrophilic subdomains of the protein exposed alternately to the cytoplasm and external milieu (Fig. 2). Such proteins often are capable of forming pores and can be involved in the movement of solutes into or out of the cell, or they can be involved in sensing external stimuli and relaying a signal into the cell (Fig. 2A). Alternatively, membrane proteins that are in contact with the surroundings and are anchored to the cytoplasmic membrane by a single domain of the protein that is rich in hydrophobic amino acids are also very common (Fig. 2B). Finally, membrane proteins can be linked to the membrane by covalent coupling to a lipid moiety, usually via a cysteine residue in the protein (Fig. 2C). These covalently linked lipoproteins have many different functions, including helping bacteria adhere to target tissues.

The outer membranes of gram-negative bacteria also harbor a variety of proteins (outer membrane proteins) that serve many different functions for the organisms, although the distribution, type, and absolute number of outer membrane proteins are highly variable between genera.

FIGURE 2 Schematic representation of a typical bacterial membrane with proteins that may be involved in transport of solutes, metabolism, environmental sensing, adherence, or other critical functions of the cell. See text for description of A, B, and C.

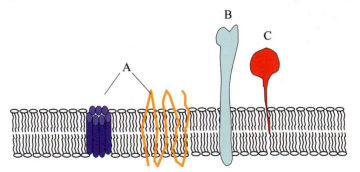

Porins are a general class of proteins that form pores in the outer membrane that allow nutrients and other small molecules to diffuse into the periplasmic space, where they can be actively transported across the cytoplasmic membrane. Porins also allow metabolic end products that are generated by the organisms to diffuse out of the periplasm so they do not accumulate to toxic levels or interfere with active transport processes. The outer membrane also contains many other types of individual proteins and complex proteinaceous structures, some of which mediate adhesion to host tissues.

Lipopolysaccharides

Only gram-negative bacteria produce lipopolysaccharide (LPS), a lipid and carbohydrate hybrid molecule that is abundant in, and adds structural integrity to, the outer membrane of the organisms. LPS consists of three major domains: a lipid A portion of the molecule, which is anchored in the outer membrane, and the core polysaccharide and O side chains, which extend from the cell into the surroundings (Fig. 3). The structure of LPS varies considerably among gram-negative bacteria, as does the length of the O side chain. Some bacteria have "rough" LPS, which lacks a repeating O side chain, whereas bacteria with "smooth" LPS have an O side chain consisting of a fairly large and variable number of repeating subunits of carbohydrate. The "rough" and "smooth" designations do not refer to the LPS molecule directly, but rather to the appearance of the colonies on agar media, with the strains with long polysaccharide O side chains appearing smooth and shiny on agar plates. The classification of bacterial strains by serotyping is frequently based on the structure and composition of the core polysaccharides and O side chains.

LPS plays major roles in the ability of the organisms to elicit diseases. A listing of some of the biological properties associated with LPS, which is sometimes referred to as endotoxin, is given in Table 3. Among the more important biological effects of LPS are the ability to elicit shock, fever, and apoptosis (programmed cell death) of host cells and the ability to stimulate potent and adverse inflammatory immune reactions through a variety of pathways that ultimately result in tissue damage. Most of the detrimental biologic activities of LPS reside in the lipid A portion of the molecule. Notably, not all bacterial LPS molecules are highly toxic, nor do all elicit the reactions described in Table 3 at biologically meaningful concentrations. Instead, there is a broad spectrum of activity of LPS depending on the organism from which it is isolated. By way of example, *Porphyromonas gingivalis*, which has been implicated in human periodontal diseases, produces an LPS that strongly stimulates bone resorption, a major problem in periodontal diseases, whereas the LPS of some strains of the common intestinal bacterium *Escherichia coli* is comparatively benign

TABLE 3 Some relevant biological activities of LPS

Lethal toxicity
Stimulation of inflammation
Complement activation
Polymorphonuclear leukocyte activation
Macrophage activation
B-cell mitogen activity
Adjuvant activity
Pyrogenicity
Stimulation of bone resorption
Stimulation of prostaglandin synthesis
Induction of tumor necrosis factor
Hypothermia
Hypotension

FIGURE 3 A schematic diagram of a typical LPS molecule of gram-negative bacteria.

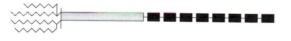

Lipid A   Core Polysaccharide   O - Side Chain

in this regard. Some of the mechanisms by which LPS exacerbates periodontal diseases are covered in greater detail in chapter 12.

Cell Wall Peptidoglycan

With few exceptions, bacteria have cell walls. The material comprising the cell wall is known as peptidoglycan or murein, which is structurally different from the cell walls of plants and fungi. Peptidoglycans consist of a repeating N-acetylglucosamine, N-acetylmuramic acid carbohydrate backbone linked to a tetrapeptide that generally contains biologically uncommon D-amino acids and diaminopimelic acid (Fig. 4). The peptides are cross-linked to various degrees, depending on the organism and growth conditions, and this cross-linking gives the peptidoglycan a meshworklike structure that is flexible, yet strong. In gram-negative bacteria, the cell wall lies between the inner and outer membrane and is held in place by covalently bound lipoproteins that anchor the wall to the outer membrane, with the protein portion bound to the wall and the lipid portion buried in the outer membrane (Fig. 5).

The cell wall is a comparatively minor architectural structure in gram-negative bacteria, although it does play key roles in the integrity of the cell by helping to prevent bacteria from bursting in hypo-osmotic conditions. The cell walls of gram-positive bacteria are much thicker and more highly cross-linked than those of gram-negatives, and are very prominent features of the cellular architecture (Fig. 6). In contrast to gram-negative bacteria, the wall of gram-positives is often the outermost structure of the cell, so it is directly exposed to the environment. Covalently linked to, or sterically anchored in, the cell wall are a diverse group of proteins, enzymes, and polysaccharides, many of which are crucial for persistent colonization of the oral cavity. In many cases, the carbohydrates in the cell wall have been useful for serological discrimination of different strains and species of bacteria, including many streptococci that elicit dental caries.

Lipoteichoic Acids

A major constituent of the outer envelope of gram-positive bacteria is lipoteichoic acid (LTA). LTAs are amphipathic molecules, i.e., they are

FIGURE 4 Schematic of peptidoglycan, with alternating N-acetylmuramic acid (M) and N-acetylglucosamine (G). A tetrapeptide is covalently linked to N-acetylmuramic acid and is cross-linked by a pentapeptide. The peptides often contain unusual amino acids such as the D-forms and diaminopimelic acid.

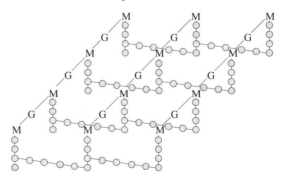

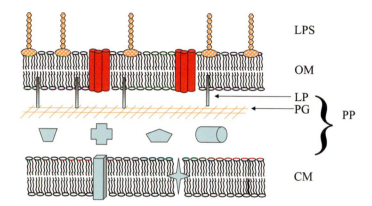

FIGURE 5 Architecture of a gram-negative surface showing the cytoplasmic membrane (CM) with transport and other proteins embedded (geometric shapes), the periplasmic space (PP) containing proteins and peptidoglycan (PG) anchored to the outer membrance (OM) by lipoproteins (LP). The outer membrane contains multiple proteins, including porins, as well as lipopolysaccharides (LPS).

composed of hydrophilic and hydrophobic constituents. LTAs consist of a lipid moiety that is generally embedded in the cytoplasmic membrane and a teichoic acid moiety, made from repeating units of phosphorylated glycerol or ribitol, which gives the teichoic acid portion of the molecule a strong net negative charge (Fig. 6). Bacteria also contain teichoic acids (TA), which are deacylated forms, i.e., lacking the lipid moiety, of LTAs. LTAs and TAs appear to contribute to the structural integrity of gram-positive bacteria, but they are also important in pathogenesis and have been implicated in such processes as adhesion to the host and avoidance of immune surveillance. Additionally, both LTAs and TAs can be shed from the cell surface into the surroundings. This can be problematic for the host because, similar to LPS, LTAs can stimulate a variety of adverse reactions, including apoptosis (programmed cell death), although the toxicity of LTAs is generally much less than that of the LPS of pathogenic gram-negative bacteria. Also like LPS, LTAs can be recognized by specific signaling molecules on the surface of host cells called Toll-like receptors,

FIGURE 6 Architecture of the exterior of a gram-positive bacterium showing the cytoplasmic membrane (CM) with transport proteins embedded. The peptidoglycan meshwork (cell wall [CW]) is anchored in the membrane. Teichoic acids (TA) and lipoteichoic acids (LTA) with a lipid moiety (LM) are illustrated, along with a surface protein (SP) anchored in the cell wall.

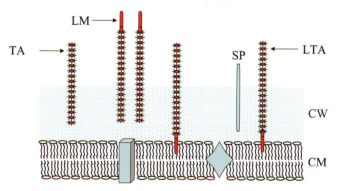

resulting in stimulation of innate and immune defenses (see chapter 2). Finally, it appears as though LTAs can be oriented in the cell wall with the lipid moiety protruding into the environment (Fig. 6). In this case, LTAs are thought to be important in conferring surface hydrophobicity to the bacteria, a trait that is strongly correlated with the ability to adhere to host tissues and saliva-coated teeth.

Some gram-positive bacteria can also produce teichuronic acids. Teichuronic acids are structurally similar to TAs, except the glycerol or ribitol phosphate backbone is replaced by a backbone of a hexuronic acid, such as glucuronic acid, or by other sugars, including N-acetyl-galactosamine. For organisms capable of producing both teichoic and teichuronic acids, growth conditions usually dictate which polymers will dominate, with availability of phosphate in the growth medium having the most profound impact. Not surprisingly, when phosphate is abundant, the formation of TAs is favored, since TAs are rich in phosphate.

Other Important Components Produced by Bacteria

CAPSULES

Capsules, which are produced by a wide variety of bacteria, are extracellular polymers that are loosely attached to the surface of the organisms. Generally, capsules are composed of polysaccharides, although there are a number of examples of nonpolysaccharide capsules, including the poly-D-glutamic acid capsule of the agent of anthrax, *Bacillus anthracis*. Capsules are high-molecular-mass polymers ($>10^5$ Da) that consist of repeating units of the same building blocks (homopolymers) or of a number of different building blocks (heteropolymers). Capsule synthesis by bacteria usually involves the production within the cell of the core repeating subunit of the capsule using nucleotide sugars, e.g., UDP-glucose. Subsequently, the core unit is translocated across the membrane(s) and polymerized at the surface of the cell. The variety in the structure and composition of bacterial capsules is remarkable. Since microorganisms spend significant amounts of energy to produce a capsule, it is not surprising that capsules provide substantial benefits to them, including protection against physical insult, serving as a source of food during starvation periods, and conferring substantial resistance to phagocytosis. Also of note, bacterial polysaccharides form a major proportion of the total mass of dental plaque.

Many oral bacteria produce extracellular polysaccharides that are not usually thought of as capsules, yet these polymers have many properties in common with true capsules. In particular, a number of cariogenic oral streptococci, including *Streptococcus mutans* and oral *Actinomyces* species, produce secreted enzymes that convert sucrose to high-molecular-mass (10^5 to 10^8 Da) homopolymers of glucose or fructose, known as glucans (or mutan) and fructans, respectively. Glucans and fructans are often responsible for the "furry" feeling on teeth after one consumes foodstuffs containing high concentrations of sucrose. Fructans and glucan polysaccharides produced by oral bacteria represent a large proportion of the dry weight of dental plaques formed in humans fed a diet containing sucrose. Glucans are produced by the action of glucosyltransferases, which are enzymes that convert sucrose to α1,3- and α1,6-linked homopolymers of glucose. Glucans serve mainly as an adhesive scaffolding to support the irreversible binding of a group of cariogenic organisms, known as mutans streptococci, to the teeth. Mutant strains of *S. mutans* that lack the ability to produce glucans are essentially devoid of the ability to cause caries on the smooth surfaces of the teeth (discussed in more detail in chapter 11). Notably, the glucans produced by *S. mutans* cannot be digested by the enzymes of any known oral organisms or by salivary amylase, so once glucans are produced in the mouth, they must be removed by mechanical forces. Fructans are also rapidly synthesized in the mouth by oral streptococci and certain strains of oral *Actinomyces*, but these polymers are probably not as important for adhesion of bacteria to the teeth. Instead, fructans function as extracellular storage compounds that allow the organisms to accumulate carbohydrates in a form that will not readily diffuse away from plaque. Then the bacteria can degrade these polysaccharides when dietary sources of sugar are exhausted.

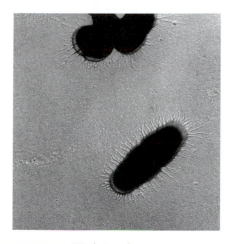

FIGURE 7 Fimbriated *A. actinomycetemcomitans*. Photo courtesy of Paula Fives-Taylor, University of Vermont.

FIMBRIAE AND PILI

The terms fimbriae and pili are often used interchangeably to refer to filamentous, or hairlike, structures on the surface of bacteria (Fig. 7). The fimbriae of many oral bacteria mediate adhesion to salivary proteins; the extracellular matrix, e.g., collagen and fibronectin; proteins in the clotting cascade; many different types of host cells; and other bacteria. In addition, pili and fimbriae mediate many functions that are detrimental to the host, like induction of programmed cell death (apoptosis), stimulation of bone resorption, and facilitation of entry of the bacteria into cells of the host (invasion). Pili can also mediate transfer of DNA from a donor bacterium to suitable recipient bacteria. Many of the fascinating aspects of pili and fimbriae biogenesis and function will be discussed in subsequent chapters.

FIBRILLAR LAYERS

Many gram-positive bacteria possess a fibrillar layer. Fibrillar layers or "fuzzy coats" are so named because they confer a fuzzy appearance to the cell surface when viewed under the electron microscope. The fibrils, which are shorter and distinct from fimbriae, are often composed of proteins that act as specific adhesins and directly mediate the binding of bacteria to host proteins or host cells. Often the fibrillar layer helps confer hydrophobicity to the cells, which, as mentioned above, is an important determinant in bacterial adhesion because it appears to stabilize the specific stereochemical interactions governed by cell surface adhesins.

FLAGELLA

Flagella are organelles of locomotion produced by many different species of bacteria, but only a relatively small subset of oral species produce flagella. In conjunction with chemotaxis systems, flagella can facilitate the directed movement of bacteria toward an attractant, such as a nutrient, or away from a repellant, such as a toxic metabolic end product. The distribution of flagella on bacteria is highly variable, but a given species of bacteria generally displays a very specific pattern of flagella. Some bacteria have a single flagellum or have one flagellum located at each end of the cell; these are known as polar flagella. Some have many flagella distributed along the body of the organisms, called peritrichous flagella. In virtually all cases, flagella are in direct contact with the surroundings and spin to propel the bacteria through the media. One notable exception to this rule is the group of organisms known as spirochetes. Some examples of spirochetes include *Treponema pallidum*, the syphilis agent, and *Treponema denticola*, an organism associated with human periodontal diseases. Although the mechanisms of rotation of spirochetal flagella are generally similar to those of other bacteria, the flagella of spirochetes are located in the periplasm of the organism between the cytoplasmic and outer membranes of the organisms, and thus are known as periplasmic flagella. In most cases, flagella and motility have not been strongly correlated with colonization or virulence of oral bacteria, but again, an exception is the spirochetes. The corkscrew shape of spirochetes and the periplasmic flagella render these organisms able to penetrate tissues. Interestingly, spirochetes are the bacteria that are most frequently found at the front of a progressing periodontal lesion, which is likely due to their unique motility characteristics.

VESICLES
Vesicle production is a characteristic of many gram-negative bacteria. Vesicles are produced by shedding or "blebbing" of the outer membrane. The small, lipid-rich vesicles that are shed can contain many or all of the components of the outer membrane, including LPS, tissue-damaging enzymes, and other virulence factors. Vesicles are thought to be relevant in oral diseases because they are very small—tens of nanometers in diameter—and can diffuse into host tissues carrying virulence factors and stimulating adverse reactions, such as inflammation and bone resorption.

S-LAYERS
Some oral bacteria can produce a surface layer known as an S-layer, which is a highly ordered proteinaceous coat that covers the surface of the bacteria. S-layers are generally composed of a single protein and can be highly effective in protecting the organisms from being phagocytized and killed by immune cells or from other inimical influences.

ENDOSPORES
Some bacteria have the ability to form endospores. Endospores, or spores as they are more commonly referred to, are dormant forms of bacteria that are highly resistant to killing by physical or chemical agents—heat, bleach, alcohol, peroxides, and so on. Under favorable conditions, spores can germinate to produce progeny organisms. Sadly, the American public became familiar with bacterial endospores when *B. anthracis* (the causative agent of anthrax) spores were used in assaults on media figures, government officials, and innocent citizens in the fall of 2001. Most oral bacteria are not able to form spores, but spore-forming bacteria are relevant to the practice of dentistry by virtue of their near ubiquity and high level of resistance to antimicrobials, disinfectants, and autoclaving. Characteristics of spores and methods for sterilization and disinfection are covered in chapter 18.

GENETIC ORGANIZATION OF BACTERIA

The Bacterial Chromosome

Bacteria have a single, covalently closed, circular chromosome, although there are some rare exceptions when the chromosomal DNA is linear. The chromosome is double-stranded and contains the same bases as human DNA—adenine (A), cytosine (C), guanine (G), and thymine (T) bases. The actual nucleotide composition and size of the chromosome vary widely among species of bacteria. For example, many of the oral streptococci have a chromosome with a combined guanine and cytosine content, or G+C content, of roughly 35%. On the other extreme, *Actinomyces* species, which are gram-positive, non-spore-forming anaerobic bacteria that are abundant colonizers of the teeth and soft tissues, have a G+C content around 68%. Now that the technology is available to sequence entire genomes, the complete sequence and, thus, the exact sizes of many bacterial chromosomes have been determined, including several oral pathogens. For example, the entire chromosome of the dental caries pathogen *S. mutans* is 2,032,327 bp, containing over 2,000 genes. It is noteworthy that the chromosomes of oral bacteria are generally smaller than those of organisms that are able both to exist in the environment and to colonize a variety of hosts. The *S. mutans* chromosome at 2.03 million base pairs (Mbp) and the chromosome of *P. gingivalis* at 2.3 Mbp are only about a third the size of the chromosome of *Pseudomonas aeruginosa* (6.2 Mbp), a bacterium that is widely disseminated in water, soil, and plants but that can also cause serious diseases in immunocompromised patients, burn victims, and persons with cystic fibrosis. For additional comparisons, the enteric bacterium and common laboratory pet *E. coli* has a chromosome of about 4.6 Mbp and the chromosome of the sporulating soil bacterium *Bacillus subtilis* is 4.2 Mbp. Thus, it appears as though oral bacteria have lost, or failed to acquire, many of the genes that environmental bacteria need to survive and thrive outside the oral cavity. In spite of the relatively small size of chromosomes of oral bacteria though, these organisms have evolved highly specialized and extremely elegant mechanisms to colonize and persist in the oral cavity. To provide a bit more perspective, the species with the smallest genome of free-living organisms is *Mycoplasma genitalium*, which has a chromosome of 580,074 bp (580 kbp), containing around 520 genes—so oral bacteria have the potential to express many more genes than may be required simply for growth and replication in a human host. As discussed in subsequent chapters, many of these genes have in fact been shown to be critical for persistence and elicitation of diseases by oral microorganisms.

Chromosome Replication in Bacteria

Replication of the bacterial chromosome begins at a single origin of replication and proceeds bidirectionally to a terminus located asymmetrically on the chromosome. DNA replication in bacteria has been studied extensively and the machinery required for replication—DNA polymerase, DNA winding and unwinding enzymes, single-stranded DNA-binding proteins, and the use of RNA primers to initiate DNA synthesis—have much in common with that found in mammalian cells. However, the processes to control initiation of replication and the machinery involved in DNA replication are somewhat streamlined in bacteria when compared with mammalian cells. Nevertheless, control of DNA replication is a carefully orchestrated process and bacteria face some interesting challenges in coordinating DNA replication with cell division. One of the problems that bacteria face is that replication of the entire chromosome can take substantially longer than it takes for a rapidly growing culture of bacteria to divide. For example, replication of the *E. coli* chromosome is predicted to take a little over 80 min, whereas rapidly growing *E. coli* can divide in less than 20 min. To overcome this problem, bacteria do something substantially different than eukaryotes—they initiate additional rounds of chromosome replication before the initial round is completed. In fact, there are multiple replication events proceeding concurrently in rapidly growing bacteria. Completed chromosomes, and those still replicating, can then be passed on to daughter cells when division takes place. The daughter cells will then have partially replicated chromosomes and can divide faster than could be accomplished if it was necessary to complete one full cycle of DNA replication before division.

Bacteria frequently harbor extrachromosomal elements, i.e., discrete DNA elements that can replicate independently of a direct association with the chromosome. The most common extrachromosomal elements of bacteria are called plasmids. Plasmids usually consist of circular double-stranded DNAs that carry an origin of replication that allows replication of the element by the host machinery. Most plasmids carry additional genetic information, including genes encoding resistance to antibiotics, genes that allow the plasmids to be transferred from one bacterium to another, genes that allow organisms to use certain types of compounds, or in some cases, genes that are crucial to the ability of the organisms to cause disease. Plasmids can be extremely small, less than 2,000 bp, or fairly large, upward of 100 kbp. Other elements that can replicate independently of the chromosome include the genetic material of bacteriophages (bacterial viruses). In these cases, bacteriophages inject their nucleic acids into the host cell, where it can be replicated using the host machinery and, in some cases, with the assistance of bacteriophage-derived enzymes. Extrachromosomal DNA elements have proven to be the essential tools of molecular biology because they allow researchers to work with manageably small DNA fragments and to easily recover engineered DNAs free of the large chromosomes of the organisms (see chapter 7).

Gene Transfer in Bacteria

Genetic exchange between bacteria can enhance the diversity of the population and allows the transfer of genes that can augment the virulence of organisms. In fact, "horizontal" gene transfer, i.e., gene transfer between organisms, appears to be the major route for acquisition of resistance to antibiotics and of certain traits that augment the virulence of the organisms. Genetic exchange by bacteria can take place in three general ways: transformation, transduction, or conjugation. These methods are covered in greater detail in chapter 7. Briefly, transformation involves the uptake of DNA from the surroundings. A variety of bacteria, including oral streptococci, are naturally competent for transformation, meaning that these cells can actively take up DNA from their surroundings. Work is ongoing to determine whether this type of genetic exchange may be occurring in natural dental plaque. Many other oral bacteria are not naturally competent, but can be induced to take up DNA. Transduction involves the transfer of genetic information from one organism to another via bacteriophages, which are bacterial viruses. Generalized transducing bacteriophages can package fairly large pieces of DNA from a donor strain and transfer that DNA by infecting a suitable recipient strain. Specialized transducing phages pick up selected segments of DNA from the donor and transfer the DNA, along with some or all of the genetic material of the virus, into a recipient cell. Conjugation involves transfer of genetic material by direct cell-cell contact. In many gram-negative bacteria, DNA transfer is mediated through a sex pilus on the surface of the cell through which DNA can be funneled to the recipient. In some gram-positive bacteria, a sophisticated pheromone system induces clumping between a donor and a compatible recipient and the close cell-cell contact allows DNA to be transferred.

BACTERIAL GROWTH AND NUTRITION

Growth

Bacteria divide by binary fission. Because one bacterium becomes two bacteria, cultures of bacteria exhibit exponential growth: 2 become 4, then 8, 16, 32, and so on. When bacteria that are not already dividing are inoculated into a liquid medium, the organisms must alter their metabolism and gene expression patterns to produce sufficient quantities of the constituents needed to grow as rapidly as is possible in the new environment. During this adjustment period, known as the lag phase (Fig. 8), the

FIGURE 8 Typical growth pattern of bacteria.

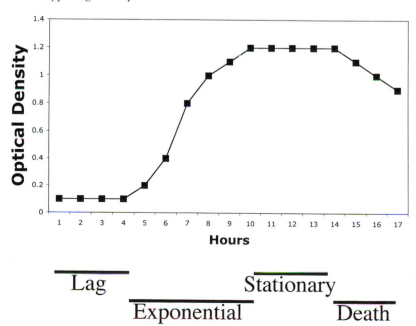

organisms begin replicating their chromosomes and synthesizing the machinery to transcribe and translate their genetic material into the building blocks of the cell. The organisms begin to grow and divide during the exponential phase of growth, sometimes called log phase, although exponential phase is the more appropriate terminology. Cells will continue to divide exponentially until nutrients begin to be exhausted or until inhibitory metabolites start to accumulate in sufficient concentrations to inhibit growth. When the culture begins to cease to grow, the organisms are said to have entered stationary phase. During this period, DNA replication largely is arrested, the number of ribosomes diminishes, and the cell slows production of the enzymes needed to catalyze the synthesis of the building blocks of the cell. Cells also start to synthesize a new subset of proteins that help to enhance survival during nutrient starvation. Stationary-phase cells are more resistant to antibiotics, since most antibiotics target exponentially growing bacteria by acting on cell wall synthesis (penicillins and cephalosporins), DNA replication (nalidixic acid), transcription (rifampin), or translation (tetracyclines and macrolides). Relating the growth phases to bacteria in dental plaque, it is easy to imagine that, during fasting periods, dental plaque bacteria are frequently limited for nutrients, especially carbohydrates. Thus, they may be in a state akin to stationary phase and their phenotypic properties in plaque and their susceptibilities to antimicrobial agents may be different from what we can observe in the laboratory using traditional methods. After some time, cells enter a death phase. This is highly variable, depending on the organisms. Some oral bacteria, like *Streptococcus gordonii*, do not survive for prolonged periods (days) without nutrients, whereas some bacteria can survive for weeks.

Another environmental factor that has a major impact on microbial growth is oxygen, which is present in near atmospheric quantities, about 20%, in the oral cavity. Oxygen itself is not toxic, but single electron reductions of oxygen catalyzed by enzymes of bacteria can lead to the generation of toxic oxygen radicals, including superoxide, peroxides, and hydroxyl radicals, which can damage membranes (lipids), proteins, and DNA. Bacteria vary dramatically in their abilities to utilize oxygen and to cope with oxygen radicals. Some bacteria actually require oxygen for growth because the organisms respire to generate energy and use oxygen as a terminal electron acceptor. These aerobic organisms consume oxygen and have high levels of the enzymes needed to detoxify oxygen radicals. There are relatively few obligately aerobic bacteria in dental plaque. Obligate anaerobes cannot grow in the presence of oxygen, largely because they create toxic oxygen radicals through metabolism, but lack sufficient quantities of, or lack altogether, the enzymes needed to cope with oxygen radicals. Many of the organisms associated with periodontal diseases, *P. gingivalis*, *Prevotella intermedia*, *Fusobacterium nucleatum*, and oral spirochetes, are obligate anaerobes. These organisms can be abundant in dental plaque, particularly subgingival plaque, and can exist there because they are protected from oxygen metabolites by other plaque microorganisms that can detoxify or consume the oxygen. Facultative or facultatively anaerobic bacteria can grow in the presence of oxygen, but also grow well when oxygen is absent. Most of the abundant species in the mouth are facultative organisms, such as oral streptococci.

Some bacteria that require but can only tolerate small amounts of oxygen are referred to as microaerophilic. Organisms that have their growth enhanced by carbon dioxide are referred to as capnophilic. Important oral capnophiles include *Actinobacillus actinomycetemcomitans* and *Capnocytophaga gingivalis*, both of which are associated with human periodontal diseases.

Nutrient Acquisition

For one bacterium to become two bacteria, it is necessary for the organisms to be able to acquire all of the nutrients needed for growth from their surroundings. In many cases, the first step in this process for oral bacteria involves the degradation of complex macromolecules in saliva and crevicular fluids, or in the diet, to compounds that are sufficiently small in size that they can diffuse through, or be transported across, the membranes of the organisms. Some of the types of extracellular enzymes that are produced by oral bacteria that assist in processing nutrients include proteinases (or proteases), which cleave proteins into peptides or individual amino acids; glycohydrolases (or glycosidases), such as amylase, which break down polysaccharides or oligo-saccharide side chains on proteins; neuraminidase, which removes sialic acid from glycoproteins; and lipases, which break down lipids. Once the oral secretions or the diet is processed to constituents that can be assimilated by bacteria, the organisms use many different types of transport proteins, which are found in the cytoplasmic membrane, to internalize the nutrients. These transporters can be divided into several different categories. Most of the transporters are "active transporters" that use energy in the form of ATP or that exploit the electrochemical gradient (Δp, the proton motive force) to move the desired compounds into the cell. Peptides and some sugars are generally taken up by high-affinity, multisubunit transporters known as ATP-binding cassette transporters, or ABC transporters. This class of transporters usually contains, at a minimum, a substrate-binding domain, a membrane-spanning domain, and an ATP hydrolysis domain that energizes movement of the compounds into the cells. Another important type of transporter for oral bacteria is a family of proteins that is part of the sugar-phosphotransferase system (PTS) (Fig. 9). The PTS consists of a general PTS protein called enzyme I, which transfers phosphate from phosphoenolpyruvate to a general phosphocarrier protein called HPr. HPr can then donate that phosphate to sugar-specific enzyme II proteins that bind the sugar outside the cell, and, with the concomitant transfer of a phosphate group to the sugar, transport the sugar phosphate into the cell. For example, an enzyme II specific for glucose binds glucose in the environment and moves it into the cell as glucose-6-phosphate, which can directly enter the glycolytic pathway. The PTS is a very high affinity system, with K_m values (the concentration of substrate at which the system operates at 50% of its maximum rate) for the cognate sugars of approximately 10 μM, which is about the same concentration of glucose that is found in the mouth during fasting periods. The PTS has many important roles in oral bacteria, but it is probably an especially critical pathway when nutrients become limiting because it will allow oral bacteria to scavenge the trace amounts of carbohydrates that are present in the mouth between periods of food consumption.

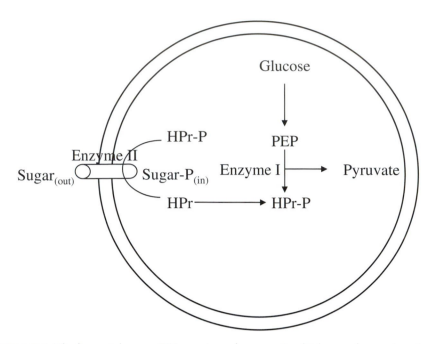

FIGURE 9 The bacterial sugar-PTS consists of enzyme I, which transfers a phosphate group from phosphoenolpyruvate (PEP) to the HPr at histidine residue 15. HPr can then donate the phosphate to a series of sugar-specific enzyme II proteins that catalyze the transport and concomitant phosphorylation of incoming sugars.

INTRODUCTION TO FUNDAMENTAL CONCEPTS OF ORAL MICROBIAL ECOLOGY

Microbial Biofilms

Much of what is currently known about the properties and metabolism of oral bacteria has been learned from studying pure cultures of individual species growing in test tubes, primarily because this was the most convenient and reliable way to study the behavior of bacteria. However, growth as suspended populations in liquid medium is not the normal mode of growth for bacteria in the mouth. Oral microorganisms instead grow as compositionally and structurally complex mixtures of species adhering to a surface. These types of populations are generally known as biofilms (Fig. 10). In fact, the simplest definition of a biofilm is "organisms colonizing a surface and embedded in a polymer-rich matrix," dental plaque being an archetypical example of a biofilm. Importantly, recognition of the oral microbiota as highly diverse, surface-adherent communities of microorganisms—biofilms—is central to understanding oral microbial ecology and oral disease development.

ADHESIVE AND COOPERATIVE INTERACTIONS HELP TO DICTATE COMMUNITY COMPOSITION AND STABILITY

From multiple studies on dental plaque, it is clear that oral bacteria exist in very close association with one another, and in many cases, oral biofilms appear to have a highly ordered structure. These apparently specific associations among various species of bacteria are believed to be driven, at least in part, by production of surface adhesins that allow groups of species to colonize the same tissues and to adhere to one another with high affinity. Notably, these interbacterial associations may have evolved

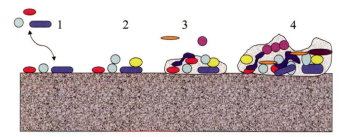

FIGURE 10 General features of biofilm formation. (1) Reversible adherence of microbes with a surface. (2) Stable adherence of the bacteria. (3) Growth, polymer production, and recruitment of new species to the biofilm through interbacterial interactions. (4) Formation of a mature biofilm, often referred to as a climax community.

because of nutritional benefits or other advantages to the two species of growing very close to one another. Such cooperative growth behavior facilitated by adhesive interactions has been seen between *S. mutans*, which produces copious amounts of lactic acid, and another important oral bacterium, *Veillonella parvula*, which consumes lactic acid. Similarly, production of certain fatty acids by *P. gingivalis* can stimulate the growth of the oral spirochete *T. denticola*. Interestingly, strong associations of *S. mutans* and *Veillonella* species with dental caries and of *P. gingivalis* and spirochetes in periodontal diseases are well documented. Thus, there is likely to be a real benefit to bacteria to grow in dense biofilms, and specific associations between certain species may be an essential factor in the persistence of those organisms in plaque.

ANTAGONISTIC INTERACTIONS INFLUENCE COMPOSITION AND PATHOGENIC POTENTIAL OF ORAL BIOFILMS

Antagonistic interactions can also influence the composition and biological activities of the oral biofilms on the teeth and soft tissue. Perhaps the simplest form of antagonism occurs when end products of one organism directly inhibit the growth of other organisms in plaque. One example of this type of antagonism can be seen during the development of dental caries. Consumption by the host of a diet that is rich in carbohydrates leads to bacterial production of organic acids, such as lactic and acetic acids, which in turn drives the pH of oral biofilms down to values of 4 and below. Acidification of plaque by cariogenic bacteria, like *S. mutans* and lactobacilli, inhibits the growth of acid-sensitive organisms. Over time, the acid-sensitive organisms can no longer compete effectively, leading to the enrichment in cariogenic biofilms of organisms that are acid tolerant, like *S. mutans* and lactobacilli. Another example of an antagonistic interaction that may influence plaque ecology is the production of hydrogen peroxide (H_2O_2) by certain streptococci. H_2O_2 is toxic to many bacteria that lack, or have low levels of, the enzymes needed to detoxify oxygen radicals. Thus, this simple diffusible compound may kill or inhibit the growth of selected organisms, making the H_2O_2-producing organism more competitive. Even more sophisticated forms of antagonism exist, such as production of compounds known as bacteriocins by bacteria in plaque. In one well-characterized case, it is known that certain strains of *S. mutans* produce bacteriocins known as mutacins, which are peptide antibiotics that specifically inhibit the growth of closely related species. Through production of bacteriocins, *S. mutans* is able to suppress the growth of other streptococci that would otherwise compete for similar nutrients.

Ecology of the Oral Microbiota and Development of Oral Diseases

The oral environment and ecology of the oral microbiota are covered in detail in chapters 3 and 5. However, it is useful to provide a brief introduction to the current concepts of biofilm homeostasis and the ecological basis of oral diseases. Why? Because the normal microbial constituents are an important contributor to tissue homeostasis in the oral cavity. These normally benign populations that colonize all the surfaces of the mouth establish shortly after birth, persist throughout the individual's lifetime, and generally are compatible with oral health. Unless there is significant perturbation from an adverse environmental stress—such as increased carbohydrates in the diet or reduction of salivary flow, both of which can lead to a sustained lowering of the pH of plaque—there is little or no obvious damage to the colonized tissues. So, the microbes of the oral cavity do not necessarily have an adverse effect on the health of the individual, nor is it predetermined that these organisms will eventually cause disease. In fact, there are many reasons that the normal microbial composition of the body is believed to have major health benefits for the host. Not surprisingly then, the concept of stabilizing a microbiota that is compatible with health is more and more frequently being embraced as a way to maintain oral health. Major challenges facing oral health researchers are how to foster a healthy microbiota and how to prevent the ecologic shifts seen during disease development in the oral cavity. But the benefits to perseverance and development of new preventive and treatment strategies for oral disease will be great. Hopefully, as you make your way through the following chapters, you will gain an appreciation for the complexity of the oral environment, the microbial inhabitants of this environment, and the host responses to disease, and you can begin to envision how to exploit this knowledge to improve overall oral health.

▮ KEY POINTS

The three primary domains of life are the *Eukarya*, which encompass all eukaryotes, and the *Bacteria* and *Archaea*, which are the prokaryotes.

Bacteria almost uniformly can be divided into two major classes based on the Gram-staining reaction. Gram-positive bacteria have only a single cell membrane and a thick, highly cross-linked cell wall. Gram-negative bacteria have a cytoplasmic and outer membrane and a thin, less highly cross-linked cell wall found in the periplasmic space between the inner and outer membranes.

A variety of bacterial factors that are relevant to the pathogenic potential of bacteria are located on the surface of the cell, including the LPS of gram-negative organisms, LTAs of gram-positive bacteria, pili, fimbriae, flagella, capsules, and S-layers.

Bacteria divide by binary fission. Replication of the circular chromosomes of bacteria is initiated at a single origin of replication and proceeds bidirectionally to a single terminus. The growth rate of some organisms can be very fast, with cells dividing as rapidly as every 15 min. Many other bacteria grow more slowly, with generation times measured in tens of hours.

The mouth has a variety of habitats, and the bacteria in the mouth exist as adherent biofilms. The biofilm lifestyle facilitates diversity in the population and allows the establishment of degradative communities, the members of which cooperate to convert the complex constituents of saliva and the diet, such as glycoproteins, into substances that can be used for growth and energy generation. Antagonistic interactions, such as acid production by species that inhibit the growth of acid-sensitive organisms or the overt production of antibiotics by certain species in oral biofilms, also help dictate the composition of dental plaque.

The vast majority of oral diseases arise from a perturbation in the homeostatic mechanisms of oral biofilms, generally driven by environmental changes, such as dietary changes or diminished salivary flow from radiation or hyposalivation-inducing drugs.

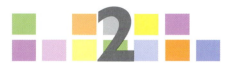

The Immune System and Host Defense

PETER M. LYDYARD AND MICHAEL F. COLE

INTRODUCTION

The human body has evolved a large variety of mechanisms to protect itself from invasion by pathogenic microorganisms. These host defenses (Fig. 1) include prevention of entry and dealing with the pathogens once they have penetrated the outer defenses of the body. Once a pathogen is inside the body, the immune system must recognize the pathogen as foreign and dispose of it. The overall immune system is divided into two separate but not mutually exclusive systems. The innate system, with which one is born, functions in the same way whether or not one has already encountered the pathogen. The adaptive system adapts to the first encounter with the pathogen (i.e., remembers it) so that the response is faster and more specific.

The innate and adaptive immune systems work in concert both in recognition and disposal of pathogens. The main differences between the two systems are the speed and fine specificity of the pathogen recognition systems and the memory capacity of the adaptive system, although the boundaries between the two are becoming more blurred as we learn more about them.

INNATE IMMUNITY

Microbes penetrating the physical barriers of the body (Fig. 2) pass across epithelial surfaces to enter the tissue. In most cases this will be across mucosal epithelial surfaces. Once in the tissues, a number of cells (Fig. 3) and molecules (Table 1) begin to function in early defense against the invading microbes.

Cells Involved in Early Defense

PHAGOCYTES

There are two main types of phagocytes, or "eating" cells. Polymorphonuclear cells (polymorphs, or PMNs) are blood borne (mobile) and make up the majority of the blood granulocytes. In contrast, macrophages derived from circulating monocytes are "tissue-associated" phagocytes and are found in the tissues and organs of the body, waiting to encounter invading microbes. On contact with the phagocyte, a susceptible microbe

23

Prevention of entry	Physical barriers	
	Creating an adverse environment	

Once inside the body

Innate immunity

First line of defense	Cells	Phagocytes (neutrophils and macrophages) Natural killer cells Mast cells (some link to adaptive immunity)
	Humoral factors	Acute-phase proteins Cytokines Complement proteins

Adaptive immunity

Second line of defense	Cells	Lymphocytes and dendritic cells
	Humoral factors	Antibodies

FIGURE 1 Summary of host defenses.

is rapidly ingested and killed inside the cell by enzymes derived from primary lysosomes. The engulfment process can be enhanced by a number of molecules that coat the microbe and bind to the phagocytes, a process called opsonization. Complement and antibodies coating the microbe act as opsonins (see later).

NK CELLS

Natural killer (NK) cells are large lymphocyte-like cells that recognize body cells that are infected with a virus. On contact with a virus-infected cell they release substances that induce the target cell to commit suicide through the process of apoptosis. In this way, the virus particles are retained inside the cell and are killed following phagocytosis of the dying cell.

MAST CELLS

Mast cells are found throughout the body and particularly at epithelial sites. Their large cytoplasmic inclusions contain pharmacologically active substances, such as histamine, that play an important role in the acute inflammatory response. They release their granular contents very rapidly on contact with activated complement proteins or with some kinds of antibodies (immunoglobulin E [IgE]) when bound to antigen (see below).

Molecules Involved in Early Defense

COMPLEMENT

Complement consists of around 20 different proteins, some of which are regulatory. Components of complement have three important roles in defense: inflammation, phagocytosis, and the lysis of susceptible microbes. Complement needs to be "activated" in order for it to function and, like blood clotting, comprises a "cascade" system (Fig. 4). The complement system can be activated directly by microbes (alternative and lectin pathways) or through antibodies bound to the microbes (classical

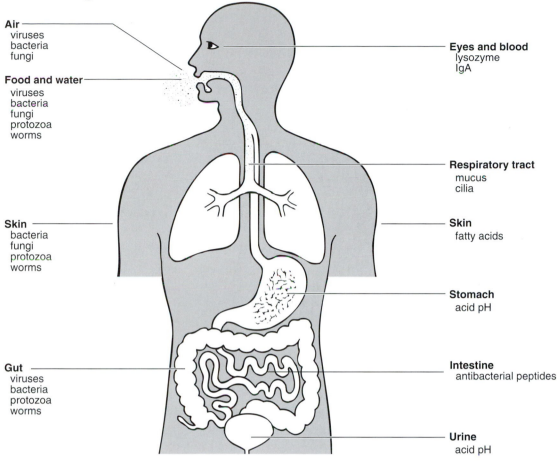

Infectious organisms

Air
viruses
bacteria
fungi

Food and water
viruses
bacteria
fungi
protozoa
worms

Skin
bacteria
fungi
protozoa
worms

Gut
viruses
bacteria
protozoa
worms

Defences

Eyes and blood
lysozyme
IgA

Respiratory tract
mucus
cilia

Skin
fatty acids

Stomach
acid pH

Intestine
antibacterial peptides

Urine
acid pH

FIGURE 2 External defenses of the body. Humans are exposed daily to large numbers of microbes (mostly bacteria and viruses) through the air they breathe and the food and drink they take in. The skin also acts as a physical barrier through its dead external layers. Bacteriocidal secretions by the skin, gastric acidity, and mucus and cilia in the respiratory tract all help prevent the attachment of microbes that is essential for colonization. Blood and secretions contain the enzyme lysozyme, which kills many bacteria by attacking their cell walls. IgA is also an important host defense mechanism at mucous membrane surfaces (see section on antibodies). Reprinted from J. H. L. Playfair and P. M. Lydyard, *Medical Immunology Made Memorable*, 2nd ed. (Churchill Livingstone, Edinburgh, United Kingdom, 2000), with permission from Elsevier Science.

FIGURE 3 Cells involved in innate immune defense. The mobile phagocytic cells, called polymorphs or PMNs (left), are present in large numbers in the bloodstream whilst macrophages (middle) police the various organs and tissues of the body. Mast cells (right) are found throughout the body but particularly at sites lining mucosal surfaces (lamina propria) and are pivotal cells in the acute inflammatory response.

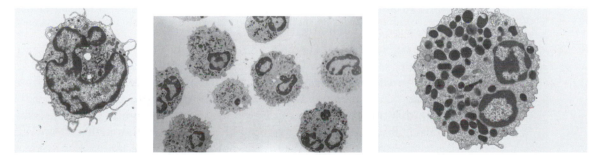

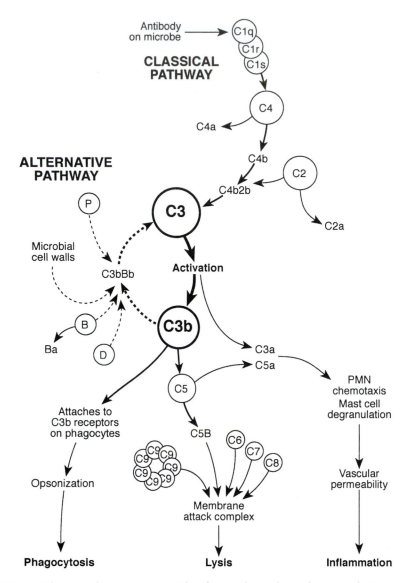

FIGURE 4 The complement system. This figure shows how the pivotal C3 complement component is cleaved into its C3a and C3b by enzymes (convertases) through the alternative and classical pathways (activation of complement). The classical pathway involves antibodies, while the alternative pathway "ticks over" slowly and is accelerated when it occurs on surfaces such as those of bacteria. The lectin pathway (not shown) is activated when the mannan-binding ligand attaches to mannose residues on the surfaces of microorganisms and it has its own convertase to cleave C3. Following cleavage of C3, a cascade of events occurs, leading to phagocytosis, lysis, and inflammation, as shown at the bottom of the figure. There are, of course, inhibitory factors that regulate the "activation" of complement and prevent it from occurring at the surface of the body's own cells. Reprinted from J. H. L. Playfair and P. M. Lydyard, *Medical Immunology Made Memorable*, 2nd ed. (Churchill Livingstone, Edinburgh, United Kingdom, 2000), with permission from Elsevier Science.

pathway [see below]). The main component of complement is C3, a major serum protein (about 1 g/liter) that is enzymatically split (in both pathways) or "activated" to give rise to two components, C3a and C3b. When this occurs at the surface of a bacterium, C3b acts as an opsonin, resulting in enhanced phagocytosis. The released C3a, together with C5a, plays an important role in activating mast cells and attracting phagocytic cells (neutrophils) to the site of the invading bacterium. Later components C5 to C9 form a membrane attack complex that punches a hole in the bacterial surface, causing lysis and the bacterium's demise.

ACUTE-PHASE PROTEINS

Acute-phase proteins are plasma proteins that are generally increased following infection with a microbe. They are not only important in host defense but also in repairing the damage caused by the invaders.

Table 2 shows the important acute-phase proteins and their function. Their production by liver cells is induced mainly through cytokines (e.g., interleukin-1 [IL-1], tumor necrosis factor alpha [TNF-α], and IL-6) secreted by macrophages following contact with the microbes. Complement components are also acute-phase proteins.

CYTOKINES

Cytokines are small proteins (usually <15 kDa) that have a variety of functions, including producing fever (IL-1) and also enhancing acute inflammatory responses (TNF-α). These chemical "messengers" or communication molecules also have important roles in the adaptive immune system (see below). Cytokines important in innate defense against viruses are the interferons. This family of proteins, most of which are produced in nucleated cells following viral infection, have the ability to prevent the growth of viruses in other cells local to the infection. Interferons (IFN) "interfere" with viral protein synthesis through inhibition of RNA translation. IFN-α and IFN-β are produced by most nucleated cells while IFN-γ is made by NK cells and T cells of the adaptive system. More recently, a group of cytokines called chemokines has been described that function to attract and activate cells including lymphocytes, macrophages, and PMNs. A large number of other molecules produced by phagocytes and epithelial cells that protect against infection are described in chapter 10 and include defensins.

RECOGNITION

The important first step in the innate early defense response is to recognize that the invader is nonself or foreign. The phagocytes recognize the invading organisms through pattern receptors. These include mannose

TABLE 2 Acute-phase proteins

Protein	Function
C-reactive protein	Binds to phosphorylcholine and activates complement (by binding to C1q); see Fig. 4.
Mannose-binding ligand	Binds to mannose on the surfaces of bacteria and viruses and activates complement via the lectin pathway; also acts as an opsonin
Complement components	Involved in chemotaxis, opsonization, and lysis (Fig. 4), e.g., C2, C3, C4, C5, C9
Metal-binding proteins	Removal of essential metal ions required for bacterial growth
α_1-Antitrypsin, α_1-antichymotrypsin	Protease inhibitors
Fibrinogen	Coagulation factor

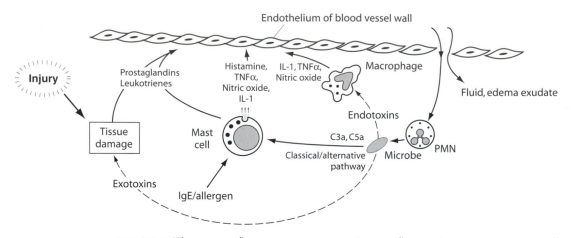

FIGURE 5 The acute inflammatory response. Acute inflammation is a response to cell injury and is a sequence of events that is similar following injury caused by invading microbes or by physical mechanisms. Thus, direct damage by injury or via exotoxins produced by microbes leads to a release of mediators, e.g., prostaglandins and leukotrienes, which increase vascular permeability. The pivotal cell in the acute inflammatory response is the mast cell. This can be activated to release inflammatory cytokines such as TNF-α by binding microbes through pattern receptors, or to release inflammatory mediators such as histamine in an explosive exocytosis when the activation is via complement components that are the result of activation by microbes through the three pathways described. IgE/allergen complexes and neuropeptides can also activate mast cells to release pharmacological mediators. Microbial endotoxins activate macrophages to produce IL-1 and TNF-α, which have vasodilatory properties. The outcome of the copious local mediator release is loosening of endothelial tight junctions, increased adhesion of PMNs and monocytes, and their migration into the surrounding tissues where they come into contact with, and are able to phagocytose, the microbes. Fluid containing fibrinogen, antibodies, etc. is released into the area from the bloodstream, and this edema protects the damaged area during repair. Reprinted from P. M. Lydyard, A. Whelan, and M. W. Fanger, *Instant Notes in Immunology*, 2nd ed. (Bios Scientific, Taylor and Francis, Oxford, United Kingdom, 2004), with permission.

receptors, scavenger receptors, and Toll-like receptors (see chapter 10). Complement "recognizes" some bacteria, for example, those lacking a capsule, and is directly activated (alternative and lectin pathways) via the bacterial surface (Fig. 4).

ACUTE INFLAMMATION

The archetypal innate immune response is that of acute inflammation and occurs very rapidly following infection. The function of this response is to rapidly bring blood-borne host defenses to bear on the invader. The acute inflammatory response is illustrated in Fig. 5.

THE LYMPHOID SYSTEM

The innate immune system operates rapidly and can often eliminate most of the invading organisms. However, usually the second level of defense—the adaptive immune system—is also alerted. The lymphocytes are the main players of the adaptive system and are found in specialized lymphoid tissues and in the bloodstream. The total mass of lymphoid tissues in an adult is about the size of a soccer ball. There are several kinds of lymphocyes that are adapted to carry out specific functions. They recirculate around the body and recognize pieces of the foreign microbes (called antigens) through specialized receptors that differ from those of the innate immune system (see below).

Lymphocyte Heterogeneity

The two major lymphocyte populations are T cells (so called because they are produced in the thymus) and B cells (so called because they are produced in the bone marrow). In the bloodstream, both B and T lymphocytes are small cells with a thin rim of cytoplasm and cannot morphologically be identified from one another. B cells develop into plasma cells, which are specialized to produce antibodies to protect against microbes that live outside body cells (extracellular). On the other hand, the T cells (helper and cytotoxic T cells) have evolved to protect against microbes that live inside cells, such as viruses and certain bacteria (intracellular). The mechanisms by which the lymphocytes carry out these functions are described later. The different lymphocytes can be distinguished from one another by the surface molecules that are important to their function. Further subsets of T cells (Th1 and Th2) can be distinguished by the spectrum of cytokines that they produce. The main "markers" identifying the different lymphocyte populations are shown in Table 3.

Lymphoid Organs and Tissues

There are around 1×10^9 to 2×10^9 lymphocytes per liter of blood (1×10^6 to 2×10^6/ml), which is 5 to 10 times fewer than the innate mobile phagocytes (the PMNs). The lymphocytes are also found in organized lymphoid tissues in the body. These are divided into systemic lymphoid organs and tissues, and lymphoid tissues associated with mucosal areas of the body that line the three main tracts (digestive, genitourinary, and respiratory). These tracts are the major sites of entry of microorganisms into the body so it is not surprising that greater than 50% of the lymphoid tissue is found associated with the mucosal epithelial surfaces. Figure 6 shows the distribution of lymphoid tissues within the body. Mucosa-associated lymphoid tissues (MALT) are covered in some detail in chapter 10.

Lymph nodes range in size from 1 to 10 mm and are found in superficial and in deep locations within the body. T and B lymphocytes are located at different sites within lymphoid tissues and associate with other cells (e.g., dendritic cells) that are important for lymphocyte function. Figure 7 shows the structure of a typical lymph node and its components. The secondary lymphoid follicles found in lymph nodes (and other lymphoid tissues) contain "germinal centers" of B lymphocyte foci that are

TABLE 3 Lymphocyte markers

Cell type	sIg	TCR	CD3	CD4	CD8	CD19/20	Cytokine(s) produced
B lymphocytes	+	−	−	−	−	+	−
T lymphocytes							
Th1 cells	−	+	+	+	−	−	IL-2, IFN-γ
Th2 cells	−	+	+	+	−	−	IL-4, -5, -6, -10
Tc cells	−	+	+	−	+	−	−

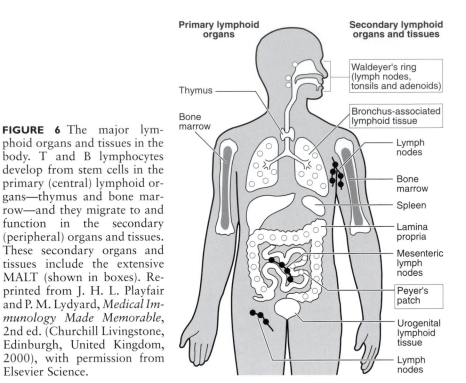

FIGURE 6 The major lymphoid organs and tissues in the body. T and B lymphocytes develop from stem cells in the primary (central) lymphoid organs—thymus and bone marrow—and they migrate to and function in the secondary (peripheral) organs and tissues. These secondary organs and tissues include the extensive MALT (shown in boxes). Reprinted from J. H. L. Playfair and P. M. Lydyard, *Medical Immunology Made Memorable*, 2nd ed. (Churchill Livingstone, Edinburgh, United Kingdom, 2000), with permission from Elsevier Science.

FIGURE 7 Lymph node structure. The outer cortical area of the node contains predominantly B lymphocytes in primary follicles. Some of these contain germinal centers (then called secondary follicles) that are the sites of B-cell proliferation, memory generation, class switching, and antibody affinity maturation. Dendritic-antigen presenting cells are found mainly in the cortical region while the medulla is rich in plasma cells. Lymph enters the node from the tissues via the afferent lymphatics and passes across the node into the medulla where it exits via the efferent lymphatics. During passage across the node, microbes are "filtered" out by an extensive network of phagocytic macrophages. The efferent lymphatics carry lymph back into the circulation via the thoracic duct. Reprinted from P. M. Lydyard, A. Whelan, and M. W. Fanger, *Instant Notes in Immunology* (Bios Scientific, Taylor and Francis, Oxford, United Kingdom, 2000), with permission.

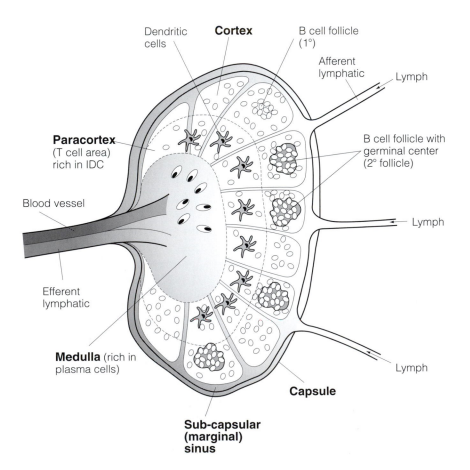

proliferating in response to antigens. These are important in the development of memory responses to antigens. As part of the lymphatic system, lymph nodes are mainly localized at the junctions of lymphatic vessels where they act as "filters," catching any microbes in the lymph and mounting an immune response to them.

The spleen has T and B lymphocytes localized in the white pulp (Fig. 8). The immunological function of the spleen is to filter microbes from the bloodstream and mount an immune response to them.

Lymphocytes are not sedentary but recirculate from the bloodstream to spleen and lymph nodes and back again. Lymphocytes stimulated by antigen in the MALT tend to migrate back to these areas (Fig. 9). Through recirculation, lymphocytes are able to "monitor" the body for invading organisms through their "antigen-specific receptors" (see below). They do this through surface adhesion molecules that allow them to bind to specialized endothelial cells of blood vessel walls. On attachment to the endothelial cells they are then able to migrate between them and gain entry into extravascular spaces. In the lymph node, these specialized endothelial cells (called high endothelial cells because of their tall morphology) are localized in the paracortical region.

ANTIBODIES: SPECIFICITIES, CLASSES, AND FUNCTIONS

Generalized Structure and Specificity

Antibodies have long been known as important molecules that protect against invading microbes. Their basic structure (Fig. 10) is two identical heavy and two identical light polypeptide chains held together with

FIGURE 8 The spleen. Lymphocytes are located in the white pulp of the spleen whereas plasma cells and macrophages are more frequent in the red pulp. The white pulp consists of T cells and B cells surrounding a branch of the splenic artery; hence it is referred to as the periarteriolar lymphoid sheath. The outer area of the periarteriolar lymphoid sheath (the marginal zone) contains macrophages (MØ) and B cells. Primary and secondary follicles are also found associated with specialized follicular dendritic cells (FDC), important in the function of B cells. Reprinted from P. M. Lydyard, A. Whelan, and M. W. Fanger, *Instant Notes in Immunology*, 2nd ed. (Bios Scientific, Taylor and Francis, Oxford, United Kingdom, 2004), with permission.

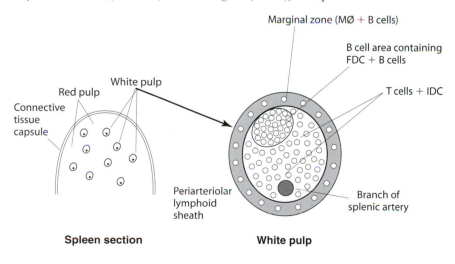

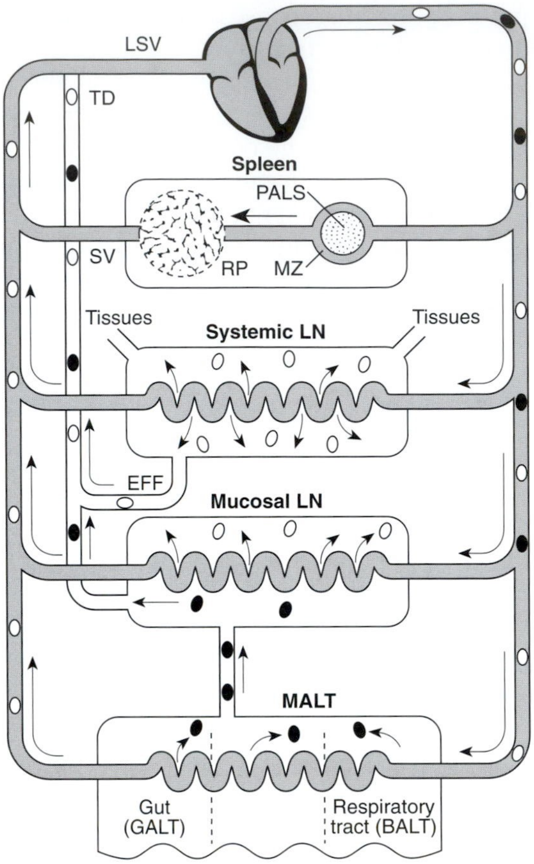

FIGURE 9 Lymphocyte recirculation. Lymphocytes (white ovals) enter the periarteriolar lymphoid sheath (PALS) through the marginal zone (MZ) and leave through the splenic vein (SV) of the red pulp (RP). Lymph node entry of lymphocytes can be from the tissues but is mainly from the bloodstream, facilitated by specialized capillary endothelial cells in the corticomedullary junction. Lymphocytes leave via the efferent lymphatics (EFF) into the thoracic duct (TD) that empties into the left subclavian vein (LSV) and hence back into the bloodstream. Recirculation through mucosa-associated tissues is unique. Lymphocytes stimulated at one site, e.g., intestine, traffic via the draining lymph nodes into the bloodstream (black ovals) and not only back to the intestine but also to other mucosal surfaces, e.g., bronchus and genitourinary tissues. Reprinted from J. H. L. Playfair and P. M. Lydyard, *Medical Immunology Made Memorable*, 2nd ed. (Churchill Livingstone, Edinburgh, United Kingdom, 2000), with permission from Elsevier Science.

FIGURE 10 Antibody structure. The basic antibody unit (here illustrated with the IgG molecule) is composed of two heavy and two light chains held together by disulfide bridges and a hinge region that gives the molecule flexibility when it binds to an antigen. The specific part of the molecule is the $F(ab)_2$ whilst the biological activity (e.g., binding to Fc receptors on phagocytes and complement-activating activity) is located in the Fc region. Reprinted from P. M. Lydyard, A. Whelan, and M. W. Fanger, *Instant Notes in Immunology* (Bios Scientific, Taylor and Francis, Oxford, United Kingdom, 2000), with permission.

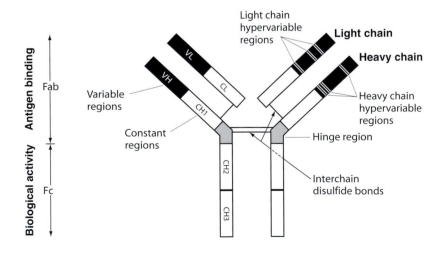

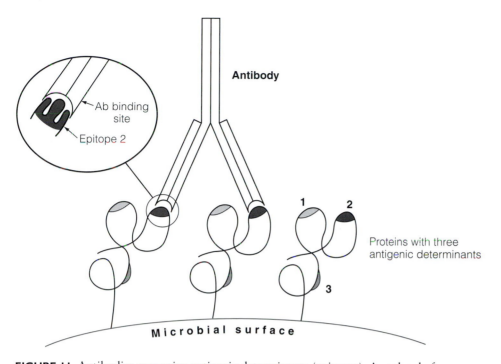

Antibody

Ab binding site

Epitope 2

1   2

Proteins with three antigenic determinants

3

M i c r o b i a l   s u r f a c e

FIGURE 11 Antibodies recognize antigenic determinants (epitopes). A molecule from a microbe will have several unique structures that will elicit an antibody and cellular immune response. An antigenic determinant (or epitope) is the smallest unit to which an antibody or cell can bind. Antibody is shown here binding through its two binding sites to antigenic determinants shared by the same protein molecules on a microbial surface. Antibodies recognize the three-dimensional shape of antigenic determinants whereas linear amino acid sequence is seen by T cells. Reprinted from P. M. Lydyard, A. Whelan, and M. W. Fanger, *Instant Notes in Immunology* (Bios Scientific, Taylor and Francis, Oxford, United Kingdom, 2000), with permission.

interchain disulfide bonds. Early studies on determining the structure of the molecule recognized two fragments, an $F(ab)_2$ fragment containing the variable part of the molecule and an Fc-crystallizable fragment. The front end (N terminus) is the part that binds to the foreign antigen while the rear end of the two heavy chains is responsible for the secondary function of the molecule (see below). In many cases the antibodies act as a "flag" to identify the foreign invader to immune cells and other molecules responsible for dealing with it. What makes an antibody specific are the different sets of amino acids in the "hypervariable" part of the heavy and light chains. Each chain, heavy and light, has a domain structure defined by intrachain disulfide bonds. Light chains have two domains and heavy chains have three or four, depending on the antibody class (see below). Each of the two N-terminal domains of the heavy and light chains contains hypervariable regions possessing two different sets of amino acids. The other domains of both heavy and light chains are constant for each antibody. The amino acids in the hypervariable region make up the antigen-binding site, each of which attaches to part of the antigen: the antigenic determinant, or epitope (Fig. 11). The reason the amino acids create different specificities is through their different properties of charge, shape, etc. In fact, the interaction of the binding site with an antigenic determinant is purely physical (Table 4), and the strength of the interaction is

TABLE 4 Physical forces between antibody molecules and antigenic determinants

Electrostatic forces
van der Waals forces
Hydrogen bonds
Hydrophobic forces

called the affinity. In practice, the binding of the two binding sites to two antigenic determinants is stronger than the sum of the two separate physical interactions. This is the avidity of the antibody for the antigen and is highest with those antibodies having several antigen-binding sites. Because of the structure of the binding sites, they are able to bind antigens in solution, giving rise to immune complexes. Immune complexes are usually cleared from the bloodstream following activation of complement (see below). In some situations these immune complexes can be deposited in blood vessels to give rise to vasculitis or glomerulonephritis. Immunopathology is the term given to tissue damage resulting from immune mechanisms.

Antibody Classes

Antibodies are called immunoglobulins because they are globular proteins with immune function. There are five major classes of antibodies built on the structure described above. Their differences lie in the types of heavy chain in the molecule. There are five different heavy chains that can produce different antibody molecules (Table 5). In addition, different classes of antibodies are of different sizes based on how many of the basic units described above are assembled to form the molecule. For example, IgG exists as a single basic unit (a monomer) (Fig. 10), whilst IgM is composed of five basic units joined together by a small polypeptide chain called J chain (Fig. 12). With regard to the light chains, a given antibody molecule can have one or another of two kinds of light chain, κ and λ, but not both.

Differential Properties of Antibodies

In general, there is a division of labor among the different classes of antibodies. Although there is overlap in their properties, they generally carry out their functions at different sites and with different consequences for the microbe.

IgM is the first antibody to be produced in an immune response. It is mainly localized in the bloodstream (Table 5) and, being a large molecule, tends to stay there and protect the body against blood-borne microbes. IgM is very efficient in activating complement through the classical pathway (Fig. 4). Indeed, it is generally believed that antibodies evolved as a specific way to target encapsulated microbes, as capsules protect microbes against complement activation via the lectin and alternative pathways. In a monomeric form, IgM occurs as an antigen receptor on the surface of B cells.

IgG is the most abundant antibody class in the bloodstream and, like IgM, can activate complement when two molecules attached to a mi-

TABLE 5 Antibody classes

Antibody class	Heavy chain	Units	Molecular mass (kDa)	Concn in adult blood (mg/ml)
IgM	μ	5	900	0.4–2
IgG	γ	1	150	8–16
IgD	δ	1	180	0.03
IgA	α	2/1	170–420	1.4–4
IgE	ε	1	190	Nanograms per milliliter

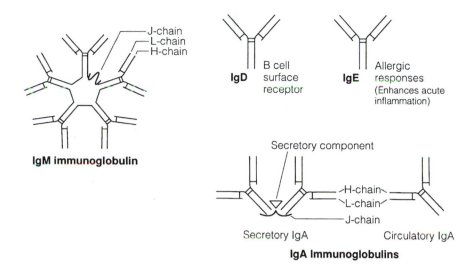

FIGURE 12 Structures of the different antibody classes. Secreted IgM has five "antibody units" (i.e., is pentameric), each made up of two heavy and two light chains held together by a small polypeptide J chain. IgD and IgE (like IgG) are single antibody units (monomeric). Blood-borne IgA exists as a single antibody unit while secretory IgA consists of two (or more) antibody units, also bound by J chains. These have a "secretory component" (polypeptide chain) attached when they are secreted across epithelial surfaces (see Fig. 13). Reprinted from P. M. Lydyard, A. Whelan, and M. W. Fanger, *Instant Notes in Immunology* (Bios Scientific, Taylor and Francis, Oxford, United Kingdom, 2000), with permission.

crobe are close enough together to bind C1q. IgG permeates the tissues of the body and is unique in that during gestation it is transported across the placenta into the bloodstream of the fetus to protect the newborn while its immune system is developing. Structures on its γ heavy chain allow it to bind to phagocytes (and some other cells) that have an Fc receptor for IgG.

IgD is mainly restricted to the surface of B cells where, with IgM, it forms an antigen receptor (Fig. 12).

IgA is present as both a monomer and dimer held together with a J chain. The latter is transported across mucosal surfaces into the lumen of the major tracts—respiratory, genitourinary, and gastrointestinal (see chapter 10)—by binding to specialized receptors on epithelial cells at luminal surfaces (Fig. 13).

IgE is an antibody that has "anaphylactic" activity. It binds to mast cells through Fc receptors and amplifies the acute inflammatory reaction (Fig. 5). It is thought that IgE evolved to protect the tracts where entry of worms is common. Enhanced traffic of blood-borne effector cells and molecules to sites of invading worms results from the binding of IgE to specific antigenic determinants on the worm and activation of mast cells.

Antibody-Mediated Protection against Microbes

ANTIBODY ALONE

Prevention of attachment of microbes and toxins to cells

Unless introduced into the tissues by a breach of the surface barriers of the skin and mucosae by trauma, insect bites, etc., pathogenic microorganisms must be able to bind to epithelial cells as a prerequisite for entry

FIGURE 13 IgA is transported across epithelial surfaces. IgA in the lamina propria beneath the epithelium attaches to poly-Ig receptors and is transported via endosomes to the luminal surface. The IgA is released into the lumen with a piece of the poly-Ig receptor (secretory component) attached. This is thought to protect the IgA molecule against the damaging effects of proteolytic enzymes. Reprinted from J. H. L. Playfair and P. M. Lydyard, *Medical Immunology Made Memorable*, 2nd ed. (Churchill Livingstone, Edinburgh, United Kingdom, 2000), with permission from Elsevier Science.

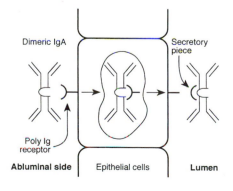

into the body. IgA antibodies that bathe the epithelial surfaces of the body lining the tracts provide an important protective mechanism by blocking the attachment of pathogenic microorganisms at these sites (Fig. 14; also see chapter 10). Viruses that traverse the surface barriers need to attach to specific surface molecules on host cells to enter. Antibody (especially IgG and IgM) recognizing the binding site on the virus prevents this (virus neutralization). In the same way, invading bacteria can be prevented from interacting with host cells. Furthermore, IgM and IgG antibodies can prevent pathogenic exotoxins produced by bacteria from binding to body cells.

Immobilization of bacteria by binding to flagella and agglutination

IgM, being pentameric, is very effective at this; IgG and IgA can also function in this way.

FIGURE 14 Antibody-mediated protection against infection. (a) Antibody alone: IgM and IgG can protect on their own by blocking attachment of viruses, bacteria, or toxins. They can also attach to the flagellae of bacteria and cause immobilization. In addition, IgM and IgG can bind to antigenic determinants on microbes and through their multiple binding sites (e.g., IgM has 10 binding sites) cause them to stick together, i.e., agglutinate. (b) Antibody plus complement: Following complement activation by antibodies, components C5 to C9, the membrane attack complex, cause lysis of bacteria. Note C3b also acts as an opsonin, to facilitate uptake by phagocytes (not shown here). (c) Antibody plus cells: Antibody (especially IgG) acts as an opsonin through binding to Fc receptors on phagocytes. Binding of IgG attached to large organisms, e.g., worms, through Fc receptors on phagocytes causes extracellular release of enzymes, etc. Reprinted from J. H. L. Playfair and P. M. Lydyard, *Medical Immunology Made Memorable*, 2nd ed. (Churchill Livingstone, Edinburgh, United Kingdom, 2000), with permission from Elsevier Science.

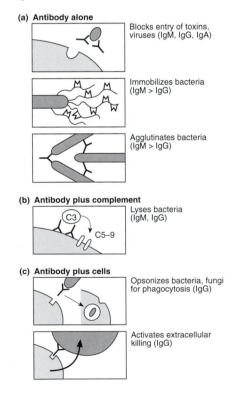

(a) **Antibody alone**

Blocks entry of toxins, viruses (IgM, IgG, IgA)

Immobilizes bacteria (IgM > IgG)

Agglutinates bacteria (IgM > IgG)

(b) **Antibody plus complement**

Lyses bacteria (IgM, IgG)

C3   C5–9

(c) **Antibody plus cells**

Opsonizes bacteria, fungi for phagocytosis (IgG)

Activates extracellular killing (IgG)

ANTIBODY ACTING WITH THE COMPLEMENT SYSTEM LEADING TO LYSIS

Complete activation of the complement system via the classical pathway leads to lysis of the bacteria via the membrane attack complex (Fig. 4).

ANTIBODY WITH CELLS

Opsonization: making microbes more tasty to phagocytes!

IgG antibodies binding to microbial cell surfaces can attach via their Fc parts to Fc receptors on phagocytes. This enhances the phagocytic process. Complement component C3b on the surface of microbes, resulting from IgG or IgM antibody-induced activation of the classical pathway, also acts as an "opsonin" since the phagocytes also have receptors for this complement component. IgA can also opsonize microbes through binding to Fc recptors but does not activate complement.

Antibody-dependent cytotoxicity

Antibody-dependent cytotoxicity occurs through extracellular release of molecules by effector cells, leading to death of an organism. The best example is protection against large worms that cannot be phagocytosed because of their size. Eosinophils attach to antibody (mainly IgG) coating the tough worm surface through Fc receptors. This causes the release of enzymes that damage the worm surface, leading to its demise. Phagocytes can then deal with broken up pieces of the dead worm.

RECOGNITION OF ANTIGEN BY LYMPHOCYTES

B Lymphocytes

To carry out their function, lymphocytes have to recognize microbial antigens through their specialized receptors. B lymphocytes use antibodies themselves as their antigen receptors. Each B lymphocyte has around 10^5 antibodies in its membrane, and each has the same hypervariable regions in its heavy and light chains, i.e., they have the same specificity. Each B lymphocyte has antibodies with different specificities, and there are probably around 10^8 or so different specific B lymphocytes. This large diversity of specific B lymphocytes is made possible by the random assortment of genes coding for the hypervariable regions during B-cell development.

Since B lymphocytes are specific, only a relatively small number (a few thousand) of B lymphocytes recognize foreign antigens from a given microbe, and only those that can bind the antigen proliferate and mature into plasma cells. This clonal selection by the antigen also requires T-helper cells (see below) and results in production of a large number of cells derived from the original cell stimulated by antigen (Fig. 15). In addition to maturation into antibody-producing plasma cells, some of the same B-cell clones will become memory cells that are important in protection against reinfection by the same microbe. As a result of the primary infection with the microbe, many more B cells (memory cells) with the same specificity will have been produced, resulting in a far larger antibody response to a second infection by the same microbe (Fig. 16). This is the basis of vaccination.

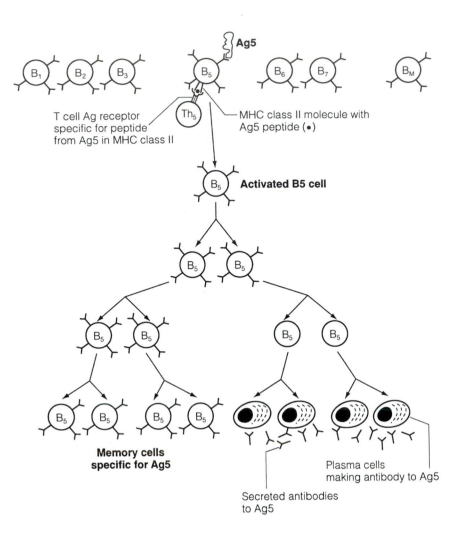

FIGURE 15 Clonal selection, memory cells, and plasma cells. Each B cell is specific for an antigenic determinant. With the help of Th cells that interact with antigenic peptides presented by the B cell through MHC class II molecules (see later), a particular B cell attaching to its specific antigenic determinant will be "activated" to divide. Some of the proliferating clonal cells are destined to become plasma cells (antibody factories) with specificity for the determinant originally recognized by the antigen receptor of the B cell. Another set of proliferating clonal cells becomes "memory" cells that are now more frequent than the original B cell and therefore able to provide a quicker response to a second encounter of the microbe. Note that a particular microbe might have a few thousand determinants recognized by different B cells, and shown here is the response of only one specific B cell. Reprinted from P. M. Lydyard, A. Whelan, and M. W. Fanger, *Instant Notes in Immunology* (Bios Scientific, Taylor and Francis, Oxford, United Kingdom, 2000), with permission.

T Lymphocytes

ANTIGEN PROCESSING AND PRESENTATION

Since the function of T cells is to protect against intracellular microbes, their receptors (TCRs) (Fig. 17) allow them to recognize components of the microbe displayed on the surface of an infected cell. If TCRs were able to bind microbial antigens directly, they would be stimulated to respond against soluble antigens, which would be useless to combat intracellular microbes. Thus, TCRs are designed not only to recognize foreign microbial antigens but also self-components that "present" antigenic pieces of microbe to them (Fig. 18). These antigen-presenting molecules are the major histocompatibility complex (MHC) molecules—called HLA (or human leukocyte antigens for historical reasons) in humans. The HLA molecules are of two major kinds: class I molecules are found on all nucleated cells of the body whereas class II molecules are normally restricted to dendritic cells, macrophages, and B cells. The distribution is necessarily different so as to direct the T cells (cytotoxic [Tc] and helper [Th] cells) to carry out their appropriate functions. Thus, Tc cells need to be directed to kill cells of the body infected with viruses, and this could be any nucleated cell. They are, therefore, programmed to recognize pieces

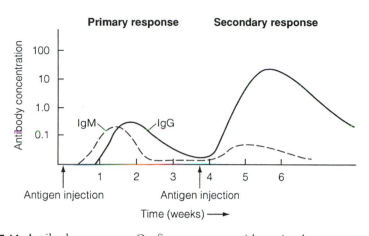

FIGURE 16 Antibody responses. On first encounter with a microbe, many specific B-cell clones will be activated to become plasma cells, first IgM and then IgG (primary antibody response). This takes time, due to the relatively few specific B cells available able to recognize the microbe. The antibody concentration rises in the circulation but drops again as the microbe is cleared from the body and the antigenic stimulation of the B cells is removed. On second encounter with the same microbe, memory cells from individual B-cell clones generated in the primary response will be stimulated by their antigenic determinants and produce more antibodies more quickly than in the primary response, together with even more clonal memory B cells (secondary response). Note that the primary antibody response is mostly IgM, while the memory response mainly results in the production of IgG and classes other than IgM. Reprinted from P. M. Lydyard, A. Whelan, and M. W. Fanger, *Instant Notes in Immunology* (Bios Scientific, Taylor and Francis, Oxford, United Kingdom, 2000), with permission.

of antigen, peptides of about 8 to 10 amino acids presented with HLA class I molecules. Th cells help macrophages to rid phagocytosed microbes growing inside them and recognize peptide antigens of 10 to 20 amino acids presented in HLA class II molecules.

For the peptides to assemble with the HLA molecules, they need to be "processed" by intracellular enzymes. Two different processing pathways determine which of the two HLA molecules display the microbial peptides for T-cell recognition. The pathway used is mainly determined by the mode of entry of the invading microbes. Thus, for viruses that enter cells and are present in the cytosol, the endogenous pathway is used to assemble viral peptides with HLA class I molecules (Fig. 19), whereas for those microbes taken in by phagocytosis, the exogenous pathway is used and the peptides are assembled with HLA class II molecules.

THE ADAPTIVE IMMUNE SYSTEM IN ACTION

Initiation of Adaptive Immune Responses: the Interface between the Innate and Adaptive Systems

Immature dendritic cells, like macrophages, are phagocytic and pick up microbes through their pattern receptors. They mature, and the processed microbial antigen is presented to antigen-specific Th cells (Fig. 20) that recognize peptides via surface HLA class II molecules on the dendritic "antigen-presenting cells" (Fig. 21). Specific Th cells also recognize peptides on macrophages in the same way. Interaction with antigen-presenting cells "activates" the T cells to proliferate in a clonal fashion, giving rise to more cells of the same specificity (memory cells), and to produce

FIGURE 17 The T-cell antigen receptor. T cells do not use antibody as their antigen receptor but instead most have two polypeptide chains—alpha and beta—held together by covalent bonds and passing across the outer membrane of the T cell. Like antibodies, the N termini of the chains—the outer domains—have variable amino acid sequences that determine their specificity for antigenic determinants. A smaller number of T cells use two different chains as their receptor—γ and δ. Reprinted from P. M. Lydyard, A. Whelan, and M. W. Fanger, *Instant Notes in Immunology* (Bios Scientific, Taylor and Francis, Oxford, United Kingdom, 2000), with permission.

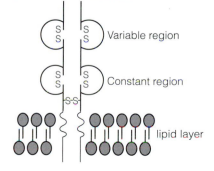

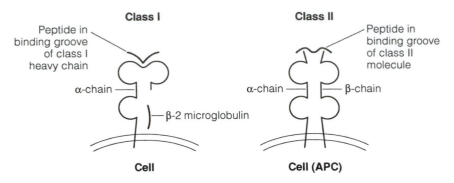

FIGURE 18 T cells recognize antigen presented by MHC class I and II molecules. MHC class I molecules are present on the surface of most nucleated cells of the body and MHC class II molecules are found on specialized antigen-presenting cells (APC) such as dendritic cells and B cells. They are composed of two polypeptide chains. The α-chain of the MHC class I and both α- and β-chains of MHC class II molecules have amino acid sequences and tertiary structures that allow them to bind (through a binding groove) microbial antigenic peptides within the cell and move to the surface. Here they "display" the peptides to be recognized by passing T cells. Reprinted from P. M. Lydyard, A. Whelan, and M. W. Fanger, *Instant Notes in Immunology* (Bios Scientific, Taylor and Francis, Oxford, United Kingdom, 2000), with permission.

FIGURE 19 Endogenous and exogenous antigen-processing pathways. Endogenous processing pathway: Viruses infecting cells enter the cytoplasm where they begin synthesizing their own peptides. Some peptides are cleaved by proteolytic enzymes and transported into the endoplasmic reticulum through specialized transporter molecules (TAP proteins). Viral peptides then attach to MHC class I molecules and are transported to the cell surface where they are displayed to T cells. Exogenous processing pathway: Microbes entering a cell through endosomes (by phagocytosis or pinocytosis) are digested in part through proteolytic enzymes. Endosomes fuse with vacuoles containing MHC class II molecules that pick up the antigenic peptides and are transported to the cell surface where they display the peptide to T cells. Reprinted from P. M. Lydyard, A. Whelan, and M. W. Fanger, *Instant Notes in Immunology* (Bios Scientific, Taylor and Francis, Oxford, United Kingdom, 2000), with permission.

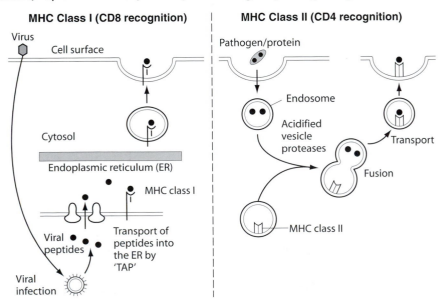

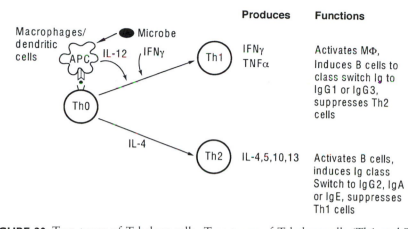

| Produces | Functions |

FIGURE 20 Two types of T helper cells. Two types of T helper cells (Th1 and Th2) differentiate from immature antigen-specific CD4⁺ T cells. Th1 and Th2 cells possess different functions depending on the cytokines they produce. Th1 cells are primarily involved in cell-mediated immunity against intracellular microbes including bacteria and viruses. Th2 cells are mainly involved in helping B cells divide and class switch to make the IgG2 subclass of antibodies and other antibody classes, i.e., IgA and IgE. Th1 cells also help in class switching to IgG1 and IgG3 antibodies. Reprinted from P. M. Lydyard, A. Whelan, and M. W. Fanger, *Instant Notes in Immunology* (Bios Scientific, Taylor and Francis, Oxford, United Kingdom, 2000), with permission.

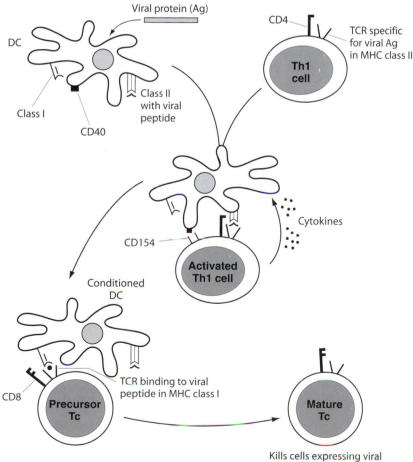

FIGURE 21 Dendritic cells (DC) at the interface between innate and adaptive immune responses. Viruses and other microbes are phagocytosed by immature dendritic cells, which then mature and are able to present antigenic peptides through MHC class II molecules to Th1 cells. These Th1 cells become activated and surface CD154 attaches to CD40 on the dendritic cells. This causes release of cytokines that "condition" the dendritic cell. This conditioning allows the microbial antigens to be processed through the endogenous pathway, and thus some antigenic peptides are presented through MHC class I molecules to cytotoxic T-cell precursors that have CD8 molecules. These precursor cells, with the aid of other cytokines, e.g., IL-2 provided by the Th1 cells, are able to proliferate and develop into mature cytotoxic cells. Reprinted from P. M. Lydyard, A. Whelan, and M. W. Fanger, *Instant Notes in Immunology* (Bios Scientific, Taylor and Francis, Oxford, United Kingdom, 2000), with permission.

cytokines—the main function of Th cells (cf. B-cell clonal activation). Two kinds of Th cells "help" different cells in host defense mainly through production of different patterns of cytokines (Fig. 20). They both express CD4 molecules that interact with part of the HLA class II molecules not binding the microbial peptides. Th1 cells are activated by peptides associated with macrophages and dendritic cells (Fig. 21). The production of IL-2 by Th1 cells stimulates proliferation of the T cells (i.e., it has autocrine function) whereas IFN-γ induces ("conditions") the dendritic cells so that they are able to present the microbial peptides with HLA class I molecules to cytotoxic CD8$^+$ T-cell precursors. Additional molecules on the surface of the Th1 cells (CD154) interact with their ligand on the surface of the dendritic cells (CD40) to enhance this conditioning process. Different kinds of dendritic cells can also suppress immune responses, for example, to food antigens entering the intestine.

Most B Cells Require Help from T Cells

B cells can directly be stimulated to develop into IgM-producing plasma cells by antigens that have repetitive sequences recognized by the specific antigen receptors on B cells. Examples of such antigens are sugars that have a backbone with multiple hexose residues. However, for most antigens T cells are required. B cells do not phagocytose large microbes but can pick up pieces of microbes or their products that attach to their specific antigen receptors. Whole viruses can also be taken into B cells in this way. Similar to phagocytosis by macrophages, B-cell entry of microbes or products via these receptors triggers the exogenous pathway of antigen processing and the microbial peptides are assembled in HLA class II molecules on the specific B-cell surface. Th2 cells that have TCRs specific for the microbial peptides assembled with HLA class II molecules will attach to the specific B cells. Cytokines produced by the Th2 cells (IL-4, -5, and -6) help the B cell to proliferate and differentiate into plasma cells (Fig. 22). Interaction of CD154 on the Th2-cell surface with CD40 on the B-cell surface results in antibody class switching so that some of the B cells develop into IgG-producing plasma cells and memory cells that on second encounter with antigen will develop into IgG-producing plasma cells.

FIGURE 22 T-cell help for B cells. B cells pick up antigen through their specific antigen receptors. Following receptor-mediated endocytosis, antigen is processed and peptides are displayed on surface MHC class II molecules to be recognized by antigen-specific Th cells. Activation of the Th2 cell results in cytokine production required for proliferation and development into plasma cells. In addition, CD154 is produced at the T-cell surface that interacts with B-cell CD40. This is necessary to induce class switching from IgM to the other antibody classes. Reprinted from P. M. Lydyard, A. Whelan, and M. W. Fanger, *Instant Notes in Immunology* (Bios Scientific, Taylor and Francis, Oxford, United Kingdom, 2000), with permission.

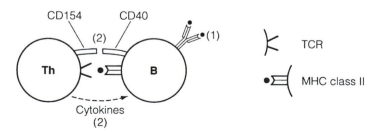

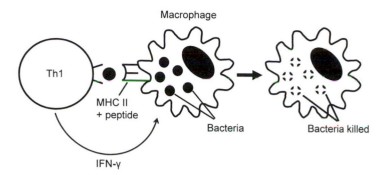

Macrophage

Th1

MHC II
+ peptide

Bacteria

Bacteria killed

IFN-γ

FIGURE 23 Th1-mediated activation of macrophages. Mycobacteria (e.g., *Mycobacterium tuberculosis* or *Mycobacterium leprae*) phagocytosed by macrophages are difficult to kill. However, antigenic pieces of the intracellular mycobacterium are processed and small peptides displayed on the surface to specific Th1 cells. Intracellular killing is enhanced by Th1 cells releasing IFN-γ that "activates" the macrophages. Reprinted from P. M. Lydyard, A. Whelan, and M. W. Fanger, *Instant Notes in Immunology*, 2nd ed. (Bios Scientific, Taylor and Francis, Oxford, United Kingdom, 2004), with permission.

Follicular germinal centers (Fig. 7) are the sites where B-cell proliferation, class switching, and memory-cell production take place in lymphoid tissues. In addition, selection of B cells that have higher affinity for antigen takes place, resulting in a progressive increase in antibody affinity in secondary and tertiary responses to the same antigen.

T-Cell Mechanisms in Host Defense: Cell-Mediated Immunity

We have already seen how Th2 cells help B cells make antibodies and the way they work in protecting against invading microbes and even large worms. Th1 cells directly interact with macrophages containing intracellular microbes that are proliferating inside them, e.g., mycobacteria. The IFN-γ produced by them is a macrophage activation factor that stimulates the macrophage to kill the intracellular invader (Fig. 23). This is not always successful and overstimulation of Th1 cells can lead to "hypersensitivity" and formation of granulomata (immunopathology). It is these granulomata that often cause death in tuberculosis since they obliterate large areas of respiratory tissues.

Mature cytotoxic cells derived from cytotoxic precursor T cells interact with virus-infected cells that are presenting viral peptides through their HLA class I molecules. Killing of the infected cells occurs via two mechanisms, both designed to induce the cells to commit suicide (apoptosis):

1. Perforin-mediated cell death: Mature Tc cells (also called cytotoxic lymphocytes, or CTL) have cytoplasmic granules containing perforin and granzymes that induce apoptosis (Fig. 24).
2. Fas-mediated apoptosis: Virus-infected cells increase a molecule called Fas (CD95) on their surface; mature activated Tc cells have the ligand for Fas on their surface, and cross-linking of the Fas leads to apoptosis (Fig. 25).

In this way the cell shrivels up without releasing the viral particles to infect further cells. The apoptotic cells are taken up by phagocytic cells and digested, the viral particles being killed by effective intracellular killing mechanisms.

FIGURE 24 Perforin-mediated cytotoxicity by Tc cells. (a) Virus-infected cells displaying viral peptides in their MHC class I molecules are recognized by mature specific cytotoxic T cells that, on contact, release lytic granules containing perforin that forms pores in the target cell membrane. (b) Enzymes (granzymes) pass into the target cell, causing the infected cell to commit suicide (apoptosis). Reprinted from P. M. Lydyard, A. Whelan, and M. W. Fanger, *Instant Notes in Immunology* (Bios Scientific, Taylor and Francis, Oxford, United Kingdom, 2000), with permission.

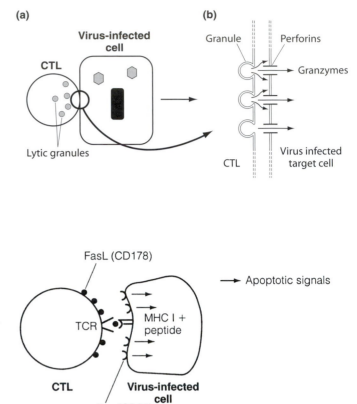

FIGURE 25 FasL-mediated cytotoxicity by cytotoxic T cells. Mature cytotoxic T cells on attachment to target infected cells become activated and express FasL. Interaction of this molecule with Fas on the surface of the infected cell also induces cell death by apoptosis. Reprinted from P. M. Lydyard, A. Whelan, and M. W. Fanger, *Instant Notes in Immunology* (Bios Scientific, Taylor and Francis, Oxford, United Kingdom, 2000), with permission.

KEY POINTS

Physical barriers such as the skin, along with antimicrobial secretions such as lysozyme, defensins, and short-chain fatty acids, are the first line of defense against microorganisms.

Microorganisms that penetrate these barriers encounter:
- Phagocytic cells that ingest and kill organisms—PMNs circulate in the blood, and macrophages are tissue associated
- NK cells that attack virus-infected cells
- Mast cells that release inflammatory mediators
- Complement that is activated by microbes or antibodies, and through a cascade of enzymatic reactions, helps initiate inflammation and produces opsonins and components that induce lysis of bacteria by punching holes in their membranes
- Acute-phase proteins that can contribute to host defense and repair damage caused by infection
- Cytokines, messenger molecules, that regulate immune activity. Interferons also have antiviral activity.

The adaptive immune response is the second level of defense.

Lymphocytes are the key cell type in the adaptive system. T cells are produced in the thymus and B cells are produced in the bone marrow.

Lymphocytes recirculate in the blood and are also found in specialized lymphoid tissues such as the lymph nodes and spleen. Lymphoid tissue associated with mucosal surfaces is known as the MALT.

B cells produce antibodies, Y-shaped molecules that bind foreign antigens through hypervariable domains in the heavy and light chains at the front end of the molecule.

There are five major classes of antibodies based on the type of heavy chain in the molecule. IgA, IgG, IgM, IgD, and IgE all have differing functional properties.

General functions of antibodies include preventing attachment of microbes and toxins; agglutination and immobilization of organisms; opsonization; activation of the complement cascade; and induction of extracellular release of antimicrobial enzymes.

B cells have antibody receptors of predetermined specificity. Binding of a complementary antigen causes proliferation and maturation into antibody-producing cells (clonal selection). Some B-cell clones will become memory cells that can react more rapidly to infection with the same organism.

T cells have receptors that recognize microbial antigens but only when the antigen is presented by an MHC molecule (called HLA molecules in humans). Cytotoxic T cells recognize and kill virus-infected nucleated cells by TCR binding to small antigenic peptides presented with HLA class I molecules. Helper T cells facilitate microbial killing inside macrophages and recognize slightly longer

KEY POINTS

(Continued from previous page)
antigenic peptides than those presented by HLA class II molecules. Differential processing inside cells directs peptides to either the HLA class I or II molecules.

The innate and adaptive immune systems interface with each other. Antigen-presenting cells such as dendritic cells and macrophages recognize antigens through their pattern recognition receptors. Processed antigen in conjunction with HLA class II molecules is presented to CD4 on Th cells. The T cells become activated and proliferate clonally to produce memory cells with the same specificity and also secrete cytokines. A subset of Th cells (Th1) produces cytokines that condition dendritic cells to present antigen with HLA class I molecules that then stimulate CD8$^+$ Tc cells. In addition, cytokines are produced that stimulate intracellular killing by macrophages. Another subset of T cells (Th2) produces cytokines that stimulate B-cell proliferation and class switching of antibodies (from IgM to IgG).

ACKNOWLEDGMENTS

We thank Elsevier Science and Bios Scientific, Taylor and Francis, for permission to reprint figures.

M. F. Cole is supported by Public Health Service grant DE08178 from the National Institute of Dental and Craniofacial Research, National Institutes of Health.

CORE READING

Lydyard, P. M., A. Whelan, and M. W. Fanger. 2000. *Instant Notes in Immunology*, 2nd ed. Bios Scientific, Taylor and Francis, Oxford, United Kingdom.

Playfair, J. H. L., and P. M. Lydyard. 2000. *Medical Immunology Made Memorable*, 2nd ed. Churchill Livingstone, Edinburgh, United Kingdom.

FURTHER READING

Janeway, C. A., P. Travers, M. Wolpert, and M. Shlomchik. 2001. *Immunobiology*, 5th ed. Garland Publishing, Taylor and Francis, New York, N.Y.

Roitt, I. M., and P. J. Delves. 2002. *Essential Immunology*, 10th ed. Blackwell Scientific, Oxford, United Kingdom.

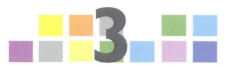

3

The Oral Environment

Frank A. Scannapieco

INTRODUCTION

Bacteria that reside in the oral cavity occupy a unique and fascinating habitat. The mouth is the only part of the body where hard tissues (the teeth) are naturally exposed to the external environment. Like barnacles attaching to a ship's hull, a diverse ensemble of bacteria firmly adhere to and grow on the teeth to form a complex biofilm known as dental plaque. The complexity of the oral microbial ecology is magnified by the fact that the mouth also possesses a variety of other surfaces, including the buccal and vestibular mucosa, hard palate, tongue, and the floor of the mouth, all of which provide unique habitats for microbial colonization. Considerable fluctuations in oral environmental parameters also occur, such as temperature, oxygen availability, pH, and variability in the composition and frequency of exposure to dietary constituents. Finally, the oral tissues are bathed in saliva, which provides physical cleansing by virtue of fluid flow and dilution effects, as well as host immune and non-immune defense factors that together have profound consequences for the microbial ecology. The goal of this chapter is to provide an overview of the environment in which oral bacteria live and to describe some host defense factors oral bacteria face and the mechanisms the bacteria use to overcome them.

GENERAL FEATURES OF THE ORAL ENVIRONMENT

Teeth

Uniquely in the mouth, the mineralized enamel surfaces of the teeth are exposed to the external environment. In a healthy person, the tooth emerges from the supporting tissues that cover the root of the tooth apical (toward the apex) of the cementoenamel junction; as such, only enamel is exposed within the oral cavity. The tooth itself is composed of four tissues: enamel, dentin, cementum, and pulp (Fig. 1). (The reader is urged to consult textbooks and reviews of oral histology for more information on the histology of these tissues. Some of these are listed at the end of this chapter.) Like bone, each of these tissues is formed from the mineralization of an organic matrix secreted by specialized cells during

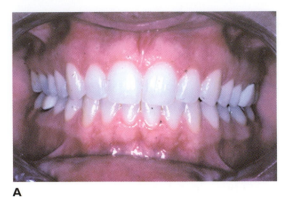

A

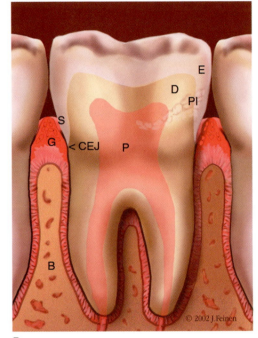

B

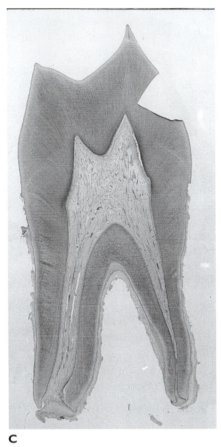

C

FIGURE 1 The mouth and teeth in health. (A) Clinical picture of a healthy mouth. Note absence of deposits on the teeth and the pink gingival tissues. (B) Artist's depiction of the structures of the healthy tooth. E, enamel; D, dentin; B, bone; P, pulp; G, gingiva; Pl, plaque; CEJ, cemento-enamel junction; S, sulcus. Connective tissue fibers of the periodontal ligament span the space between the cementum and the supporting bone. (C)Axial section through maxillary first molar showing prominent pulp space surrounded by dentin. (Courtesy of H. E. Schroeder, Institute of Oral Structural Biology, University of Zurich, Zurich, Switzerland.)

the process of development. This matrix is composed of proteins involved in extracellular mineralization. They include amelogenins, tuftelins, ameloblastins, enamelins, and proteinases.

The crown of the tooth is composed of enamel, which is the most highly mineralized tissue in the body (containing 96% inorganic material). As the result of developmental processes, enamel displays a variety of structural features conspicuous on the surface of tooth crowns. For example, horizontal lines across the crown, called perikymata, can lend an undulation to the tooth surface. Each type of tooth (anterior, premolar, and molar) has unique patterns of fissures and grooves specific to each tooth type. These grooves can be shallow or deep, depending on the individual. Enamel itself is composed of an assemblage of numerous rods that extend at roughly right angles from the dentoenamel junction toward the outer surface of the tooth. The average diameter of each rod is about 4 μm. Each enamel rod, itself the product of the ameloblast, a specialized cell responsible for the development of the enamel and tooth crown, is organized as arrays of hydroxyapatite crystals. The outline form of each keyhole-shaped rod is visible on a slightly demineralized enamel surface. Taken together, these diverse structures may have clinical significance insofar as they may subtly influence dental plaque development and susceptibility to dental caries and periodontal disease.

The surface of the enamel is covered by the pellicle, a film composed of salivary and other proteins. This pellicle plays an important role in the interaction of bacteria with the tooth surface and in preventing mineral loss from the tooth, and is discussed in greater detail below.

Dentin, which is 70% mineral and 30% water and organic matrix, comprises the bulk of each tooth. It underlies the enamel and surrounds the tooth pulp. Dentin is not exposed in the oral cavity of a healthy individual. Dentin develops as the odontoblast secretes a set of matrix proteins at the mineralization front that becomes calcified. This matrix is composed of collagen and other proteins common to mineralized tissues such as osteopontin, acidic glycoprotein-75, dentin matrix protein 1, bone sialoprotein, decorin, and biglycan. The odontoblast also produces proteins unique to dentin, including dentin phosphoprotein and dentin sialoprotein. Certain oral bacteria, especially those implicated in the process of dental caries, can interact specifically with dentinal proteins such as collagen. This interaction may assist bacterial invasion of dentin during the process of dental caries.

As a result of development, the odontoblast produces a dentinal tubule that extends from the pulp to the dentinoenamel or cementoenamel junction of the tooth. In health, each tubule is filled with the odontoblastic process, an extension of the odontoblast. The odontoblast is also responsible for the formation of secondary or reparative dentin. During the process of dental caries, bacteria can invade the dentinal tubules to injure the odontoblast (for a more complete discussion of dental caries, see chapter 11). Reparative dentin is often produced in response to such chronic infection in order to isolate the bacteria from the pulp. Should the bacteria spread into the pulp, the resulting infection and inflammation are often the cause of serious pain and the possible spread of infection into the bone surrounding and supporting the teeth. In most cases, pulpitis requires root canal therapy or tooth extraction. Before the advent of antibiotic use, such dental infections could cause a severe and sometimes fatal infection.

The pulp space is filled with soft tissues that are enclosed in dentin. The pulp is the only nonmineralized tissue of the tooth. It contains several types of cells, including fibroblasts, macrophages, monocytes and other immune competent cells, mesenchymal cells, and odontoblasts. The latter cells line the pulp-dentin interface and project the odontoblast processes into the dentinal tubules. The intercellular space within the pulp is composed of collagen fibrils and a variety of proteins and proteoglycans. The pulp also contains nerve fibers and blood vessels that provide sensory innervation, nutrition, and metabolite disposal. The pulp under normal circumstances is sterile, but could be invaded by bacteria during the process of dental caries (see chapter 11).

The Oral Soft Tissues (Periodontium, Oral Mucosa, and Tongue)

The gingiva surrounds the teeth to provide a seal that prevents microbial invasion into the underlying tissues. The surface of the gingiva is covered by stratified squamous keratinized epithelium. Underlying the epithelium is fibrous connective tissue (the lamina propria) that is directly attached to the underlying alveolar bone via collagen fibrils.

The gingiva forms a collar around the teeth that defines the gingival sulcus. The portion of the gingiva not attached to the tooth is called the free gingiva. The inner wall of the sulcus is the tooth surface. The outer wall is the sulcular epithelium that is continuous with the outer epithelial surface of the gingiva. The base (toward the tooth apex) of the gingival sulcus is continuous with the junctional epithelium that is directly attached to the tooth surface. It is the junctional epithelium that seals the external environment from the underlying tissues that support the teeth. The junctional epithelium attaches to the tooth surface by structures (hemidesmosomes) that resemble those that attach the epithelial basal cell membrane to the basement lamina. In health, the depth of the gingival sulcus rarely exceeds 2 mm. As an individual ages, the teeth slowly but continuously erupt and the gingival tissues may migrate slowly apically. The tissues that cover the tooth root can become exposed to the oral cavity environment as a result of physical abrasion of the gingival tissues (for example, by aggressive oral hygiene procedures) or as a consequence of the pathological process of periodontal disease that results in loss of the tooth's connective tissue attachment and supporting alveolar bone (see chapter 12).

The cementum and periodontal ligament are specialized tissues that surround and support the root surface of each tooth. Cementum is a mineralized tissue that overlies and is attached to the root dentin. Collagen fibers (Sharpey's fibers) from the periodontal ligament extend into the cementum. It is these Sharpey's fibers that are responsible for the attachment of the tooth root via the cementum to the periodontal ligament and the tooth socket of the alveolus. Cells within the cementum (cementoblasts) also provide reparative functions following trauma. The periodontal ligament is a layer of connective tissue that surrounds the tooth root between the cementum and alveolar bone. It is composed of cells (mostly fibroblasts, with some nerve cells, macrophages, and lymphocytes), connective tissues (primarily collagen), blood vessels, and interstitial fluids.

The tissues lining the buccal mucosa and vestibule, floor of the mouth, hard and soft palate, and tongue in many ways resemble skin from a histologic point of view. The surface of the oral mucosa is covered by epithelium, which is supported by an underlying connective tissue (or lamina propria). Interspersed throughout the oral mucosa are numerous minor salivary glands of the mucous type. Oral mucosa differs from skin in that the epithelium is not keratinized (except on the tongue, gingiva, and palate), and it is kept moist by saliva rather than by sebaceous oils and sweat. Passing through the oral mucosa are ducts of the major salivary glands (parotid, submandibular, sublingual) as well as the minor glands.

The surface of the tongue is different from other oral epithelia in that it demonstrates a complicated surface, with a variety of structures including filliform, fungiform, and circumvallate papillae and lingual tonsils that furnish numerous crypts, trenches, and other protected sites providing sheltered habitats for bacterial colonization.

All oral surfaces are covered with a layer of components mostly derived from the salivary glands. These oral pellicles serve to lubricate and hydrate the tissues and modulate the microbial flora. Of added significance to the microbiology of the mouth, the epithelial cells also express a variety of potential bacterial receptors, such as glycolipids, on their surfaces. As described below, the pellicle and cell surface proteins may provide adhesion receptors to which oral bacteria may attach. Epithelial cells also respond to bacterially induced inflammation by producing a variety of antimicrobial peptides, such as human beta-defensins, adrenomedullin, and calprotectin that likely limit bacterial invasion of the soft tissues.

PHYSICAL AND HOST PARAMETERS AFFECTING ORAL MICROBIAL COLONIZATION

Temperature

The temperature in the mouth of a healthy person may vary considerably. For example, during a standardized drinking regimen of hot black coffee (72.5°C) followed by cold orange juice, a maximum intraoral temperature of 68.0°C and a minimum of 15.4°C were recorded. The maximal intraoral temperature differences between upper and lower extremes following such a regimen were measured to be 29.6°C at the base of a coronal restoration, 27.1°C on the facial surface of teeth, and 11.8°C within the root canal. Localized inflammatory processes may also modulate oral tissue temperature. The mean temperature of healthy gingival sulci has been measured to range from 33.7 to 36.6°C, depending on the tooth, whereas the temperature within a diseased periodontal pocket may be several degrees higher. These temperature fluctuations may influence oral microbes since it is known that such fluctuations can influence the synthesis of global regulators of gene expression in bacteria known as transcriptional regulators (for example, sigma factors). These regulatory proteins can then direct the expression of the so-called heat shock proteins. It is thought that heat shock proteins may modulate the virulence of certain pathogens subjected to temperature stress, as occurs during the process of infection.

pH

It is well known that bacteria in dental plaque are capable of producing copious amounts of lactic and other organic acids from the metabolism of simple dietary sugars. This is discussed in greater detail in the context of the pathogenesis of dental caries in chapter 11. The classic studies of Robert Stephan in the 1940s illustrate the central role of dental plaque acid in the caries process. Those studies showed that resting plaque pH of caries-free subjects is slightly alkaline (~7.2). However, the resting plaque pH of subjects with severe caries could be measured to be as low as 5.5. Stephan also found that plaques of caries-susceptible subjects challenged with a glucose rinse reduce pH levels from above 6 to well below 5 within 10 min, presumably due to the effects of bacterial metabolism of the sugar to organic acids. These shifts in dental plaque pH have profound effects on plaque ecology. When a person frequently eats foods rich in carbohydrates (especially simple sugars such as sucrose), acid-sensitive bacteria are eliminated and acid-tolerant bacteria such as the mutans group streptococci and lactobacilli are enriched within the plaque microbiota. This ecologic shift likely causes an increase of the pH-lowering and cariogenic potential of plaque.

Acid-resistant (aciduric) bacteria such as oral streptococci and lactobacilli possess interesting mechanisms to maintain appropriate intracellular pH levels in the face of very low extracellular pH. For example, *Streptococcus mutans* has been shown to have a membrane proton-translocating ATPase, a pump that exports H^+ ions out of the cell. Bacteria such as *S. mutans* can also grow at low pH, a property not seen in other more acid-sensitive species. Other bacteria may also protect themselves from low pH conditions by producing compounds that can buffer acid. For example, *Streptococcus salivarius* is capable of producing significant amounts of the basic compound urea.

Oxygen

The concentration of oxygen varies enormously in the mouth, depending on the location in which it is measured. Obviously, inspirated gases contain the same concentration of O_2 as does ambient air. However, its concentration rapidly diminishes as it approaches the oral surfaces. Early dental plaque is relatively rich in oxygen, but mature plaque is relatively anaerobic. More important to the colonization of the mouth by bacteria than the oxygen content of breathed air are the production and metabolism of highly reactive oxygen species by the bacteria and the host. They include the superoxide radical (O_2^-), hydrogen peroxide (H_2O_2), and hydroxyl radical (OH^-). Such reactive species are highly toxic to bacteria, causing irreversible damage to membranes and proteins. The plaque biofilm, however, adjusts environmental conditions to allow anaerobic bacteria to flourish. These anaerobes also possess mechanisms to remove toxic oxygen for example, enzymes such as superoxide dismutase, catalase, and NAD oxidase.

Mechanical Abrasive Forces

Inspection of the typical pattern of dental plaque on teeth reveals that plaques are not homogeneously spread over the teeth but appear to be localized to interproximal, buccal, and lingual tooth surfaces adjacent to the gingival margin. Typically, buccal and lingual surfaces of teeth at or above the height of contour are free of plaque, even in patients with very poor oral hygiene habits. This is due to the potent abrasive cleansing action of the movement of the lips, buccal mucosa, and tongue over the surfaces of the teeth. This leads to desquamation of the surface cells of the epithelia, explaining why plaque does not form to a great extent on mucosal surfaces.

Fluid Flow

It is clear that saliva is important in the control of dental plaque formation and in the pathogenesis of dental caries and periodontal disease. Subjects with compromised salivary function display enhanced plaque formation and have a greater risk for oral diseases such as dental caries and periodontitis. One of the most important functions of saliva is the physical cleansing action of the fluid on the oral cavity.

The contribution of each gland to whole saliva is quite variable (Table 1). Normal flow rates for whole saliva have been calculated to be 0.3 ml/min unstimulated and ≥1.0 ml/min stimulated. Most of the saliva is secreted from the major glands, with minor glands contributing <5% of the volume of whole saliva. Frequent swallowing combined with continuous salivary flow constantly replenishes the fluids in the oral cavity and promotes the dilution and clearance of acid and bacterial toxins from plaque into saliva and eventually away from the oral cavity.

Host Age

A variety of studies have suggested that the mouth is susceptible to colonization by different bacterial species at different times over the course of the human life span. For example, early studies suggested that anaerobic bacteria such as *Porphyromonas gingivalis* do not colonize the mouths of children in appreciable numbers. These organisms begin to colonize the mouth around the time of adolescence. Recent longitudinal studies of transmission and acquisition of oral bacteria within mother-infant pairs found that the permanent colonization of the mouth by oral streptococci occurs during a discrete "window of infectivity" (around 9 months of age). This group of bacteria, which includes the mutans group streptococci, requires the presence of teeth or other nonshedding surfaces (for example, a denture) to colonize the mouth. Thus, these bacteria are found only transiently in the mouth of children before tooth eruption.

THE ORAL MICROBIOTA

Tooth (Dental) Plaque: Early Determinants of Plaque Formation

Dental plaque is a dense bacterial mass (also known as a biofilm) that is tightly adherent to the tooth surface. Bacterial attachment to the tooth is mediated by receptors in the thin salivary coating of the tooth, termed the

TABLE I Mean flow rates from various salivary glands[d]

Gland	Unstimulated flow rate[a]	Stimulated flow rate[a]
Parotid[b]	47.0 ± 1.2 μl/min/gland	619 ± 56 μl/min/gland
Submandibular[c]	58 ± 9 μl/min/gland	254 ± 25 μl/min/gland
Palatal	0.74 ± 0.35 μl/min	0.75 ± 0.30 μl/min
Labial	0.96 ± 0.55 μl/min	1.00 ± 0.39 μl/min
Buccal	2.64 ± 0.98 μl/min	2.52 ± 0.92 μl/min
Whole saliva	300 μl/min (range, 250–350)	1,500 μl/min (range, 1,000–3,000)

[a]Mean ± standard deviation.

[b]Data for middle-aged males.

[c]Data for young males.

[d]Information from B. J. Baum, p. 126–134, *in* D. B. Ferguson (ed.), *The Aging Mouth* (Karger, Basel, Switzerland, 1987); I. L. Shannon et al., *Saliva: Composition and Secretion* (Karger, Basel, Switzerland, 1974); and R. J. Shern et al., *J. Dent. Res.* **69:**1146–1149, 1990.

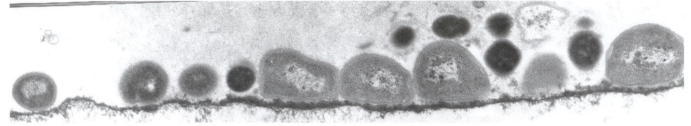

A

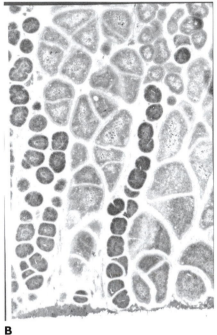

FIGURE 2 (A) Transmission electron micrograph of the initial adhesion of cocci to supragingival enamel pellicle. The dark line of material is the salivary pellicle adsorbed to enamel. (B) Growth of the initial layer of adherent bacteria on the tooth to form columnar microcolonies. (Courtesy of H. E. Schroeder, Institute of Oral Structural Biology, University of Zurich, Zurich, Switzerland.)

B

acquired pellicle (Fig. 2). The pellicle and plaque matrices are composed of host-derived and bacterial products. The tightly adherent dental plaque should be differentiated from the so-called materia alba, a loosely adherent soft, white material composed of food debris, bacteria, leukocytes, and desquamated oral epithelial cells that accumulates on the oral surfaces of an unclean mouth and that is easily removed from the oral surfaces by a strong water spray.

A critical determinant of bacterial colonization to any surface is the ability of the bacteria to adhere to that surface. Bacterial adhesion to host tissues may occur by a variety of mechanisms. One general mechanism involves nonspecific forces (e.g., ionic, hydrophobic, hydrogen bonding, and van der Waals) between the microbial and host surfaces. Another mechanism involves specific or stereochemical interactions between bacterial surface adhesins and the host components in pellicle. The latter interactions, similar to antibody-antigen or enzyme-substrate interactions, depend on recognition of molecular shapes between proteins. These interactions are highly specific and, when superimposed on the nonspecific forces, account in part for selective colonization of the host tissues. Specific adherent interactions are mediated by specialized bacterial surface proteins, or adhesins, that bind to receptors on the host surface. The receptor may be another protein or a carbohydrate (often attached to a glycoprotein or glycolipid).

Dental plaque maturation, the stage of plaque development following initial bacterial adhesion, is thought to depend to a large extent on the adsorption of bacteria in saliva to bacteria already adherent to the tooth. This phenomenon has been studied in vitro by allowing two or more strains of different species to interact, which results in clumping together of the two cell types. This can occur between two species in solution ("coaggregation") or between one bacterium in solution adhering to an already adherent bacterium ("coadhesion").

Plaque maturation also depends on bacterial growth and multiplication. Plaque bacteria derive their nutrition from metabolism of host products (for example, salivary proteins) or dietary constituents (for example, sugar or amino acids from foods) to grow and divide to form microcolonies on the tooth surface. Often, these bacteria produce products that can injure the host tissues. Thus, the bacteria in plaque can ferment sugar to form lactic acid, which can then cause demineralization of the tooth substance, resulting in dental caries.

Following thorough mechanical cleansing of the tooth (thus removing all plaque deposits), the first morphologically identifiable structure to immediately form on the tooth surface is the acquired enamel pellicle. Bacteria then adhere to the pellicle and proliferate. The first bacteria to adhere are usually cocci. With time, plaque becomes morphologically diverse, with filaments, flagellated and motile forms, and spirochetes all taking up residence in plaque. In all cases, an amorphous substance, or interbacterial matrix, surrounds bacteria in plaque. This matrix is composed of both bacterial and host products.

Histomorphologic, electron microscopic, culture, and molecular biological investigations of dental plaque have together provided important information on the microbiologic composition of plaque associated with health and a variety of disease states. It is now estimated that over 700 species have the potential to inhabit the human oral cavity. The bacterial taxa found in the mouth are listed in Table 2, and species commonly associated with oral health and various disease states are presented in Table 3. It should be noted that recent studies that use culture-independent molecular methods suggest that many of the genetic types are not cultivable.

This approach has also suggested that bacteria heretofore not recognized as human pathogens may be involved in the pathogenesis of oral disease. For example, members of the TM7 group, a recently described division of the bacteria known only from environmental 16S ribosomal DNA sequence studies, have been identified as prominent members of subgingival dental plaque. This phylotype was originally found in sludge wastewater treatment systems. Such findings suggest that many of the older experiments that identified only cultivable bacteria associated with health and disease conditions may not have provided an accurate picture of the microbial diversity associated with these clinical states.

The initial or early colonizers of plaque are primarily commensal species such as streptococci (S. sanguis, S. gordonii, and S. oralis) and actinomyces. Oral health begins to deteriorate as plaque becomes colonized with other species. Gingivitis is defined as inflammation of the

TABLE 2 Some common bacterial taxa in the oral cavity[a]

Bacterial phylum	Representative species
Obsidian pool OP11	
TM7	
Deferribacteres	
Spirochetes	*Treponema medium, T. denticola, T. maltophilum, T. socranskii*
Fusobacteria	*Fusobacterium naviforme, F. animalis, F. nucleatum, Leptotrichia buccalis*
Actinobacteria	*Actinomyces naeslundii, A. israelii, A. odontolyticus, Rothia dentocriosa, Atopobium, Bifidobacterium dentium, Corynebacterium matruchotii, Propionibacterium propionicus*
Firmicutes	Class "Bacilli": *Streptococcus oralis, S. mitis, S. gordonii, S. mutans, S. sobrinus, S. sanguis, S. parasanguis, S. salivarius, S. intermedius, S. constellatus, S. anginosus; Abiotrophia adiacens, A. defectiva, Gemella haemolysans*
	Class "Mollicutes": *Mycoplasma; Solobacterium moorei*
	Class "Clostridia": *Catonella morbi, Dialister, Eubacterium brachy, E. saburreum, Megasphaera, Peptostreptococcus anaerobius, P. micros, Selenomonas, Veillonella dispar, V. parvula, Eubacterium saphenum,* clone PUS9.170, *Filifactor alocis, Catonella morbi, Megasphaera elsdenii, Dialister pneumocintes, Selenomonas sputigena*
Proteobacteria	*Haemophilus parainfluenzae, Campylobacter rectus, C. gracilis, C. concisus, Neisseria mucosa, Desulfobulbus* oral clone R004, *Actinobacillus actinomycetemcomitans, Eikenella corrodens,* enteric species *(Escherichia coli), Pseudomonas aeruginosa*
Bacteroidetes	*Porphyromonas gingivalis, P. endodontalis, Bacteroides forsythus, Prevotella denticola, P. oris, P. tannerae, Capnocytophaga ochracea, C. gingivalis*

[a]Information from W. E. C. Moore and L. V. H. Moore, *Periodontol. 2000* **5:**66–77, 1994; B. J. Paster et al., *J. Bacteriol.* **183:**3770–3783, 2001; and J. M. Tanzer et al., *J. Dent. Educ.* **65:**1028–1037, 2001.

TABLE 3 Microbiota of the human mouth in health and disease[a]

Health	Gingivitis *(continued)*	Chronic periodontitis *(continued)*
Teeth	*Actinomyces viscosus*	*Porphyromonas endodontalis*
Streptococci	*S. sanguis*	*Wolinella recta*
Streptococcus mitis bv. 1	*Fusobacterium nucleatum*	*Treponema* sp. strain 1:G:T21
Streptococcus gordonii	*Selenomonas sputigena*	*F. nucleatum*
Veillonellae	*Haemophilus parainfluenzae*	*Atopobium rimae*
Streptococcus sanguis	*Actinomyces israelii*	*Megasphaera* sp. clone BB166
Streptococcus oralis	*S. mitis*	*Catonella morbi*
Actinomyces	*Peptostreptococcus*	*Eubacterium saphenum*
Tongue	*Prevotella intermedia*	*Gemella haemolysans*
S. mitis bv. 2	*Campylobacter sputorum*	*Streptococcus anginosus*
Streptococcus salivarius	*Veillonella* species	*Campylobacter gracilis*
	Chronic periodontitis	*H. parainfluenzae*
Disease	Clone I025	*Prevotella tannerae*
Dental caries	TM7	*Porphyromonas gingivalis*
S. sanguis	*Fusobacterium animalis*	*Peptostreptococcus micros*
S. oralis	*Atopobium parvulum*	Localized aggressive periodontitis
Mutans streptococci	*Eubacterium* sp. strain PUS9.170	*Eikenella corrodens*
Veillonellae	*Abiotrophia adiacens*	*Capnocytophaga sputigena*
S. mitis bv. 1	*Dialister pneumosintes*	*Actinobacillus actinomycetemcomitans*
S. gordonii	*Filifactor alocis*	*P. intermedia*
Actinomyces	*Selenomonas* sp. strain GAA14	
Lactobacilli	*Streptococcus constellatus*	
Gingivitis	*Campylobacter rectus*	
Actinomyces naeslundii	*Tannerella forsythia*	

[a]Information from L. R. Brown et al., *Infect. Immun.* **51:**765–770, 1986; W. E. C. Moore and L. V. H. Moore, *Periodontol. 2000* **5:**66–77, 1994; B. J. Paster et al., *J. Bacteriol.* **183:**3770–3783, 2001; and J. Slots et al., *Scand. J. Dent. Res.* **86:**174–181, 1978.

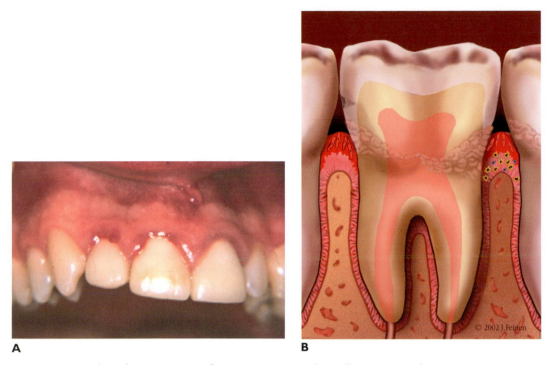

A   **B**

FIGURE 3 (A) Clinical presentation of gingivitis. Note red, swollen gingiva adjacent to crown restorations of maxillary anterior teeth. (B) Artist's depiction of gingivitis and initial interproximal caries formation. Plaque formation has become extensive. Gingival tissues are infiltrated with inflammatory cells (right gingival tissues). Incipient carious lesion is found in enamel under the left interproximal contact point.

epithelial and connective tissues around the teeth, but without loss of the connective tissue attachment or alveolar bone supporting the tooth. Plaque associated with gingivitis appears somewhat thicker than that from normal healthy sites (Fig. 3). Bacteria in deeper layers often appear lysed ("ghosts"). Mineralized deposits within these plaques are common (eventually developing into dental calculus or tartar). Greater proportions of filamentous and gram-negative bacteria (for example, *Fusobacterium nucleatum, Prevotella intermedia, Selenomonas sputigena, Campylobacter sputorum*, and *Haemophilus parainfluenzae*) reside in these plaques.

Chronic periodontitis is defined as the loss of connective tissue and alveolar bone support of the teeth that is the result of both the direct activity of pathogenic bacteria and plaque-induced inflammation. Periodontitis-associated plaque, by definition, always extends onto the cementum. Plaques are as thick as or thicker than those associated with gingivitis (Fig. 4). Filamentous gram-positive and motile gram-negative bacteria and spirochetes predominate. Many distinct configurations of bacterial interactions occur in subgingival plaque, including interesting interactions between bacteria of different species resulting in "corncob" and "test-tube brush"–like formations (Fig. 5). These interactions occur between a central filamentous bacterium and numerous bacterial cells of a different species that adhere along the length of the filament. Anaerobic species such as *P. gingivalis, P. intermedia, Tannerella forsythia*, and spirochetes are common in the subgingival plaque of periodontitis

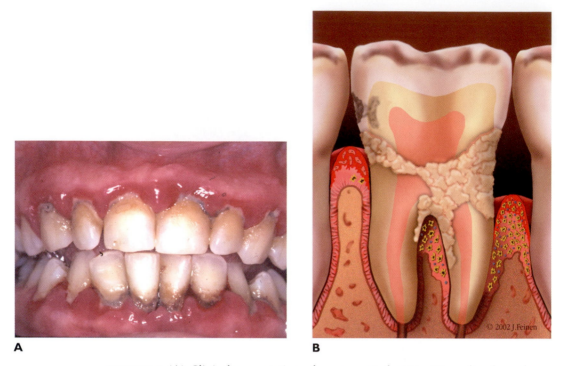

A   **B**

FIGURE 4 (A) Clinical presentation of severe periodontitis. Note abundant plaque deposits, that have, in many places, mineralized to form stained calculus (tartar). (B) Artist's depiction of severe periodontitis and dentinal caries. Plaque has become mineralized calculus. The action of plaque and of the host inflammatory response has resulted in severe alveolar bone destruction. Caries has penetrated the dentinal-enamel junction and is spreading through the dentinal tubules toward the pulp.

patients. A transitional zone is noted between supra- and subgingival plaque, with filamentous and flagellar forms in greater proportions in subgingival plaque. This plaque displays all of the features of a climax community with a stable, mature habitat.

The plaque of patients with aggressive periodontitis (such as localized aggressive periodontitis) appears much different from that seen in chronic periodontitis. The plaque associated with localized aggressive periodontitis is relatively sparse and morphologically simple. The predominant bacterial morphologic type appears to be small gram-negative coccoid forms. Clinical microbiological findings indicate that the primary pathogen associated with this disease is *Actinobacillus actinomycetemcomitans*.

The dental plaque associated with acute necrotizing ulcerative gingivitis presents a unique morphology. It appears that spirochetes, fusobacteria, and other microorganisms invade the nonnecrotic lamina propria of the gingiva of patients demonstrating symptoms of acute necrotizing ulcerative gingivitis. Similar findings have been described for the necrotizing gingiva seen in patients with human immunodeficiency virus (HIV) infections.

Calculus

Dental calculus is calcified dental plaque, composed primarily of calcium phosphate mineral salts deposited between and within remnants of formerly viable microorganisms. Viable bacteria cover calculus deposits

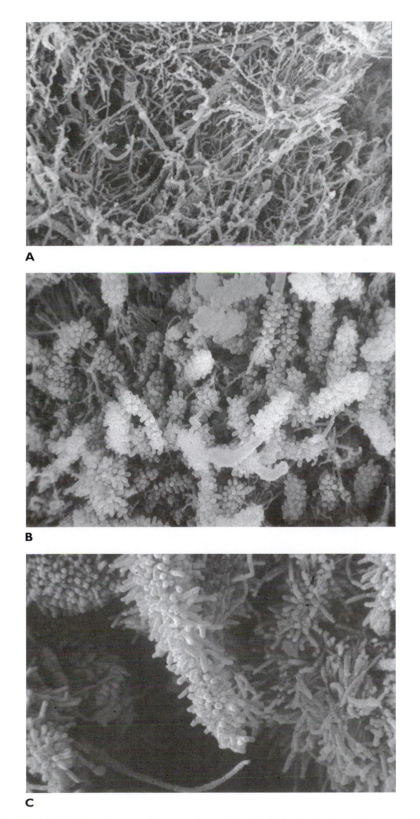

A

B

C

FIGURE 5 Scanning electron micrographic study of subgingival plaque from a patient with severe periodontitis. (A) Spirochetes and filamentous bacteria; (B) "corncobs"; (C) "test-tube brushes." (Courtesy of H. E. Schroeder, Institute of Oral Structural Biology, University of Zurich, Zurich, Switzerland.)

(Fig. 6). Supragingival calculus is that which forms coronal to the gingival margin, and subgingival calculus forms below the gingival margin. In patients who do not practice regular hygiene and who do not have access to professional care, supragingival calculus often is present throughout the dentition and can be extreme. Although calculus itself is not thought to cause periodontal disease (it is the viable bacteria growing on the surface of the calculus that incite the disease), removal of subgingival plaque and calculus remains the cornerstone of periodontal therapy since good oral hygiene can only be maintained on calculus-free teeth.

Calculus formation can be controlled by inhibitors of biomineralization. It is known that certain salivary proteins are effective inhibitors of mineralization in dental plaque. Such mineralization is also affected by changes in plaque pH, as well as by fluctuations in the concentrations of ions and molecules in the solution phase of the plaque. How these

FIGURE 6 (A) Clinical presentation of supragingival calculus (at end of arrow), which often forms on the lingual surfaces of the mandibular anterior teeth. These tooth surfaces are in close proximity to Wharton's duct that drains the submandibular and submaxillary glands to deliver mineral-laden saliva to the teeth. (B) Transmission electron micrograph of calcified bacteria and a portion of a crystal aggregate in supragingival calculus (Courtesy of H. E. Schroeder, Institute of Oral Structural Biology, University of Zurich, Zurich, Switzerland.)

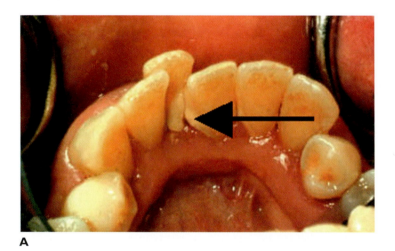

A

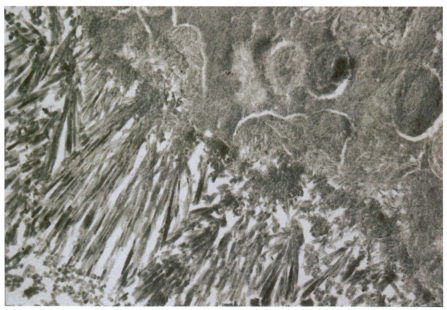

B

salivary proteins function in the process of mineralization is not yet completely understood, especially in subjects in whom heavy calculus forms.

The Mucosal Microbiota

The epithelium covering the gingival, buccal, and palatal tissues is also a habitat for microbes. Because the surface cells of epithelia desquamate at a regular rate (thus shedding attached bacteria), the soft tissues do not support the voluminous microbiota seen on the surface of the teeth. Stable colonization of the mucosa therefore requires a continuous process of attachment, growth, and generation of daughter cells that detach and readhere to freshly exposed epithelial cells. An interesting recent study that used fluorescent in situ hybridization with probes to conserved and variable regions in the ribosomal 16S subunit suggests that human buccal epithelial cells contain intracellular bacteria, including the periodontal pathogens *A. actinomycetemcomitans* and *P. gingivalis*, as well as other species of bacteria (Fig. 7). The invasion of these epithelial cells may allow bacteria to establish themselves in the mouth and find a habitat protected from host defense factors such as salivary antimicrobial systems.

The tongue offers another unique habitat for bacterial growth. Because the tongue surface is covered with papillae, there are numerous protected sites that provide sheltered habitats for bacterial colonization. Indeed, with the exception of the teeth and gingival sulcus, the dorsum of the tongue harbors a greater microbial biomass than any other site in the mouth. It is therefore interesting that relatively few comprehensive studies of the microbiology of the tongue have been reported. From the few studies that are available, it appears that the tongue microbiota includes bacterial species that also colonize the teeth, as well as those that are relatively selective for the tongue. Thus, the dorsum of the tongue harbors streptococci such as *Streptococcus mitis* that typically colonize teeth, as well as organisms such as *S. salivarius*, whose primary habitat in the mouth appears to be the tongue. The tongue of medically compromised subjects, for example, patients with Sjögren's syndrome who suffer from dry mouth (xerostomia), may be more susceptible to colonization by potential pathogens such as *Candida albicans*, *Staphylococcus aureus*, enteric gram-negatives, and enterococci than normal subjects are.

RECENT CONCEPTS OF DENTAL BIOFILM FORMATION

Our conception of dental plaque formation has expanded in recent years as a consequence of the development of several powerful methodologies to study microbial ecosystems. The development of confocal scanning laser microscopy and other advanced microscopic techniques, as well as molecular approaches to identify and quantify noncultivable bacterial species, has revolutionized the study of dental plaque. The confocal microscope allows computer analysis of confocal laser images and can produce repeated three-dimensional reconstruction of microbial systems over time (Fig. 8). Morphologic, biochemical, and molecular biologic studies demonstrate that dental plaque is an example of a biofilm, a polymer-encased community of microbes that accumulates at a surface

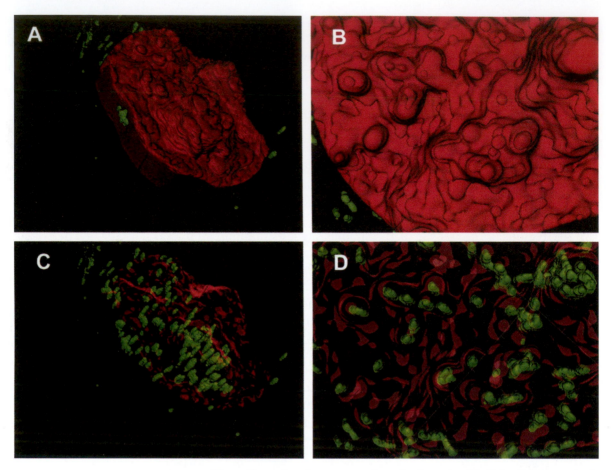

FIGURE 7 Three-dimensional reconstruction of a buccal epithelial cell from a single subject. (A) Surface contour of the target cell, with the surface rendered opaque in red. Green bacteria, which appear to be extracellular, were in fact contained within the cells that were edited out. (B) A close-up view of the opaque host cell surface reveals a very irregular contour. (C) The surface of the target cell is rendered transparent with red highlights. This reveals clusters of green bacteria, which appear to be intracellular, since they cannot be seen otherwise. (D) The close-up transparent view shows that some surface protuberances were associated with bacterial clusters. However, bacteria in those clusters seemed to be located below the surface. Reprinted from J. D. Rudney et al., *Infect. Immun.* **69:**2700–2707, 2001, with permission.

interface. Microbial biofilms are complicated structures that appear to undergo specific developmental events as they mature. It has been suggested that most bacteria do not survive in nature as unicellular organisms, but as biofilms. The bacteria within the biofilm organize to distribute metabolic activities among the different members of the biofilm. In addition, many bacteria use small soluble molecules to signal the expression of multiple target genes in neighboring cells and this coordinates metabolic activities (see chapter 5). It is also clear that biofilms demonstrate intrinsic resistance to antibiotics and host defense systems. Thus, biofilm-induced diseases are difficult to treat. This antibiotic resistance may be due to slow bacterial cell growth and/or induction of a genetically directed stress response. Bacterial exopolysaccharides or other aspects of biofilm architecture could also confer resistance by exclusion of antibiotics from the bacteria.

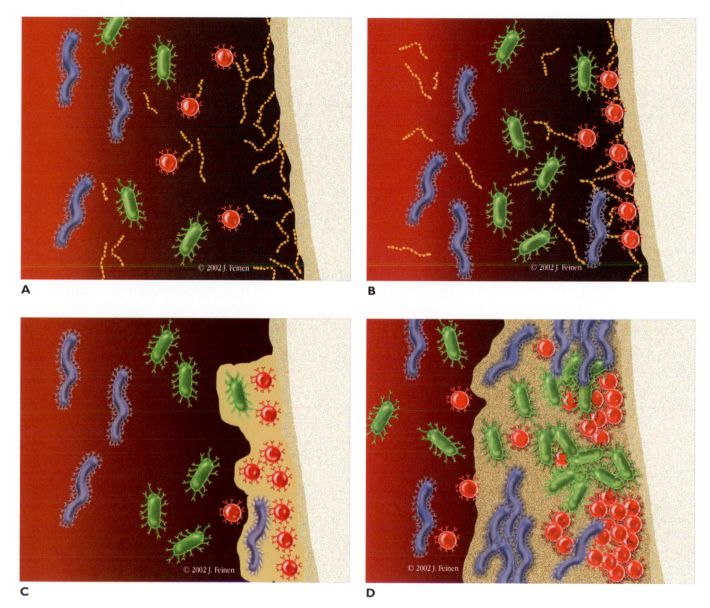

A   B

C   D

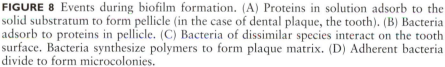

FIGURE 8 Events during biofilm formation. (A) Proteins in solution adsorb to the solid substratum to form pellicle (in the case of dental plaque, the tooth). (B) Bacteria adsorb to proteins in pellicle. (C) Bacteria of dissimilar species interact on the tooth surface. Bacteria synthesize polymers to form plaque matrix. (D) Adherent bacteria divide to form microcolonies.

ORAL FLUIDS: SALIVA AND SALIVA-BACTERIUM INTERACTIONS

Whole saliva ("spit") is actually a mixture of fluids from several sources. Per unit volume, the bulk of whole saliva is derived from salivary gland secretions. The major salivary glands are the paired parotid, submaxillary, and sublingual glands. In addition, a multitude of minor glands scattered within the oral mucosa (labial, buccal, glossopalatine, palatine, lingual) contribute substantially to the total output of whole saliva. The saliva of most people, especially those with periodontal disease, also contains constituents of gingival crevicular fluid (GCF), which is derived from serum and whose flow rate from the gingival sulcus is related to the severity of gingival inflammation. Degradation products of bacterial and oral cells along with components from gastric and respiratory reflux can also be found in whole saliva.

The relative concentration of various components in saliva varies with their source. Some components, such as mucin glycoproteins, are produced for the most part by mucous glands (e.g., the submaxillary, sublingual, and minor glands). Mucins are essentially absent in parotid secretions. In contrast, parotid secretions have higher concentrations of serous proteins, such as amylase, parotid agglutinin, and proline-rich proteins, than do secretions from mucous glands.

Once saliva exits the gland ducts, the distribution of its components within the oral cavity is probably not homogeneous. For example, parotid components released into unstimulated whole saliva are distributed primarily within the region vestibular to the maxillary molars (where roughly 61% of all saliva is from the parotid glands). Only 7% of whole saliva found vestibular to the upper incisors is from the parotid glands. This localization of specific salivary components within the mouth may have subtle but real effects on bacterial interactions that are responsible for dental plaque formation at different anatomical sites within the mouth.

Saliva is involved in a diverse range of functions (Table 4). It plays a role in food digestion by solubilizing food components to facilitate taste, by preparing the food bolus for swallowing, and by providing enzymes to initiate digestion. Saliva is also thought to function, in part, by forming tenacious films, or pellicles, on the oral surfaces such as the tooth (enamel, dentin, and cementum), the epithelium (oral, lingual, alveolar, and palatal mucosa, gingiva, etc.), and plaque itself. Salivary pellicles help maintain a balance between tooth demineralization and remineralization. The salivary molecules controlling these processes have high affinities for the tooth surface through possession of negatively charged domains. These molecules appear to function by inhibiting the precipitation of calcium phosphate salts from solution and thus maintaining calcium and phosphate in a supersaturated state in saliva.

TABLE 4 Functions of salivary molecules with reference to dental plaque formation

Molecule	Microbial agglutination	Promotion or inhibition of microbial adhesion	Antimicrobial	Microbial nutrition
Amylase	−	+	−	+
β₂-Microglobulin	+	?	?	?
Fibronectin	−	+	−	?
Lysozyme	+	+	+	?
Mucin	+	+	+	+
Parotid agglutinin	+	+	−	?
Proline-rich proteins	−	+	−	?
S-IgA	+	+	+	?
Statherin	−	+	−	?

The adsorbed salivary molecules also lubricate tissues to facilitate chewing, speaking, and swallowing and prevent the oral tissues from drying. Other important functions of salivary molecules include buffering of acids and neutralization of toxic products produced by oral microorganisms.

The function of individual salivary molecules is dependent on their conformation or molecular shape. For example, proline-rich proteins only promote bacterial adhesion when they are adsorbed onto a surface. Interestingly, when these proteins are in solution, they do not interact with bacteria. This suggests that the adsorption of these molecules to a surface causes a shape change that exposes otherwise hidden domains capable of interacting with bacteria. Another interesting molecule with conformational requirements is human salivary amylase. This relatively large protein contains 496 amino acids with 5 interchain disulfide bonds that are distributed over the overall length of the molecule. Its biological activities include the enzymatic digestion of starch, interaction with oral streptococci, and binding to hydroxyapatite tooth surfaces. Cleavage of this enzyme's disulfide bonds results in the disruption of its suprastructure and loss of all biological activities.

The protective functions of saliva are enhanced by its built-in redundancies. In other words, many of the molecules in saliva have overlapping functions. Indeed, most salivary molecules are multifunctional. Thus, mucins play a role in lubrication, tissue coating, digestion, and agglutination of microorganisms. This results in functional compensation and may explain why most cross-sectional studies find a high degree of variability in the concentration of individual salivary molecules within study populations and often no correlation with the prevalence of oral disease. A single salivary molecule may have both protective and detrimental properties ("amphifunctionality"). For example, statherin and acidic proline-rich proteins work at the enamel surface by inhibiting the formation of primary and secondary calcium phosphate salts. However, when adsorbed to the enamel surface, these components may also promote adhesion of potentially cariogenic microorganisms to the tooth surface.

Comparisons of purified salivary molecules with intact secretions have shown that functional relationships must exist between different molecules in saliva. These functional relationships are likely predicated on complexing between molecules. Two types of complexing can occur: homotypic ones between similar molecules and heterotypic ones between different molecules. Complexes can occur by either covalent or noncovalent interactions. Mucins provide an interesting example. These molecules may form homotypic complexes, or end-to-end oligomers, with themselves via interchain disulfide bonds. Mucin oligomer formation is required for this molecule to exert its lubrication and viscoelastic properties. Mucins that coat the various oral tissue surfaces can also form heterotypic complexes with other salivary molecules, including antimicrobials such as secretory immunoglobulin A (S-IgA), lysozyme, and cystatins. These complexes are mediated primarily by noncovalent ionic forces and function to concentrate these antimicrobials at the saliva-tissue interface. It is possible that the complexes themselves may have additional functions over and above those of the individual molecules comprising the complex.

Covalent bonding can be important in other salivary complexing mechanisms. Proline-rich proteins can cross-link into higher-molecular-mass complexes by the action of buccal epithelial cell transglutaminase on the lysine residues of proline-rich proteins. This enzyme also cross-links statherin to proline-rich proteins. These observations suggest that such cross-linking reactions may permit other proteins in the oral cavity to be incorporated into oral pellicles.

Many salivary components have been shown to interact with oral microorganisms. The interactions between bacteria and salivary components can be divided into four major categories: (i) interactions causing aggregation or agglutination of bacteria, (ii) interactions that foster adhesion of bacteria to surfaces, (iii) interactions that kill or inhibit the growth of microorganisms, and (iv) interactions that contribute to microbial nutrition. Together, these interactions probably control to a considerable extent the microbial ecology of the oral cavity. The following discussion provides examples of individual salivary molecules that display each of these four general functions (Table 4).

CLEARANCE OF BACTERIA FROM THE ORAL CAVITY: AGGLUTININS

Forces that promote bacterial clearance from the oral cavity are powerful. When suspensions of pure cultures of bacteria are experimentally introduced into the oral cavity, most are soon removed, with only a small fraction able to attach and persist. Clearance occurs by mechanical flushing due to physiologic movements (e.g., swallowing, chewing, and speaking) and dilution effects by continuous salivary flow. In addition, many species of bacteria are rapidly agglutinated (that is, clumped or aggregated) when suspended in saliva (Fig. 9). It is thought that agglutination promotes bacterial clearance from the oral cavity. The binding of salivary components to the bacterial surface may block the adhesion of bacteria to the tooth, mucosa, or plaque. Salivary molecules that have been shown to agglutinate bacteria include mucins, S-IgA, parotid agglutinin, lysozyme, β_2-microglobulin, and Ca^{2+} ions.

Salivary mucins are large-molecular-weight glycoproteins originating from mucous acinar cells. By definition, mucin glycoproteins contain 30 to 80% carbohydrate. Several mucins in human submandibular-sublingual saliva have been identified. Initial biochemical studies identified two mucins: mucin-glycoprotein 1 (MG1, also known as MUC5B) and mucin-glycoprotein 2 (MG2, also known as MUC7). MG1 was found to be composed of monomers having a molecular mass greater than 1×10^6 kDa, whereas MG2 was found to have a molecular mass of about 200 kDa. More recent molecular and genetic studies have clarified the chemical nature of these mucins. It is now recognized that human salivary glands make membrane-bound mucins, MUC1 and MUC4, in addition to the gel-forming mucin MUC5B. MG1 has been shown to be composed mostly of MUC5B, which appears to be the major subunit secreted from sublingual and submandibular glands, as well by gallbladder, colon, female reproductive tract, and respiratory tract epithelium. MUC5B monomers interact to form dimers via disulfide linkages between cysteine residues in the C-terminal cysteine knot motif. The

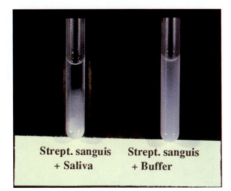

FIGURE 9 Incubation of *S. sanguis* with parotid saliva (left tube) or buffer (right tube). Agglutinins in parotid saliva cause the bacteria to clump and fall to the bottom of the test tube within minutes. Bacteria remain suspended in buffer.

dimers are then O glycosylated in the *cis*-Golgi and form trimers during passage to the secretory granules. Tissue-bound MUC1 is expressed as a single polypeptide chain that is cleaved in the endoplasmic reticulum into two subunits, one the extracellular portion and the other the membrane-spanning and C-terminal cytoplasmic domains. The extracellular portion is probably shed to form the soluble form of MUC1. MUC4 is the largest mucin gene product so far described. Like MUC1, MUC4 is synthesized as a single polypeptide that is cleaved and reassembled into extracellular and membrane-spanning domains. Both MUC1 and MUC4 are also expressed by minor glands and, surprisingly, in low amounts by parotid gland and buccal epithelial cells. It is likely that these forms of mucin are involved in the physical protection of the epithelial surfaces from which they are secreted.

High-molecular-weight salivary glycoproteins, including mucins, can aggregate oral bacteria. Removal of the terminal sialic acid of the mucin oligosaccharide side chains abolishes its interaction with some, but not all, species of oral streptococci. The interaction of these bacteria with mucin is thus mediated by a sialic acid-binding protein, or lectin, on the bacterial surface.

If mucins participate in clearance of bacteria from the oral cavity, it would make sense that people with higher mucin concentrations in their saliva would have fewer bacteria in their mouth. This hypothesis was tested with respect to the relationships between the number of *S. mutans* in the oral cavity and mucin concentrations in saliva. The results of this study suggested that an elevated level of *S. mutans* is significantly associated with diminished concentrations of MG2 in unstimulated whole saliva. This suggests that *S. mutans* may not be cleared from the mouth due to low concentrations of MG2 in saliva.

Another important agglutinin in saliva is S-IgA. S-IgA is the predominant immunoglobulin found in all mucosal secretions, including saliva. S-IgA is composed of an IgA dimer (300 kDa), J chain (15 kDa), and secretory component (70 kDa). J chain is a glycoprotein that polymerizes the two IgA molecules into a dimer. Polymeric IgA (pIgA) containing the J chain is secreted by local plasma cells. pIgA is taken up by the polyimmunoglobulin receptor, which is expressed on the basolateral surface of the secretory epithelial cells in the glands. The complex is transported in membrane vesicles through the epithelial cells, and the membrane part of the receptor is cleaved off when the complex reaches the surface. The remaining part of the receptor is secretory component. Secretory component functions to protect the molecule from attack by acids or proteases in the oral environment.

A major function of S-IgA appears to be the inhibition of microbial adherence to the host surface, thus preventing colonization. Inhibition is usually specific, requiring that S-IgA be directed against antigenic determinants on the microbial surface. Indeed, like other antibody species, S-IgA in saliva is a mixture of many S-IgA molecules, each synthesized by a B-cell clone and directed to a specific antigen. It is this function that forms the basis for a number of proposed mucosal vaccines, the immunogens being various components of pathogenic bacteria such as the cariogenic mutans group streptococci (see chapter 10). It is also possible that certain bacteria may interact with S-IgA through lectin binding to the oligosaccharide structures of the immunoglobulins. It has also been suggested that bacteria may subvert the inhibitory function of S-IgA via specific proteases. Indeed, several oral bacteria, including important initial colonizers of tooth surfaces, produce an IgA1 protease similar to that produced by the bacterial species that are the three principal causes of bacterial meningitis. However, the exact role of the S-IgA-cleaving enzymes in the pathogenesis of oral disease remains to be determined.

Another high-molecular-weight salivary glycoprotein agglutinin is the parotid agglutinin that is identical to lung (lavage) gp340, a member of the scavenger receptor cysteine-rich protein family. This glycoprotein binds to the surface of oral streptococci through the interaction of its sialic acid residues with a lectin protein on the bacterium's surface. This lectin is a high-affinity calcium-binding protein that binds 1 mol of calcium per mole of protein.

PELLICLE ADHESION RECEPTORS

Saliva influences the attachment of bacteria to the tooth surface via the enamel, cemental, or dentinal pellicle. Such surfaces have been modeled in vitro using experimental pellicles formed by incubating saliva with beads of hydroxyapatite (HA), enamel, or dentin powders. The adhesion of bacteria to saliva-coated hydroxyapatite (sHA) has been shown to be complex. Whereas some species of bacteria adhere in similar numbers to naked HA, coating HA with saliva markedly alters the adhesion of other species. *S. mutans*, for example, adheres in lower numbers to sHA than to uncoated HA. Furthermore, *S. mutans* first suspended in saliva will attach in even lower numbers to sHA than untreated *S. mutans*. In contrast, *S. gordonii* and *Actinomyces viscosus* attach in higher numbers to sHA than to bare HA. These in vitro investigations must, however, be interpreted with some caution. For example, pellicles formed on HA in vitro have been shown to differ from those formed in vivo. As an example, albumin is found in greater amounts in in vivo pellicles compared to in vitro pellicles (probably contributed from periodontal inflammation through GCF). There appears to be less proline in in vivo pellicle compared to in vitro pellicle, probably due to a reduction in the content of acidic proline-rich proteins in the in vivo pellicles. Thus, constituents of the oral environment, such as enzymes released from GCF into whole saliva, may alter oral surfaces to account for the differences in bacterial adhesion observed between in vivo and in vitro systems.

Despite these limitations, the few studies that have attempted to study these phenomena in vivo support the modulatory role of saliva in bacterial colonization. Thus, the implantation of *S. mutans* in the oral cavity of humans is modified by pretreatment of the bacteria with saliva. Saliva from caries-active individuals enhanced the implantation of *S. mutans* in volunteers compared to *S. mutans* suspended in saliva from caries-free controls. This suggests that there may be a component in the saliva of some individuals that promotes the colonization of *S. mutans*.

Cataloging the salivary components in pellicles has consistently identified several components, including proline-rich proteins, lysozyme, albumin, histatins, statherin, mucins, S-IgA, and α-amylase. Each of these proteins probably serves as a pellicle receptor for one or more species of oral bacteria that adhere to the tooth surface. It is also interesting that enamel pellicles display a distinctive structure consisting of a spongelike meshwork of microglobules.

Salivary components do not, however, appear to be homogeneously distributed within pellicles sampled in different parts of the oral cavity. In fact, enamel pellicles eluted from the premolar teeth (bathed mostly by saliva from the parotid glands) are qualitatively different from pellicles that form on mandibular anterior teeth (bathed primarily by secretions from the submandibular/sublingual glands). Thus, parotid agglutinin is found in maxillary premolar pellicles in greater amounts than in mandibular anterior pellicles, whereas mucins show the opposite pattern of localization. The observed variations in salivary protein localization might be important to the establishment of microbiota and tooth-related disease patterns in various parts of the dentition. A more complete discussion of bacterial adhesion to receptors in salivary pellicle can be found in chapter 5.

ANTIMICROBIAL COMPONENTS IN SALIVA

Several salivary components have been shown to kill or inhibit the growth of bacteria in vitro. Lysozyme, one of the first salivary antimicrobial components to be described, is a 14-kDa protein that hydrolyzes the β-1,4 glucosidic linkages between *N*-acetylmuramic acid and *N*-acetylglucosamine in the peptidoglycan of the bacterial cell wall (see chapter 1). The resultant weakening of the cell wall of susceptible bacterial species, mostly gram-positive bacteria, results in the lysis of the bacteria. Interestingly, many oral species are insensitive to the action of lysozyme. However, other mechanisms of lysozyme bacteriocidal activity have been described. One involves the activation of endogenous bacterial enzyme(s) by lysozyme, which can kill bacteria that are insensitive to the muramidase activity of lysozyme. Lysozyme can also bind to oral bacteria and aggregate them, thus facilitating their clearance from the oral cavity. Finally, lysozyme possesses small amphipathic sequences within the C terminus that have antimicrobial effects.

Histatins (also known as histidine-rich proteins) comprise an interesting family of cationic low-molecular-weight proteins found in abundance in submandibular/sublingual and parotid salivas (~10 to 150 μg/ml of saliva, depending on the source and degree of stimulation). At least a dozen human salivary molecules with similar properties have been described, all of which have large amounts of the basic amino acid histidine (up to 41%). Variants of histatins differ with respect to primary sequence, chain length, and phosphorylation. A variety of functions have been ascribed to the histatins, including histamine release from mast cells, inhibition of HA crystal growth, and tanin binding. However, the function paid most attention by investigators is the antimicrobial activity of these peptides. The first antimicrobial property described for histatin was antifungal; however, these peptides also have less potent but measurable antibacterial properties and have been noted to prevent bacterial coaggregation. Additionally, histatins may serve as a competitive inhibitor of several proteinases, including cysteine proteinases from mammals and bacteria. By inhibiting such enzymes, the histatins may affect the course of diseases such as periodontitis where there is extensive proteolytic destruction of the periodontal tissues.

Salivary peroxidase and thiocyanate act together with hydrogen peroxide (produced by bacteria) to generate oxidized thiocyanate ion derivatives, which inhibit the growth of bacteria as well as inhibit acid formation by oral streptococci. Recent evidence also suggests that the lactoperoxidase-hydrogen peroxide-thiocyanate antimicrobial system inhibits respiration in gram-negative species such as *Escherichia coli* by inhibiting membrane dehydrogenases. Together with lysozyme, lactoperoxidase may also inhibit the adhesion of bacteria to teeth.

Lactoferrin (Lf) is a glycoprotein of 75 kDa synthesized by glandular acinar and epithelial as well as inflammatory cells. Lf binds two atoms of iron per molecule, with the simultaneous binding of two molecules of bicarbonate. The primary function of Lf may thus be to bind and sequester iron from bacteria. In addition, iron-free (apo)-lactoferrin (apoLf) may also possess a direct, iron-independent, bacteriocidal effect on various strains of oral bacteria such as *P. gingivalis*. It is possible that apoLf forms a complex with essential iron-containing nutrients such as hemin. Moreover, the 25-residue N-terminal peptide from Lf, called lactoferricin, itself has antimicrobial activity. Functional studies suggest that this peptide causes a depolarization of bacterial cytoplasmic membranes, loss of the pH gradient, and a resultant bactericidal effect. In addition to this bacteriocidal activity, apoLf may also serve to inhibit the adhesion of bacteria to oral surfaces such as hydroxyapatite.

Saliva also appears to possess potent antiviral factors. For example, the infectivity of HIV has been shown to be significantly suppressed in the presence of human saliva, and antiviral factors have been isolated from saliva. The protein secretory leukocyte protease inhibitor appears to possess substantial anti-HIV-1 activity at physiological concentrations. The human parotid basic proline-rich proteins also inhibit HIV-1 activity. The mechanism of action may involve the binding of the basic proline-rich proteins to the HIV-1 gp120 coat of the virus before the interaction of the virus with host target cells.

SALIVA AS A SOURCE OF BACTERIAL NUTRITION

Some bacteria such as certain oral streptococci and actinomyces are able to grow on chemically defined medium supplemented with saliva. A number of protein components of saliva are degraded following growth of these bacteria, suggesting that these bacteria are unable to utilize free amino acids in saliva for growth but instead metabolize salivary proteins. Bacteria grown in saliva also appear to have elevated levels of cell-associated hydrolytic activities, including glycosidases, exo- and endopeptidases, esterases, and neuraminidase. The bacteria may therefore obtain nutrients by the enzymatic breakdown and subsequent metabolism of oligosaccharides and peptides from salivary glycoproteins. Other studies have extended these findings by demonstrating that the utilization of salivary peptides may be more dependent on their physical properties (hydrophobicity) than their size. That is, hydrophilic peptides stimulated growth of streptococci far better than hydrophobic peptides.

Another example of how saliva may influence bacterial nutrition involves amylase. Salivary amylase binds with high affinity to certain species of oral streptococci that are abundant in dental plaque. It appears that the bound enzyme remains enzymatically active and thus may facilitate dietary starch hydrolysis to provide additional glucose for metabolism by plaque microorganisms in close proximity to the tooth surface.

GINGIVAL CREVICULAR FLUID

GCF is an inflammatory exudate that can be collected at the gingival margin or within the gingival crevice. When the gum tissues are absolutely healthy, the flow of crevicular fluid from the sulcus is so low that it can hardly be measured. However, GCF flow increases as gingival inflammation increases, and significant amounts of GCF can be collected from patients with severe disease. GCF is a mixture of plasma proteins such as albumin, inflammatory products, and constituents released from phagocytic cells. Many attempts have been made to relate the presence or amount of certain proteins in GCF with the progression or activity of periodontal disease. Inflammatory mediators such as prostaglandin E_2, beta-glucuronidase, neutrophil elastase, aspartate aminotransferase, and matrix metalloproteinases, especially collagenase-2 (matrix metalloproteinase 8), have all been studied in this regard, although thus far none have proved to be reliable markers of the disease. The significance of GCF in the context of oral microbiology relates to the role of GCF constituents in oral bacterial colonization. For example, a variety of plasma proteins such as intact fibrin, as well as degradation products of fibrin and fibronectin, were seen in both healthy and diseased GCF samples. These proteins are known to interact with oral bacteria, and such interactions may influence bacterial colonization of host surfaces.

KEY POINTS

The oral cavity contains the mineralized hard tissues of the teeth along with the soft tissues of the oral mucosa, all of which are continuously bathed in saliva. The environment of the oral cavity experiences fluctuations in temperature, pH, oxygen levels, and availability of nutritional substrates.

The crown of the tooth (that part above the gum) is composed of enamel, a highly mineralized, substituted hydroxyapatite. Beneath the enamel is located dentin, which is less mineralized and surrounds the pulp chamber. The tooth root is anchored in the gum and has a cementum surface.

The gum (gingiva) forms a collar around the tooth with a gap (sulcus) between the root and the sulcular epithelium. Junctional epithelium attaches the inner surface of the sulcus to the cementum of the root. The periodontal ligament attaches the tooth to the underlying alveolar bone. A serum exudate called GCF collects in the gingival sulcus.

To first colonize teeth, bacteria must attach to salivary receptors in the pellicle of salivary molecules that coats the enamel surface. This allows bacteria to resist the mechanical shearing forces that would tend to dislodge them. Shearing forces arise from tongue and lip movement and from salivary fluid flow.

Primary colonizers of the tooth are mainly streptococci and actinomycetes. Subsequently, more actinomycetes and related organisms arrive. Finally, increasing numbers of gram-negative anaerobes and spirochetes colonize. The pattern of plaque accumulation is driven by bacterial adherence to host surfaces and to other bacteria, nutrient availability that will modulate multiplication, and environmental factors such as oxygen levels.

Bacterial colonization of mucosal surfaces is less abundant as the epithelial cells are continually dying and sloughing off, thus removing the attached bacteria.

Saliva contains numerous components that can either promote or inhibit bacterial colonization. Salivary receptors for bacterial adherence, along with molecules that can act as a carbon and nitrogen source for bacteria, will assist bacterial colonization. Antibacterial components include agglutinins, lysozyme, histatins, peroxidase and thiocyanate, and lactoferrin.

FURTHER READING

Avery, J. K. 2000. *Essentials of Oral Histology and Embryology: a Clinical Approach*, 2nd ed. Mosby, St. Louis, Mo.

Baum, B. J. 1987. Saliva secretion and composition, p. 126–134. *In* D. B. Ferguson (ed.), *The Aging Mouth*. Karger, Basel, Switzerland.

Gibbons, R. J., and J. van Houte. 1980. Bacterial adherence and the formation of dental plaques, p. 62–104. *In* E. H. Beachey (ed.), *Bacterial Adherence*. Chapman and Hall, Ltd., London, United Kingdom.

Scannapieco, F. A. 1994. Saliva-bacterium interactions in oral microbial ecology. *Crit. Rev. Oral Biol. Med.* **5:**203–248.

Socransky, S. S., and A. D. Haffajee. 2005. Periodontal microbial ecology. *Periodontol. 2000* **38:**135–187.

Ten Cate, A. R. 1998. *Oral Histology: Development, Structure, and Function*, 5th ed. Mosby, St. Louis, Mo.

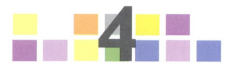

Isolation, Classification, and Identification of Oral Microorganisms

EUGENE J. LEYS, ANN L. GRIFFEN, PURNIMA S. KUMAR, AND MARK F. MAIDEN

INTRODUCTION

The title of this chapter, "Isolation, Classification, and Identification of Oral Microorganisms," until very recently would have reflected a general approach to oral microbiology where oral samples were taken and the bacteria were dispersed and plated on various media. Those bacteria that grew were isolated and characterized, while species unable to grow on the media were overlooked. Today, using molecular techniques, we have seen a glimpse of many more species than were apparent by culture. Therefore, a common scheme today is to first identify bacteria by analyzing the DNA present in an oral sample, and then to use molecular methods to characterize the new bacteria by determining where it grows in the mouth (subgingival, supragingival, etc.) and when and under what conditions (health or disease). Attempts can then be made to grow these new species, although this can be very difficult, especially considering that most of the easily cultivable species have been isolated. At this time there are a large number of species of interest to oral microbiologists that have yet to be cultured, and the number is growing, much faster than the number of cultured species is growing.

DIVERSITY OF THE ORAL MICROBIOTA

The bacterial community in the oral cavity is one of the most complex mixtures of bacteria known. More than 100 species are likely to be found in any oral site, and the profile varies greatly from site to site, depending on the local environment. Also, the bacterial composition can be radically different from person to person even though they have similar oral health. More than 700 bacterial species have been identified from the oral cavity; over half of those have not been cultivated and more species are continuing to be discovered. There have been attempts to estimate the number of species that could potentially be found; however, with the wide variety seen from sample to sample, the number appears to be open ended. It is likely at this time that all or almost all of the common species have been observed.

Because of the complexity of bacteria in the oral cavity, it has been necessary to use a large number of technical approaches to analyze oral samples. Many of these approaches have been developed by oral microbiologists to study the unique features found in the oral cavity. Microbiologists studying complex mixtures of bacteria in other environments have developed additional techniques. At this time, there is no one technique that can be used to obtain a comprehensive list of all bacteria in a sample. Therefore, a variety of techniques have been used to get a better picture of the bacterial community in oral health and disease. With these techniques, a new picture of the bacterial composition is emerging. Bacterial communities are complex organizations composed of many species, and consortia of several species may be required for disease. Many of the traditional "pathogens" that were first identified because they grow readily in culture are not the predominant species and may be present at very low levels.

THE RIBOSOMAL 16S GENE AND BACTERIAL IDENTIFICATION AND CLASSIFICATION

The most powerful techniques for bacterial identification are based on comparisons of an essential gene, the ribosomal 16S gene. This gene codes for the RNA present in the small subunit of the ribosome. Ribosomes are the machinery that translates DNA sequence into proteins using the universal genetic code. Because fidelity and maintenance of this translation function are critical, some regions of the rDNA are so highly conserved that they can be used to align genes from dissimilar organisms. Other regions less critical to translation of the code are under less selective pressure and show enough variation so that each species has a unique sequence. This variation allows similar species to be distinguished. Currently over 125,000 bacterial 16S sequences have been deposited in the major public DNA databases, GenBank and the Ribosomal Database Project. An unknown bacterium can be identified by obtaining its 16S gene DNA sequence and comparing it to sequences in these databases with a search engine called BLAST. The process is commonly referred to as "BLASTing."

The conserved and variable regions of the 16S gene provide targets for PCR (see chapters 7 and 8). The 16S DNA from all bacteria can be amplified using primers homologous to the conserved regions of the 16S gene. This allows previously unknown bacteria to be studied. Species-specific primers homologous to variable regions can also be designed to allow the detection of specific bacteria in clinical samples.

16S and Phylogeny

Comparison of 16S gene sequences allows more than just the identification of bacteria. The longer two species have diverged over their evolutionary history, the greater will be the difference between their 16S genes. The 16S sequences from multiple species can be aligned based on conserved regions, and computations based on the number of differences found in variable regions used to construct a tree diagram of evolutionary relationships. This technique is the basis for modern bacterial phylogeny. Figure 1 shows a tree diagram of the nine bacterial phyla (also called divi-

FIGURE 1 Phylogenetic tree of the nine bacterial phyla that have been detected in the human oral cavity. (Adapted from B. J. Paster et al., *J. Bacteriol.* **183:** 3770–3783, 2001.)

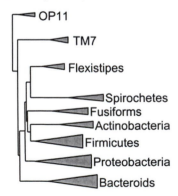

sions) commonly found in the oral cavity. With this approach the relationship among bacteria at the genus and species level can also be determined. This phylogenetic information is useful in designing PCR primers for groups of bacteria, for example, a primer that is homologous to all species of a genus such as *Streptococcus*.

Ribosomal 16S phylogeny is the most widely applicable technique currently available, but the inference of evolutionary relationships based on ribosomal genes has some limitations. Ribosomal gene-based phylogeny traces direct lines of descent, but bacteria often undergo lateral transfer of genes. Mixed ancestry from lateral transfer of distant genes may not be reflected in 16S-based phylogeny, and these genes could be critical determinants of important functions such as virulence factors. Complete genome sequences are known for a number of bacteria (see chapter 7), and as the list expands, ultimately genomic comparisons will provide a more comprehensive basis for phylogenic classification of bacteria.

SAMPLING ORAL BACTERIA

The oral cavity contains a variety of different niches that harbor distinctive communities of bacteria. For example, the gingival sulcus is a mechanically protected environment bathed in gingival crevicular fluid, and the supragingival surface of the tooth is bathed in saliva and periodically washed with ingested food. As a result of these environmental determinants, the bacterial communities found in the sulcus and on the crown of the tooth are distinct. One feature they do share, however, is that they are biofilms (made up of sessile bacteria). Unattached (planktonic) bacteria are quickly lost from the oral cavity due to the constant washing of biological fluids. Studies of various niches in the oral cavity have shown distinctive microbial profiles for the tongue, the tooth, the sulcus, the buccal mucosa, and the gingival crevice. Saliva is easily sampled, but it contains a mix of bacteria shed from these many ecosystems. Having patients chew paraffin prior to collecting saliva in order to dislodge bacteria from the tooth surface is commonly used to enrich the tooth-derived bacteria in a saliva sample. When patients are too young to provide a stimulated saliva sample, a sterile tongue blade may be applied to the dorsum of the tongue to collect a bacterial sample. These approaches are often used for convenience in large studies, but collecting the biofilm (dental plaque) from specific sites yields a more representative sample.

There are two commonly used techniques for sampling dental plaque. One approach is to use a curette to scrape the biofilm off the tooth. This is the most commonly used technique for sampling supragingival plaque. For subgingival plaque, the curette method is frequently used, but there are difficulties in sampling deep pockets in patients with periodontal disease. The curette cannot physically be inserted deeper than about 6 mm. The alternative approach is to use an endodontic paper point that consists of a very thin paper rolled into a tapered stick. The paper point can be inserted into a periodontal pocket where it wicks up fluid containing bacteria. A large number of bacteria can be recovered with this approach, and the paper point has the potential to obtain material from even the deepest pocket. This approach may obtain more of the planktonic (or free-floating) bacteria than the bacteria within the biofilm. At this time, very little work has been done to compare these two methods.

IDENTIFYING ORAL BACTERIA

Approaches to identifying and classifying oral bacteria can be grouped into two major categories: techniques that require culturing of the organisms and molecular techniques that do not require culturing. Over the last 2 decades, molecular techniques have acquired a more prominent role in the analysis of oral bacteria and they have become the standard. This approach has resulted in the identification of hundreds of new species that have yet to be cultured. With the identification of these new bacteria, many of which could play important roles in oral health or disease, it is time for the reemergence of culturing as an important tool for furthering our understanding of oral microbiology. The culturing of these potentially important bacteria may require the development of new methods or media.

At present, there is no one technique that can be used to characterize the full complement of organisms in an oral sample; therefore, a variety of techniques have been used to give us the picture of the microbial community that we have today. All of these techniques offer their own advantages, drawbacks, and biases. Both molecular and cultivation approaches provide vital information for understanding oral bacteria.

Molecular Techniques for Bacterial Identification

The accurate identification and quantitation of complex mixtures of bacteria like those found in the oral cavity are difficult processes. All techniques that are used for the characterization of mixed cultures of bacteria are potentially subject to some experimental bias. Many of the molecular techniques involve the analysis of DNA isolated directly from oral samples without culturing. Although this will circumvent the bias introduced by culturing, which will overlook more than 50% of the species present in the sample, it can introduce bias due to differential recovery of DNA from the hundreds of different organisms in the sample.

RECOVERY OF BACTERIAL DNA FROM CLINICAL SAMPLES

To extract the DNA from the bacterial cell so it can be analyzed, the bacterial cell wall must be lysed without damage to the DNA. There are several methods used to lyse bacteria, and these methods can result in relative differences in yields from different organisms. Methods that result in high recovery of one group of bacteria may not recover similar amounts of DNA from other groups of bacteria. There are a number of commercially available "kits" for isolating bacterial DNA, using a variety of methods to lyse the cells. These kits often target specific types of bacteria (i.e., gram negative). A common approach is to use detergent and proteinase K to lyse bacterial cell walls. This approach generally lyses a wide spectrum of bacteria, but there is evidence suggesting that gram-positives such as the streptococci are resistant to this method. For this reason it is used primarily for subgingival samples. Over the past few years, the use of bead-beating has become more popular. Bacteria are mixed with a slurry of tiny glass beads. The beads are projected through the bacteria by vibration in an apparatus much like an amalgam triturator. The duration of vibrating and the composition of the beads can be varied to make the process more or less severe. This procedure will lyse even the most sturdy bacteria, but fragile bacterial species such as spirochetes may be lost due to destruction of the DNA by the bead-beating process. Bead-beating has become the method of choice for isolating DNA from supragingival samples that are likely to contain high levels of streptococci. It is likely that new methods will continue to be developed in an effort to obtain a more representative DNA profile of complex oral bacterial samples.

Preparation of bacterial DNA for molecular analysis after lysis can be accomplished in a number of ways. The simplest approach is to use the lysate directly in PCR or some alternative analysis. But the use of crude preparations can be problematic, so the DNA is usually purified. Commercial kits for isolation of DNA from small sample volumes are available and are widely used. Many of them rely on adhering DNA to ground glass and removong impurities by washing.

PCR DETECTION

Almost every DNA-based method that does not require culturing uses PCR at some point during the procedure. The amplification of DNA with PCR has allowed the detection of bacteria that are present in very low levels, theoretically as low as one bacterial cell. PCR has also made it possible to do extensive, detailed analysis with very small samples.

One of the simplest approaches to identifying bacteria is to use species-specific primers in a PCR. This allows the specific amplification of DNA from a target species even in the presence of the hundreds of species of bacteria in an oral sample. It can be used to detect cultivable and yet-to-be cultivated species.

Primer design

With the availability of DNA sequence data for the 16S genes from thousands of bacteria, it is possible to design species-specific primers without any laboratory work and to do a virtual test of their specificity. First, sequences from closely related species are downloaded from a database such as GenBank and aligned, and regions that are unique to the species of interest are identified. The candidate sequence for primer construction can then be checked against the entire GenBank database to confirm its uniqueness. The likelihood of there being undiscovered bacteria that contain the presumed unique sequence is becoming smaller each day with the availability of 16S sequences from more species. However, it is still possible that unknown species may cross-hybridize with the chosen primers.

PCR assay

The presence or absence of a species-specific PCR product from a sample is generally determined by agarose gel electrophoresis (Fig. 2). Very rapid detection for clinical assays can also be obtained with monitored or "real-time" PCR systems that detect the appearance of amplification product during the reaction. Real-time PCR is described in more detail in the next section.

It is also common to develop PCR assays based on genes other than 16S by targeting other genes that are unique to an individual bacterium.

FIGURE 2 An agarose gel showing the results of PCRs with ribosomal 16S primers specific for *Porphyromonas gingivalis* on five clinical samples and positive and negative controls. Size markers are shown in lane λ. *P. gingivalis* was detected in samples 2 and 5.

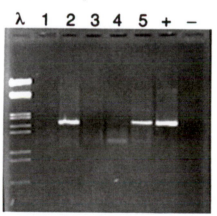

An example is the leukotoxin gene of *Actinobacillus actinomycetemcomitans*, a bacterium associated with localized forms of aggressive periodontitis. A PCR assay based on the leukotoxin gene allows the detection of *A. actinomycetemcomitans*.

PCR provides an extremely sensitive and efficient approach to identifying oral bacteria. Once unique primers are identified and tested, large numbers of samples can be analyzed. At this time it is the fastest, simplest, and most sensitive method for detecting the presence of bacteria. This approach, however, does not provide quantitative information. Quantitative (or real-time) PCR, an adaptation of PCR using specialized monitoring technology, allows the monitoring of bacterial levels.

QUANTITATIVE PCR

PCR can be used to determine whether an oral sample contains a bacterial species, but it normally does not give quantitative information. This is because the final amount of product in a PCR is not directly dependent on the amount of target DNA in the original sample. However, with the addition of a fluorescent indicator dye, the progress of the reaction can be monitored in real time and quantitative information obtained. Quantitative PCR (qPCR) is often referred to as real-time PCR. One commonly used qPCR approach is the TaqMan system (Fig. 3). For the TaqMan assay, in addition to the two primers needed for PCR, an oligonucleotide probe is added. This probe binds to the template internal to the two primers. The probe has two fluorescent dyes attached, a reporter dye at the 5′ end and a quencher at the 3′ end. When the probe is intact, because of the proximity of the two dyes, fluorescence by the reporter is quenched. The TaqMan system relies on the 5′ to 3′ exonuclease activity

FIGURE 3 The TaqMan method for real-time PCR. See the text for a description of the method.

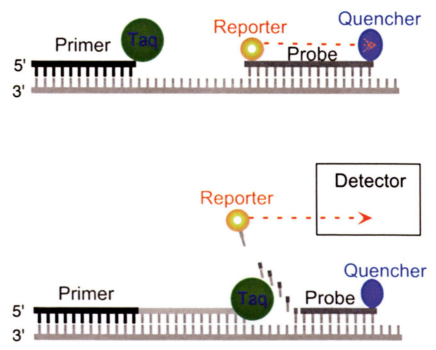

of *Taq* DNA polymerase, the enzyme used in PCR. During the extension phase of PCR, the probe that is hybridized downstream of the primer is cleaved into nucleotides, releasing the reporter dye from the quencher. The resulting fluorescent signal, which is proportional to the amount of DNA synthesis, is measured by a fluorometer attached to the PCR thermocycler. Samples with unknown amounts of bacteria can be compared to a standard curve to determine the amount of target sequence that was present in the original sample (Fig. 4). Real-time PCR thermocyclers can measure fluorescence in 96 samples simultaneously.

An alternative to the TaqMan qPCR approach is to use a dye that fluoresces only when it is bound to double-stranded DNA, such as SYBR green. By adding this dye to the PCR and monitoring the appearance of fluorescent signal during PCR, the amount of synthesis of new DNA can be measured. Standard curves are generated from known amounts of the target DNA. While easier to carry out and less expensive than the TaqMan method, the SYBR green method is more subject to artifacts resulting from the amplification of extraneous DNA. Therefore, the TaqMan approach is more often used, especially for complex mixtures of DNA, like oral samples.

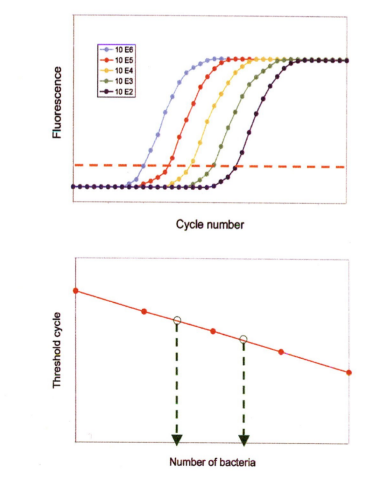

FIGURE 4 (A) Real-time PCR measurement of fluorescence from five 10-fold serial dilutions of bacterial DNA. Fluorescence is monitored at every cycle during the PCR. The number of cycles it takes for the fluorescence to reach the threshold level shown by the dashed line (threshold cycle) is proportional to the quantity of DNA in the standard. Fluorescence is detected earliest in the samples with the most DNA. (B) A standard curve obtained from plotting the number of bacteria in the serially diluted standards against the threshold cycle determined in panel A. This standard curve is used to determine the DNA concentration in samples. The threshold cycle for samples (green circles) is fit to the line and used to calculate the number of bacteria in the sample (green arrows).

DNA HYBRIDIZATION ASSAYS

Because of the complexity of the oral microbial community, in order to study the bacterial etiology of oral infections it is necessary to identify many species of bacteria from a single sample. Checkerboard analysis is a DNA hybridization assay that was developed to identify many bacterial species from a sample at the same time.

Whole-genomic checkerboard analysis

Whole-genomic, species-specific hybridization probes are used for this analysis. DNA from bacterial samples is attached to nylon membranes in long strips. Species-specific probes constructed from whole-genomic DNA are labeled and hybridized in long strips at right angles to the samples, creating a checkerboard pattern. With this approach, 30 to 40 samples can be analyzed for the presence of 30 to 40 species at the same time. By using controls containing known amounts of DNA, this technique can be semiquantitative.

Only cultivated species can be analyzed with this type of checkerboard analysis, since whole-genomic DNA probes must be constructed. This technique can also be subject to cross-reactivity with species that are closely related to the target species, due to the presence of sequences in the probe that are not species specific, despite the care taken in making the original probes to minimize cross-reactivity. With the checkerboard technique, it is possible to generate large amounts of data in a relatively short time, allowing the comparison of multiple species in studies that involve very large sample sizes.

Oligonucleotide checkerboard analysis

In this modification of the original checkerboard technique, oligonucleotides homologous to 16S ribosomal genes are used as hybridization probes instead of the whole-genomic probes (Fig. 5). Because the probe rather than the sample is attached first to the membrane, this approach is sometimes called "reverse capture checkerboard." PCR is used to amplify and label samples before hybridization. Labeled universal 16S primers are used for this amplification. This approach has the potential to be more specific than the original checkerboard method. However, finding hybridization conditions that work well for the many different probes used in an assay can be difficult. The reverse capture technique offers the advantage that probes can be made for species that have never been cultivated, as long as the sequence of the 16S gene has been determined.

Microarrays

Several research groups are currently developing DNA microarrays containing oligonucleotide probes to a large range of oral species. Microarrays are essentially a miniaturization of the checkerboard approach, potentially allowing investigators to probe for extremely large numbers of species at the same time. Microarrays have the potential to identify almost unlimited numbers of species in complex oral samples. The ultimate goal is to establish arrays containing probes to every species found in the oral cavity. Microarrays are likely to continue to evolve as technical challenges are overcome.

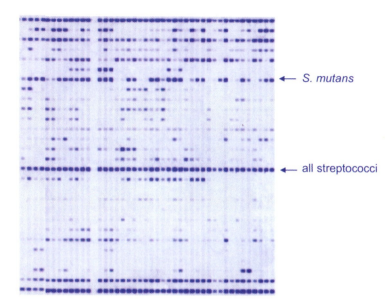

← *S. mutans*

← all streptococci

FIGURE 5 Reverse capture checkerboard hybridization blot. Probes were applied in horizontal rows, and samples and standards were then hybridized in vertical columns. Each spot on the blot represents hybridization of one probe to one sample. The intensity of the spot is proportional to the amount of DNA in the sample. The rows indicated by the arrows represent an *S. mutans* probe that gave positive results for most samples, and a multiple-species streptococcal probe that gave a positive result for every sample tested. (From M. R. Becker et al., *J. Clin. Microbiol.* **40**:1001–1009, 2002.)

Of the approaches to bacterial detection discussed so far, both PCR and checkerboard allow the detection of species that have not been cultivated. As long as the sequence of the 16S gene or another unique gene is known, probes or primers can be constructed for the assays. However, neither technique allows the discovery of new species or the detection of unexpected species. To detect new species another technique, 16S cloning and sequencing, is used.

RIBOSOMAL 16S CLONING AND SEQUENCE ANALYSIS

Ribosomal 16S cloning and sequence analysis (Fig. 6) is an open-ended molecular technique that allows the identification of any bacterium present in a sample, regardless of whether it can be cultivated or has been previously discovered. This approach relies on PCR amplification of bacterial community DNA with universal bacterial 16S primers that hybridize to all eubacteria. The amplified product, containing 16S sequences from all the bacteria present in the sample, is ligated into an *Escherichia coli* plasmid (vector), and *E. coli* cells are transfected with the plasmid. Each successfully transformed *E. coli* cell now includes the 16S gene from one bacterium. The transformed *E. coli* cells are plated onto media and grown. The vector contains a reporter gene system so that colonies with successful integration of a bacterial 16S gene appear white (those without inserts are blue). DNA from the *E. coli* colonies with inserts of bacterial 16S DNA is sequenced. Sequences are matched to 16S profiles in public databases such as GenBank for identification of bacterial species.

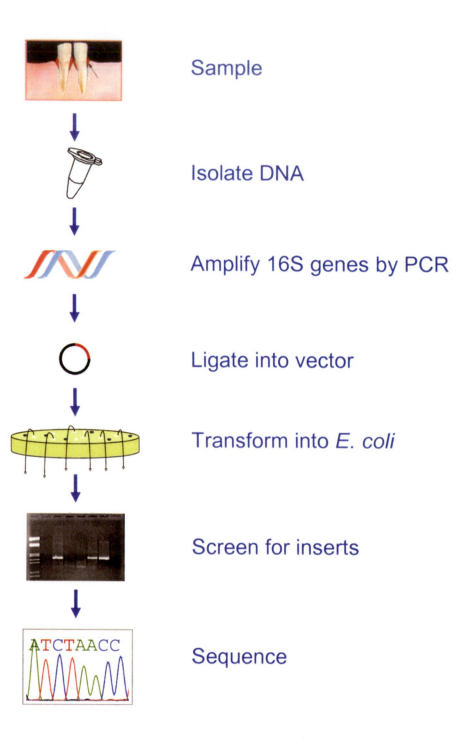

Sample

Isolate DNA

Amplify 16S genes by PCR

Ligate into vector

Transform into *E. coli*

Screen for inserts

Sequence

FIGURE 6 Cloning and sequencing of bacterial 16S genes. DNA is isolated from samples, and 16S rDNA is amplified from all the bacteria present in the sample. The 16S fragments are ligated into an *E. coli* plasmid (vector), and *E. coli* cells are transfected with the plasmid. Each successfully transformed *E. coli* cell now includes the 16S gene from one bacterium. The transformed *E. coli* cells are plated onto media and grown. The vector contains a reporter gene system so that colonies with successful integration of a bacterial 16S gene appear white (those without inserts are blue). DNA from the *E. coli* colonies with inserts of bacterial 16S DNA is sequenced for identification of bacterial species.

Sequences that do not match any sequence in a public database may indicate the discovery of a new species. The number of bacteria that have been found in the oral cavity has more than doubled from the results of this approach. It is possible to use 16S cloning and sequencing as a quantitative technique if conditions that maintain the original composition of the 16S genes are used.

Subgroups of bacteria can be targeted for cloning and sequencing by using a subgroup-specific primer prior to cloning. This is analogous to using selective media to culture specific groups of bacteria. The targeted technique has been useful in identifying many of the *Bacteroides* spp. and treponemes that are present at low levels in the subgingival biofilm.

NAMING OF BACTERIA AND MOLECULAR ANALYSIS

The classification and naming of bacteria are ongoing processes that are continually being refined and updated. There is a Judicial Commission that decides on any changes or additions to the current list of known bacteria, and proposed changes in the classification of bacteria are continuously being considered and acted on. Official recognition of a bacterium occurs when it has been described in the *International Journal of Systematic and Evolutionary Microbiology*, based on observations of it in culture.

The many species of bacteria that have been detected based only on their DNA sequence do not have official names. So uncultivated bacteria are unofficially named, usually with the genus of their closest neighbor and a letter and number code, such as *Veillonella* sp. oral clone X042.

Bacterial names are often changed when new information about genetic lineage is discovered. For example, *Fusobacterium alocis* was originally named on the basis of its phenotypic similarity to the fusobacteria. It was later given a genus of its own, *Filifactor alocis*, when 16S sequencing showed it should be placed in a different phylum from the fusobacteria.

DIRECT OBSERVATION OF ORAL BACTERIA

Oral bacteria can be directly observed by microscopy. Basic morphotypes and motile and nonmotile bacteria can be distinguished in unstained specimens viewed under phase-contrast or dark-field microscopy. The Gram stain further divides bacteria into two groups based on cell wall structure. Species-specific stains are used to label bacteria so that individual species or groups of bacteria can be visualized and identified.

Antibodies raised by injecting cultured bacteria into animals can be fluorescently tagged and used to label bacteria for visualization by microscopy. Bacteria can even be counted as a method of quantitation. This approach is very sensitive to variations in technique, and since the development of oligonucleotide probes, it is seldom used.

Fluorescent in situ hybridization (FISH) is a technique that allows targeted labeling of bacterial cells with fluorescently labeled oligonucleotide probes (Fig. 7). Probes that hybridize to ribosomal 16S RNA are most commonly used. The 16S rRNA is an excellent target for labeling since there are many ribosomes in a cell, and the 16S sequence has variable regions that can be used for construction of probes that are unique for individual bacteria or groups of bacteria. FISH is performed on glass slides or microscopic wells, and the labeled cells are visualized under a microscope. Conventional epifluorescence microscopes are used to visualize monolayer slides. However, thicker samples, such as biofilms, can be viewed using confocal laser scanning microscopy. Serial optical sections are collected from a thick specimen, and the serial images are used to reconstruct a three-dimensional image. Multiple species-specific probes, each labeled with differently colored fluorescing compounds, can be used

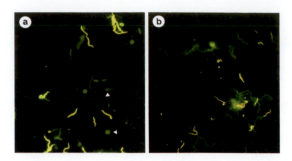

FIGURE 7 FISH of subgingival plaque material. Multiple colors can be used simultaneously, and the specificity of probes can be controlled. (a) Microphotograph showing simultaneous hybridization of a universal eubacterial probe (green) and a spirochete-specific probe (yellow). (b) Microphotograph showing hybridization with two different spirochete probes, one yellow and one green. (From A. Moter et al., *J. Clin. Microbiol.* **36**:1399–1403, 1998, with permission.)

at the same time. This approach is useful for determining the relationship of multiple species or groups of bacteria in a biofilm. The specificity of the probe is critical to the accuracy of FISH, and it can be challenging to differentiate closely related species.

CULTIVATION OF ORAL BACTERIA

The oral cavity harbors a diverse group of bacteria with a broad spectrum of physical and chemical requirements. To successfully grow bacteria in the laboratory, cultivation conditions must be adjusted to suit these varied requirements.

The general scheme for the cultivation of oral bacteria (Fig. 8) is to collect a sample and place it immediately into a transport medium. The medium is taken to the laboratory for processing. Bacteria tend to clump together, so they are usually dispersed by agitation or sonication prior to plating onto petri dishes. There are many more bacteria in an oral sample than could be grown on one plate, so serial dilutions are generally carried out before plating to obtain discrete colonies rather than a solid lawn of bacteria. The natural habitat of oral species is approximately 37°C, so oral bacteria are usually grown in incubators. Further specific conditions for cultivation are described below. Once bacteria are grown from a clinical specimen, they may be isolated for growth in pure culture by picking out a colony and subculturing it.

Oxygen Requirements

The amount of oxygen in the atmosphere is a critical determinant of bacterial growth. Most bacteria in the oral cavity are either facultative anaerobes that can grow in the presence or absence of oxygen or anaerobes that can grow only in a reduced oxygen atmosphere. Strict anaerobes cannot tolerate any oxygen, and microaerophilic anaerobes require low levels of oxygen. In addition, many capnophilic bacteria, such as the periodontal pathogen *A. actinomycetemcomitans*, require carbon dioxide in the atmosphere.

Many facultative bacteria important in dental caries, such as *Streptococcus mutans* and lactobacilli, can be grown in normal atmospheric con-

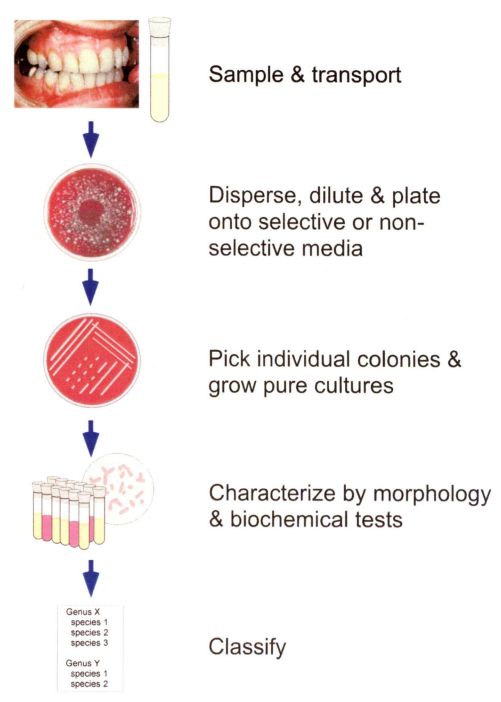

Sample & transport

Disperse, dilute & plate onto selective or non-selective media

Pick individual colonies & grow pure cultures

Characterize by morphology & biochemical tests

Genus X
species 1
species 2
species 3

Genus Y
species 1
species 2

Classify

FIGURE 8 Process for identification and classification of bacteria by culturing. Samples are collected and placed immediately into a transport medium. Bacteria are dispersed by agitation or sonication prior to plating onto petri dishes. There are many more bacteria in an oral sample than can be grown on one plate, so serial dilutions are generally carried out before plating to obtain discrete colonies rather than a solid lawn of bacteria. Bacteria may be isolated for growth in pure culture by picking out a colony and subculturing it. Bacteria are characterized and classified by biochemical tests and other methods.

ditions. But subgingival species are almost exclusively anaerobic and must be grown in special chambers that provide a reduced oxygen environment. Most anaerobic growth chambers contain low levels of CO_2 to promote the growth of capnophilic bacteria.

Care is often taken to remove oxygen from the media used to transport the bacteria from the mouth to the anaerobic chamber. This is accomplished by boiling the media or flushing it with oxygen-free gas. Pre-reduced media may be purchased from commercial sources for prepared media. Many oral anaerobes will grow even after being stored in transport fluid for hours.

There are several methods for creating and maintaining an oxygen-free environment. After inoculation, plates can be placed into an anaerobic jar or bag. The container is sealed and the oxygen is removed with a chemical reaction involving hydrogen generation and formation of water from hydrogen and oxygen in the presence of a palladium catalyst. Indicator strips are generally used to monitor for oxygen. The jar or bag is placed in a 37°C incubator. The use of small containers to grow anaerobic bacteria requires that any manipulations that need to be done be carried out on the bench top in an aerobic environment. This is generally not a problem for all but the most fastidious anaerobes. Anaerobic chambers are also available for manipulation and growth of anaerobic bacteria. Flexible plastic bags that are big enough to contain a small 37°C incubator can be used. These are entered through gloves attached to the chamber. This makes it easy to manipulate cultures without disturbing the atmosphere. Rigid gastight cabinets can also be used (Fig. 9). These cabinets are often heated to 37°C and can therefore serve as an incubator as well as a place to work on the bacteria. They also may contain gloveless sleeves that seal around the operator's arms. This eliminates the dexterity problem associated with gloves that tend to be cumbersome. The glove-less cabinet requires that the air in the sleeves be evacuated before opening the entrance to the chamber.

To maximize recovery of the greatest number of bacteria, both aerobic and anaerobic cultures can be established from the same samples.

Culture Media

Cultivation on broad-spectrum, nonselective media such as blood agar supports the growth of many oral species. An oral sample typically produces a bewildering array of colony morphologies. It can be difficult to sort out individual species from the mix, and species that comprise only a

FIGURE 9 An anaerobic chamber. This rigid gastight cabinet is heated to 37°C and serves as an incubator as well as a place to work on the bacteria. It contains gloveless sleeves that seal around the operator's arms. This eliminates the dexterity problem associated with gloves that tend to be cumbersome. The gloveless cabinet requires that the air in the sleeves be evacuated before opening the entrance to the chamber. The airlock doors are open and visible in the picture.

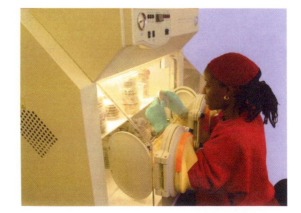

small percentage of total bacteria may not even be seen. Selective media that contain ingredients that inhibit the growth of all but a few species can be very useful for isolating individual species. For example, mitis salivarius agar with the addition of the antibiotic bacitracin (MSB agar) is highly selective for mutans group streptococci. This or similar selective media are the basis for commercial chair-side tests for mutans streptococci. The use of selective media to enhance recovery is often necessary for the detection of bacteria, such as *Bacteroides* spp., that are present in low levels.

Some bacteria have specific requirements for nutrients and can be difficult to culture until those requirements are determined and the media are supplemented. *Tannerella forsythia* (formerly *Bacteroides forsythus*) is strongly associated with periodontitis. It was not until it was discovered that *T. forsythia* has a metabolic requirement for N-acetylmuramic acid (NAM), a component of the cell wall that most other bacteria synthesize, that it was possible to isolate it in culture. The particular nutritional requirements of many species have so far eluded oral microbiologists; based on data from 16S cloning and sequencing, less than half of known oral bacteria have been cultured.

Classification of Cultured Bacteria

Prior to the development of molecular approaches to bacterial classification and phylogeny, bacteria were classified exclusively based on a series of morphological and biochemical tests. These tests are still an important part of the classification process. After a new bacterium is obtained in pure culture, it is first described morphologically. Colony morphology is documented; the size, shape, and color of colonies are noted. Growth of the bacterium on a different medium, however, can produce a totally different morphology. Microscopic examination is used to determine the shape of individual cells (rods, spheres, etc.) and whether the bacterium is positive or negative by Gram staining.

Bacteria are also characterized based on their biochemical profiles. One method is to test for the presence of metabolites using gas chromatography (GC analysis). As with colony morphology, the results may be influenced by the culture conditions. This method is less commonly used today, partially because specialized equipment is needed to perform the analysis. Other approaches test for activity of several enzymes or the ability to ferment various sugars. Commercial kits are sold for these purposes. The biochemical profiles of even closely related species may differ, and individual species can be characterized by their distinctive fingerprints.

Using cultivation-based techniques, microbiologists were able to make tremendous progress in characterizing and classifying bacteria. The advent of molecular techniques has allowed the refinement of bacterial classifications based on phylogeny, and has revealed a whole new world of bacteria that have not yet been cultivated. Now new cultivation techniques are needed to move ahead with the study of these yet-to-be-cultivated species.

Antibiotic Susceptibility

Antibiotic susceptibility tests can be performed on cultured bacteria. Most commonly the disk diffusion test is used. Disks impregnated with antibiotic are applied to a petri dish that has been inoculated with the bacterium to be tested and the plate is incubated. The zone of growth inhibition around the disk is proportional to susceptibility to the antimicrobial agent. Antibiotic susceptibility testing is used only rarely in dentistry, usually for patients with serious odontogenic infections that are refractory to empirical antibiotic therapy.

KEY POINTS

The oral flora is one of the most diverse microbe communities known. More than 700 species of bacteria have been identified in the oral cavity. Over half of known oral species have never been grown in culture.

Bacteria can be identified with both culture-based and molecular techniques. Of course, only molecular techniques allow the detection of yet-to-be-cultivated species.

Molecular identification methods for bacteria are most often based on sequence analysis of the ribosomal 16S genes. Ribosomal gene analysis also allows evolutionary relationships to be inferred and so is useful for bacterial classification.

Common techniques for molecular detection of bacteria:
- PCR with specific primers
- Quantitative PCR
- DNA hybridization assays (checkerboards)
- Ribosomal 16S cloning and sequence analysis
- FISH and microscopy

Cultivation of many oral species requires special conditions such as an anaerobic environment, CO_2 in the atmosphere, and incubation at 37°C. Some oral bacteria have specialized nutritional requirements, and this may be the reason many have not yet been cultivated. New culture techniques must be developed to grow the many species that have been identified but not yet cultured.

Cultivated bacteria may be identified and classified based on morphology and biochemical tests.

FURTHER READING

Jousimies-Somer, H., and V. L. Sutter. 2002. *Wadsworth-KTL Anaerobic Bacteriology Manual*, 6th ed. Star Publishing, Belmont, Calif.

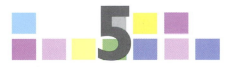

Oral Microbial Ecology

HOWARD F. JENKINSON AND RICHARD J. LAMONT

INTRODUCTION

An eclectic and diverse assemblage of microorganisms call the oral cavity home. At least 500 species of bacteria are supported by the habitats within the mouth, such as the surfaces of the teeth and oral mucosa. Distinct microbial communities accumulate on these surfaces through successive colonization events. On the tooth surfaces, for example, early or primary colonizers are mainly streptococci and actinomyces. Over time, the proportions of these gram-positive facultatively anaerobic bacteria decrease and eventually gram-negative anaerobes become more established, especially at the interface of the teeth and gums (gingival margins). The resulting mixed species community, familiar as dental plaque, is a complex and dynamic entity, and populational shifts within plaque contribute to oral diseases. Overrepresentation of bacteria tolerating more acidic conditions (acidophiles) increases susceptibility to caries, whereas elevated numbers of gram-negative obligately anaerobic bacteria, particularly in the gingival crevice, can lead to periodontal disease.

Although an immense variety of organisms are displayed in the oral microbiota, many more bacteria pass through the oral cavity than are retained. A cursory comparison between the bacterial inhabitants of the mouth and those within the small intestine will attest to this. Successful colonizers of the oral cavity must, therefore, possess certain attributes that allow them to survive and thrive in this unique environment (Fig. 1). The ability of microorganisms to adhere to oral surfaces is especially important in the oral system. Continuous flow of saliva together with the mechanical shearing actions of the tongue and lips act to dislodge and expel bacteria, so adhesion is essential for retention. Furthermore, the mouth can experience rapid and dramatic changes in physical parameters such as temperature, oxygen tension, pH, osmolarity, and nutrient availability. Bacteria that are capable of sensing and responding to these stresses have a selective advantage over those that are less adaptable and are more likely to increase in number. Bacteria that lack a critical number of these survival attributes are likely to be present in the mouth only temporarily.

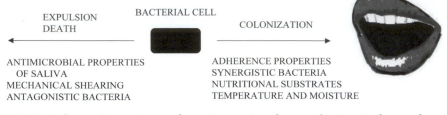

EXPULSION
DEATH

BACTERIAL CELL

COLONIZATION

ANTIMICROBIAL PROPERTIES
OF SALIVA
MECHANICAL SHEARING
ANTAGONISTIC BACTERIA

ADHERENCE PROPERTIES
SYNERGISTIC BACTERIA
NUTRITIONAL SUBSTRATES
TEMPERATURE AND MOISTURE

FIGURE I Constraints acting on bacteria entering the mouth. Certain factors favor colonization while others tend to eliminate bacterial cells.

ACQUISITION OF ORAL BACTERIA

The oral cavity generally lacks significant bacterial colonization at birth. However, beginning shortly after birth, bacteria are continually being introduced into the mouth from contaminated animate and inanimate objects. While the majority of these bacteria are transients, successful oral colonizers will be obtained from exogenous saliva. Primary caregivers or other close contacts, such as siblings, are usually the source of this bacteria-containing saliva. After a few months, most mouths possess a microbiota consisting of recognizable oral organisms. The next major ecological event is the eruption of the deciduous teeth at around 6 months of age. The appearance of these hard nonshedding surfaces allows the colonization of organisms that are exquisitely adapted to this environment. Bacteria such as the oral streptococci and actinomyces thus comprise a significant proportion of the organisms in dental plaque on tooth surfaces. The oral microbiota continues to develop, changing with age in composition and overall activity. Hormonal changes during puberty can contribute to increased colonization by groups of gram-negative anaerobes and spirochetes, with some hormones possibly acting as nutritional sources. In adults, gradual age-related changes, physical exercise levels, and psychological stress can all influence the numbers or proportions of oral bacteria, often through effects on immune function or salivary flow rate. Similarly, lifestyle events such as smoking, frequency of carbohydrate consumption, or pregnancy can affect the microbial composition. In later years the decline in salivary flow rate and in general health status leads to changes in microbial colonization, such as increased carriage of the yeast *Candida albicans*, with subsequent higher risk of oral candidiasis.

The excessive buildup of dental plaque is unsightly and malodorous and causes inflammation of the gingival tissues (gums). Moreover, among the oral microbiota there are a number of bacterial species that are considered undesirable because they clearly contribute to oral disease. Nonetheless, many of the microorganisms present within plaque may not be especially undesirable and in fact provide a protective function for the host. There are many examples of how nonpathogenic resident (commensal) bacteria can restrict establishment and growth of pathogenic organisms in microbial communities, such as by competing for adhesion receptors and by producing toxic metabolic products. The temporal acquisition of oral streptococcal species by infants provides an excellent example of how components of the normal microbiota can be beneficial to the host. Shortly after birth, the infant acquires an oral microbiota on the mucosa that after some weeks consists generally of *Streptococcus*, *Haemophilus*, and *Neisseria* species. Many of these species, e.g., *Streptococcus mitis*, *Streptococcus oralis*, etc., produce immunoglobulin A (IgA) proteases that specifically cleave secretory IgA (S-IgA) antibodies. It is speculated that this provides an early selective advantage for survival of these bacteria in an environment rich in S-IgA from the mother's milk. These species of bacteria are able to colonize the mucosal surfaces. It is not until after the emergence of the first teeth that species such as *Streptococcus sanguis* and *Streptococcus mutans* are found in the oral cavity. Colonization by *S. sanguis* is dependent on the presence of teeth and occurs at a median age of about 9 months. This is referred to as the window of infectivity, and levels of these bacteria increase with age of the infant, as more teeth emerge. Colonization by *S. mutans*, the principal agent associated with dental caries, generally occurs much later (around 26 months) and is associated with a decline in *S. sanguis* numbers. Thus, these two bacteria antagonize or compete with each other. Early colonization of infants with *S. sanguis* results in delayed colonization by *S. mutans* and reduces the incidence of carious lesions. This is an important concept because it implies that initial adhesion events (primary colonization) during the acquisition phase can shape the microbial plaque community and directly influence oral disease potential.

COLONIZATION BY ORAL BACTERIA

A microorganism first entering the oral cavity is all at sea, buffeted in the waves and currents of saliva that continually flow through the mouth and across the oral surfaces. As discussed in chapter 3, saliva contains direct antimicrobial components as well as molecules (agglutinins) that can aggregate or clump bacterial cells such that they are more readily removed from the mouth by expectoration or swallowing. To resist this innate host protective mechanism, and to resist physical dislodgement by mechanical shearing forces, oral bacteria adhere to the available surfaces. Localization at surfaces provides the additional advantage that such sites often concentrate nutrients and so will promote bacterial growth. In this regard, a tooth in the mouth is similar to a rock in a stream; both sites favor bacterial colonization and the accumulation of cells into multiple-species communities that are known as biofilms.

The oral cavity provides a variety of surfaces for bacterial attachment and colonization. These include the saliva-coated surfaces of the teeth, along with the epithelium of the cheeks, gums, and tongue. Moreover, as these surfaces become colonized by bacteria, adhesion between cells of different species becomes important. Such interbacterial coaggregation (or coadhesion) drives the temporal development of mixed-species biofilms on oral surfaces and facilitates nutritional relationships among organisms. To fully appreciate the genesis and development of the oral ecosystem, it is necessary to consider what bacteria stick with, how they stick, what they stick to, and what happens after they are stuck.

Surface Structures and Molecules Involved in Adhesion

The surfaces of both gram-positive and -negative bacteria are structurally complex (see chapter 1). Proteins, glycoproteins, lipoproteins, lipopolysaccharides (gram-negative), and lipoteichoic acids (gram-positive) can all be present to varying degrees. Protein subunits can be assembled into flagella, which provide motility, while other subunits (called fimbrillins) can be assembled into threadlike appendages known as fimbriae or fibrils. Fibrils are common on oral streptococci and are usually much shorter than fimbriae and extend only 200 nm from the cell surface, as opposed to fimbriae that are up to 1 mm in length. Fibrils have tapered ends and may be peritrichous (evenly distributed over the bacterial cell surface) or localized to a lateral crust or polar tuft. Some bacteria are also closely surrounded by a loose polysaccharide layer called a capsule. The question then arises: which of these surface-exposed molecules or structures are responsible for bacterial adhesion? The answer, unfortunately, is not a simple one. Adhesion is unlike motility, for example, because it is not usually defined by one specific surface component. Rather, bacteria utilize different and often multiple surface structures for adhesion, and any of the surface available components can be involved in the adhesive process. The contribution of an individual component to the overall binding process can involve a physicochemical aspect, often charge or hydrophobicity dependent, or a more specific ligand-receptor type aspect (as discussed in more detail below). From a bacterial perspective, the presence of multiple adhesion-mediating molecules (designated "adhesins") with distinct binding partners ("receptors") on host surfaces is likely to both improve the chances of adhesion occurring and result in stronger binding.

Although all bacterial surface components could potentially be involved in adhesion, certain trends have emerged for the well-studied oral bacteria. Major adhesins are often fimbriae or major outer membrane proteins in gram-negative bacteria; and fibrils, fimbriae, or prominent cell-wall linked surface proteins in gram-positive bacteria. *Actinomyces naeslundii*, for example, possesses two major classes of fimbriae, type 1 and type 2. Type 1 fimbriae are associated with adhesion to the tooth surfaces through interactions with salivary acidic proline-rich proteins and statherin deposited within the salivary pellicle that coats enamel. Adhesion may not be mediated by the fimbrial subunit protein itself, but instead by accessory proteins displayed on the fimbrial support structure. The adherence-promoting activity of the proline-rich proteins is enhanced after deposition on the enamel surface, probably through conformation changes exposing previously hidden binding domains (cryptitopes). Type 2 fimbriae are involved in adhesion through a lectin-like mechanism to glycosidic (sugar) receptors on epithelial cells.

Streptococcal adhesion is also a complex process and streptococcal cell surfaces are decorated with multiple adhesins with differing specificities. Many of these adhesins are conserved across species, a testament to their importance to the organisms. *Streptococcus parasanguis* fimbriae (composed of a protein called Fap) and *Streptococcus gordonii* fibrils (composed of a protein called CshA) are involved in adhesion. The CshA protein forms the fibrillar component in several species of mitis group streptococci and also mediates attachment of these cells to some other oral bacteria and to human fibronectin. The tufts of fibrils on *Streptococcus cristatus* are associated with the binding of these bacteria to *Fusobacterium nucleatum* to form characteristic corncob aggregates of bacteria seen in mature dental plaque (Fig. 2). *S. mutans* adhesion to the salivary

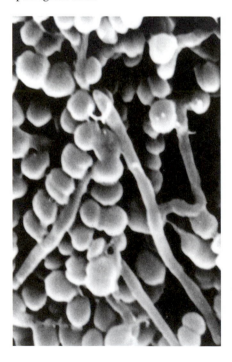

FIGURE 2 Scanning electron micrograph of "corncob" bacterial aggregates often seen in mature dental plaque. A number of coccal *Streptococcus crista* cells bind along the surface of a central *F. nucleatum* rod-shaped cell. Such adhesive interactions are thought to aid colonization and retention of the participating bacteria.

pellicle appears to involve a major surface protein of the antigen (Ag) I/II family. This protein is well conserved across a number of streptococcal species and possesses multifunctional domains that have been adapted by different species for binding to salivary pellicle receptors, salivary agglutinins, and other bacteria. They thus provide a pivotal role in the development of dental plaque that is usually initiated by the primary colonizing streptococci. The AgI/II protein of mitis group streptococci is responsible, in part, for initial adhesion to the salivary pellicle, and it also allows streptococci to bind to collagen present in dentin that can be exposed after carious destruction of the enamel. This can lead to bacteria penetrating the dentinal tubules and infecting the tooth root canals and pulpal tissues. AgI/II polypeptides also provide a mechanism for binding the salivary agglutinin glycoprotein to the streptococcal cell surface. This in turn generates a receptor to which other bacteria can adhere (Fig. 3). The AgI/II protein also participates in the direct binding of some bacteria, such as the gram-negative pathogenic *Porphyromonas gingivalis*, to streptococci, thus enabling these secondary colonizing organisms to become incorporated into plaque communities (Fig. 3).

Another example of streptococcal adhesion to salivary receptors, again illustrating the multiplicity of adhesion mechanisms, involves the salivary starch-degrading enzyme amylase. Amylase, which is abundant in saliva, binds to several species of oral streptococci by at least two specific amylase-binding proteins (called AbpA and AbpB) on the bacterial surface. Mutant strains of bacteria deficient in amylase binding adhere less well to amylase-coated enamel than do wild-type strains. While the wild-type strain produced large microcolonies in a flow cell biofilm model, a mutant strain made deficient in AbpA (and shown not to bind

FIGURE 3 Microbial adhesion in the development of oral microbial plaque communities. Primary colonizers (e.g., mitis group streptococci and *A. naeslundii*) adhere with high affinity to salivary components (SC), such as proline-rich proteins, statherin, α-amylase, and mucin glycoproteins, that are bound to the enamel surface (1). Glucan polysaccharides (GPS), generated by the activities of bacterial glucosyltransferase enzymes, also become incorporated into the salivary pellicle and provide adhesion receptors for bacteria expressing glucan-binding proteins (2). Secondary colonizers (e.g., *F. nucleatum*, *P. gingivalis*, and *T. forsythia*), which do not effectively compete with the primary colonizers in binding to the tooth surface, adhere to SC and GPS that are deposited onto the surfaces of the primary colonizers (3, 4). Direct cell-to-cell adhesion (coaggregation) of secondary and primary colonizers (5), often through protein-carbohydrate (lectinlike) interactions, promotes the development of spatially defined groups of microorganisms.

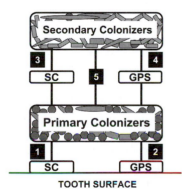

TOOTH SURFACE

amylase) grew much more poorly and produced relatively small micro-colonies. It is possible that in addition to a role in adhesion, amylase may support microbial nutrition by degrading dietary starch in proximity to the cell surface. The starch metabolites can be rapidly transported into the cell to be used as a source of energy.

Many streptococcal species, as well as *A. naeslundii*, have the ability to synthesize extracellular polysaccharides. Glucans, which are synthesized from sucrose through the activities of secreted glucosyltransferase enzymes, are thought to play a key role in the formation of plaque because they adhere to smooth surfaces and mediate the coadhesion of bacterial cells (see chapter 11). The accumulation of mutans group streptococci within plaque is enhanced through the activities of cell surface-associated glucan-binding proteins. These proteins act as adhesins mediating attachment of streptococci to glucans incorporated into the salivary pellicle, as well as mediating coadhesion of streptococci (Fig. 3). Since the glucan-binding proteins and AgI/II proteins are so important for the adhesion of streptococci, there is considerable interest in developing inhibitors of their functions, such as adhesin or substrate analogues, or specific antibodies, that might be utilized in the future to control plaque development.

Mechanisms of Adhesion

To adhere to an oral surface, bacteria that are initially suspended in saliva must first come in close proximity to the substratum. Many factors contribute to the approach of a microorganism to a surface. When salivary flow is high, convective transport by fluid dynamic forces causes accumulation of bacteria at solid-liquid interfaces where there is a viscous boundary layer. Frictional drag and turbulent downsweeps also assist contact with the surface. Irregularities present on surfaces provide shelters in which the bacteria can be protected from shear forces. When salivary flow is low, diffusive transport resulting from Brownian motion can serve, albeit more slowly, to concentrate suspended bacteria at a surface. Some bacterial species, such as the spirochetes (e.g., *Treponema denticola*), can actively participate in their surface localization by chemotactic motile responses.

Following arrival at a surface, the next challenge is to avoid displacement. It is instructive, although an oversimplification, at this point to consider bacteria as inert negatively charged particles and the host surface as similarly inert and negatively charged. The physical interaction between two such entities can then be predicted by the Derjaguin-Landau-Verwey-Overbeek (DLVO) theory of energetic interactions in biocolloidal systems. Simply put, the tendency for two negatively charged surfaces to repel each other can be overcome by fluctuating dipoles (van der Waals attraction) within individual molecules on the approaching surfaces. If the surfaces become too close, there will again be a repulsive force due to overlapping electron layers. Although the DLVO theory provides a theoretical framework for initial attachment, it is unable to fully accommodate the complexity of bacterial adhesion. Other factors that contribute to this early attachment phase include bridging by divalent cations (e.g., Ca^{2+}) in saliva, hydrophobic interactions between nonpolar regions of molecules on the surfaces, and hydrogen bonding (Fig. 4).

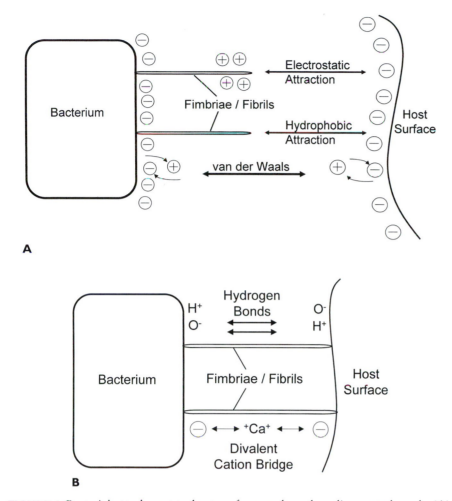

FIGURE 4 Bacterial attachment to host surfaces such as the saliva-coated tooth. (A) The bacteria first localize at sites on the salivary pellicle that are most thermodynamically favorable. This depends on interactions between the bacterial surface and the tooth surface that include van der Waals forces, along with electrostatic and hydrophobic interactions. Bacteria can concentrate positively charged or hydrophobic amino acids on their fimbriae/fibrils in order to strengthen the adhesive forces. (B) As the bacterial cells get closer to the surface, hydrogen bonds and divalent cation bridges can also stabilize the interaction. The sum total of all these weak interactions allows initial attachment but is not enough to retain the bacteria on the surface for long periods. Thus, after initial localization at the surface, bacteria must then form a higher-affinity bond between complementary adhesins and receptors (see text for details). The figure is not to scale.

The sum total of these forces still produces only a relatively weak association of bacteria and substratum, and the bacteria cycle on and off the surfaces. To remain more firmly attached for an extended period, bacteria need to form higher-affinity bonds utilizing specific surface molecules that interact stereochemically with cognate receptors, much as in an antibody-antigen interaction. The common arrangement whereby such adhesins are localized on fimbriae or fibrils that can extend several microns out from the bacterial wall facilitates engagement of a receptor while keeping the bacteria at an optimal distance from the host surface. These stronger, essentially irreversible, short-range associations can be mediated by protein-carbohydrate (lectinlike) interactions and by protein-protein interactions, as mentioned above. In either event, the requirement for complementary adhesins and receptor imparts a high degree of specificity to the adhesion mechanism. This is the basis for the tissue-specific binding (tropism) demonstrated by many oral bacteria. For example, a major reason that *S. sanguis* is found almost exclusively on the tooth surface, whereas the closely related *Streptococcus salivarius* resides on the dorsum of the tongue, is due to the specificity of the adhesins displayed by these organisms. Coordinated expression of a number of bacterial cell activities may be required for optimal adhesion. For example, partial degradation of host cell receptors by bacterial proteinases can expose binding domains that would otherwise remain hidden within the molecule and unavailable for attachment purposes.

Host Surface-Specific Constraints on Bacterial Adhesion

Teeth are highly mineralized structures that reside for extended periods, if not permanently, in the oral cavity. A newly erupted or professionally cleaned tooth becomes coated with a layer or pellicle of salivary proteins and glycoproteins within minutes. It is to this saliva-coated surface, rather than enamel itself, that bacteria adhere. Once established, pioneer colonizers of the tooth (such as streptococci, which can account for up to 80% of early plaque, and *A. naeslundii*) become long-term inhabitants. These organisms, together with their products such as insoluble polysaccharides, provide adhesion substrates for secondary colonizers. Epithelial surfaces, in contrast, continuously turn over, and cells along with their attached bacteria are lost from the mouth. As living cells, the epithelial layer expresses surface molecules and is embedded in a matrix that comprises fibronectin and laminin, along with other proteins and proteoglycans. Given these discrete challenges, it is not surprising that the microbiota of the oral epithelia differs from that of tooth surfaces, both qualitatively and quantitatively. Moreover, there are distinct consequences of adhesion to living epithelial cells in that bacterial and host cells can both sense and respond to each other, as discussed below. The multiplicity of adhesins displayed by oral bacteria thus increases the likelihood and strength of receptor binding and provides the means by which bacteria can manipulate host cell signaling pathways that are stimulated through individual receptor engagements.

Adhesion and Metabolism

There is an enormous diversity of substrates present within the oral cavity that provide receptors for bacterial adhesion. There is also an equally large, or larger, diversity of substrates for bacteria to metabolize. These two processes, adhesion and metabolism, are not often considered together, but they are intricately linked. The composition and activities of oral microbial communities are shaped by environmental (extrinsic) influences, such as temperature, shear forces, nutrient supply, etc., and by intrinsic influences from both adherence capabilities and microbial metabolism. These intrinsic effects may result in the establishment of close metabolic, usually nutritional, interrelationships between groups of microorganisms. The interrelationships in catabolism develop mainly through differences in the efficiency of substrate utilization. Thus, it becomes beneficial for bacteria to assemble into groups that can utilize a complex substrate to maximum efficiency. Many metabolic interactions between bacterial pairs or groups have now been defined, and it is of considerable significance that these interactions are often associated with specific coadhesion (or coaggregation) of the bacteria involved. The outcome is a close physical association of microorganisms that comprises a more efficient, and thus more successful, metabolic unit.

The complex streptococcal microbiota of the nasopharynx provides an example of how diversity in metabolic function benefits a community. It is thought that the availability of sugars for utilization is scarce on the mucosal surfaces, in contrast to the oral cavity where sugars are often readily available from dietary food intake. Sugar utilization by streptococci in the nasopharynx may depend to a considerable extent on the abilities of bacteria to cleave, and then metabolize, sugar residues from oligosaccharide substitutions on host glycoproteins or from mucins. Cleavage of sugars from these substrates is achieved through the production of secreted enzymes known as glycan hydrolases. These enzymes include sialidase (neuraminidase), galactosidase, and fucosidase that cleave sialic acid, galactose, or fucose residues, respectively, from oligosaccharides. Not all streptococci produce all of these enzymes, so defined groups of organisms become established that can assist, and feed off, each other to make most efficient use of the complex oligosaccharide substrates. Not only do different species of streptococci come together in these associations, but other bacteria such as *Haemophilus*, *Neisseria,* and *Staphylococcus* species benefit from metabolic synergies. Moreover, the modification of oligosaccharide structures on the mucosal cell surfaces continually provides new adhesion receptors for many of these bacteria.

Coaggregation itself may facilitate metabolic interactions between microorganisms. Perhaps the most frequently cited example is the utilization by *Veillonella* species of organic acids, e.g., lactic acid, produced by streptococci. Removal of lactate from the immediate environment results in a transient rise in pH that then drives more carbohydrate fermentation by the streptococci and more lactate production. High lactate-producing streptococci, such as *S. mutans*, coaggregate with *Veillonella* species, and communities of these two species are found in carious lesions. *Veillonella* species are also found in associations with *S. salivarius* on the dorsum of the tongue.

Gram-negative anaerobic bacteria such as *F. nucleatum, P. gingivalis,* and *Tannerella forsythia* demonstrate a variety of associations with each other and with gram-positive bacteria. These associations can be theorized to provide multiple benefits for the nutritionally and metabolically fastidious gram-negative bacteria. For example, *P. gingivalis* binds only weakly to *S. gordonii* cells in suspension but adheres avidly to *S. gordonii* cells when they are deposited onto a surface. Once attached to the streptococci, *P. gingivalis* cells can accumulate rapidly into a biofilm. Since *P. gingivalis* is an obligate anaerobe, it will only survive at sites where the redox potential is low and oxygen is scarce. Regions of plaque composed of streptococci provide such sites. These kinds of interactions can form the basis for more complex interbridging events (Table 1), each generating a perceived benefit for one or more bacteria within the community.

TABLE 1 Mutually beneficial adhesion and nutritional interactions among oral bacteria

Interaction	Benefits
S. gordonii-P. gingivalis	Adhesion, reduced oxygen and redox potential for *P. gingivalis*
S. gordonii-F. nucleatum	Adhesion, reduced redox potential, and tricarboxylic and fatty acids for *F. nucleatum*
F. nucleatum-T. forsythia	Growth factors, e.g., N-acetylmuramic acid, for *T. forsythia*
P. gingivalis-T. forsythia	Peptides and hemin for *T. forsythia*

GENE REGULATION

The ever-changing environment of the oral cavity provides an impetus for bacteria to regulate gene expression in order to maintain optimal phenotypic properties. Consider the journey an organism can undertake in the mouth (Fig. 5). Upon first entry, bacteria encounter the prevailing conditions of saliva with temperatures, pH, and osmolarity less than the levels in blood and tissues. In addition, there are extremes of nutrient availability depending on host feeding patterns. Once in the gingival crevice, the amount of oxygen decreases, osmolarity and pH increase, and nutrients can be obtained from gingival crevicular fluid. During periodontal disease progression the temperature increases as a result of inflammation and there is elevated iron (or heme) availability because of bleeding. In addition to the changes in parameters in the oral cavity, bacteria that gain access systemically (see chapter 16) face a new set of challenges. The ideal numbers and types of adhesins, for example, expressed in the mouth may not be the most advantageous configuration in the tissues where such adhesion might promote uptake by the host professional phagocytic cells. To survive in different host environments, therefore, a successful oral organism has to rapidly sense and respond to the prevailing environmental circumstances. The mechanistic basis of gene regulation in oral bacteria remains to be determined in most cases. In general, however, bacteria often regulate gene expression at the level of transcription. This can occur through transcriptional activators that bind to DNA in or near the promoter regions of genes and then interact with RNA polymerase to stimulate the rate of initiation of transcription. Conversely, transcriptional repressors prevent transcription, usually by binding to DNA in the promoter region and physically impeding the action of RNA polymerase. Both activators and repressors often have active and inactive forms, depending on the binding of a ligand. For example, repressors for iron (Fe)-regulated genes may only bind DNA when complexed with Fe^{2+} or Fe^{3+} ions. Transcriptional activators are often turned on by phosphorylation, frequently as the result of a series or cascade of effector molecules. In this manner gene regulation can be connected to events at the cell surface where signaling is initiated by phosphorylation of a sensor molecule. Many other means and levels of gene regulation are also available to bacteria that will allow both fine-tuning of gene expression and rapid on/off responses to major environmental changes.

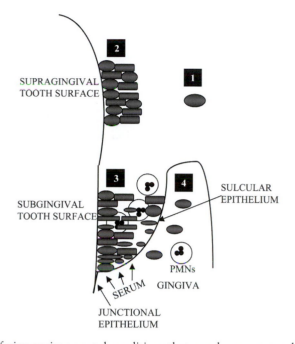

FIGURE 5 Differing environmental conditions that may be encountered by bacteria in the various oral niches. (1) Upon entry into the mouth, bacteria are suspended in saliva and experience lower pH, osmolarity, and temperature than internal body levels. Saliva also contains antimicrobial factors including antibodies, along with proteins and glycoproteins that can be metabolized by bacteria that express the necessary enzymes. (2) Once attached to the salivary pellicle coating the supragingival tooth surface, bacteria accumulate in a densely packed multispecies biofilm containing the metabolic products and signaling molecules of these organisms, and host dietary components. Temperature varies between extremes, for example, when one drinks hot coffee or eats ice cream. (3) Bacteria that colonize the gingival crevice are bathed in crevicular fluid that is a serum exudate. Host polymorphonuclear leukocytes (PMNs) and other immune cells are present. As inflammatory periodontal disease progresses, there is an increase in temperature and bleeding into the periodontal pocket, which increases the levels of, among other things, heme-containing proteins. (4) Certain oral bacteria are able to invade the host tissues, both intercellularly and intracellularly. Within the gingival tissue there are normal body physiologic conditions, and the bacteria are also challenged with host immune cells and immune effector molecules.

BACTERIAL COMMUNICATION

Bacteria in complex communities such as biofilms communicate with one another through a variety of chemical signaling molecules. Intercellular communication blurs the distinction between single- and multicellular organisms and allows bacteria to coordinate gene expression and thus the behavior of the entire community. In this way bacteria in biofilms such as plaque can derive benefits from their physical proximity that would not be available to organisms suspended in flowing fluids such as saliva.

One means by which bacterial cells communicate is through quorum sensing: cell density-dependent regulation of gene expression. This process involves the production and secretion of a signaling molecule called an autoinducer (AI). Upon reaching a threshold concentration, the AI triggers a change in gene expression. Quorum sensing can control a broad range of bacterial activities, including virulence, competence, conjugation, antibiotic production, motility, sporulation, and biofilm formation. There are three major classes of quorum-sensing systems. Gram-negative bacteria use acylated homoserine lactones as autoinducers (AI-1), whereas gram-positive bacteria utilize oligopeptides (discussed below). Both gram-negative and gram-positive bacteria can also use an autoinducer-2 (AI-2) molecule. AI-2 is formed chemically from 4,5-dihydroxy-2,3-pentanedione that is generated by the action of LuxS autoinducer synthase on *S*-ribosylhomocysteine. AI-1 signaling has not been detected among oral gram-negative bacteria; however, many oral organisms possess AI-2 signaling. In *P. gingivalis* and *Actinobacillus actinomycetemcomitans*, LuxS-based signaling regulates expression of iron acquisition systems and/or virulence factors such as proteases in *P. gingivalis* and leukotoxin in *A. actinomycetemcomitans*. In *S. gordonii*, aspects of carbohydrate metabolism are controlled through this pathway. The AI-2 signal also transmits information between bacterial species, as *P. gingivalis* genes respond to *A. actinomycetemcomitans* AI-2. The extent to which AI-2 signaling truly represents quorum sensing (i.e., is strictly cell density dependent) or is partially a reflection of the metabolic state of the cell remains to be determined. In either event, since plaque bacteria accumulate to high cell density in metabolically synergistic communities (discussed above), AI-2 signaling can be expected to play a role in plaque development.

A feature of many species of oral streptococci is that they are able to exchange segments of genetic material (DNA) with high frequency. This leads to considerable adaptability because new populations of cells that have a selective advantage may arise relatively quickly. The process of uptake and incorporation, by one cell, of DNA extruded by another is termed transformation, and streptococci are able to undergo this process in the natural environment only when they are in a state of competence. Competence is generated through a signaling mechanism involving an extracellular peptide pheromone designated competence-stimulating peptide (CSP). CSPs are produced by a wide range of oral streptococci and by *Streptococcus pneumoniae*. Cells in a population secrete low levels of CSP during growth, and CSP gradually accumulates in the environment to reach a critical threshold level. Once the bacteria sense this threshold level, the expression of genes that are involved in CSP production are upregulated (so that the population as a whole is stimulated) and so are genes involved in the processes of DNA uptake and recombination. Different species of streptococci produce slightly different pheromone peptides, so that more closely related strains or species are better stimulated than those more distantly related. Originally, it was thought that CSP production was uniquely involved in competence development. However, it was discovered later that competence pheromones promote other intracellular changes not necessarily linked to DNA uptake and recombination. Many of these changes occur through induction of expression of an alternate RNA polymerase sigma factor that transcribes new sets of genes. Thus, CSP production and sensing by *S. mutans* in biofilms have been found to be necessary for the bacteria to express proteins necessary for the cells to tolerate acid stress and adapt to low pH. In mitis group streptococci, it is possible that CSP-mediated induction of the DNA-repair enzymes, including RecA, may be part of a general stress or SOS response. These observations allow speculation that competence pheromones may actually be alarm signals that prime whole bacterial communities to oncoming stress conditions.

Oral streptococci also secrete a wide range of peptides (called bacteriocins) that are inhibitory to bacterial growth. Generally, bacteriocins are able to kill competing organisms by forming pores in the cytoplasmic membrane of sensitive gram-positive bacterial cells but do little or no harm to human cells. Bacteriocins that contain the thioether amino acid lanthionine are termed lantibiotics and tend to be synthesized and secreted through a complex machinery of proteins encoded by a number of genes. These genes are clustered on the streptococcal chromosome and include the structural gene for the bacteriocin (lantibiotic) precursor, genes encoding modification and transport proteins, genes for immunity, and sensor and regulatory protein genes. Immunity peptides provide protection for the producing strain against its own lantibiotic, while the sensor and regulatory proteins provide a mechanism for sensing and responding to the presence of lantibiotic. In this way, lantibiotics may also act as signaling molecules between streptococci. While sensing of CSP may signal impending general stress conditions, sensing of lantibiotic may signal the presence of competing streptococci and stimulate a defensive response within the population. Strains of *S. mutans* and *S. salivarius* produce potent lantibiotics, called mutacin and salivaricin, respectively, that act on other species of oral streptococci. These lantibiotics may thus play important roles in determining the composition of oral microbial communities.

Hence, bacteria that find themselves neighbors as a result of specific adhesion mechanisms and nutritional requirements also have means by which they can communicate. Different species may be able to effectively talk to each other, but the extent to which this occurs is unknown. Cross-talking between similar organisms clearly may help promote subpopulations or societies of organisms that then have a growth advantage over individual cells. In addition, the killing effects of some signaling molecules will be likely to provide an added advantage to those bacteria that are resistant.

COMMUNICATION WITH HOST CELLS

The epithelial cells that line the gingival crevice provide an important barrier function and physically prevent the ingress of bacteria into the highly vascularized gingival tissues. In addition to this mechanical role, the epithelial cells are capable of sensing and responding to the presence of bacteria and there exists an elaborate communication network between bacterial and host cells. This molecular dialogue conveys information among the bacteria, epithelial cells, and underlying immune and inflammatory cells in the mucosa. The results of this communication have a significant effect on the overall health status of the gingiva. Processes that can be affected by host-bacteria cross-talk range from the production of immune effector molecules such as cytokines to cell life-or-death decisions through both necrotic and apoptotic pathways.

One of the most visible and dramatic outcomes of the intimate association between bacteria and epithelial cells is internalization of the organisms into the host cells. As epithelial cells are not professional phagocytes, the bacteria themselves provide the molecular instructions to allow membrane invaginations of the host cells that accommodate bacterial cell uptake. An intracellular location may benefit bacteria by providing a nutritionally rich environment that is partially sheltered from the ravages of the immune system. The role of intracellular invasion as a virulence factor for enteric pathogens such as *Salmonella* and *Shigella* is well established and is emerging as an important aspect of the pathophysiology of oral organisms such as *P. gingivalis* and *A. actinomycetemcomitans*.

In the case of *P. gingivalis*, invasion is initiated through fimbriae-mediated adhesion to epithelial cell receptors. A series of signal transduction events then occur that lead to reorganization of both actin microfilament and microtubule cytoskeletal components, facilitating subsequent bacterial entry into the cytoplasm (Fig. 6A). Both bacterial and epithelial cells remain viable following internalization, indicating that this is a long-term stable association. The phenotypic results of *P. gingivalis* having seized control of a variety of epithelial cell intracellular pathways have immediate relevance to the disease process. Regulation of matrix metalloproteinase production by gingival epithelial cells is disrupted following contact with the organism, and this interferes with extracellular matrix repair and reorganization. Invasion of *P. gingivalis* also has implications for innate host immunity. Secretion of interleukin-8 by gingival epithelial cells is inhibited following *P. gingivalis* invasion. Inhibition of interleukin-8 accumulation by *P. gingivalis* at sites of bacterial invasion could have a debilitating effect on innate host defense in the periodontium where bacterial exposure is constant. The host would no longer be able to

FIGURE 6 Schematic (not to scale) representation of the interactions between oral bacteria and gingival epithelial cells. (A) *P. gingivalis* cells bind through adhesins such as fimbriae to integrins on gingival cells. FAK and paxillin are recruited, and microtubules and microfilaments are rearranged to facilitate invagination of the membrane that results in the engulfment of bacterial cells. *P. gingivalis* cells rapidly locate in the perinuclear area where they replicate. Calcium ions are released from intracellular stores that may regulate calcium-gated pores in the cytoplasmic membrane. Other signaling molecules such as the mitogen-activated protein (MAP) kinase family can be phosphorylated/dephosphorylated or degraded. Gene expression in the epithelial cells is ultimately affected. Ca, calcium; CM, cytoplasmic membrane; IL-8, interleukin 8; MF, actin microfilaments; MT, tubulin microtubules; NM, nuclear membrane; P, phosphate; solid arrow, pathway with potential intermediate steps; dashed arrow, release; two-headed arrow, reversible association. (B) *A. actinomycetemcomitans* cells bind through adhesins, such as fimbriae and outer membrane proteins, to surface receptors on gingival cells. The epithelial cell membrane ruffles and effaces, and invaginations engulf the bacteria, which then become internalized within a membrane vesicle. Invasion can be actin-dependent, resulting in a focus of actin microfilaments around the bacteria. The bacterial cells destroy the membrane vesicles (possibly by secretion of phospholipase C), releasing bacteria into the cytoplasm where they grow and divide rapidly. Bacteria become localized at membrane protrusions through which they enter adjoining epithelial cells in a microtubule-dependent process. MF, actin microfilaments; MT, tubulin microtubules; dashed arrow, release. (C) *T. denticola* cells do not enter the epithelial cells; however, they secrete a chymotrypsinlike enzyme (open circles) that can degrade junctional complexes (JC) and can be transported into the cell where it disturbs the actin cytoskeleton (MF). A major surface protein of *T. denticola* (ovals) can be translocated into the epithelial cell membrane where it forms a conductance ion channel and depolarizes the membrane. The result is a loss of cell-cell adhesion and substratum detachment, allowing the spirochetes to gain access to the protein-rich gingival tissues.

detect the presence of bacteria and direct leukocytes for their removal. The ensuing overgrowth of bacteria could then contribute to an episodic recurrence of periodontal disease activity.

A. *actinomycetemcomitans* invades epithelial cells by a similar dynamic multistep process. Initial attachment induces effacement of the microvilli and the bacteria enter through ruffled apertures in the cell membrane (Fig. 6B). Internal bacteria are initially constrained within a host-derived membrane vacuole, but this membrane is soon broken down and the bacteria are released into the cytoplasm where they can replicate. What then follows is a remarkable example of bacterial orchestration of host cell function. A. *actinomycetemcomitans* induces the formation of surface

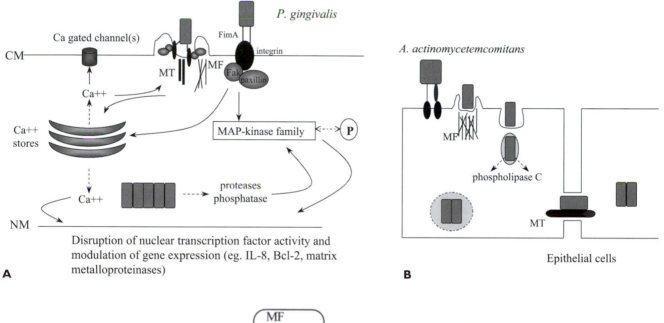

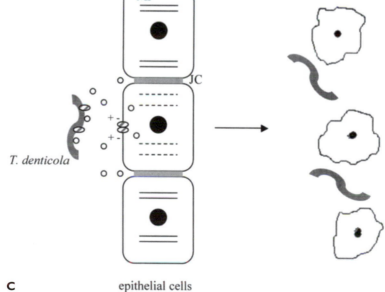

membrane protrusions through which the organism can migrate and enter into adjacent cells. The formation of these protrusions is consequent to bacterial interaction with the plus-ends of microtubules, and movement through them may depend on bacterial cell division. Cell-to-cell spread results in the organisms gaining access deeper in the tissue and may allow the organisms to avoid immune responses targeted to infected cells.

Internalization is not always an outcome of bacterial-host cell cross-talk. For example, the oral spirochete *T. denticola* does not invade live epithelial cells but does induce depolymerization and rearrangement of actin microfilaments along with a loss of cell-cell adhesion and substratum detachment (Fig. 6C). In addition, a spirochetal chymotrypsinlike enzyme can degrade junctional complexes and can be transported into the cell where it disturbs the actin cytoskeleton. A major surface protein of *T. denticola* can also be translocated into the epithelial cell membrane where it forms a conductance ion channel and depolarizes the membrane. In light of this onslaught on normal epithelial cell physiology, it is unsurprising that elevated numbers of treponemes are associated with periodontal disease.

Oral bacteria and host cells can be seen to be involved in an intricate and orchestrated series of interactive events. Both sets of cells maneuver and manipulate each other in order to obtain a physiological advantage. The adaptability of host cells to encroachment by bacteria plays a large part in determining whether the bacteria will be constrained or will evade host innate defenses and cause tissue destruction.

KEY POINTS

Dental plaque that develops on tooth surfaces is a diverse and complex microbial community (biofilm) containing more than 500 species.

Colonization of bacteria is ordered and sequential. Initially plaque is rich in commensals such as streptococci and actinomycetes. Populational shifts ultimately result in higher levels of gram-negative potential periodontal pathogens such as *P. gingivalis*, *A. actinomycetemcomitans*, and *T. denticola*.

Bacterial binding to host surfaces and to other oral bacteria is important in the development of plaque. Lower-affinity attachment occurs through physicochemical forces such as van der Waals, hydrophobic, and electrostatic. Higher-affinity adhesion occurs through complementary adhesin-receptor interactions. These closely fitting molecules can be on the surfaces of bacteria, in the salivary pellicle on the enamel surface, or on the surfaces of host cells. Hence, bacteria can form stable associations with themselves and with the oral hard and soft tissues. The pattern of expression of bacterial and host cell adhesive molecules imparts specificity of adhesion and colonization.

Complexes of bacteria often participate in complementary metabolic interactions that ensure optimal substrate utilization.

Bacteria can also be antagonistic to one another through competition for nutritional substrates and attachment sites and by the production of toxic metabolites and bacteriocins.

Bacteria in close proximity can communicate with one another, resulting in modulation of phenotypic properties and, potentially, coordination of gene expression throughout multispecies communities. One such signaling system is mediated by AI-2, produced through the action of the LuxS enzyme. Gram-positive bacteria also signal through short peptides such as the CSPs and lantibiotics.

Certain oral bacteria such as *P. gingivalis* and *A. actinomycetemcomitans* can manipulate host cell signal transduction pathways and locate intracellularly within epithelial cells. Internalized bacteria are protected from the immune system and can affect host immune status by modulating cytokine expression. Bacteria within host cells may serve as a reservoir of infection. Other organisms such as *T. denticola* utilize secreted bacterial components to interfere with host cell functions without invading the cells.

FURTHER READING

Kuramitsu, H. K., and R. P. Ellen (ed.). 2000. *Oral Bacterial Ecology: the Molecular Basis*. Horizon Scientific Press, Wymondham, United Kingdom.

Lamont, R. J. (ed.). 2004. *Bacterial Invasion of Host Cells*. Cambridge University Press, Cambridge, United Kingdom.

Wilson, M. (ed.). 2002. *Bacterial Adhesion to Host Tissues*. Cambridge University Press, Cambridge, United Kingdom.

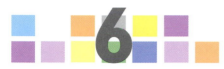

Oral Microbial Physiology

ROBERT E. MARQUIS

OVERVIEW

The physiology of most of the organisms in the oral cavity is geared to their need to adapt to life in crowded conditions and to the stresses associated with existence in biofilms. There are exceptions. For example, surfaces of epithelial cells of the buccal mucosa are only sparsely colonized by oral bacteria. The epithelial surface environment is less competitive in regard to crowding and also more buffered against stresses such as acidification. However, the organisms there have a limited existence because of regular shedding of the mucosa into saliva and then passage of the shed cells, plus their microorganisms, into the gut after swallowing or into the environment after expectoration. In the gut, the environment is hostile with pH values in the stomach as low as 1. Relatively few oral bacteria survive the rigors of the passage and competition with intestinal microbes to emerge viable in the feces.

The majority of oral bacteria are not well equipped to deal with the world outside the mouth. They are specifically adapted oral organisms, that is, they are specialists designed for a specific lifestyle. Bacteria such as *Streptococcus mutans* are prime examples. Not only is *S. mutans* adapted to life in the mouth, it is more narrowly adapted to life only on hard surfaces in the mouth. Prior to eruption of the teeth, it is not usually a permanent member of the oral microbiota. If there is loss of all the teeth and no implant or denture replacement, it vacates the premises. Like other streptococci, *S. mutans* has multiple nutritional dependencies and derives needed nutrients from the host, either from saliva or from the diet. It is multiply auxotrophic, that is, it does not have genes coding for enzymes required for synthesis of many required nutrients, including many amino acids and vitamins. The commonly used, defined, minimal medium for growth of *S. mutans* contains some 42 separate ingredients, plus trace minerals, to meet minimal nutritional needs for growth.

Organisms such as *Treponema denticola* are even more dependent on their host. There is a defined, minimal medium on which *T. denticola* can grow. However, the spirochete requires very specialized growth conditions, including an anaerobic environment. Its physiology is adapted specifically to life in periodontal pockets or along inflamed gingival margins. It appears from sequence analyses of genes for 16S ribosomal RNA in extracts from periodontal plaque that many of the spirochete relatives of *T. denticola* have never been cultivated. Thus, there is currently no medium that provides their required nutrition for in vitro growth, and our knowledge of these other organisms is scant. Of the 500 or more species of bacteria detectable in the mouth by means of modern analyses of 16S rRNA gene sequences in extracted DNA, only a limited number have been cultivated in the laboratory.

There are also transient organisms in the mouth, but unless there is fairly severe physiological upset of the host, they are only temporary colonizers not capable of competing with the specialized organisms of the autochthonous microbiota.

Oral bacteria regularly enter the circulatory system of the human body. Bacteremia occurs as a result of activities such as brushing the teeth, flossing, dental prophylaxis, other dental procedures, or minor daily traumas. The seeding does not generally lead to septicemia (growth of microbes in the bloodstream) but only bacteremia (presence of bacteria in the bloodstream). However, oral bacteria may lodge in specific sites in the body, such as defective heart valves, or may be involved in mixed-organism abscesses. Currently, there are also questions regarding whether oral bacteria can be involved in long-term colonization of the host, for example, in blood vessel walls associated with atherosclerotic plaques (see chapter 16). In all these situations, adaptation of the oral organisms to growth in biofilms associated with surfaces enhances their abilities to colonize the host and evade normal host defenses such as phagocytosis or the complement-antibody-mediated lytic system.

Saliva has a moderately dense microbiota with some 10^6 to 10^8 organisms/ml dependent on how long it has been in the mouth and how much shedding from surfaces has occurred. As indicated above, saliva provides only a very transitory home for microbes. At the other extreme of the spectrum is plaque in protected regions, for example, in pits and fissures or interproximal regions. In these protected sites, the organisms can look forward to long-term coexistence with the host, but life can be tough because of slow inward movement of nutrients and slow outward movement of toxic wastes. In these protected environments, organisms such as *Lactobacillus* bacteria can compete, and because of their high levels of acid tolerance, probably cause major damage to the teeth in pit and fissure caries. Our knowledge of the physiology of plaque bacteria in these protected sites in the mouth is very limited, but fissure caries is important because it currently makes up a major part of the total caries of humans and appears to be less amenable than smooth-surface caries to the anticaries actions of fluoride.

In this chapter, no attempt is made to consider all aspects of the physiology of oral microorganisms. Instead, focus is on specific aspects of physiology considered to be important for oral diseases, which are predominantly infectious diseases.

ACID-BASE PHYSIOLOGY OF ORAL MICROORGANISMS

Acid-Base Cycling in the Mouth

Acid-base physiology of oral bacteria is of particular significance in relation to dental caries. To be cariogenic, a bacterium such as *S. mutans* must be able to colonize plaque, mainly preexisting plaque. *S. mutans* is a secondary colonizer rather than a pioneer. After initial attachment, it must be able to become sufficiently well established in plaque to make up a significant fraction of the total population. Finally, it must be able to function at low pH values. Caries occurs only at acid pH values, below about 5, especially when acidification is prolonged. The range of pH in the mouth is from values somewhat below 4 in plaque in pits or fissures of the teeth or near contact points between teeth to close to 8 in periodontal pockets. The harmful effects of acid to teeth in causing demineralization are well known. There appear also to be harmful effects of alkali in regard to calculus formation and in gingivitis or periodontal diseases. In the latter diseases, a major harmful factor may be specifically ammonia, which can be cytotoxic, rather than just alkaline conditions.

The Range of Acid Tolerance among Oral Bacteria Related to Oral Ecology

The range of acid tolerance among oral bacteria extends from certain strains of *Actinomyces naeslundii* or many periodontal organisms, which cannot function at pH values much below about 6, to *Lactobacillus* organisms able to carry out glycolysis at pH values close to 3. Even within a single genus or species, there can be an ecologically significant range of tolerance. For example, one well-studied strain (NCTC 10904) of *Streptococcus sanguinis* (*S. sanguis*) has low acid tolerance and does not function well at pH values much below 5. In contrast, other strains of *S. sanguis* have sufficient acid tolerance to compete with *S. mutans* at pH values as low as 4 and are considered to be cariogenic organisms. Fungi in general are adapted to function best in acidified environments, and organisms such as *Candida albicans* can survive in the confines of denture plaque, where acids can build up because of poor diffusion into the oral cavity and low local salivary flow.

Periodontal pockets generally have nearly neutral pH or are slightly alkaline, in part because the microbiota is not highly acidogenic and in part because crevicular fluid is buffering. Although some periodontal organisms, including *Fusobacterium nucleatum*, *T. denticola* and others, can degrade sugars to produce acids, many are asaccharolytic and cannot catabolize sugars. Organisms in subgingival plaque catabolize amino acids to produce the ATP they need to grow and function. Oral bacteria have a variety of known pathways for catabolism of amino acids. Our knowledge of specific pathways for periodontal organisms is currently sketchy. Many of the organisms have the arginine deiminase system (ADS) from which ATP can be derived, as depicted in Fig. 1. There is also a variant of the usual arginine deiminase enzyme described for *Porphyromonas gingivalis*. This variant enzyme acts on the N-terminal arginine residues of proteins and peptides to release ammonia and leave a citrulline residue. Other catabolic systems include the Stickland reaction for fermentation of certain amino acids, such as proline or ornithine. *T. denticola* also has the ADS, and in addition, can ferment glycine, alanine, cysteine, and serine. Unfortunately, our knowledge of the overall metabolism of periodontal organisms still has many gaps.

Catabolism of amino acids generally results in a rise in pH. The CO_2 produced diffuses away. The pK_a for the reaction $HCO_3^- + H^+ \rightarrow H_2CO_3$ is about 6.5, and H_2CO_3 readily dissociates into $CO_2 + H_2O$. In contrast, the ammonia produced is generally retained as ammonium

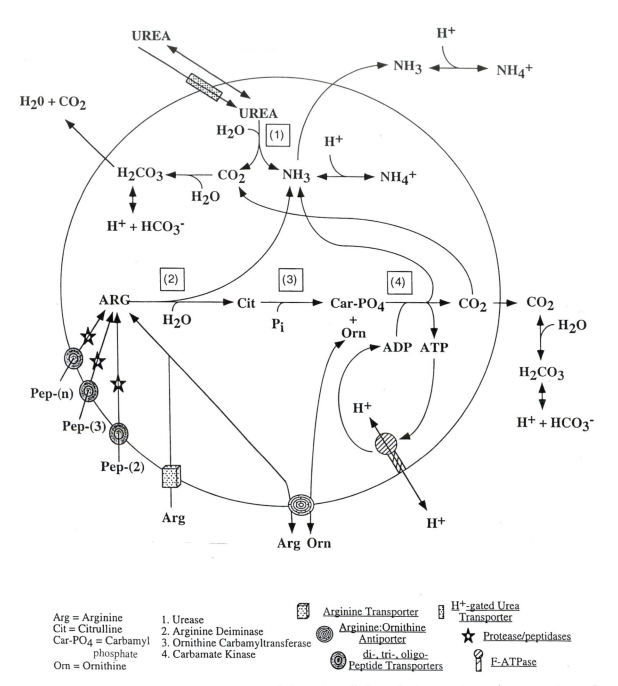

FIGURE 1 Overview of the major alkali-producing reactions of a composite oral streptococcus. (From R. A. Burne and R. E. Marquis, *FEMS Microbiol. Lett.* **193:** 1–6, 2000.)

because the pK_a for the reaction $NH_3 + H^+ \rightarrow NH_4^+$ is about 9.6. Thus, the organisms of subgingival plaque have not had to adapt to compete in acidified environments and generally are not major components of the microbiota of supragingival plaque, although they can be detected regularly in small numbers in supragingival plaque, especially near the contact points of teeth. In general, supragingival plaque is made up mainly of gram-positive, facultative anaerobes, while subgingival plaque is very much enriched for gram-negative anaerobes. A commonly accepted sequence for development of periodontal disease starts with accumulation of supragingival plaque at the gingival margin leading to irritation. Subsequent host responses, involving inflammation, lead to a shift in the microbial population to include anaerobic, gram-negative rods and spirochetes, and finally, development of periodontal pockets and outright disease.

Acid Tolerance Related to Specific Functions

The terms acid tolerance or aciduricity are relative terms—one organism is more or less acid tolerant than another. Highly acid-tolerant bacteria, such as *Thiobacillus* organisms, can function at pH values as low as 0. They are commonly obligate acidophiles not able to function well at pH values close to neutrality. Most of the organisms in the mouth are neutrophiles, that is, they operate best at pH values close to neutrality. However, the more acid-tolerant organisms, especially *Lactobacillus* strains and fungi, function better at lower pH values of 3 to 4, and can be considered moderate acidophiles. Bacteria such as *S. mutans* generally function better at pH values on the acid side at a pH value of about 6, but can carry out glycolysis even at pH values somewhat below 4.

The term acid tolerance is relative in another sense in that it pertains to specific functions. Most of the organisms of the mouth cannot grow at pH values much below about 5 with a few exceptions, such as *Lactobacillus* strains or yeasts. Even *S. mutans* strains do not grow at pH values lower than about 5. The key acid tolerance in relation to virulence and disease is the capacity of a plaque bacterium to carry out glycolysis at low pH values. *S. mutans* can catabolize sugars at pH values close to 4, but it cannot use the ATP produced for growth at this low pH value. Thus, the metabolism of the organism is uncoupled—catabolism is uncoupled from anabolism. The organism continues to carry out glycolysis and to synthesize ATP but then simply degrades it, mainly catalyzed by the F-ATPase of the cell membrane. This breakdown of ATP is not a waste of resources because the F-ATPase excretes protons across the cell membrane in association with ATP hydrolysis. The pumping out of protons prevents severe acidification of the cytoplasm, which would result in inactivation of key enzymes by acid. In fact, most of the glycolytic enzymes are severely inhibited at pH values much below about 6. Thus, the only way the organism can carry out glycolysis in an environment at pH as low as 4 is to maintain a cytoplasmic pH higher than the environmental pH. The difference in pH between the cytoplasm and the environment is termed ΔpH, which may be one full pH unit or even greater when the bacteria are operating in acidified plaque. Clearly, the proton-pumping activity of the F-ATPase is key to acid tolerance and, therefore, to cariogenicity because the cariogenic potential of plaque is highly and inversely correlated with pH value. The damage to tooth mineral is exponentially related to pH drop in plaque. The solubility of tooth mineral in aqueous solutions is exponentially related to the fall in pH in plaque during sugar metabolism. Since the relation is exponential, small reductions of plaque pH can have major effects.

The acidification of plaque by bacteria such as the mutans group streptococci also gives them an advantage over less acid-tolerant organisms. In the extreme, organisms with low acid tolerance can be killed or severely compromised in acidified plaque. Prolonged acidification of plaque favors the more acid-tolerant organisms of the community. However, it should be realized that this growth of these organisms occurs mainly during the more alkaline phases of the plaque pH cycle, above pH values of about 5. Organisms disabled as a result of acid damage are less likely to be able to grow rapidly when plaque pH rises to levels allowing for growth of undamaged organisms.

Constitutive and Adaptive Acid Tolerance

Not only are organisms such as the mutans group streptococci constitutively acid tolerant, but they also can respond to acidification adaptively. In other words, when they grow in acidified media at a pH value of 5, they become even more acid tolerant than when they grow in environments at pH close to neutrality. Constitutive acid tolerance depends on a number of physiologic characteristics of the organism, but the most important is the level of F-ATPase activity. Acid-adapted cells have higher levels of F-ATPase activity and higher capacities to pump protons out of the cytoplasm and reduce internal acidification during glycolysis. Adaptive acid tolerance involves up-regulation of genes not only for F-ATPase but also a variety of other genes, including those responsible for changes in membrane fatty acid composition, for synthesis of chaperonin proteins involved in renaturation and proteolysis of damaged proteins, and for increased activities of DNA or protein repair systems. These changes enhance the capacities of the organisms to produce acid at low pH values and increase their cariogenic potentials. Therefore, continued acid challenge in the mouth associated with activities of the host, such as snacking on hard candies, would serve not only to select for the more acid-tolerant bacteria in plaque, but also would enhance the caries-producing potential of the selected organisms by inducing adaptive increases in acid tolerance.

Newly synthesized F-ATPase units cannot be inserted into old membrane, but need to be incorporated into growing membranes. Therefore, for acid adaptation, new membrane has to be synthesized by the organisms, and full adaptation takes a number of generations. F-ATPases in their fully functional state are actually aggregates of proteins and lipids. The lipids associate mainly with the F_o part of the enzyme, which is embedded in the membrane and contains a pore through which protons move into or out of the cell. The diagram in Fig. 2 shows the basic structure of an F-ATPase. The older name for the enzyme was F_1F_o ATPase. The enzyme is often called the H^+-ATPase to distinguish it from ATPases that function to transport metal cations, rather than H^+, across the cell membrane. The F_1 component sticks out from the membrane into the cytoplasm and can catalyze either hydrolysis or synthesis of ATP. It consists of three α subunits, three β subunits, and single copies of the γ, δ, and ε subunits. The β subunits have the active sites for ATP hydrolysis or synthesis. The F_1 complex when separated from the cell membrane can catalyze hydrolysis of ATP but cannot carry out coupled proton transport. The F_o part of the enzyme in the membrane consists of one a, two b, and usually about 12 c subunits. The enzyme is the major energy-transfer agent in living cells. It is able to transform electrical energy, associated with transmembrane electrical potentials, into mechanical energy involved in enzyme rotation, and then into chemical energy involved in ATP synthesis or hydrolysis. In respiration, protons are excreted across

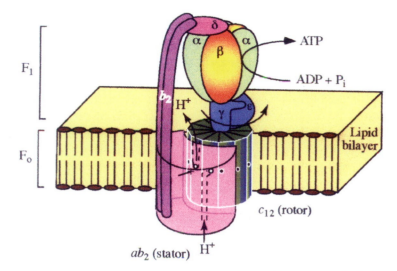

FIGURE 2 Rotary model for F_1F_o ATPase. (From R. H. Fillingame et al., *J. Exp. Biol.* 203:9–17, 2000, with permission.)

the cell membrane by respiratory catalysts to acidify the environment. The protons then move back in across the membrane through the ATPase, and this movement is coupled to ATP synthesis. The movement involves a mechanical process in which the c subunits rotate in relation to a stator made up of ab_2 subunits. The γ and ε subunits spin with the c rotator and translate the spin to the complex of alternating α and β subunits. This movement results in transfer of energy with synthesis of ATP from ADP and P_i. In the oral streptococci, the enzyme functions mainly in the reverse direction. ATP is synthesized at the substrate level, primarily through glycolysis, and can be hydrolyzed by the F-ATPase with concomitant movement of protons out of the cell and maintenance of a cytoplasmic pH higher than the environmental pH.

Acid-tolerance responses are of the global type, that is, many genes are up-regulated and many others are down-regulated in response to growth in acidified environments. Often in stress responses of microorganisms, cells become more resistant not only to the inducing stress, but also to other stresses. A good example here is the stress response of *S. mutans* to acidification, which results in the organism becoming more tolerant not only to acidification but also to oxidative stresses, such as those associated with exposure to peroxides, which are frequently in oral care products. Acid adaptation also leads to increased levels of long-chain and unsaturated fatty acids in the cell membrane and changes in general membrane physiology. Thus, the acid-adaptive response is a complicated response involving global regulators, multiple genes, multiple proteins, and lipids.

Most organisms in plaque undergo stress adaptation, notably to acid but also to other stresses associated with life in crowded conditions. In addition, many plaque bacteria are capable of what is called quorum sensing (see chapter 5). They can sense crowded conditions and respond by up-regulating certain genes and down-regulating others. For oral streptococci, the biofilm state results in enhanced genetic exchange among cells, and this enhancement appears also to be related to quorum sensing and to responses to environmental stress.

Alkali Production and Tolerance

Much of the focus of interest on bacterial metabolism in relation to caries has been on acid production. However, many people feel that alkali production may be important also, but for moderation of caries. In the standard Stephan curve for changes in plaque pH after a sugar challenge, there is generally a rapid pH drop followed by a slow rise back to the original pH for resting or fasting plaque or even to somewhat higher values (Fig. 3). The rise in pH is thought to involve multiple factors, including the washing action of saliva, buffering by salivary bicarbonate, and alkali production by plaque bacteria. The washing effect may be moderated because of the slow, diffusion-controlled movement of acids out of plaque. In addition, bicarbonate in saliva is not a very good buffer for plaque, again because of diffusion problems. However, plaque itself has high buffering capacity, mainly because of the high concentration of bacteria embedded in the plaque matrix. The bacteria are buffering against acid drop because of their content of phosphate ($pK_a = 6.5$) and of side chain carboxyl groups such as those of aspartyl or glutamyl residues ($pK_a = 4.5$). A significant part of the pH rise is considered to be due to production of ammonia from arginine via the ADS (Fig. 1) and from urea through the action of urease. Prominent ADS-positive bacteria include *Streptococcus gordonii, S. sanguis, Streptococcus rattus, Streptococcus anginosus, A. naeslundii, Lactobacillus fermentum, P. gingivalis,* and *T. denticola.*

The major urease-positive bacteria in supragingival plaque are the actinomycetes and organisms such as *Haemophilus parainfluenzae.* However, other oral bacteria not so prominent in plaque, such as *Streptococcus salivarius* and *Streptococcus vestibularis,* are also urease-positive and

FIGURE 3 Representative pH changes in plaque following ingestion of a carbohydrate source. Time periods involving demineralization of enamel by low pH and subsequent remineralization as the pH rises are indicated. Note that in addition to a more acidic resting pH, plaque from caries-susceptible individuals drops to a lower pH value and has a slower recovery time compared to plaque from caries-resistant individuals. Adaptation of Stephan curve provided by Ann Griswold, University of Florida.

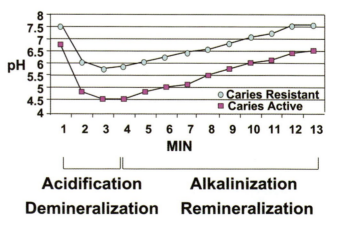

may degrade urea in saliva rather than in plaque. Saliva contains high levels of urea, from 3 to 10 mM, approximately the same as those in serum. Arginine is present as the free amino acid at average levels of only about 50 μM in saliva. However, the major source of arginine for oral bacteria is considered to be in peptides and proteins, which can be degraded by proteases and peptidases of saliva and those secreted by oral bacteria. Many oral bacteria have multiple transport systems for uptake of peptides from proteolysis, including those as large as octapeptides.

Acid-Base Physiology, Virulence, and Disease

The main reactions involved in ammonia production by oral bacteria are shown in Fig. 1. There are other reactions that can release ammonia in plaque, including reduction of proline or ornithine to 5-aminovalerate via Stickland reactions and reactions catalyzed by deaminases. However, urease and ADS are considered the main agents for ammonia release. Base production and the associated pH rise are considered to be beneficial in supragingival plaque in relation to dental caries. Base production in plaque is considered to have beneficial ecological effects in favoring the survival of less acid-tolerant organisms in the oral microbiota. The effect then would be to lower the cariogenic potential of plaque.

Alkali production can also have negative influences on oral health. It is thought to enhance production of calculus or tartar because of enhanced precipitation of calcium salts at higher pH values. Ammonia may also be damaging in gingivitis and periodontal disease, but more information is needed to have a better view of the damaging actions.

OXYGEN METABOLISM, OXIDATIVE STRESS, AND ADAPTATION

Sources of Oxygen for Oral Bacteria

There are two main sources of O_2 for oral bacteria. The one is the gas atmosphere in the mouth, which is basically air with periodic depletion of O_2 and enrichment in CO_2 as a result of respiratory exchange. The gases in the mouth are important for the physiology of supragingival plaque and of the organisms on the soft tissues of the mouth, including the tongue, which is a major site for microbial growth and metabolism. Saliva can be a direct source of O_2 because of oxygen it contains when secreted, or an indirect source because it transfers O_2 from the gas phase in the mouth to tissues and biofilms it bathes. The other source of O_2 for the mouth is crevicular fluid. This fluid has approximately serum levels of O_2 (1.3 ppm of O_2, 0.04 μmol of O_2/ml, or an average P_{O2} of about 30 mm Hg, values similar to those for venous blood) and supplies oxygen to subgingival plaque. The presence of subgingival plaque during the development of periodontal disease is a stimulus for enhanced flow of crevicular fluid as the host attempts to respond to inflammatory products of bacteria and to rid itself of invaders. Host-produced inflammatory molecules also play important roles in enhancing crevicular fluid flow. The situation in gingivitis is intermediate with some inflammation and fluid flow but also some access to the gas in the mouth.

Oxygen Levels and Oxidation-Reduction Potentials in Dental Plaque

Mature dental plaque is often considered to be highly anaerobic because of its dense biomass. However, plaque is actually a thin film with a large surface-to-volume ratio so that O_2 can diffuse readily into it. Electrode measurements of O_2 levels in periodontal pockets indicate P_{O2} at some 10% of the value for air-saturated water, or an average partial pressure of 13.3 mm Hg. Thus, even subgingival plaque is not highly anaerobic. Measurements have been made also of oxidation-reduction potentials (E_h) of supragingival plaque as it develops on the teeth. As shown in Fig. 4, the E_h value drops as plaque ages but not to a very low value indicative of highly anaerobic conditions. E_h is a measure of oxidation or reduction state, somewhat analogous to pH as a measure of acid or base state. The pH value indicates the activity of protons in the system under study, whereas E_h indicates the potential in the system for electrons to be transferred, that is, the potential for oxidation or reduction. Figure 4 shows what are called E_0' values for biologically important oxidation-reduction couples. These values are similar to pK values for acids and bases, only they indicate the E_h value at which the concentration of the oxidized form is equal to that of the reduced form. Thus, for the lactate/pyruvate couple, the E_0' is the E_h value at which the lactate and pyruvate concentrations are equal. Positive values for E_0' indicate an oxidizing couple, for example, the O_2/H_2O couple ($E_0' = +818$ mV), whereas negative values indicate more reducing couples, for example, the NAD/NADH couple ($E_0' = -320$ mV). In cells, NADH can serve to transfer electrons to O_2, that is, NADH can serve to reduce O_2. This reduction may involve cytochromes and an electron transport system coupled to oxidative phosphorylation. For many oral bacteria, including the oral streptococci, respiration involves mainly NADH oxidases, which are flavin enzymes able to catalyze transfer of reducing equivalents from NADH through sulfenic acid and flavin to O_2 to produce either H_2O_2 or H_2O. Flavin enzymes typically transfer single electrons, and so there is a propensity for formation of superoxide radicals ($O_2^{\cdot-}$) during catalysis.

FIGURE 4 E_h drop in developing supragingival plaque and E_0' values for some of the oxidation-reduction couples pertinent to plaque.

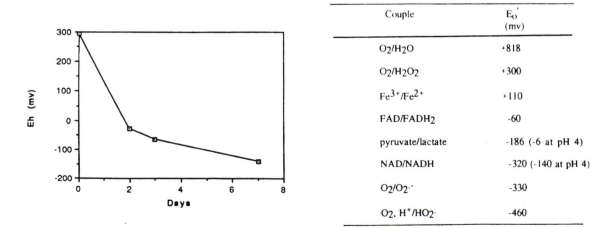

Couple	E_0' (mv)
O_2/H_2O	+818
O_2/H_2O_2	+300
Fe^{3+}/Fe^{2+}	+110
$FAD/FADH_2$	-60
pyruvate/lactate	-186 (-6 at pH 4)
NAD/NADH	-320 (-140 at pH 4)
$O_2/O_2^{\cdot-}$	-330
$\cdot O_2, H^+/HO_2^{\cdot}$	-460

Even in mature plaque, the E_h value falls only to about -100 mV, close to the E_0' value for the pyruvate/lactate couple. Highly anaerobic systems have E_h values in the range of -400 to -500 mV. Thus, plaque is a reducing system overall, but not highly reducing. However, it should be realized that the plaque biofilm is stratified. The general finding is that the outer strata are more aerobic and the deeper strata more anaerobic. Thus, E_h in plaque would be expected to decrease with depth away from the saliva-plaque interface or the boundary between plaque and crevicular fluid.

Another oral malady associated with the development of an environment conducive to growth and metabolism of anaerobic bacteria is halitosis or oral malodor. It is associated particularly with conditions such as gingivitis and periodontitis. Malodor can occur without these inflammatory states but is related to metabolism of the tongue microbiota. Malodor is due mainly to putrefactive actions of bacteria on endogenous or exogenous proteins and peptides. The major offending compounds are hydrogen sulfide (H_2S), methyl mercaptan (CH_3SH), and to a lesser extent, dimethylmercaptan (CH_3SSCH_3). These sulfides are produced mainly from cysteine, cystine, and methionine by enzymes such as L-cysteine desulfhydrase, which catalyzes cysteine hydrolysis with production of H_2S, ammonia, and pyruvate. The enzyme is produced by gram-positive bacteria, such as *S. anginosus*, or by *F. nucleatum*, which is commonly associated with gingivitis. *T. denticola* and other gram-negative anaerobes prominent in periodontal disease also produce the enzyme. In addition, compounds such as indol and skatol may contribute to malodor. Currently, there are no good inhibitors of sulfide production for use in the mouth. Control measures, such as brushing of the tongue, are mainly oriented to general plaque reduction. However, there is need for effective antimicrobials against malodor organisms to extend the time between mechanical removal of organisms and regrowth.

Oxygen Metabolism in Oral Bacteria, Reactive Oxygen Species, and Oxidative Damage

In a biological system such as dental plaque, the residual O_2 is not the biologically most important O_2 other than serving as an indicator that not all of the incoming O_2 is metabolized. The important O_2 is that which is metabolized by the cells. This respiratory metabolism is of importance in transferring energy for the various functions of oral microbes. Respiration involving O_2 as a terminal electron acceptor and that involving alternative acceptors such as nitrate, fumarate, and sulfide can occur in the mouth. Estimates of O_2 flow into plaque with a 1-cm^2 surface area and 0.1-cm thickness are about 15 μmol of O_2/ml/min. This flux can be compared with measured respiratory capacities of 2 to 5 μmol of O_2/ml of wet cells/min for organisms such as *S. mutans*. Anaerobes in plaque also are able to respire. In fact, if anaerobes did not metabolize O_2, they would not likely be anaerobes. It is mainly when O_2 is metabolized that it becomes toxic through production of reactive oxygen species (ROS), such as hydrogen peroxide (H_2O_2), superoxide radical, perhydroxyl radical (HO_2·), and hydroxyl radical (HO·), which are capable of causing oxidative damage. The indicated ROS can be produced directly during oxygen metabolism except for hydroxyl radical, which is thought to be produced mainly through the Fenton reactions indicated below involving hydrogen peroxide and reduced transition metal cations, mainly Fe^{2+} and Cu^+ in biological systems. As shown in reaction 1, the oxidized forms of the metal cations can be reduced through reaction with superoxide radical. Then, the reduced cations react with H_2O_2 produced by metabolism or added from outside the mouth to yield hydroxyl anion and hydroxyl radical.

$$O_2^{\cdot -} + Fe^{3+} \rightarrow O_2 + Fe^{2+} \tag{1}$$

$$Fe^{2+} + H_2O_2 \rightarrow Fe^{3+} + OH^- + OH^{\cdot} \tag{2}$$

The example here is with iron cations, but copper cations in biological systems are also involved commonly. Nickel and cobalt cations are generally at low levels in biological systems, but they also can take part in Fenton reactions. $OH^{\cdot}$ is considered to be one of the most damaging radicals produced as a result of O_2 metabolism. To avoid having it formed in significant amounts, most cells, especially those of organisms able to grow aerobically, produce catalases and peroxidases to catalyze degradation of H_2O_2 and superoxide dismutases to catalyze removal of the superoxide radical. In addition, levels of free transition-metal cations are highly regulated by means of various binding proteins so that free Fe and Cu cations do not occur in the cytoplasm. Nitrogen-based radicals, such as peroxynitric acid (HOONO), or organic radicals can also be produced secondarily through reactions involving ROS. They also can be major agents of oxidative damage.

By definition, anaerobes cannot grow in the presence of air in which O_2 is present at a level of 0.21 atm (ca. 160 mm Hg) because they metabolize the gas at a level that overwhelms their limited defense mechanisms against ROS stress. While anaerobes generally have protective enzymes and other mechanisms against oxidative damage, the problem is that they do not have sufficient protection to allow for growth or survival in the presence of the 0.21 atm of O_2 in air. There are also microaerophilic organisms in plaque. They require O_2 for growth but cannot manage the stress of the full 0.21 atm of O_2 in air.

Plaque appears to be stratified in regard to aerobic and anaerobic organisms. There are very few, if any, strict aerobes in plaque. Most of the oral organisms able to grow aerobically are actually facultative anaerobes. The main possible exceptions are the neisseriae, although even they can carry out functions such as glycolysis under conditions of restricted oxygen supply. Most of the organisms in supragingival plaque are facultatively anaerobic, including oral streptococci, most *Actinomyces* and related organisms, *Haemophilus*, *Actinobacillus*, etc. Strictly anaerobic bacteria can routinely be isolated from supragingival plaque, including *Veillonella* organisms, which have a close nutritional relationship with lactate-producing organisms because lactate is their major catabolite. Gram-negative anaerobes can also be isolated, especially in interproximal areas and deep plaque, presumably in part because of restricted access to O_2 in these areas. In addition, facultative anaerobes can protect strict anaerobes against damage by ROS. For example, many facultative organisms produce catalases, which are highly effective in degrading H_2O_2. Catalase-positive bacteria can protect catalase-negative bacteria against

H_2O_2 damage. Still, in supragingival plaque the gram-negative anaerobes are generally only a minority population.

In subgingival plaque, anaerobes flourish. They include organisms of the genera *Porphyromonas*, *Prevotella*, and *Fusobacterium*, many *Actinomyces* organisms, and a variety of oral spirochetes. It was once thought that oral anaerobes such as *T. denticola* were among the most extremely anaerobic organisms. However, the results of more recent work with improved culturing methods suggest that they actually are not all that extreme. Although they cannot grow when cultures are aerated, they can grow in complex media in static cultures under an atmosphere of air. They do have protective mechanisms against oxidative damage, including enzymes such as superoxide dismutase. Moreover, in mixed cultures they can be protected against peroxide damage by other bacteria capable of rapidly degrading peroxides.

In the mouth, there are relatively high levels of thiocyanate (SCN^-), which can react with H_2O_2 in reactions catalyzed by peroxidases to produce hypothiocyanite ($OSCN^-$). Hypothiocyanite can be highly damaging for oral bacteria, and the thiocyanate-H_2O_2-peroxidase system is considered to be a major defense against infection. There are questions about which is more toxic—hypothiocyanite or hydrogen peroxide. Conceivably, production of hypothiocyanite by peroxidases could be protective for bacteria because it reduces the level of H_2O_2. Moreover, many oral bacteria produce the protective enzyme hypothiocyanite reductase (Table 1).

In environments where halogens are in greater supply than thiocyanate, peroxidases can couple peroxide degradation to form compounds such as hypochlorite or hypoiodite. These compounds are toxic to microorganisms, and their formation is part of the innate immune response of the host. As mentioned above, nitric oxide (NO) produced by phagocytes and other host cells from arginine can induce oxidative damage. It can also react with superoxide radical to produce toxic HOONO, which can be lethal for bacterial cells. HOONO is a weak acid with a pK_a value of 6.8. It can move readily across membranes in the protonated state and then dissociate in the relatively alkaline cytoplasm to yield H^+ and $OONO^-$.

ROS and other highly reactive radicals can react with lipids, nucleic acids, and proteins to yield a variety of damaged products. Lipid peroxidation is important in damage to eukaryotic organisms and involves peroxidation of polyunsaturated fatty acids with possible formation of secondary lipid radicals. Bacteria generally do not produce polyunsaturated fatty acids, with only a few exceptions, for example, certain deep-sea bacteria. Therefore, damage to lipids is not likely to be major for oral bacteria. However, damage to proteins and to nucleic acids does occur. In fact, ROS can be mutagenic as a result of damage to DNA, which the cell then attempts to repair by means of multiple repair systems, many of which are error-prone and introduce genetic changes. Many sites in nucleic acids are sensitive to oxidative damage with many products, including those resulting from double-strand breaks. Oxygen metabolism presents a mutagenic challenge to organisms and is a major force for variation leading to evolution and biodiversity.

Damage to enzymes and other proteins has also been well documented. For example, the glycolytic enzyme glyceraldehyde-3-phosphate dehydrogenase is highly sensitive to H_2O_2, and damage is enhanced by the presence of reduced transition-metal cations. The enzymes or proteins usually most sensitive to oxidative damage are those to which transition-metal cations can bind and those with disulfide bonds, especially in the form of Fe-S clusters. Many amino acid residues can be damaged by ROS, and so the products of damage are multiple. However, the range of sensitivity to damage among proteins is wide with high sensitivity, say, among dehydratase enzymes, related particularly to their metal-binding sites, which often involve iron-sulfur clusters.

Repair Systems

There may be questions about just how important oxidative stress and damage are in a system such as dental plaque. The physiology of plaque bacteria tells us clearly how important they are. Oral microbes possess an impressive array of defense systems against oxidative damage. They would not have multiple systems for protection if oxidative stress were not a part of day-to-day life, either because of their own oxidative metabolism or a need to neutralize oxidative products secreted by their neighbors or produced by the host. Moreover, as indicated earlier, oral bacteria are generally specifically adapted to life in the mouth and do not have much of a life outside of the mouth. Therefore, their protective mechanisms against oxidative stress are indicative of stress conditions in the mouth.

Table 1 presents examples of some of the protective systems of oral bacteria against oxidative damage. Basically, there are two prominent modes of protection, either getting rid of the damaging species by reduction or dismutation and repairing the damage after it has already been done. There are other possible protective strategies, one of which is just not to metabolize O_2. As discussed earlier, this avoidance does not seem

TABLE 1 Examples of enzymes and proteins of oral bacteria protective against oxidative damage[a]

Enzyme or protein	Protective reaction or function
Catalases	$2H_2O_2 \rightarrow 2H_2O_2 + O_2$
Mn-peroxidase	$2Mn^{2+} + H_2O_2 \rightarrow 2Mn^{3+} + H_2O + 0.5O_2$
NADH peroxidases	$NADH + H^+ + H_2O_2 \rightarrow NAD + 2H_2O$
Alkyl hydroperoxidases	$NADH + H^+ + ROOH \rightarrow NAD^+ + H_2O + ROH$
Superoxide dismutases	$2O_2^{\cdot-} + 2H^+ \rightarrow H_2O_2 + O_2$
Hypothiocyanite reductase	$NADPH + H^+ + OSCN^- \rightarrow NAD^+ + H_2O + SCN^-$
Peroxynitrite reductase (AhpC)	$HOONO + NADH \rightarrow NO_2^- + H_2O$
Glutathione reductase	$NADPH + H^+ + GSSG \rightarrow NADP^+ + 2GSH$[b]
Disulfide reductase	$NADPH + H^+ + protein (S-S) \rightarrow NADP^+ protein(SH)_2$
Iron-binding proteins, such as Dpr protein	Bind iron cations
Copper-binding proteins	Bind copper cations
Endonuclease IV, exonuclease III	Apurinic/apyrimidinic endonucleases
Endonuclease III	Removes thymine glycols
Excision nuclease	Excision of damaged DNA
DNA polymerase	DNA synthesis after excision
Glucose-6-P-dehydrogenase	Production of NADPH
SoxRS, OxyR, RpoS, RecA	Regulators of oxidative stress genes

[a]From R. E. Marquis, *Sci. Prog.* **87:**153–177, 2004.

[b]GSH, glutathione (glutamyl-cysteinyl-glycine); GSSG, oxidized glutathione.

to be a common strategy. Another is to develop metabolic pathways that do not result in production of ROS. The usual sort of cytochrome aa_3 oxidase is a good example. It catalyzes a 4-electron reduction of O_2 with little or no production of ROS. In contrast, many flavin-based enzymes carry out 1-electron reductions of O_2 and are prone to produce superoxide radicals. When the metabolic systems are under stress or when compounds such as the herbicide paraquat are present, normal electron transport can be disrupted and the production of ROS increased. Many oral bacteria produce H_2O_2, for example, as a result of NADH oxidase action. Then the H_2O_2 can react with reduced transition-metal cations to yield the highly toxic hydroxyl radical. Oral bacteria may also produce NADH oxidases that yield water instead of hydrogen peroxide, and these enzymes are considered protective against peroxide damage.

PHYSIOLOGY OF ORAL BIOFILMS

As mentioned previously and discussed in chapters 3 and 5, the microorganisms of the mouth exist generally in closely knit communities. They adhere to pellicle on tooth surfaces, to cells of soft tissues, especially on the dorsum of the tongue, or in the gingival crevice, which in periodontal disease may be enlarged to form pockets filled with aggregates and biofilms of oral microbes. The most common surfaces in the mouth for adherence are those of other microbial cells. Bacteria stick to each other by means of a wide variety of mechanisms. It is key to our understanding of the workings of oral microbes and of their roles in health and disease that we understand better the nature and workings of biofilms associated with oral surfaces. The study of biofilms is not new, but it has become more popular during the last decade or so. Oral microbiology has been a leader in this field because of many decades of research on dental plaque, much of it before the term biofilm was widely used to describe dental plaque.

Physicochemical Gradients in Oral Biofilms and Concentrative Capacities of Biofilms for Fluoride and Other Antimicrobials

Entry and exit of solutes into and out of plaque biofilms tend to be diffusion limited, especially for larger solutes. Very large solutes, such as biopolymers from the environment, are generally excluded from biofilms. Slow diffusion can limit metabolism in biofilms by restricting supplies of nutrients and allowing buildup of inhibitory products such as lactic acid. However, it appears from analysis of biofilms by confocal microscopy using fluorescent beads that there are abundant water channels penetrating deep into biofilms. These channels increase the surface-to-volume ratio of biofilms and enhance diffusion. However, water channels do not appear to be quite as prominent in plaque as in biofilms of organisms such as *Pseudomonas aeruginosa*. Nutrients coming into plaque from saliva or crevicular fluids are at their greatest concentrations at the biofilm surface exposed to the environment. Nutrient levels then decrease with depth in the biofilms as the nutrients are metabolized initially by surface organisms. Products of metabolism by more superficial organisms may then diffuse out of plaque but also into the depth of plaque, where metabolism is thought to be of a more anaerobic nature. Thus, damaging molecules such as organic acids can move into deep plaque to affect the tooth. In caries development, dissolution of tooth enamel generally initiates below, rather than at, the tooth surface, probably because pellicle can act as a buffer, as well as a modulator of solute movement into and out of the tooth. The mineral ions released through acid dissolution of tooth structure also tend to be concentrated deeper in the plaque biofilm and diffuse only slowly to the surface. In general, salivary influences are separated from the tooth surface by the plaque biofilm but also by pellicle. The dynamics of solute movements through biofilms clearly are of major importance in terms of oral disease. The picture of biofilm or aggregate dynamics in relation to gingivitis and periodontal disease has not been well developed, and we are still very short on knowledge, although it has been found that multiple nutritional interactions occur among microbes in subgingival plaque.

Biofilms are noted for being resistant to a variety of antimicrobials. It appears that there are multiple mechanisms for their resistance. Some types of resistance, for example, to higher-molecular-weight antibiotics, appear to depend on diffusion barriers in the biofilms. Other types of resistance can depend simply on the high biomass concentration within the biofilms, especially for many disinfectants for which cells have many binding sites not involved in the damage done to the cell by the agent. Typically, the potency of these agents is very biomass dependent with potency inversely related to biomass concentration. Still other types of resistance depend on the physiology of the biofilm organisms. For example, biofilm cells tend to be resistant to β-lactam antibiotics simply because they are growing so slowly, and β-lactams target peptidoglycan synthesis by growing cells. Moreover, biofilms have microenvironments in which microbes are in nongrowing or stationary-phase states, which generally lead to enhanced levels of protective resistance against environmental stresses, including those caused by antimicrobials. Growth in biofilms is thought to occur predominantly in peripheral regions where nutrient levels are highest. Thus, there is heterogeneity within the population that can affect overall sensitivity to antimicrobials and can also result in high levels of persistor organisms not greatly damaged by the agents. However, long-term exposure of plaque to agents such as fluoride has not resulted in development of a resistant microbiota, probably because of the constant fluctuations and turnover of organisms in the mouth.

Biofilms also have a tendency to concentrate many chemicals. This concentrative action can be of advantage to biofilm organisms especially in the early stages of biofilm formation because nutrients are concentrated in the developing film, mainly through adsorption. However, these concentrative effects can also be negative, for example, in terms of concentration of heavy-metal ions in biofilms. A concentrative action of oral biofilms significant in relation to disease is that of fluoride, which is concentrated in dental plaque to levels some 100 times those in saliva. It appears that the concentration of fluoride is mainly related to its weak-acid character (pK_a = ca. 3.15). Fluoride moves into bacterial cells in relation to ΔpH across the cell membrane with the cytoplasm alkaline relative to the environment. In the relatively acidified environment outside of a cell, fluoride becomes protonated to yield HF. The cell membrane is highly permeable to HF, some 10^7 times more permeable than it is to F^-. Therefore, HF moves readily into the cell where the pH value is higher than that of the environment. Once in the relatively alkaline cytoplasm, HF dissociates to yield F^-, which may act as an enzyme poison, but also H^+, which acts to acidify the cytoplasm. Cytoplasmic acidification is inhibitory for many cytoplasmic enzymes, including those of glycolysis. As long as there is ATP in the cell, and the F-ATPase can function to move protons back out of the cell, some level of ΔpH across the membrane will be maintained, and fluoride will remain concentrated within bacterial cells. Thus, fluoride acts to thwart the action of the F-ATPase in moving protons out of the cell by bringing extruded protons back across the membrane with HF acting as a carrier. This return of protons to the cytoplasm reduces the acid tolerance of the cell and, presumably, also the cariogenicity of organisms such as S. mutans. Other weak acids also are concentrated by dental plaque biofilms including food preservative weak acids, such as benzoate and sorbate, and weak-acid, nonsteroidal, anti-inflammatory agents, such as ibuprofen or indomethacin.

Fluoride may under certain conditions precipitate on plaque as calcium fluoride. This type of concentration is relatively short term but is considered important for increasing the levels of fluoride associated with plaque.

Plaque Nutrition Related to Biofilm Physiology

As mentioned, many nutritional interactions occur in plaque biofilms. A well-known example is production of lactic acid by oral streptococci and its subsequent use as a major catabolite by Veillonella organisms. Another major example involves hydrolysis by certain oral streptococci and Actinomyces organisms of salivary glycoproteins with release of sugars, which can then be used by pathogenic organisms such as S. mutans for catabolism and acid production. In subgingival plaque, cross-feeding interactions involving oral spirochetes and P. gingivalis have been well demonstrated. In addition to the cooperative interactions, many interactions in plaque are antagonistic. For example, organisms such as S. sanguis are able to produce H_2O_2 and can be antagonistic to nonproducers such as S. mutans, which generally are more peroxide sensitive. It appears also that production of bacteriocins such as the lantibiotic, mutacin, can result in damage to nonproducing organisms. A very important point when considering the physiology of oral biofilms is that a biofilm truly is an integrated community. Its physiology and, therefore, its capacities to cause disease or to protect against disease are related to the entire community and not just to one of the members. This community view can be important in terms of strategies to control oral infectious diseases and highlights the roles for the so-called good oral microbes in maintaining oral health.

KEY POINTS

A variety of challenging conditions are faced by the oral microbiota—from the need for the capacity to catabolize a wide variety of substrates in saliva and the diet, to tolerance of major fluctuations in environmental conditions that place considerable stress on the populations.

The pH of the mouth fluctuates often and to a great extent. Oral bacteria have multiple physiologic and genetic mechanisms to cope with sudden drops in pH and in sustained acidification, which favor the growth of aciduric, cariogenic plaque bacteria.

Pumping protons to maintain a cytoplasmic pH that is neutral relative to the outside, production of ammonia, for example, by arginine deiminase, and adaptive acid tolerance are critical factors in low pH tolerance.

A primary mechanism of action of fluoride is to dissipate the proton gradient ($pH_{out} < pH_{in}$) by carrying protons into the cell as HF at low plaque pH values.

Oxygen itself is not particularly toxic for bacteria. Instead, it is the single electron reductions of oxygen by the oxidative enzymes of bacteria that generate ROS that can damage lipids, proteins, and DNA. Anaerobes cannot tolerate oxygen because they either have very low levels of, or lack, the enzymes needed to detoxify ROS.

Growth of oral bacteria in biofilms, which have an ordered three-dimensional structure that creates gradients of nutrients, end products, and stressors, fosters biodiversity and allows complex, degradative communities of bacteria to persist in the mouth. Growth in biofilms offers bacteria considerable protection from host immune and nonimmune defenses and from antimicrobial agents.

FURTHER READING

Doyle, R. J. (ed.). 1999. *Methods in Enzymology,* vol. 310. Academic Press, San Diego, Calif.

Doyle, R. J. (ed.). 2001. *Methods in Enzymology,* vol. 336. Academic Press, San Diego, Calif.

Doyle, R. J. (ed.). 2001. *Methods in Enzymology,* vol. 337. Academic Press, San Diego, Calif.

Marquis, R. E. 2004. Applied and ecological aspects of oxidative-stress damage to bacterial spores and to oral microbes. *Sci. Prog.* **87:**153–177.

Marsh, P., and M. V. Marshall. 1999. *Oral Microbiology.* Butterworth-Heinemann, Oxford, United Kingdom.

Slots, J., and T. E. Rams. 1992. Microbiology of periodontal diseases, p. 425–443. *In* J. Slots and M. A. Taubman (ed.), *Contemporary Oral Microbiology and Immunology.* Mosby-Year Book, St. Louis, Mo.

Tanzer, J. 1992. Microbiology of dental caries, p. 377–424. *In* J. Slots and M. A. Taubman (ed.), *Contemporary Oral Microbiology and Immunology.* Mosby-Year Book, St. Louis, Mo.

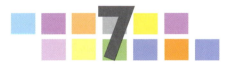

Genetics and Molecular Biology of Oral Microorganisms

SUSAN KINDER HAAKE AND DONALD J. LEBLANC

INTRODUCTION

The genetics of oral microorganisms as an area of study, relative to the broader field of microbial genetics, is still very much in its infancy. With the exception of reports in the early 1960s on the development by some strains of oral streptococcal species of natural competence for transformation, genetic analysis of the oral microbiota only began in earnest in 1973 with the first report of the presence of plasmid DNA in a strain of *Streptococcus mutans*. This was followed, throughout the remainder of the decade and into the 1980s, by a flurry of papers on the exchange of genetic information between oral streptococcal species, on the isolation and characterization of naturally occurring plasmids from them, on the development of molecular tools based on such plasmids, and on the application of those tools to studies of oral streptococcal traits. By the late 1980s, reports began to emerge that described the results of genetic and/or molecular analyses of such oral microorganisms as *Actinomyces* spp., *Actinobacillus actinomycetemcomitans*, and *Porphyromonas gingivalis*. Then, as we entered the 1990s, such studies were being extended to strains of *Treponema denticola*, soon followed by genetic and molecular analyses of *Fusobacterium nucleatum* and *Prevotella intermedia* strains. Many of these studies, and the impact that they have had or are expected to have on our understanding of the oral microbiota, are described in this chapter and chapter 8.

It is assumed that the reader has at least a basic understanding of the fundamentals of genetics. Some terms, as they apply specifically to microorganisms, and more specifically to bacteria, are defined below. For a more thorough review of microbial genetics and molecular biology, the reader is referred to chapters 14 through 20 in J. W. Lengeler et al. (ed.), *Biology of the Prokaryotes* (Blackwell Science, Malden, Mass., 1999). The term microbial genetics refers to studies of the processes by which all the qualities of a microbial species are transmitted from one generation to another by mechanisms associated with DNA replication and with the expression of the information contained in that DNA. The genotype of a microbial strain is the total complement of genetic information that is carried by that strain on the chromosomal, plasmid, or viral DNA molecules that comprise its total genome. The phenotype of a strain refers to those characteristics encoded by the genome that are actually expressed at any one time, and under a particular set of environmental conditions, as observable or measurable traits. The genetic information of bacteria is organized in operons, which are contiguous segments of DNA that encode single mRNA molecules containing one or more structural genes and a single set of regulatory elements that coordinate the expression of all the genes within an operon. A structural gene is a segment of DNA, also referred to as an open reading frame, that encodes a protein, and the segment of an mRNA transcript from which the protein will be translated is referred to as a cistron. Thus, an operon may yield a monocistronic or polycistronic mRNA. The expression of structural genes within an operon is governed by regulatory elements that may be *cis*-acting nucleotide base sequences in the DNA or RNA, or *trans*-acting molecules such as proteins. The more common regulatory elements that may be associated with operon expression include a promoter, or region of DNA at which RNA polymerase binds and initiates transcription, and a sigma factor, which is a subunit of RNA polymerase that ensures proper recognition of a specific promoter sequence. An operator is the region of DNA at the 5′ end of an operon at which either a repressor that inhibits transcription (negative control) or an activator, which potentiates transcription (positive control), binds for control of operon expression. An operon inducer may be a molecule or environmental condition that serves to remove a repressor from an operator to allow transcription, or converts a repressor to an activator of transcription. Groups of operons, some of which are induced while others are repressed by the same environmental stimuli, are referred to as regulons. Operons that are part of the same regulon need not be adjacent to each other on the chromosome, and the expression of an operon may be influenced through more than one regulon. Progress toward a more comprehensive understanding of the genetics of microorganisms, as well as correlations between genotypes and phenotypes under a variety of environmental conditions, has been accelerated by the development of recombinant DNA technology and the publication of the nucleotide base sequences of an ever increasing number of bacterial genomes. The application of these technologies and advances to studies of the oral microbiota is the topic of this chapter and chapter 8.

GENOMES AND GENETIC TRANSFER IN NATURE

Analyses of the genomic DNA sequences of oral microorganisms (Table 1) provide important information for investigation of microbial taxonomy, metabolism, and virulence mechanisms. Comparative sequence analyses of microbial genomes led to recognition of the tremendous diversity in genetic composition among species and the importance of horizontal gene transfer in the evolution of microorganisms. For example, sequence analyses of enteric bacteria indicate that they harbor substantial amounts of foreign DNA and that the newly acquired DNA is central to bacterial diversity and pathogenesis. Mechanisms of horizontal gene transfer are also of interest in the development of systems that enable molecular manipulation of pathogenic microorganisms.

DNA can be acquired by either vertical or horizontal (also referred to as lateral) transmission (Fig. 1). Vertical transmission (Fig. 1A) refers to

TABLE I Genome data on oral microorganisms

Microorganism	Strain	Genome size (Mb)	Avg. % G+C[a]	URL sequence data[b]
A. actinomycetemcomitans	HK1651	2.2	(42.7)	http://www.genome.ou.edu/act.html
F. nucleatum subsp. polymorphum	ATCC 10953	2.4[c]	(27–28)	http://hgsc.bcm.tmc.edu/microbial/Fnucleatum/
F. nucleatum subsp. nucleatum	ATCC 25586	2.17	27	http://www.integratedgenomics.com/genomereleases.html or http://www.tigr.org/tigr-scripts/CMR2/GenomePage3.spl?database=ntfn01
F. nucleatum subsp. vincentii	ATCC 49256	2.12	(27–28)	http://www.integratedgenomics.com/genomereleases.html
P. gingivalis	W83	2.34	48.3	http://www.tigr.org/tigr-scripts/CMR2/GenomePage3.spl?database=gpg
P. intermedia	17	3.3	(41–44)	http://tigrblast.tigr.org/ufmg/index.cgi?database=p_intermedia|seq
S. gordonii	Challis	2.21	42	http://tigrblast.tigr.org/ufmg/index.cgi?database=s_gordonii|seq
S. mitis	NCTC 12261	2.11	(39.5)	http://tigrblast.tigr.org/ufmg/index.cgi?database=s_mitis|seq
S. mutans	UA159	2.03	37.54	http://www.genome.ou.edu/smutans.html or http://www.tigr.org/tigr-scripts/CMR2/GenomePage3.spl?database=ntsm02
S. sanguis	SK36	2.2	(40–46.4)	http://www.sanguis.mic.vcu.edu/
S. sobrinus	6715	3.53	(44–46)	http://tigrblast.tigr.org/ufmg/index.cgi?database=s_sobrinus|seq
Tannerella forsythensis (Bacteroides forsythus)	ATCC 43037	3.4	(44–48)	http://tigrblast.tigr.org/ufmg/index.cgi?database=b_forsythus|seq
T. denticola	ATCC 35405	3.06	(37–38)	http://hgsc.bcm.tmc.edu/microbial/Tdenticola/

[a]Figures for % G+C are from analysis of genomic DNA sequence, except those in parentheses, which are estimates described for the species.

[b]Sites for comparative analyses of oral pathogens may be found at The Institute for Genomic Research (TIGR) Comprehensive Microbial Resource site (http://www.tigr.org/tigr-scripts/CMR2/CMRHomePage.spl) and the Los Alamos National Laboratory Bioscience Division Oral Pathogens Sequence Databases (http://www.oralgen.lanl.gov/).

[c]Estimated.

the transfer of a copy of the parental DNA to daughter cells upon cell division. DNA acquired by vertical transmission is generally identical to that of the parental cell, and the daughter cells are most often phenotypically indistinguishable from the parental cells. However, phenotypic alteration can occur in the context of vertical DNA transmission, for example, in the acquisition of antibiotic resistance resulting from the occurrence of one or more point mutations.

Horizontal transmission refers to the acquisition of foreign DNA, which can occur between clones of the same species or related and even diverse species (Fig. 1B). The significance of lateral gene transfer became evident in the 1960s when the spread of antibiotic resistance among bacterial pathogens was correlated with the acquisition of plasmid DNA by resistant strains. At a molecular level, two basic approaches are used to identify regions of DNA acquired by horizontal transmission. Phylogenetic analyses involve molecular characterization of specific genes and DNA or amino acid sequence comparisons. These analyses reveal identity or similarity of genes with homologues in other strains or species and provide evidence for horizontal transfer. Mosaic genes, which demonstrate blocks of DNA that appear to have arisen by lateral transfer of DNA from homologous genes in related species based on sequence analyses, have also

A.

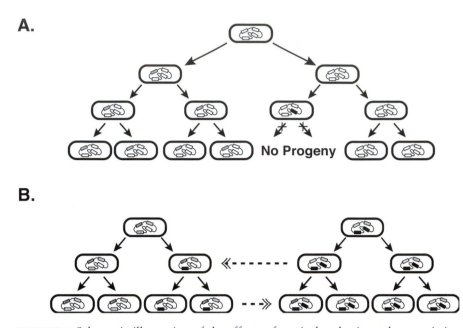

B.

FIGURE 1 Schematic illustration of the effects of vertical or horizontal transmission of genes. (A) Vertical transmission involves the transfer of a duplicate copy of the parental DNA to each of the daughter cells. Genetic diversity is dependent on mutations (hatched and black blocks) that yield variants of a given gene, which follow a clonal distribution. Selective pressures that can influence the population distribution include lethal mutations; cells receiving such lethal mutations do not produce progeny. (B) Horizontal transmission involves the transfer of DNA between cells of a population, enabling a shuffling of genes or DNA segments. The occurrence of a given genetic variant does not follow a clonal pattern of distribution when transfer is by horizontal transmission. (Adapted from Fig. 1 in M. C. J. Maiden, *FEMS Microbiol. Lett.* **112**:243–250, 1993, with permission from Elsevier.)

been described (Fig. 2). More recently, sequence-based parametric analyses have been used to examine DNA regions in the context of the genome in which they occur. Bacterial genomes have a characteristic average percentage of G+C content, which can range from approximately 25 to 75%. For example, the *P. gingivalis* genome has a G+C content of 48%, whereas *F. nucleatum* strain genomes range from 27 to 28% and *Actinomyces naeslundii* genomes range from 59 to 69.9% (Table 1). Within the chromosome of a given species, genes are typically relatively uniform in the distribution of DNA base composition. Thus identification of a gene or region of DNA with a base composition markedly different from that of the genome as a whole suggests that the atypical region of DNA may have been acquired by horizontal transmission. Similar analyses are conducted using codon bias and dinucleotide frequencies. The identification of segments of DNA specifically associated with mobile genetic elements, such as plasmids, bacteriophage, or transposons, and flanking genes with disparate base composition provides additional evidence of a foreign origin of the DNA.

Horizontal gene transfer requires the uptake and establishment of the DNA in the recipient cell, either by integration into and subsequent replication as part of the chromosome or as an extrachromosomally replicating element, such as a plasmid or bacteriophage. The known mechanisms

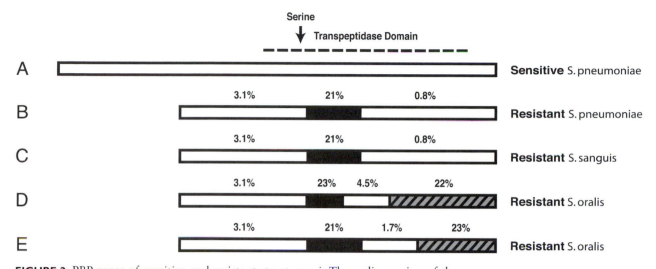

FIGURE 2 PBP genes of sensitive and resistant streptococci. The coding region of the PBP2B gene of penicillin-sensitive *S. pneumoniae* strain R6 is represented by the open bar in A, with the transpeptidase domain and active site serine residue indicated above the bar. The sequenced regions of the PBP2B genes from penicillin-resistant streptococci are represented in bars B to E. Two distinct blocks, one black and one hatched, each represent homologous DNA sequences that are highly diverged from the sequence of the penicillin-sensitive wild-type strain. The percentage divergence from the sequence of the gene from the penicillin-sensitive strain is indicated above the relevant region of the gene. The distribution of homologous blocks of divergent DNA in the resistant strains, forming "mosaic genes," indicates horizontal transfer of DNA as a mechanism of resistance development. (Adapted from C. G. Dowson et al., *Proc. Natl. Acad. Sci. USA* 87:5858–5862, 1990.)

responsible for horizontal gene transfer are transformation, conjugation, and transduction. Transformation involves the uptake of naked (cell-free) DNA by the recipient cell. The ability of a bacterium to take up DNA is referred to as "competence," and specific environmental conditions influence competence development. Transduction refers to the introduction of DNA into a bacterial cell by a bacteriophage (bacterial virus). Bacteriophage have been found in a variety of bacterial species. Bacteriophage are produced within a bacterial cell and then released from this donor cell for subsequent infection of a new recipient strain. However, transduction requires specific receptors on the recipient strain that are recognized by the bacteriophage, and this requirement limits the bacterial host range of bacteriophage. Transduction, like transformation, does not require contact between the donor and recipient bacterial cells. The third mechanism, conjugation, involves the transfer of DNA in a process that requires cell-to-cell contact. A DNA element that possesses all the genes necessary for transferring itself is referred to as "conjugative." In some cases plasmids are "mobilizable," possessing one or more properties necessary for conjugative transfer, but with most of the genes required for conjugation encoded by another coresident conjugative plasmid or on the host chromosome. DNA elements transferred by conjugation may be conjugative or mobilizable plasmids or conjugative transposons. Most plasmids transferred by conjugation remain as extrachromosomally replicating elements upon transfer to a new host. Transposons and some plasmids integrate into the recipient cell chromosome and are replicated along with the chromosomal DNA. Conjugation is responsible for the transfer of genetic elements between similar microbial species, as well as between organisms as diverse as bacteria and plants.

Gene Transfer in Nature

Evidence of gene transfer involving oral microorganisms consists of documentation of the acquisition and spread of phenotypic properties such as antibiotic resistance, documentation of DNA sequences in different strains and species consistent with horizontal transfer, and demonstration of naturally occurring mechanisms of gene transfer in oral species. Issues regarding antibiotic resistance are discussed in chapter 17, and are not discussed in detail here. The discussion below focuses on natural mechanisms of gene transfer and evidence for gene transfer based on analyses of DNA sequence.

Natural transformation is widespread in bacteria. The details of naturally occurring transformation have been described for many oral streptococci (Table 2) and *Streptococcus pneumoniae*, and it appears that there is significant similarity in their mechanisms. In streptococci, competence develops during the early to mid-logarithmic phase of growth, and there are considerable differences in the optimal conditions for any specific strain or species. The development of competence involves a quorum-sensing process encoded by three genes, *comC*, *comD*, and *comE* (Fig. 3). The *comC* gene encodes a small peptide precursor of the signaling molecule responsible for cell-to-cell communication. The precursor molecule is cleaved during export out of the bacterial cell by the products of *comA* and *comB*. This mature signaling peptide is a 19-amino-acid competence factor in *Streptococcus gordonii*, and 17- or 21-amino-acid competence-stimulating peptides in *S. mutans* and *S. pneumoniae*, respectively. Concentrations of competence factors or competence-stimulating peptides in the extracellular milieu above a threshold level are detected by neighboring bacterial cells by a sensor kinase (histidine kinase) encoded by *comD*, which then phosphorylates a response regulator encoded by *comE* within the bacterial cell. Phosphorylated ComE interacts with a specific DNA sequence upstream of genes involved in transformation, thereby upregulating their expression and inducing a signaling cascade within the

TABLE 2 Natural transformation in oral microorganisms

Microorganism	Strains	Mechanisms involved in competence and DNA uptake
A. actinomycetemcomitans	D7S	Competence induced by cAMP; preferential uptake of DNA possessing USS
Streptococcus crista	CC5a, CR3, CR311, PSH1a, PSH1b	Competence induced by competence factor
S. gordonii	Wicky, M5, DL1[a]	Competence induced by competence factor
S. mutans	UA159, NG8, JH1005, BM77, GB14, CT11	Competence induced by competence factor; 10- to 600-fold increased transformation efficiency in biofilm cells as compared to planktonic cells
S. oralis	CN3410	Competence induced by competence factor
S. sanguis	ATCC 10556	Competence induced by competence factor

[a]*S. gordonii* DL1 was previously classified as *S. sanguis* Challis.

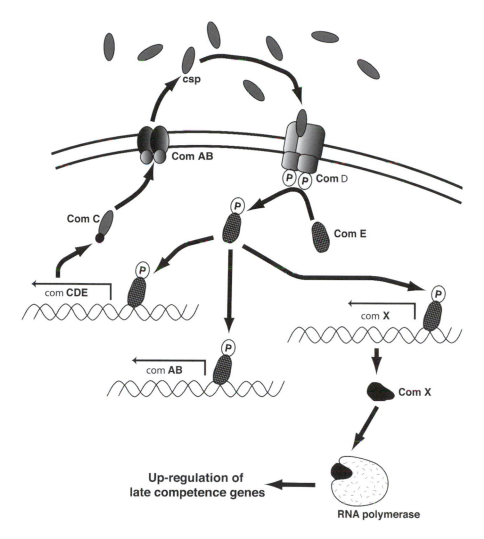

FIGURE 3 Schematic illustration of pathways involved in competence development in streptococci. The pathway of competence development in *S. pneumoniae* is illustrated. Homologues of many of the specific genes and gene products involved have been identified in the chromosomes of competent oral streptococci, including *S. mutans*. (Adapted from Fig. 2 in D. G. Cvitkovitch, *Crit. Rev. Oral Biol. Med.* **12:**217–243, 2001.) See text for details of pathways.

bacterium. These include early-competence genes such as *comCDE* whose products function in cell-to-cell signaling, as well as an alternate sigma factor gene *comX*, which up-regulates late-competence genes with gene products involved in DNA uptake and recombination.

The transformation process is initiated with binding of double-stranded DNA to the bacterial cell surface. This binding is not dependent on the DNA sequence and is sensitive to DNase treatment. Following nicking of the DNA, one strand is transported into the bacterial cell in a 3' to 5' direction, while the other strand is degraded. Within the bacterial cell the DNA may incorporate into the recipient cell chromosome in a RecA-dependent process if it contains a sufficient region of homologous DNA. Plasmid DNA may circularize and become established as an extra-chromosomally replicating element, but this process is limited in efficiency due to the recircularization requirement. Recent results obtained with *S. pneumoniae* demonstrate that DNA is released from a subfraction of cells simultaneously with the development of competence. Thus, natural competence development in streptococci appears to involve a complex coordination of mechanisms providing a pool of donor DNA as well as the uptake of environmental DNA.

Natural transformation in several gram-negative species, including *Haemophilus* species and *A. actinomycetemcomitans*, differs from that found in the streptococci. Two key differences are the existence of specificity in the uptake of DNA and regulation of competence development. The presence of an uptake signal sequence (USS) in the DNA confers specificity as to which DNA molecules will be taken up. The USS of *Haemophilus influenzae* and *A. actinomycetemcomitans*, characterized by a 9-bp core sequence (5′-AAGTGCGTT), is found at much greater frequency in the genome than would be expected if its occurrence were random. Competent cells efficiently and preferentially take up DNA molecules possessing the USS sequence. The addition of a cytoplasmic regulatory molecule, adenosine 3′5′ cyclic monophosphate (cAMP), to cultures of these gram-negative species stimulates the development of competence in both species, suggesting that catabolite repression regulates competence development. Catabolite repression is a metabolic sensing system, in which an abundance of nutrient substrate is linked to low levels of cAMP and minimal expression of the regulated metabolic pathways. In the relative absence of nutrients, increased levels of cAMP result in increased expression of selected backup metabolic pathways. In *H. influenzae*, only a small fraction of cells become competent in late exponential or early stationary-phase cultures in rich medium, whereas all cells become competent by shifting the culture to starvation conditions, and competence is inhibited by providing nucleic acid precursors.

Bacterial competence and the uptake of environmental DNA are a highly regulated process. It has been speculated that competence functions as a mechanism for acquisition of DNA as a nutrient as well as a mechanism for ensuring genetic diversity. Documentation of mosaic genes and demonstrations in vitro of transformation processes contributing to gene rearrangement support the latter hypothesis. A well-characterized example involves penicillin-binding proteins (PBP) in oral streptococci. Resistance to penicillin in *S. pneumoniae* was first reported in the 1960s and is now evident in strains worldwide. Penicillin resistance is found in strains harboring low-affinity variants of the PBPs. The variant PBP genes demonstrate discrete blocks of DNA responsible for resistance, with sequences nearly identical to homologous genes of commensal streptococci including *Streptococcus mitis* and *Streptococcus oralis* (Fig. 2). In vitro studies demonstrating transformation of *S. pneumoniae* with DNA from *S. mitis* or *S. oralis* yielded transformants with increased penicillin resistance and recombination in the PBP gene consistent with the pattern seen in mosaic genes in nature. Analyses suggest that in vivo resistance develops in commensal species prior to lateral transfer to pneumococci by transformation. There is also evidence of the transfer of a mosaic PBP gene conferring resistance from *S. pneumoniae* to *Streptococcus sanguis*, another member of the normal oral microbiota. These results demonstrate the relevance of transformation in normal ecology and pathogenesis, and the importance of commensal microorganisms as a "repository" for genetic determinants.

Evidence of genetic exchange by transduction among oral microorganisms is limited. Bacteriophages have been detected in a number of oral microorganisms, and the ability of many to replicate in their respective hosts has been demonstrated (Table 3). Bacteriophages are

TABLE 3 Bacteriophages of oral microorganisms

Microorganism	Phage designation	Phage distribution	Phage properties	Phage structure	Nucleic acid composition
A. actinomycetemcomitans	AaΦ23 (type strain of predominant class of bacteriophage), others[a]	Bacteriophages are detected in 33–54% of strains examined; the majority of bacteriophages are related to AaΦ23 and the majority of strains harboring AaΦ23 phage are serotype a	Temperate phage; generalized transducing phage	Isometric head, 60-nm diameter; contractile tail of 115 nm	Linear dsDNA, 44 kb; prophage is integrated into the host chromosome
Actinomyces viscosus, A. naeslundii	Multiple bacteriophages have been isolated, including Av-1, CT2, BF307, and Φ224	Bacteriophages isolated from dental plaque (10% of samples tested) and sewage	Temperate (Φ224) and virulent bacteriophages	Av-1, CT2, and BF307: polyhedral head 40 nm in diameter, tail of 26 nm	dsDNA ranging from 16 to 60 kb; Φ224 replicates in strain MG-1 as a plasmid
S. mutans	ΦPK 1	Bacteriophage isolated from S. mutans PK 1	Temperate bacteriophage	Hexagonal head with contractile tail	DNA, 27–29 kb
E. faecalis	No designation	Isolated from saliva (22% of samples tested) or swabs of tongue and teeth	Virulent and temperate bacteriophages	Spherical, enveloped, spiked structure, 70-nm diameter	Undetermined

[a]Numerous temperate bacteriophages have been isolated from *A. actinomycetemcomitans*. AaΦ23 appears to predominate, but the genetic relationship of AaΦ23 with others such as ΦAa has not been determined.

termed "virulent" or "temperate" depending on characteristics of their life cycle in the host bacterial cell (Fig. 4A). Virulent bacteriophages uniformly lyse the infected bacterial cell and release phage particles in what is termed lytic growth. Temperate bacteriophages are also capable of lytic growth, but alternatively may exist in a quiescent phase when the DNA integrates into the bacterial chromosome or replicates extra-chromosomally. This quiescent "prophage" DNA may be induced to lytic growth with subsequent production of phage particles and bacterial cell lysis. Bacteriophages may transfer bacterial DNA from one host to another by one of two mechanisms, i.e., either generalized or specialized transduction. In generalized transduction, virtually any segment of host cell DNA becomes incorporated into the phage head in place of the phage genome. When a phage particle containing such bacterial DNA injects its nucleic acid into a new host following attachment, some or all of the DNA may then become part of that cell's genomic makeup. In specialized transduction, a temperate phage excises imprecisely from the bacterial host chromosome. In this manner, a segment of phage DNA is left behind and a segment of chromosomal DNA adjacent to either end of the specific site of integration of the phage DNA may be excised along with the remaining phage DNA, and become packaged in new phage heads during the lytic phase. Following release of phage particles during cell lysis, if such a phage particle attaches to a bacterial cell, the excised segment of the previous host's chromosome will be injected into the new host as part of the phage DNA, and incorporated into the new host's chromosome during the formation of a prophage state (lysogeny). Among oral bacteria, prophages harbored in strains of *A. actinomycetemcomitans* and *S. mutans* have been isolated (Table 3).

FIGURE 4 (A) Schematic illustration of transduction pathways. Bacterial recipients of bacteriophage DNA enter lytic or lysogenic phases. Virulent bacteriophages use lytic growth (left side), which involves the replication and assembly of progeny bacteriophage followed by their release upon lysis of the host bacterial cell. Temperate bacteriophages may use the lytic phase or the lysogenic phase. In the lysogenic phase (right side) the bacteriophage DNA is replicated within the host cell, either integrated within the chromosomal DNA (illustrated) or extrachromosomally (not illustrated). Bacterial cells in the lysogenic phase do not undergo lysis, but may be induced to enter the lytic phase (asterisk). However, when temperate phages enter into a lytic phase, during the maturation process fragments from virtually any part of the host chromosome may be packaged into new heads in place of the phage genome (generalized transducing phage), or a segment of host chromosome adjacent to the specific site of insertion of the prophage may be excised along with the phage DNA and subsequently packaged into new heads (specialized transducing phage). In either case, bacterial DNA from one bacterial host may be transferred to a new bacterial host during subsequent rounds of phage infection (transduction). (B) Phage with contractile sheath (Bradley [1967] group A) isolated from *A. actinomycetemcomitans* from sites undergoing rapid periodontal destruction in patients with Papillon-Lefèvre syndrome. The head of the phage is 60 nm in diameter. Image kindly provided by E. Namork, Norwegian Institute of Public Health, and H. R. Preus, Faculty of Dentistry, University of Oslo, Norway. (C) Electron micrograph of *E. faecalis* bacteriophage ÆEf that was isolated from an *E. faecalis* strain originating in an infected root canal. The negative staining reveals the phage head and long tail structures. Image kindly provided by R. H. Stevens, O. D. Porras, and A. L. Delisle.

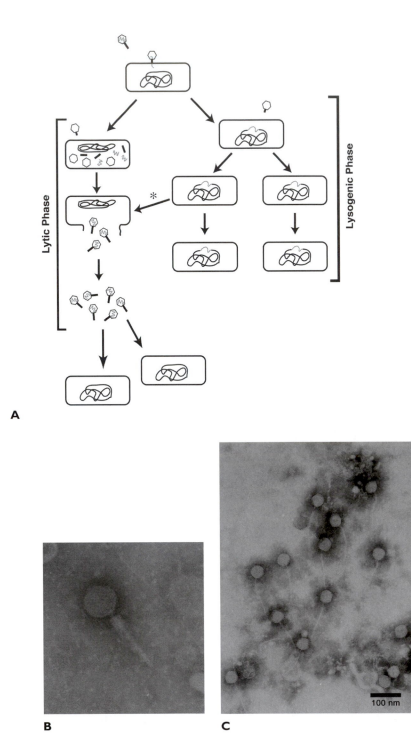

In addition, bacteriophage specific to *A. naeslundii* and *Enterococcus faecalis* have been isolated from dental plaque, saliva, oral swabs, and sewage samples (Table 3). Temperate bacteriophages are common in strains of *A. actinomycetemcomitans*, with detection rates from 33 to 54% of strains examined. The commonly isolated bacteriophage in European studies comprise a genetically related family with AaΦ23 representing the type strain (Fig. 4B). AaΦ23 is a temperate phage containing a linear 44-kb double-stranded DNA molecule that integrates into the bacterial host chromosome in the prophage state. When induced, the bacteriophage enters a lytic phase with production of phage particles that are released upon lysis of the bacterial cell. Temperate bacteriophages are found in isolates of *A. actinomycetemcomitans* from healthy and diseased sites, and their occurrence does not appear to correlate with virulence. Results of in vitro experiments reveal that AaΦ23-like bacteriophages are capable of transferring antibiotic resistance determinants to nonresistant strains, indicating that they may contribute to lateral gene transfer among strains of *A. actinomycetemcomitans*.

A third mechanism of bacterial genetic transfer is conjugation, a complex process involving intercellular contact, DNA replication, and DNA transport (Fig. 5). Evidence for gene transfer by conjugation in oral species includes the demonstration in oral bacterial isolates of genetic elements capable of conjugative transfer and demonstrations of conjugation in vitro in which donor, recipient, or both have been oral species. Among the types of genetic elements transferable by conjugation are plasmids. Many gram-negative bacteria harbor plasmids that encode the production of sex pili that initiate contact between recipient and donor cells, leading to the formation of aggregates possessing an intercellular membrane pore that enables DNA transport. The initial phase at the DNA level involves a single-strand cleavage at the origin of transfer mediated by a relaxase enzyme complex. This is followed by transport of the nicked strand of DNA from the donor to the recipient cell and synthesis of complementary DNA in both cells to yield a double-stranded product. In some gram-positive bacteria, e.g., strains of *E. faecalis*, the initial contact involves aggregation factors other than pili. A large number of gram-positive, and some gram-negative, bacterial species harbor conjugative plasmids that mediate their own DNA transfer to and replication in a recipient host but do not encode functions required for the formation of donor-recipient pairs or aggregates. For these plasmids to be transferred from a donor to a recipient cell, it is necessary that potential donors and recipients come into contact incidentally on a solid surface. In nature such incidental contact might occur in a biofilm, whereas in the laboratory it may occur on an agar-based medium or on a filter membrane subsequently placed on an agar-based medium.

Plasmids are extrachromosomally replicating genetic elements. The vast majority of plasmids are present in their host cells as double-stranded covalently closed circular DNA molecules, although linear double-stranded plasmids have been described in a few bacterial species. The first plasmid to be studied to any great extent was the F factor, a conjugative genetic element that may exist in its host as an extrachromosomal element, or it may be integrated into the host chromosome. However, most studies that led to an understanding of the molecular and genetic nature of plasmids were initiated in bacterial strains with recently acquired antibiotic resistance, underscoring their significance in horizontal gene transfer. Plasmids have been found, or shown to replicate, in a number of oral species (Table 4), although surveys of oral isolates for plasmids generally document a relatively low rate of occurrence. For example, plasmids have been reported to occur in approximately 5% of

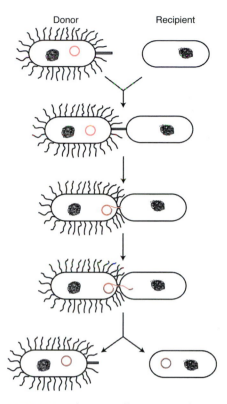

FIGURE 5 Schematic illustration of conjugative DNA transfer. The donor bacterium on the left possesses a double-stranded conjugative plasmid, which is transferred to the recipient bacterium on the right via a single-stranded DNA intermediate, after contact between the donor and recipient bacteria is established. The double-stranded conjugative plasmid is established in both donor and recipient cell following replication of a second strand.

TABLE 4 Selected native plasmids

Host species of origin	Plasmid	Plasmid size (kb)	% G+C if known	Mode of replication (if known)	Relevant phenotype and other properties of interest	Host range
E. faecalis	pAMβ1	26.5		Theta replication	MLS resistance (macrolides, lincosamides, streptogramin B alpha) Conjugative, broad-host-range, low-copy-number plasmid; replicon related to that of pIP501	11 genera including such oral species as E. faecalis, S. sanguis, S. salivarius, S. mutans, S. sobrinus
Streptococcus agalactiae	pIP501	30.2		Theta replication	Resistance to chloramphenicol and erythromycin Conjugative, broad-host-range plasmid; replicon related to that of pAMβ1	7 genera including such oral species as E. faecalis,[a] S. sanguis[a]
S. ferus (previously S. mutans)	pVA380-1	4.2	37.0	RC replication	Cryptic, mobilizable	S. sobrinus,[a] E. faecalis,[a] S. gordonii,[a] S. pyogenes,[a] S. sanguis,[a] S. agalactiae[a]
S. mutans	pUA140	5.6	32.7	RC replication	Cryptic	S. mutans
P. intermedia	pYHBil	5.1	38		Cryptic, mobilizable	P. intermedia, E. coli[a]
F. nucleatum	pFN1	5.9	23		Cryptic	F. nucleatum, E. coli[a]
A. actinomycetemcomitans	pVT736-1	2.0	38.3	RC replication	Cryptic	A. actinomycetemcomitans[a]
	pVT745	25.1	39.0		Cryptic, conjugative	A. actinomycetemcomitans, E. coli[a]
E. corrodens	pFM739	9.4			Resistance to streptomycin, penicillin and sulfonamide, RSF1010 replicon, mobilizable	Neisseria spp., E. corrodens, E. coli
T. denticola, Treponema socranskii	pTS1	3.7	34.2		Cryptic	T. denticola,[a] E. coli[a]

[a]Plasmid derived from the native plasmid.

strains of *S. mutans*, *P. intermedia*, and *A. actinomycetemcomitans*. Further, native plasmids have not been detected in strains of *Actinomyces* spp. or *P. gingivalis*. Plasmid DNA was detected in 18% of *F. nucleatum* strains examined, and in oral *Treponema* spp. reports of plasmid detection range from 13 to 44%. The occurrence of related or identical plasmids in distinct strains and species from geographically diverse sources is evident in several oral species, including *F. nucleatum*, *Treponema* spp., *S. mutans*, and *Eikenella corrodens*. These findings may reflect the presence of natural genetic transfer systems within these species, or may have resulted from vertical transfer prior to the evolutionary divergence of these species.

To ensure their survival, plasmids must encode the elements required for autonomous replication, including an origin of replication and a contiguous gene(s) encoding replication proteins and other controlling elements. Some native plasmids encode genes that confer host strain resistance to antibiotics, and selective pressures associated with the use of antibiotics may facilitate the spread of these plasmids. Other phenotypes that may be encoded by plasmids include virulence traits that contribute to the bacterium's ability to cause disease, metabolic capabilities, and the production of bacteriocins. Some plasmids have no detectable phenotype other than autonomous replication and are referred to as "cryptic." Plasmids may also be either conjugative or mobilizable. Conjugative plasmids are large, due to the requirement for genes sufficient to confer all the properties involved in conjugative transfer. For example, the conjugative plasmid pVT745 from *A. actinomycetemcomitans* is 25.4 kb in size, and the genes necessary for DNA processing and mating are encoded in two gene clusters (Fig. 6A). The *E. faecalis* plasmid pAMβ1 is a broad-host-range conjugative plasmid of 26.5 kb that has been introduced into a number of distinct oral *Streptococcus* spp. (Table 4). Several smaller plasmids can be transferred by conjugation when the genes encoding conjugative functions are provided by another plasmid or chromosomally located genes. These plasmids are termed "mobilizable," and examples include pYHBil from *P. intermedia* (Fig. 6B) and pVA380-1 from *Streptococcus ferus*.

Another type of bacterial genetic element is the transposon. Some transposons may also be transferred by conjugation. Transposons are

FIGURE 6 Representative native conjugative and mobilizable plasmids. (A) The *A. actinomycetemcomitans* plasmid pVT745 is self-transmissible by conjugation. Analysis of the pVT745 DNA sequence identified 36 putative open reading frames. Two clusters of mating-associated genes, designated *mag*A (black) and *mag*B (gray), were identified on the basis of homology to genes of known function found in other bacterial species. The *mag*A genes are predicted to be involved in DNA processing functions, including genes encoding a DNA nicking enzyme and a protein that recognizes the origin of transfer (*ori*T). The *mag*B genes are predicted to function in mating aggregate formation, including mating pore formation and pilus assembly. The orientation of the genes in the clusters is indicated by the arrow. The putative origin of replication (*ori*V) is indicated. (Adapted from Fig. 1 in D. M. Galli et al., *J. Bacteriol.* **183:**1585–1594, 2001.) (B) The *P. intermedia* plasmid pYHBil is mobilizable by conjugation. Analysis of the pYHBil DNA sequence identified two genes, *rep* and *mob*, that are predicted to encode replication and mobilization proteins, respectively. The *mob* gene of pYHBil is essential for conjugal transfer of the plasmid. Mobilization proteins are responsible for nicking of the plasmid DNA as an initial step in the process of DNA transfer, and other functions required for conjugation are provided in *trans*. The plasmids illustrated in Fig. 6 are not drawn to scale. (Adapted from Fig. 1 in K. P. Leung et al., *Plasmid* **48:**64–72, 2002, with permission from Elsevier.)

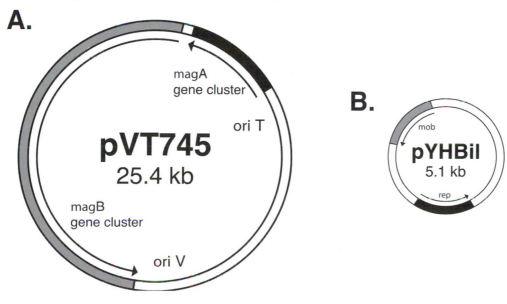

discrete nonreplicative segments of DNA capable of inserting into and being replicated as part of a bacterial replicon, such as a chromosome, plasmid, or bacteriophage genome. They may also move from one site in a DNA molecule to another. Insertion of a transposon into DNA is mediated by insertion sequence elements, which are located at the ends of transposons and encode enzymes termed transposases that catalyze the insertion events. Transposon insertion is usually random, i.e., may occur at virtually any site on a DNA molecule, independent of extensive homology, and can occur in a recombination-deficient (*recA*) host cell. DNA between the insertion sequence elements of a transposon may encode virtually any type of bacterial trait, such as antibiotic resistance, metabolic activity, etc. The conjugative transposons are additionally characterized by their ability to efficiently transfer intercellularly, as long as donor and recipient cells are brought together on a solid surface, since they do not encode the elements that would mediate the cell-to-cell contact required for conjugation. One of the best characterized of the conjugative transposons is Tn*916*, which is an 18-kb element first isolated from *E. faecalis* DS16. Tn*916* possesses a *tet*M gene, which confers tetracycline resistance to the host bacterium. Conjugative transfer begins with excision of Tn*916* from a donor host replicon and formation of a circular intermediate, which is transferred to a recipient cell and is replicated as part of the new host's genome following insertion into a replicon. In the recipient cell the transposon reinserts into the host DNA preferentially at sites that are AT rich. Relatively little is known about the conjugation process, but regions of Tn*916* required for intercellular transposition have been identified. Tn*916* is an example of a promiscuous element based on its tremendously broad host range. Tn*916*-like elements have been identified in a number of oral species, including *Streptococcus* spp., *Enterococcus* spp., *E. corrodens*, *F. nucleatum*, and *Veillonella parvula*. Other broad-host-range transposons, related to Tn*916*, encode resistance to tetracycline as well as other antibiotics, such as erythromycin.

Conjugative transfer of plasmids and transposons is important in lateral gene transfer, as exemplified by the spread of antibiotic resistance genes. Natural transformation and transduction in specific groups of oral species are also likely to be important. The acquisition of new DNA may contribute to environmental and evolutionary diversification, allowing the bacterium to survive under a wider range of environmental conditions and to evolve over time. Among oral microorganisms the increased incidence of antibiotic-resistant strains, demonstration of gene transfer in vitro, and identification of elements involved in gene transfer support the role of these processes in genetic transfer in the natural environment. These findings additionally indicate that members of the normal oral microbiota may provide a reservoir for resistance and other virulence-related determinants.

MOLECULAR ANALYSIS OF ORAL MICROORGANISMS

Examination of two isolates of a bacterial strain, one that expresses a gene of interest, i.e., the wild-type parent, and one that does not, helps define the contribution of the corresponding gene to the bacterial phenotype. A bacterial mutant in which only a defined gene has been altered is termed an isogenic mutant, and a change in sequence, total inactivation, or deletion of a gene from its native host background will lead to a change or loss of function specific to that gene. Restoration of the gene and/or its expression, referred to as complementation of the mutant, should restore function. Complementation serves as an important control in ruling out the possibility that a loss of function occurred from effects of the insertion or deletion on downstream genes, or from an undetected spontaneous mutation in another gene. Studies in *Escherichia coli* and other enteric species led the field in achieving these goals through the development of systems for the introduction of DNA into bacterial hosts that were not naturally competent, for the construction of DNA molecules that could be used to inactivate chromosomal genes, and for the complementation of inactivated genes. These technologies also facilitated studies of gene regulation, particularly with respect to gaining an understanding of how a bacterium responds to different environmental stimuli and conditions. In this regard, however, cellular functions encoded by bacterial genes, the expression of which may be regulated by such stimuli, are generally not easy to assay. Thus another important aspect of molecular analysis has involved the use of reporter genes, which encode proteins that are easily assayed. DNA molecules are constructed in such a way that the expression of a reporter gene will be controlled by the particular regulatory element under study following its introduction into a bacterial host. The most commonly used reporter genes encode the proteins β-galactosidase (detected with a colorimetric substrate), luciferase (detected by luminescence), and the green fluorescent protein or its derivates (detected with fluorescence).

The genetic manipulations required to construct the types of bacterial strains described above became possible with the emergence of recombinant DNA technology, which began in the 1970s following the discovery that restriction endonucleases are enzymes that reproducibly cleave DNA at specific sites. Bacteria produce restriction endonucleases, typically in association with a modification enzyme responsible for methylation of specific nucleotides that prevents cleavage of the host cell DNA. The ability of a bacterial system to target "nonself" DNA for degradation is postulated to function in protection against invading DNA, but may also provide a nutrient pool for synthesis of host cell nucleic acids. The percentage of bacterial strains that encode restriction endonucleases may be as high as 80%, and restriction endonucleases have been identified in all the bacterial genomes of oral species published on to date. Multiple restriction modification systems may occur in a single strain. For example, up to seven possible restriction modification systems were identified in the genome sequence of one strain of *F. nucleatum*. The existence of restriction endonucleases can be a significant barrier to the development of efficient genetic transfer in specific bacterial strains.

The type II restriction endonucleases are commonly used in recombinant DNA techniques. These enzymes are characterized by their ability to cleave DNA within, or close to, a specific recognition sequence of 4 to 8 bp (Table 5). The ability to reproducibly cleave DNA at a defined base pair sequence provided the necessary foundation for the development of DNA mapping and sequencing techniques. In addition, each enzyme leaves characteristic ends on the cleaved DNA molecule, which may be

TABLE 5 Selected restriction endonucleases

Restriction endonuclease[a]	Microorganism from which restriction enzyme was originally isolated	Recognition sequence and cleavage pattern[b]	Comments
FnuDII	*F. nucleatum*	5′...CGCG...3′ 3′...GCGC...5′	FnuDII has a 4-bp recognition sequence and cleavage leaves blunt ends. Religation of DNA with blunt ends is less efficient than religation of DNA with compatible cohesive ends.
EcoRV	*E. coli*	5′...GATATC...3′ 3′...CTATAG...5′	EcoRV has a 6-bp recognition sequence and cleavage leaves blunt ends.
FseI	*Frankia* spp.	5′...GGCCGGCC...3′ 3′...CCGGCCGG...5′	FseI has an 8-bp recognition sequence and cleavage leaves a 3′ overhang "GGCC"
XbaI	*Xanthomonas badrii*	5′...TCTAGA...3′ 3′...AGATCT...5′	XbaI has a 6-bp recognition sequence and cleavage leaves a 5′ cohesive end "CTAG" that is compatible with that of SpeI. Ligation of XbaI- and SpeI-cleaved DNA is not recleavable with either enzyme, but may be cleaved with BfaI.
SpeI	*Sphaerotilus* spp.	5′...ACTAGT...3′ 3′...TGATCA...5′	SpeI has a 6-bp recognition sequence and cleavage leaves a 5′ cohesive end "CTAG" that is compatible with that of XbaI. Ligation of XbaI- and SpeI-cleaved DNA is not recleavable with either enzyme, but may be cleaved with BfaI.
BfaI	*B. fragilis*	5′...CTAG...3′ 3′...GATC...5′	BfaI has a 4-bp recognition sequence and cleavage leaves a 5′ cohesive end "TA." The recognition sequence corresponds to the cohesive overhang generated by digestion with XbaI or SpeI. A site generated from one XbaI-digested and one SpeI-digested DNA fragment can be cleaved with BfaI.
StsI	*S. sanguis*	5′...GGATGNNNNNNNNNNNNNNNNN...3′ 3′...CCTACNNNNNNNNNNNNNNNNN...5′	StsI has a 5-bp recognition sequence and cleaves the DNA at 10 and 14 bp from this sequence as indicated, leaving a 5′ overhang of unspecified sequence.
SmuEI	*S. mutans*	5′...GGWCC...3′ 3′...CCWGG...5′	SmuEI has a 5-bp recognition sequence with the central residue as either an A or T. Cleavage leaves a 5′ cohesive end of "GACC" or "GTCC."
Fnu4HI	*F. nucleatum*	5′...GCNGC...3′ 3′...CGNCG...5′	Fnu4HI has a 4-bp recognition sequence with a central residue that may be any base. Cleavage leaves a 5′ cohesive end with the specificity of the central residue.

[a]By convention, the first three letters of the restriction endonuclease derive from the first letter of the genus followed by the first two letters of the species designation of the microorganism from which the restriction endonuclease originates. The designation StsI is an exception to this convention.

[b]Cleavage pattern is indicated by shading. Abbreviations: N = A, C, G, or T; W = A or T.

blunt or overhanging with extensions of either 3′ or 5′ ends. The overhanging ends, referred to as "sticky" or "cohesive" ends, provide a powerful template for reannealing of the DNA based on the specificity of the base pair sequence. Recognition of the utility of cohesive ends led to recombinant DNA technology. The insertion of heterologous DNA into a plasmid and its propagation in *E. coli*, in the process known as cloning, was first reported in 1972. A description of the general steps involved in recombinant DNA technology (cloning) can be found in chapter 8. The cloning and characterization of genes and gene products of oral bacteria were first reported in the early 1980s (Table 6).

Early recombinant DNA technology relied to a large extent on naturally occurring restriction endonuclease sites. This proved cumbersome when convenient sites were not present, but this limitation has largely been overcome with a major technological advance in the 1980s, the development of the PCR. PCR is a process by which millions of copies of a specific region of DNA can be synthesized using a minute quantity of DNA template, a pool of the four individual deoxyribonucleotides, and short oligonucleotide primers complementary to DNA sequence flanking the region of interest (see Fig. 3 in chapter 8). The desired DNA fragment is amplified in a cyclical thermal process of denaturation, annealing of oligonucleotide primers, and synthesis of complementary DNA with incorporation of nucleotides using a thermostable DNA polymerase. A single DNA fragment can be amplified to hundreds of millions of copies in 30 to 40 cycles, and the resulting DNA molecule is referred to as an "amplicon." A powerful use of PCR technology involves the addition of novel base pairs into the oligonucleotide primers, and thus the amplicon. This can be done to introduce new restriction endonuclease sites or regions of homology to facilitate subsequent molecular manipulations. One example of this approach is the construction of an erythromycin resistance cassette that has been widely used in the transformation of oral bacterial species (Fig. 7). Today the basic processes of specific DNA cleavage and religation in combination with PCR allow the design and engineering of almost unlimited combinations of DNA fragments of diverse biological or synthetic origin.

Molecular analyses in the native bacterial cell also require a means by which to introduce and establish DNA molecules in the bacterium. The natural processes of transformation, conjugation, and transduction have been successfully used for these purposes in many bacterial species and strains (Table 6). Another option for delivery of DNA into bacterial cells is to make them competent for transformation by some artificial means, such as electroporation. Electroporation is a process in which a brief high-voltage pulse is applied to a suspension of bacterial cells and DNA, resulting in reversible membrane permeability and DNA uptake by a fraction of the surviving cells. This technique has been widely used for both gram-negative and gram-positive bacteria.

The need for molecular analyses has only increased with the emergence of genomic information, both for confirmation of gene function initially inferred by DNA sequence homology or phenotypic analyses and for investigation of genes of unknown function. The importance of these systems in the study of microbial ecology and pathogenesis is further illustrated in chapter 8 that focuses on applied molecular biology in oral microorganisms. The remainder of this chapter focuses on molecular tools, such as vectors, designed specifically for the development of and use with genetic transfer systems in oral microorganisms, and on the use of transposons for generalized mutagenesis in oral species.

VECTORS AND THEIR UTILITY

The cloning and characterization of DNA from oral bacterial species in *E. coli* can provide considerable information regarding individual genes and, in some cases, their gene products. Ultimately, however, it is critical to be able to conduct molecular manipulations in the bacterial species of interest so that gene function can be evaluated in the native host

TABLE 6 Milestones in the development of genetic systems for oral species

Species	Development	Description
S. mutans, S. sanguis/gordonii	Gene cloned	1982: Cloning of S. mutans aspartate-semialdehyde dehydrogenase gene, asd
		1982: Cloning of S. mutans surface protein antigen gene, spaA
		1982: Cloning of S. mutans tetracycline resistance determinant in S. sanguis
	Native plasmids identified	1973: Plasmid isolated from S. mutans strain LM-7
		1978: Plasmid isolated from S. sanguis encoding resistance to erythromycin and lincomycin
	Transformation	1976: Natural transformation of S. sanguis strain Challis with plasmid DNA from S. faecalis
		1976: Natural transformation of S. sanguis strain Challis with DNA from heterologous streptococcal strains
		1981: Natural transformation of S. mutans with DNA from homologous and heterologous strains
	Conjugation	1978: Transfer to S. mutans and S. sanguis/gordonii of pAMβ from S. faecalis by conjugation
	Shuttle plasmid	1982: Streptococcus-E. coli shuttle plasmid pVA838
		1982: Streptococcus-E. coli shuttle plasmid pVA856
	Site-directed mutagenesis	1986: Defined mutation of glucosyltransferase gene of S. mutans
		1990: Defined mutation of a 76-kDa cell surface protein of S. gordonii
	Transposon mutagenesis	1988: Tn916 used to generate mutations in S. mutans chromosome, with auxotrophs identified
		1995: Tn4001 used to generate lactose-negative mutants in S. gordonii
		1996: Tn917 used to generate mutations in genes involved in acid tolerence, nutrition, and bacteriocin production
	Complementation	1992: Low glucosyltransferase activity in S. gordonii complemented with a chimeric plasmid, pAM5010, possessing the regulatory gene rgg
		1996: Complementation of lactate dehydrogenase deficiency in S. mutans with heterologous alcohol dehydrogenase on plasmid pCR3-8
Actinomyces spp.	Gene cloned	1987: Cloning and expression of the type I fimbrial subunit gene, fimP, of Actinomyces viscosus
	Native plasmids identified	Native plasmids have not been found
	Bacteriophage identified	1978: A lytic phage for A. viscosus was isolated from sewage
	Transformation	1994: Transformation of A. viscosus and A. naeslundii with broad-host-range plasmid pJDR215
	Transfection	1997: Transfection of A. viscosus and A. naeslundii strains with phage isolated from dental plaque
	Conjugation	Not reported
	Shuttle plasmid	1994: Transformation of A. viscosus and A. naeslundii with broad-host-range plasmid pJDR215
	Site-directed mutagenesis	1995: Defined mutation in the fimP gene of A. viscosus
	Transposon mutagenesis	Not reported
	Complementation	Not reported
P. intermedia	Gene cloned	1999: Cloning of P. intermedia DNA conferring hemolytic activity in E. coli
	Native plasmids identified	1990: Identification of multiple cryptic plasmids, including the 5-kb pYHBil
	Transformation	Not reported
	Conjugation	2002: Conjugation with chimeric shuttle plasmid pDRD5904
	Shuttle plasmid	2002: Shuttle plasmid pDRD5904 engineered using the native plasmid pYHBil and a kanamycin resistance determinant
	Site-directed mutagenesis	Not reported
	Transposon mutagenesis	Not reported
	Complementation	Not reported
F. nucleatum	Gene cloned	1996: Cloning and expression of the major outer membrane protein gene, fomA
	Native plasmids identified	1995: Identification of cryptic homologous plasmids, including pSG2717 and pSG4544
	Transformation	2000: Transformation by electroporation with shuttle plasmid pHS17
	Conjugation	1990: Transfer of tetracycline resistance and tetM-like DNA sequences to F. nucleatum strains

Organism	Method	Description
	Shuttle plasmid	2000: Shuttle plasmid pHS17 engineered using the native plasmid pFN1 and an erythromycin resistance cassette 2003: Shuttle plasmid engineered using the native plasmid pKH9
	Site-directed mutagenesis	2003: Defined chromosomal insertion in the *rnr* (exoribonuclease R) gene
	Transposon mutagenesis	Not reported
	Complementation	Not reported
A. actinomycetemcomitans	Gene cloned	1989: Cloning of the leukotoxin gene, *ltxA*
	Native plasmids identified	1989: Multiple plasmids identified ranging in size from 4 to 20 megadaltons
	Transformation	1990: Natural transformation 1991: Transformation via electroporation with pDL282
	Conjugation	1993: Conjugation with broad-host-range IncP and IncQ plasmids 2001: Conjugation with native plasmid pVT745
	Shuttle plasmid	1991: Shuttle plasmid pDL282 constructed from native plasmids
	Site-directed mutagenesis	1995: Defined mutations in the genes of the leukotoxin operon
	Transposon mutagenesis	1992: Tn916 mutagenesis to isolate mutants lacking serotype b-specific polysaccharide antigen 1995: Tn5 mutagenesis 1999: IS903φkan mutagenesis to isolate catalase-negative mutants
P. gingivalis	Complementation	2000: Complemented a *tad* gene mutation with a broad-host-range IncQ expression vector, pJAK16
	Gene cloned	1988: Cloning of the fimbrial subunit gene, *fimA*, in *E. coli*
	Native plasmids identified	Native plasmids have not been found
	Transformation	1993: Transformation by electroporation with pE5-2 and derivate pYT7
	Conjugation	1989: Conjugation with plasmid pE5-2
	Shuttle plasmid	1989: Shuttle plasmid pE5-2 with *E. coli* and *Bacteroides eggerthii* replicons 1997: Shuttle plasmid pYH400, engineered with *P. asaccharolytica* replicon
	Site-directed mutagenesis	1993: Defined mutation in a protase gene (*tpr*) of strain W83
	Transposon mutagenesis	1998: Tn4351 mutagenesis to isolate nonhemolytic and nonpigmented mutants 2000: Tn4400 mutagenesis shown to yield large numbers of mutants with simple insertions
T. denticola	Complementation	1997: Complemented *tpr* gene mutation in strain W83 using *Bacteroides* shuttle plasmid pNJR12 with intact *tpr* gene
	Gene cloned	1990: Cloning of a chymotrypsinlike protease gene, *prtA* (Que and Kuramitsu)
	Native plasmids identified	1991: Isolated 2.6-kb plasmid pTD1 1996: Isolated 4.2-kb plasmid pTS1
	Transformation	1996: Transformation by electroporation with broad-host-range plasmid pKT210
	Conjugation	Not reported
	Shuttle plasmid	1996: Transformation by electroporation with broad-host-range plasmid pKT210 2002: Novel shuttle plasmid pKMCou conferring coumermycin resistance
	Site-directed mutagenesis	1996: Defined mutation of the flagellar hook protein FlgE
	Transposon mutagenesis	Not reported
	Complementation	2002: Complementation of *flgE* mutant by using novel shuttle plasmid pKMCou

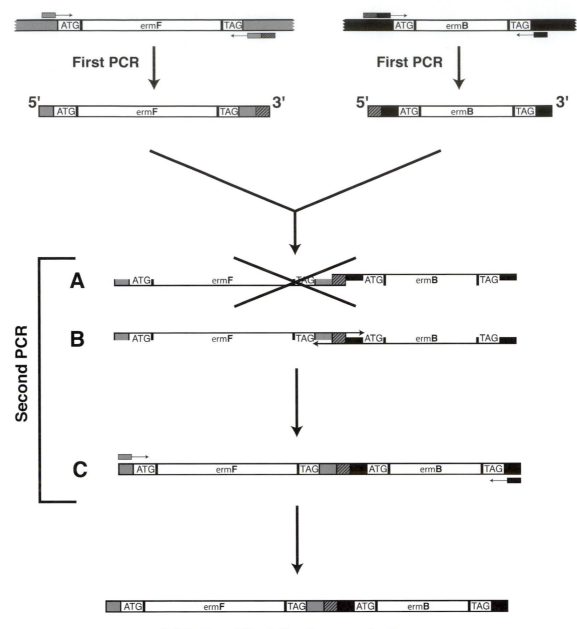

First PCR   **First PCR**

Second PCR

A

B

C

PCR Amplified Erythromycin Cassette

FIGURE 7 Construction of an erythromycin resistance cassette using the PCR-based overlap extension method. The erythromycin resistance cassette was constructed using a fusion PCR approach to combine erythromycin resistance genes that would function in *E. coli* (*erm*B gene [previously designated as *erm*AM]) and in *P. gingivalis* (*erm*F). PCR was first used to amplify the individual erythromycin resistance genes, including their regulatory regions. The 3′ primer for the *erm*F amplicon and the 5′ primer for the *erm*B amplicon incorporated a complementary overlapping sequence (indicated by the shaded box with hatch marks). The products of the first PCR were purified and combined along with primers for the 5′ region of the *erm*F amplicon and the 3′ region of the *erm*B amplicon. In the second PCR, denatured amplicons from the first reaction may hybridize with the homologous amplicon (not illustrated) or with the heterologous amplicon (A and B) due to annealing of the inserted overlapping sequence (hatched box). The combination of annealed strands illustrated in panel A was not amplified because DNA polymerase functions in a 3′ to 5′ direction. The combination of strands as seen in panel B enabled DNA synthesis complementary to the annealed strand to proceed from the free 3′ end of the overlapping region. The resulting product yielded a DNA molecule possessing both the *erm*F and *erm*B, further amplified by the flanking primers (C). (Adapted from H. M. Fletcher et al., *Infect. Immun.* **63:**1521–1528, 1995.)

background. One requirement for the majority of such studies is the availability of vectors onto which DNA can be added, introduced into the host of choice, and expressed by that host. The most basic property of such a vector is its ability to function as a replicon in the host(s) of interest. Other properties common to vectors include the presence of at least one, and preferably several, unique restriction endonuclease recognition sequences, i.e., a cloning site, for the introduction of homologous or heterologous DNA, and a selectable trait, such as resistance to an antibiotic, to detect the presence of the vector in a host into which it has been introduced. Another feature might include a gene flanking the cloning site, the function of which would be interrupted by the insertion of DNA, for the screening of selected transformants for those carrying the vector with inserts, and in some instances, the inclusion of a transcriptional terminator downstream of the insertion site to prevent readthrough beyond the cloned DNA and overexpression of potentially lethal vector-encoded traits. Another desirable feature of a vector, depending on the specific purpose, might be an inducible promoter by which the expression of cloned genes can be regulated when introduced downstream of it, or for the overexpression of the gene, particularly if the purpose is to obtain large quantities of the gene product. Finally, if the purpose is to study conditions that modulate the expression of a cloned promoter, then it may be useful to have on the vector, downstream of the cloning site, a promoterless reporter gene for the easy quantitation of promoter activity.

Extrachromosomally replicating elements, particularly plasmids, that have been isolated directly from oral species, or at least shown to replicate in them, have provided the starting points in the development of new molecular and genetic systems for several oral bacterial species. One important application of plasmids has involved the development of genetic transfer systems for species in which natural mechanisms either do not exist or have not been identified. For example, the transformation with a plasmid of a species in which that plasmid will replicate enables optimization of the methodology for introducing DNA into the microorganism, for the testing of selectable markers and reporter genes, and ultimately for the construction of a useful vector molecule based on the plasmid. Data from such experiments also provide a foundation for all other molecular analyses in the native host, such as the mutagenesis of specific chromosomal genes as a means to examine the function of the gene and its gene product, i.e., the construction of isogenic mutants. A common approach to generating isogenic mutants is to use a vector that does not replicate in the bacterium of interest (i.e., a "suicide" vector), but into which has been cloned (e.g., in *E. coli*) DNA homologous to a region of the targeted gene as well as a resistance determinant that provides a marker for selection. Phenotypic analyses are then used to evaluate the effect of the gene disruption. As mentioned earlier, when a chromosomal gene disruption (knockout) blocks gene function as assessed phenotypically, it is important to rule out the possibility that the loss of function actually occurred because of a "polar effect," or inactivation of a downstream gene due to the insertion in the upstream gene. In such an experiment, an intact copy of the disrupted gene would be provided on a replicating vector in the mutant strain to demonstrate that it can restore the lost function, a process described above as complementation. Unless a gene is the only or last one in an operon, a specific function can be attributed to that gene only if the loss is restorable by complementation. In addition, if the gene function under study is essential to the bacterial strain, then complementation would have to precede its knockout. Vectors that function in oral species also enable the cloning and expression of genes in the native host background for assessment of the phenotypic properties. This is particularly critical for genes that are not expressed or the products of which are not functional in *E. coli*, including, for example, many antibiotic resistance genes found in oral species. Additionally, extrachromosomal replicating elements provide a vehicle for delivery of reporter genes to the host species, which may be used in studies of gene regulation or as a biological marker for the microorganism in multispecies systems such as biofilms and in interactions with host tissue cells.

Features of Plasmids Essential for Vector Construction

The only absolutely essential feature of a plasmid is its ability to self-replicate, i.e., to function as an independent replicon, and the most useful component of a plasmid in terms of its potential as a vector is the region required for extrachromosomal replication, referred to as the minimal replicon (see discussion below).

Initially, plasmids were categorized on the basis of their inability to coexist within a single bacterium, referred to as "incompatibility groups" (e.g., IncP and IncQ group plasmids). In essence, plasmids in a given incompatibility group cannot survive as extrachromosomal elements in the same bacterial host due to similar mechanisms controlling their propagation. More recently, plasmids have been categorized according to the particular mechanism by which they replicate. Two general modes of replication identified for circular plasmids are theta (also the mechanism used by most bacteria for replication of their chromosomes) and rolling-circle (RC) replication. Historically, theta-replicating plasmids from gram-negative bacteria and RC-replicating plasmids from gram-positive bacteria were isolated and studied in depth. However, either mechanism of replication can be employed by plasmids from both gram-positive and gram-negative bacteria, but any given plasmid replicates by one mode or the other. The features of a minimal replicon are typically contiguous on the plasmid and include an origin of replication and a gene encoding a replication initiation protein. Additional elements of importance involve regulation of replication termination, regulation of the number of copies of the plasmid per bacterial chromosome (termed the "copy number"), and mechanisms to ensure that as the bacterial cells divide each of the progeny inherits at least one copy of the plasmid (referred to as "partitioning" or segregational stability). The origin of replication, termed ori, is characteristic of the replicon and includes the site at which DNA replication is initiated. Many plasmids encode a replication initiation protein, termed a Rep protein, which binds to a DNA sequence in the corresponding ori that is characteristic of that replicon. Host proteins required for replication are provided in *trans* from genes on the host bacterial chromosome. A wide array of systems within the broad grouping of theta and RC replication are found in bacterial plasmids. Comprehensive reviews are available elsewhere, and the discussion below highlights several plasmids of interest in oral microbiology that are representative of theta- and RC-replicating plasmids.

Basic processes in the initiation of theta replication include binding of a plasmid-encoded replication protein (Rep) and the melting of an AT-rich region of the parental DNA strands to form an "open complex," followed by initiation of DNA synthesis. Once initiated, DNA synthesis is continuous on one strand ("leading strand") and discontinuous on the other ("lagging strand"), and replication may proceed in one or both directions. The term "theta replication" derives from the θ (theta)-like appearance of replication intermediates viewed by electron microscopy (Fig. 8A).

Iteron-regulated replicons, a subgroup of theta-replicating plasmids, are commonly found in gram-negative bacteria but may also be found in gram-positive species. These plasmids are characterized by a series of tandem repeats, or "iterons," in the *ori*, which provide binding sites for the corresponding plasmid-encoded Rep proteins (Fig. 8A). Additional DNA sequences in the *ori*, known as DnaA boxes, provide specific binding sites for the host-encoded DnaA protein. Oligomerization of the Rep proteins that are bound to the iterons leads to local distortion of the DNA molecule and melting of the adjacent adenine- and thymine-rich DNA region to form the open complex. This is followed, with contributions from additional host replication proteins, by initiation of DNA synthesis. One example of a native plasmid demonstrating features consistent with iteron-regulated plasmids is pFN1, isolated from a strain of *F. nucleatum*. The structural features of the putative pFN1 *ori* include six identical tandem repeats or iterons, an adjacent AT-rich region, and several putative DnaA boxes. The adjacent *rep*A is homologous with a plasmid replication initiation gene, the protein product of which is known to initiate theta replication (Fig. 8B). Experimental evidence of theta replication involves analysis of replication intermediates by either electron microscopy or two-dimensional gel electrophoretic analysis of restriction enzyme-digested replication intermediates.

The broad-host-range plasmid pAMβ1, which replicates in numerous streptococcal species including *S. mutans*, *S. sanguis*, and *Streptococcus salivarius*, utilizes a unidirectional theta mechanism that is distinct from the iteron-regulated plasmids. The basic replicon of pAMβ1 consists of a Rep protein gene, its upstream promoter (P_{repE}), and a small *ori* located downstream of the *rep* gene (Fig. 8B). The pAMβ1 *ori* does not possess repeat sequences but provides a binding site for the cognate Rep protein (RepE), and also contains a 16-bp AT-rich region. Transcription from P_{repE}, located 2 kb upstream of the *ori*, leads to expression of *rep*E. The binding of RepE to the double-stranded *ori* induces DNA melting and open complex formation. RepE additionally binds to single-stranded DNA in the open complex, and RNA transcription through the origin is required for replication initiation, possibly by providing the RNA primer needed for initiation of DNA replication.

Plasmid replication by the RC mechanism is distinct from theta replication. RC replication is described as asymmetric due to the uncoupling of leading and lagging strand synthesis, which results in the presence of a single-stranded DNA intermediate. Replication is initiated by the Rep protein (Fig. 9), which nicks the supercoiled DNA at a site known as the

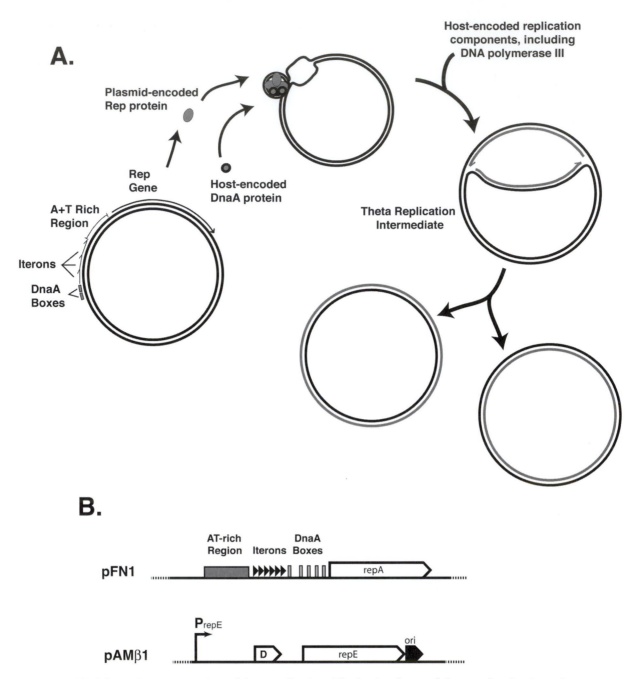

FIGURE 8 (A) Schematic representation of theta replication. The basic scheme of theta replication in an iteron-regulated plasmid is illustrated schematically. The *ori* of iteron-regulated plasmids typically possesses a series of tandem repeats at 22-bp intervals known as iterons, an A-T rich region, and DnaA-binding sequences. The plasmid-encoded Rep proteins and host-encoded DnaA proteins bind to specific DNA sequences within the iteron, inducing a melting of the parental DNA strands in the adjacent AT-rich region, and forming a pre-initiation complex. The DnaA and/or Rep protein facilitates the incorporation of additional host replication components needed for initiation. Replication proceeds in one or both directions, and leads to the characteristic theta replication intermediate structure that can be observed on examination by electron microscopy. (B) Structural features of plasmid replicons. The features of the pFN1 replicon (based on Fig. 2B in S. Kinder Haake et al., *J. Bacteriol.* **182:**1176–1180, 2000) are consistent with those of iteron-regulated plasmids. The putative *ori* contains an AT-rich region, six perfect 22-bp repeats (iterons), and several DnaA-binding sites (DnaA boxes); the downstream *rep*A homologue is related to a known theta-replication initiation protein. The features of the theta-replicating plasmid pAMβ (based on Fig. 8 in D. R. Helinski et al., p. 2295–2324, *in* F. C. Neidhardt et al. [ed.], Escherichia coli *and* Salmonella: *Cellular and Molecular Biology*, 2nd ed., vol. 2 [ASM Press, Washington, D.C., 1996]) include the *rep*E gene encoding the replication initiation protein RepE, the upstream *rep*E promoter, and the small *ori* located downstream of the *rep*E gene. See text for details of pAMβ replication initiation.

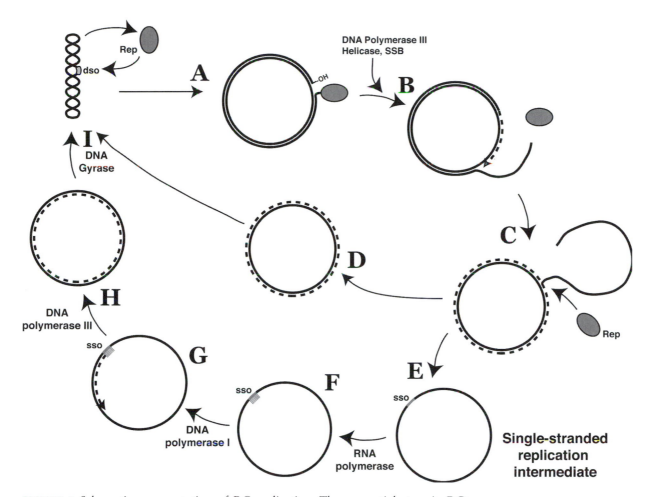

FIGURE 9 Schematic representation of RC replication. The sequential steps in RC replication are illustrated schematically. One strand of the supercoiled plasmid DNA is nicked (A) at the double-strand origin (*dso*) by the plasmid-encoded Rep protein, leaving a 3'hydroxyl end, which serves as a primer site for the initiation of DNA synthesis (B) by host cell enzymes. DNA synthesis progresses while displacing the nicked DNA strand (C) until the newly formed *dso* is reached. The Rep protein mediates cleavage and rejoining of DNA ends to yield one double-stranded plasmid (D), consisting of one parental and one newly synthesized strand, and one single-stranded DNA intermediate (E). An RNA primer is synthesized at the single-strand origin (*sso*) site (F) that provides a primer for DNA synthesis (G), which proceeds to yield a second double-stranded plasmid product (H). The double-stranded DNA is converted to the supercoiled form by DNA gyrase (I). (Adapted from Fig. 6 of G. del Solar et al., *Microbiol. Mol. Biol. Rev.* **62**:434–464, 1998.)

double-stranded origin (dso). This cleavage leaves a DNA strand with a free 3' hydroxyl that provides a primer for leading strand DNA synthesis by the host DNA polymerase III. As the newly synthesized DNA strand is elongated, the parental nicked strand is progressively displaced. Elongation continues to the newly synthesized *dso* site where the Rep protein cleaves and rejoins DNA strands, yielding one double-stranded product and one single-stranded intermediate. The single-stranded intermediate is converted to a double-stranded product by synthesis of an RNA primer at the single-stranded origin (*sso*), which is physically distinct from the *dso*, followed by DNA synthesis of the complementary strand. The conversion of the single-stranded intermediate to the double-stranded product is accomplished with host-encoded enzymes.

An RC-replicating plasmid that has proved valuable in studies of oral streptococci is pVA380-1 (Fig. 10A). This is a small plasmid of 4.24 kb that has been used extensively for cloning of streptococcal antibiotic resistance genes, construction of shuttle vectors, and mutagenesis in streptococci. The minimal replicon, for stable maintenance of the plasmid at the copy number consistent with the native plasmid, includes the contiguous region of the plasmid encoding the *dso*, *rep* gene, and *sso*. The *sso* is not essential to maintenance, but deletion of this element results in accumulation of the single-stranded replication intermediate and a loss of segregational stability (i.e., a significant portion, but not all, of the bacterial cells lose the plasmid during growth under nonselective conditions).

Both theta- and RC-replicating plasmids have been isolated from and used in molecular analyses of oral microorganisms. Plasmids that replicate by the RC mechanism are typically smaller than 10 kb in size. However, small size does not mean that a plasmid uses a RC replication mechanism, as theta-replicating plasmids less than 10 kb have also been identified. Large plasmids, such as the 25.4-kb conjugative plasmid pVT745 from *A. actinomycetemcomitans* (Fig. 6), are believed to repli-

FIGURE 10 Schematic illustration of plasmids used in molecular mutagenesis of *S. sobrinus*. (A) Native streptococcal plasmid pVA380-1. This native plasmid was isolated from a strain of *S. ferus*. It uses an RC mechanism for replication and the *dso*, *sso*, and *rep* genes are indicated. The plasmid also possesses a mobilization gene (*mob*) and is able to be mobilized to several streptococcal species when the conjugative plasmid pAMβ1 is also present in the donor bacterium. (Adapted from Fig. 1 in D. J. LeBlanc et al., *Plasmid* 30:296–302, 1993, with permission from Elsevier.) (B) Shuttle vector pDL289Δ202. The *E. coli-Streptococcus* shuttle vector was constructed by using ΔpVA380-1 (gray region), which has a 202-bp fragment of the *sso* deleted (Δ*sso*), an *E. coli* replicon from the plasmid pSC101 (black region), a kanamycin resistance determinant (*kan*), and the *lacZ*-MSC from pGEM7. Specific regions of ΔpVA380-1 are indicated with the open bars inside the plasmid. pDL289Δ202 has been transferred to several strains of streptococci, including *S. gordonii*, *S. mutans*, and *S. sobrinus*, when the conjugative plasmid pAMβ1 is also present in the donor bacterium. (Adapted from Fig. 1 in D. J. LeBlanc et al., *Methods Cell Sci.* 20:85–93, 1998, with kind permission of Springer Science and Business Media.)

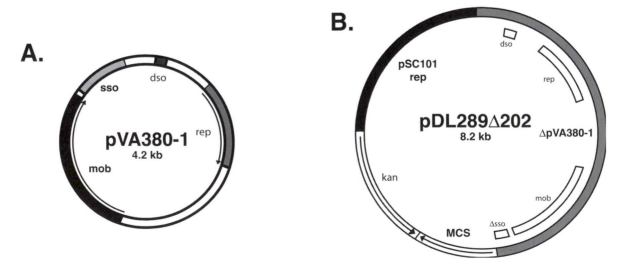

cate by a theta mechanism. Future investigations of plasmid ecology in the oral microbiota are likely to result in the identification of other types of extrachromosomal elements, e.g., linear plasmids.

The second most important feature of a vector is the presence of a marker that enables selection for cells that possess it. Quite often, the presence on a plasmid of a selectable marker is what has led to its discovery. Useful selectable markers typically encode resistance to antimicrobial agents that can be incorporated into media. This enables growth of cells harboring the resistance determinant while inhibiting the growth of cells lacking the element. The most common selectable markers encode resistance to antibiotics, but resistance to other agents toxic to bacteria, such as heavy metals, may also be plasmid-encoded. The choice of a selectable marker to use in vector development is based on consideration of several factors: the susceptibility profile of the host species and strain, as well as the known occurrence of resistance and resistance determinants in the species. If native selectable markers are not available for a given species, a reasonable alternative is to test markers that are known to function in related species. However, ethical considerations prevent the de novo introduction of determinants encoding resistance to antimicrobial agents that are used in the clinical treatment of infections involving the target species. Antibiotic resistance in the oral microbiota is discussed in detail in chapter 17 and will not be discussed further here.

Use of Native Plasmids in Molecular Analyses

Understanding the fundamental mechanisms of plasmid biology facilitates the development of genetic tools for molecular analysis of bacterial species. Results of studies on one plasmid in particular, pVA380-1 (Fig. 10A), have had a major influence on the development of molecular and genetic tools for the analysis of the lactic acid bacteria in general and of members of the oral streptococci in particular. This 4.2-kb cryptic plasmid was originally isolated from a strain of *S. ferus*. The construction of a restriction endonuclease map of pVA380-1 revealed the presence of several unique sites on the molecule, e.g., for such enzymes as EcoRI, HindIII, and EcoRV, a feature that was exploited subsequently in the cloning into pVA380-1 of several antibiotic resistance determinants from oral streptococcal isolates. The antibiotic resistance containing derivations of pVA380-1 were then introduced directly in the Challis strain of *S. gordonii* by natural transformation. Results of these early cloning experiments indicated that while cloning of genes into the native strains was essential to identifying resistance determinants phenotypically, the efficiency of cloning directly into the native strain proved cumbersome. As a result, a chimeric plasmid that combined features enabling replication in both streptococci and *E. coli* was constructed. This *E. coli-Streptococcus* shuttle vector, pVA838, is able to replicate in both *E. coli* and *S. gordonii*. Construction of pVA838 involved combining the *E. coli* plasmid pACYC184 and the streptococcal plasmid pVA749. The ability of pVA838 to replicate in *E. coli* was provided by pACYC184, which could be selected by propagation in the presence of chloramphenicol or tetracycline, resistance to each being encoded by pACYC184. The ability of pVA838 to replicate in streptococci was provided by pVA749, which had previously been constructed by the cloning of an erythromycin resistance gene, selectable in either streptococci or *E. coli*, onto intact pVA380-1, the native streptococcal plasmid. The availability of pVA838 made it possible, at least theoretically, to clone virtually any streptococcal gene, selectable or not, directly in *E. coli,* in which cloning is considerably more efficient than in most other bacterial species. The resultant recombinant molecule could be isolated from *E. coli*, and the cloned gene, and any traits encoded by it, could then be studied in a streptococcal host. Results of additional studies on pVA380-1 and on antibiotic resistance in gram-positive bacteria led to the construction of more efficient *E. coli-Streptococcus* shuttle vectors, such as pDL276 and pDL278. These vectors were smaller, 6.9 kb (pDL276) and 6.6 kb (pDL278), being composed of the basic replicon (<2.5 kb) of pVA380-1, than pVA838 (9.2 kb), and thus able to accommodate larger segments of cloned DNA. They each had only one antibiotic resistance gene, encoding resistance to either kanamycin (pDL276) or spectinomycin (pDL278), which was expressed in most gram-negative (such as *E. coli*) and gram-positive (such as streptococci) bacteria. The *E. coli* replicon of each was from one of the high-copy number pUC plasmids, and the site for cloning, derived from a pGEM vector, contained many more single restriction endonuclease sites than pVA838, and was flanked by transcriptional terminators to prevent readthrough into the vector.

The availability of *E. coli-Streptococcus* shuttle vectors was not enough to permit genetic and molecular analyses of all oral streptococcal species. An example illustrating this point relates to the acidogenic oral bacterium *Streptococcus sobrinus*, which was known in the early 1990s to be cariogenic but was not amenable to molecular analyses using existing approaches and tools, because members of this species were not transformable, either by natural competence or by electroporation. However, results of the analyses of pVA380-1 had defined not only the plasmid replicon and its basic elements, but also a mobilization gene homologue (*mob*). As mentioned earlier in this chapter, small plasmids that cannot mediate their own interbacterial transfer via conjugation may be mobilized in the presence of the gene products of larger conjugative plasmids. Typically the small plasmid encodes a mobilization protein responsible for nicking its DNA strand at a site referred to as the origin of transfer (*ori*T). With the gene products necessary for conjugation provided by the coresident larger plasmid, the nicked single-stranded DNA strand is subsequently transferred to the recipient cell. The small size of a mobilizable plasmid provides an advantage in molecular manipulations, in contrast to a larger conjugative plasmid. The smaller plasmids are more likely to have a greater number of unique restriction enzyme sites for use in cloning and, in general, larger DNA fragments can be cloned into them. In addition, conjugative transfer of DNA involves the introduction of single-stranded DNA into the recipient bacterial cell. Because restriction endonucleases typically digest double-stranded DNA, conjugative transfer may provide a means of bypassing a host cell restriction barrier. Thus gene transfer using conjugation may be possible with bacterial strains and species that are not naturally competent and not amenable to electroporation-based transformation.

Genetic transfer of DNA to *S. sobrinus* was accomplished using conjugative mechanisms. Identification of the pVA380-1 mobilization gene homologue and a putative *ori*T led to recognition that derivates of pVA380-1 can be mobilized by the coresident conjugative plasmid pAMβ1, which had been shown in the late 1970s to transfer to numerous streptococcal species, including *S. sobrinus*. *S. gordonii* harboring a pVA380-1 derivative and pAMβ1 functions as a donor strain, transferring the pVA380-1 derivative to other recipient streptococci, including *S. sobrinus*. Consequently, an *E. coli-Streptococcus* shuttle plasmid was constructed (pDL289Δ202 [Fig. 10B]) using pVA380-1 as the source of the streptococcal replicon and the *mob* gene, a replicon from the plasmid pSC101 to enable replication in *E. coli*, a gene conferring resistance to kanamycin, and a multicloning site from the *E. coli* vector pGEM7 providing unique restriction enzyme sites for cloning. In pDL289Δ202, the *sso* of pVA380-1 was partially deleted (ΔpVA380-1 [Fig. 10B]) as a strategy to promote recombination of homologous DNA inserted into the shuttle plasmid due to the loss of the replicative plasmid along with an increase in the single-stranded replication intermediate. This shuttle plasmid was then used to create an isogenic mutant of *S. sobrinus* with an insertion in the *scrA* gene, a permease important in sugar transport. A portion of the *scrA* gene, disrupted with a spectinomycin resistance gene, was cloned into pDL289Δ202 and used to generate a mutation in the chromosomal *scrA* gene by allelic exchange (Fig. 11). This process required two "crossover" or recombination events between the identical DNA regions of the plasmid (*scrA'* and *scr''* [Fig. 11]) and the chromosome. Host cell mechanisms and gene products mediate the recombination. Characterization of native streptococcal plasmids in this case led to the use of the conjugative plasmid pAMβ1 to mobilize the smaller pVA380-1-derived shuttle plasmid, establishing gene transfer to *S. sobrinus* for the first time and thus commencing molecular analysis in an important pathogenic oral bacterium.

Native plasmids have also been important in studies of the oral spirochetes, a group of microorganisms involved in disease processes that have proved difficult to study. A major handicap has been that many of the oral, as well as significant nonoral, spirochetes cannot be cultivated in the laboratory. In addition, spirochetes differ structurally and physiologically from *E. coli*, limiting the functional studies of spirochete gene products in *E. coli*. One of the distinctive features of spirochetes is their mobility. Spirochete motility is mediated by endoflagella, which reside in the periplasmic space between the cytoplasmic membrane and the outer sheath of the bacterium, and are connected to components in the cytoplasmic membrane by a flagellar hook protein. Mutation of the chromosomal *flg*E gene, which encodes the flagellar hook protein, was accomplished in an oral spirochete, *T. denticola*, a species that can be cultivated in vitro. A plasmid unable to replicate in *T. denticola*, but containing a portion of *flg*E interrupted by the erythromycin resistance cassette (pHLfE [Fig. 12]), was used to create the mutant by allelic exchange. Because pHLfE lacked a *T. denticola* replicon (thus referred to as a "suicide plasmid"), erythromycin-resistant transformants could only arise by recombination of the plasmid DNA into the bacterial chromosome. Analysis of transformants demonstrated disruption of the chromosomal *flg*E gene with the erythromycin resistance cassette and loss of the periplasmic endoflagella (Fig. 13). This

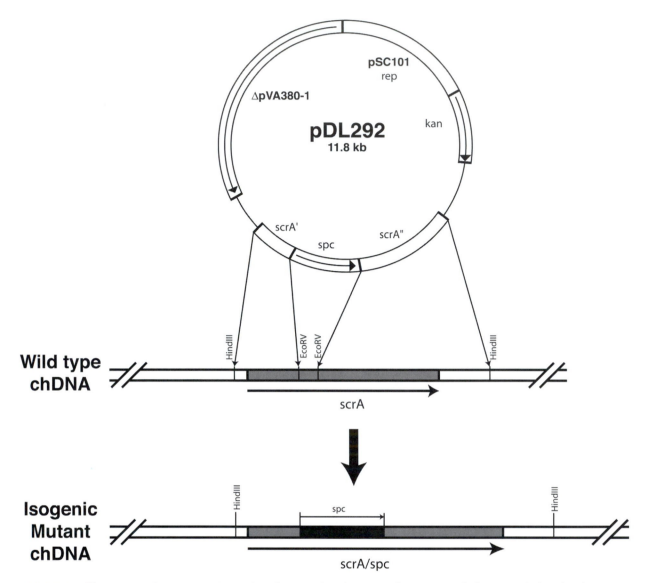

FIGURE 11 Chromosomal mutagenesis in *S. sobrinus*. A schematic illustration of the use of the shuttle vector pDL289Δ202 to introduce a chromosomal mutation in *S. sobrinus* is shown. A segment of *S. sobrinus* chromosomal DNA encoding the *scrA* gene was cloned, and a spectinomycin resistance gene inserted into an *EcoRV* fragment within *scrA* to interrupt the gene. The interrupted *scrA* gene was then cloned into pDL289Δ202 to generate pDL292. This plasmid was first transferred to *S. gordonii*, and then the conjugative plasmid pAMβ1 was transferred to the same strain. The donor strain, harboring both plasmids, was used to mobilize pDL292 to *S. sobrinus*. Homologous regions providing sites for DNA recombination between pDL292 and the chromosomal DNA are indicated (arrows). Transconjugants, in which the wild-type chromosomal *scrA* gene was replaced, were identified by their resistance to spectinomycin (indicating the presence of *spc*) and susceptibility to kanamycin (indicating the loss of pDL289Δ202). (Adapted from Fig. 3 of N. D. Buckley et al., *J. Bacteriol.* **177**:5028–5034, 1995.)

FIGURE 12 Schematic illustration of plasmids constructed for use in *T. denticola*. The pHLfE plasmid was constructed to use in allelic replacement of a fragment of the *T. denticola* chromosomal flagellar hook protein gene, *flgE*, with a mutant copy possessing an internal erythromycin resistance cassette to disrupt the gene. pHLfE includes an *E. coli ori* but not a *T. denticola ori*, so that the plasmid cannot exist in *T. denticola* as an extrachromosomal replicating element. The erythromycin resistance cassette, consisting of *ermF* and *ermB*, was cloned into a site within a cloned *flgE* fragment, leaving the two gene fragments *flgEI* and *flgEII* flanking the resistance cassette. (Adapted from Fig. 1 of H. Li et al., *J. Bacteriol.* **178**:3664–3667, 1996.) pTS1 is a cryptic native plasmid isolated from *T. denticola* strain U9b. DNA sequence analysis revealed putative *rep* and *mob* gene homologues and two additional overlapping open reading

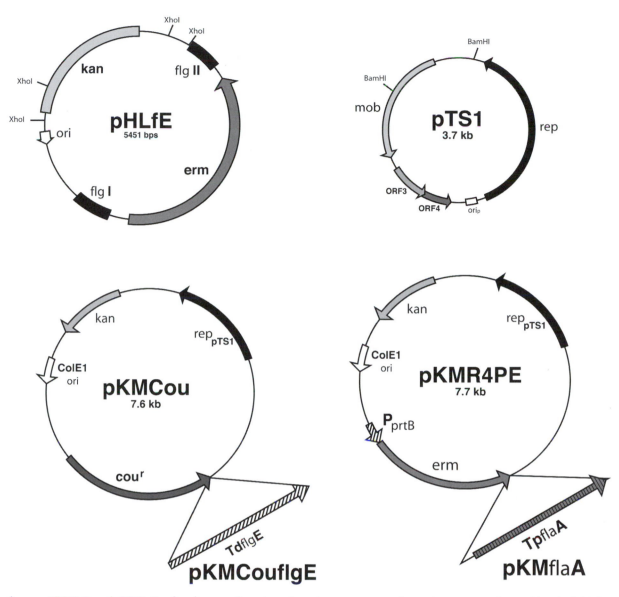

frames (ORF 3 and ORF 4) of unknown function. A region upstream of *rep* demonstrated two identical 22-bp repeats and overlapping inverted repeats, suggestive of iteron-like features of a putative origin (*ori$_p$*). A 2.7-kb fragment of pTS1 including *ori$_p$* and *rep*, isolated by digestion with BamHI, was used as a source of a native replicon in the construction of *E. coli-T. denticola* shuttle plasmids (pKMCou and pKMR4PE). (Adapted from Fig. 1 in S. Chauhan and H. K. Kuramitsu, *Plasmid* **51**:61–65, 2004, with permission from Elsevier.) pKMCou, a shuttle plasmid, is designed to replicate in *E. coli* using the ColE1 *ori* and in *T. denticola* using the pTS1 replicon. The *kan* gene provides selection in *E. coli*, and the coumermycin (Cou^r) resistance gene provides selection in *T. denticola*. Coumermycin is an antibiotic that inhibits a host cell enzyme, DNA gyrase, which is important in DNA function. The Cou^r determinant consists of a spontaneous mutant of the *T. denticola* DNA gyrase subunit GyrB that confers resistance to coumermycin. The *T. denticola flg*E gene (Td*flg*E) was cloned into pKMCou, forming pKMCou*flg*E, which was then used to complement a chromosomal mutation in the *flg*E gene in *T. denticola* (see text for further details). Note that the chromosomal *flg*E mutation includes the erythromycin resistance cassette, necessitating the use of an alternate selectable marker in the plasmids used for complementation. (Adapted from Fig. 1 in B. Chi et al., *Infect. Immun.* **70**:2233–2237, 2002.) pKMR4PE is another *E. coli-T. denticola* shuttle plasmid, in this case using the erythromycin cassette for selection in *T. denticola*. A native *T. denticola* promoter, P$_{prtB}$ from the *prt*B protease gene, was cloned upstream of the erythromycin cassette to ensure its transcription in *T. denticola*. This shuttle plasmid was used for expression of the heterologous *fla*A gene of *T. pallidum* in *T. denticola*. The *T. pallidum fla*A gene (Tp*fla*A) was cloned downstream of the erythromycin cassette and used to transform *T. denticola*. The erythromycin-resistant transformant strain was shown to express the *T. pallidum* FlaA protein. (Adapted from Fig. 1 of B. Chi et al., *Infect. Immun.* **67**:3653–3656, 1999.)

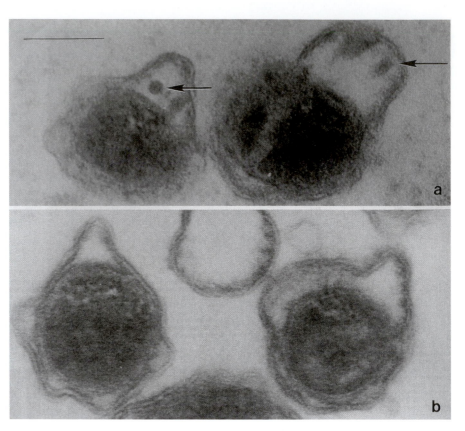

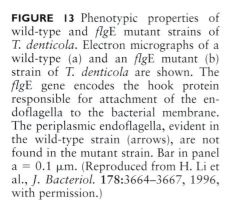

FIGURE 13 Phenotypic properties of wild-type and *flg*E mutant strains of *T. denticola*. Electron micrographs of a wild-type (a) and an *flg*E mutant (b) strain of *T. denticola* are shown. The *flg*E gene encodes the hook protein responsible for attachment of the endoflagella to the bacterial membrane. The periplasmic endoflagella, evident in the wild-type strain (arrows), are not found in the mutant strain. Bar in panel a = 0.1 μm. (Reproduced from H. Li et al., *J. Bacteriol.* **178**:3664–3667, 1996, with permission.)

chromosomal mutation was complemented using an *E. coli-T. denticola* shuttle vector (pKMCou*flg*E [Fig. 12]) possessing a replicon from the native *T. denticola* plasmid pTS1 (Fig. 12) and an intact copy of the *flg*E gene. The mutant strain was shown to be nonmotile, in contrast to both the wild-type strain and the complemented mutant. Demonstration that disruption of the *flg*E gene caused a loss of motility and that complementation of the chromosomal mutation restored motility confirms that the loss of motility is due to the disruption of the *flg*E gene.

A second shuttle vector constructed using the *T. denticola* pTS1 replicon has been used for expression of a gene from a heterologous nonoral pathogenic spirochete, *Treponema pallidum*. *T. pallidum*, the causative agent of syphilis, can be grown in rabbit testes, but no systems of genetic transfer are available for this species. The *E. coli-T. denticola* shuttle vector, pKMR4PE, was constructed using the ColE1 replicon for *E. coli*, the pTS1 replicon, and the erythromycin resistance cassette (Fig. 12). The *T. pallidum fla*A gene, which encodes the endoflagellin protein, was cloned into the shuttle vector (pKM*fla*A) and used to transform *T. denticola* by electroporation. Erythromycin-resistant transformants were shown to possess the plasmid and to express the *T. pallidum* FlaA protein. The expression of a heterologous spirochete gene in *T. denticola* demonstrates that this system may be valuable in molecular analysis of genes from other spirochetes, potentially including noncultivable oral spirochetes.

Use of Nonnative or Broad-Host-Range Plasmids in Molecular Analyses

The use of native plasmids in the development of systems for gene transfer provides the advantage of a replicon known to function in the species of interest by virtue of the isolation of the plasmid from that species. However, there may be specific applications for which the properties of native plasmids are not desirable. In addition, native plasmids may not be found in some species of interest, such as *P. gingivalis*. In these instances, the use of plasmids known to function in a broad range of species may be of benefit. There are a substantial number of broad-host-range plasmids from nonoral species that function in oral microorganisms. *A. actinomycetemcomitans* is an example of an oral pathogen for which both native and broad-host-range plasmids have been used. *P. gingivalis* provides an example of an oral pathogen found to be lacking in native plasmids but amenable to the use of selected plasmids from related bacterial species.

The first reports of transformation of *A. actinomycetemcomitans* used broad-host-range conjugative (pRK2525 and pRK212.2) and mobilizable (pBK1) plasmids (Table 7). Although these plasmids are stable in *A. actinomycetemcomitans*, they are large and thus cumbersome for use as cloning or shuttle plasmids. The native plasmid pVT736-1 is a 2-kb element that provides an *A. actinomycetemcomitans*-specific replicon that has been used in the construction of several vectors designed for cloning in *A. actinomycetemcomitans* (pDMG1 and pDMG2 in Table 7). However, the *E. coli*-*A. actinomycetemcomitans* shuttle plasmid pDL282 using the pVT736-1 replicon was found to be structurally unstable, suffering deletion on passage without antibiotics. pDL282 was additionally unstable segregationally, meaning that the plasmid did not efficiently segregate into daughter cells and was lost from the population after passage without antibiotics. Due to these difficulties a systematic investigation of replicons functioning in *A. actinomycetemcomitans* was undertaken. Alternate replicons, including p15A from the *E. coli* vector pACYC184 and the replicon of pWV01 from *Lactococcus lactis*, were found to function in *A. actinomycetemcomitans*. The shuttle plasmid pDMG4 was of particular interest based on its small size (3.4 kb), with a single replicon (p15A) that functions in both *A. actinomycetemcomitans* and *E. coli*. pDMG4 proved to be structurally and segregationally stable with selection, and was demonstrated to function in cloning of *A. actinomycetemcomitans* DNA in both species. Thus, pDMG4, which possesses the heterologous p15A replicon, appears to be better suited for use as a shuttle plasmid than constructs using the native *A. actinomycetemcomitans* plasmid replicon.

P. gingivalis has been the focus of intensive investigation of putative virulence determinants due to its strong association with periodontitis. The cloning of *P. gingivalis* genes encoding proteases and adhesins has led to investigation of their properties in the heterologous *E. coli* host system, and targeted mutations in selected genes in strains of *P. gingivalis* have greatly enhanced our understanding of the properties of the gene products in the native host environment. A limitation of many of these studies, however, has been the lack of complementation of the chromosomal

TABLE 7 Selected plasmids for use in *A. actinomycetemcomitans* and *P. gingivalis*

Bacterial host	Plasmid(s)	Relevant properties	Replicon[a]	Plasmid size	Plasmid stability	Comments
A. actinomycetemcomitans (Aa)	pRK2525, pRK212.2	Ampicillin and kanamycin resistance; conjugative	RK2	60 (pRK2525) to 67 (pRK212.2) kb	Structurally stable	Transformation of *Aa* with these IncP plasmids provided proof of principle for conjugal transfer to *Aa* and functioning of the RK2 replicon; the large size of these plasmids limits their use as vector systems
	pBKI	Chloramphenicol and ampicillin resistance; mobilizable	RSF1010	12.5 kb	Structurally stable	Mobilization of pBKI (an IncQ plasmid) by a chromosomally integrated IncP plasmid in *E. coli* SM10; large size in comparison with other plasmids a potential disadvantage
	pDL282	Spectinomycin resistance	ColEI/ replicon from *Aa* plasmid pVT736-I	5.8 kb	Structurally and segregationally stable with selection	Potential use in *Aa* and *E. coli*, but without selection plasmid is structurally and segregationally unstable
	pDMGI[b]	Erythromycin resistance	pVT736-I replicon	3.7 kb	Structurally and segregationally stable	Potential use in cloning directly in *Aa* (does not replicate in *E. coli*)
	pDMG3[b]	Spectinomycin resistance	pVT736-I replicon	3.1 kb	Structurally and segregationally stable	Potential use in cloning directly in *Aa* (does not replicate in *E. coli*)
	pDMG4	Spectinomycin resistance	p15A	3.4 kb	Structurally and segregationally stable with selection	Demonstrated use in cloning of *Aa* DNA in *E. coli*, and stable maintenance of the recombinant molecule in *Aa*
	pGA14/spc	Spectinomycin resistance	pVVOI	5.6 kb	Structurally and segregationally stable with selection	May be of use, but attempts to clone into the plasmid have not yielded positive results
	pDL293	Spectinomycin resistance	RSF1010	9.9 kb	Structurally and segregationally stable	Large size in comparison with other plasmids a potential disadvantage
P. gingivalis	pE5-2	Erythromycin and clindamycin resistance; mobilizable	RSF1010/ replicon from *Bacteroides* plasmid pB8-51	17.1 kb	Structurally and segregationally unstable	This plasmid is mobilized from *E. coli* by a coresident plasmid R751 to *P. gingivalis*. pE5-2 harbors a transposon, Tn435I, that is observed to insert in the chromosome in a significant percentage of transconjugants.
	pYH400	Ampicillin and erythromycin resistance	ColEI/ replicon from *P. asaccharolytica* plasmid pYHBAI	12.8 kb	Structurally and segregationally stable	High rates of transformation in selected recipient strains. Large size and limited convenient restriction endonuclease sites may limit utility.
	pYH420[c]	Erythromycin resistance	pYHBAI replicon	8.9 kb	Structurally and segregationally stable	Smaller size and unique cloning sites provide some advantages. High rates of transformation in selected recipient strains.

[a] Notes on replicons: RK2 is a broad-host-range conjugative plasmid of the IncP family; RSF1010 is found on broad-host-range plasmids of the IncQ family that are not conjugative but are mobilizable; pVT736-I is a 2-kb plasmid native to *A. actinomycetemcomitans*; ColEI is an *E. coli* replicon; p15A is replicon from the *E. coli* cloning vector pACYC184, which is compatible with ColEI; pVVOI is a native plasmid of *L. lactis*.

[b] Note that pDMGI and pDMG3 possess only the replicon from the *A. actinomycetemcomitans* native plasmid pVT736-I, which does not function in *E. coli*.

[c] Note that pYH420 lacks the *E. coli* replicon.

mutation to demonstrate restoration of function with the intact gene. Numerous studies have failed to detect plasmids in strains of *P. gingivalis*, and the development of plasmids that function in this species has relied on the use of native plasmids from closely related species (Table 7). The *E. coli-Bacteroides* shuttle plasmid pE5-2 was mobilized to *P. gingivalis* but is not stably maintained. pE5-2 possesses a transposon that inserts into the host cell chromosome under selective conditions, and the plasmid is lost under nonselective conditions. Studies with pE5-2 clearly demonstrated that plasmid DNA isolated from *P. gingivalis* was much more efficient in transforming *P. gingivalis* than plasmid DNA isolated from *E. coli*. This presumably is due to an indigenous restriction-modification system, so that the methylation of DNA in *P. gingivalis* protects it from cleavage by the host cell restriction endonuclease. However, *P. gingivalis* strains amenable to transformation with DNA from any source, presumed to be deficient in restriction endonuclease activity, have been isolated. These strains were then used to identify replicons that would function in *P. gingivalis* from plasmids of related species. A native plasmid of the related species *Porphyromonas asaccharolytica* was successfully used to generate the *E. coli-P. gingivalis* plasmid pYH400 and the *P. gingivalis* plasmid pYH420. These plasmids, which are stably maintained in *P. gingivalis*, along with the selected strains amenable to transformation, provide a feasible host vector system for investigation of this oral pathogen. More recently, pT-COW, based on the *Bacteroides-E. coli* shuttle vector pVAL1, has successfully been used for complementation in *P. gingivalis*.

Integration Vectors

The recombinant DNA vectors and shuttle plasmids described above, able to replicate in the oral bacterial species of interest or in both *E. coli* and the species of interest, facilitated the cloning of oral bacterial DNA and made possible the study of oral bacterial gene functions in their native host species. Descriptions of vectors that either are improvements on existing molecules or extend the spectrum of oral bacterial species amenable to genetic analysis continue to appear in the literature. However, certain types of studies cannot be conducted with genes of interest that have been cloned onto replicating plasmids. For instance, one may wish to conduct studies on a bacterial species in the absence of a particular gene product to learn more about the contribution of that product to the overall phenotype of the species. It may also be advantageous to determine if the product of a gene is essential for survival of the bacterial cell, as in the case of potential targets for new antimicrobial agents. One approach to eliminating a gene function is to attempt to interrupt or delete the gene, i.e., construct a functional knockout. If this can be done, then the gene clearly is not essential and studies on its contributions to the host species phenotype can be pursued. If attempts to knock out the gene fail, it can only be considered putatively essential, since failure to knock it out may have been due to faulty experimental design or the essentiality of a downstream gene on the same operon. Therefore, it is necessary to add to the strain a second, complementing copy of the gene, e.g., on a vector, and then show that under these circumstances the chromosomal copy can be knocked out by conducting the original knockout experiment on the strain carrying the complementing gene copy.

How would an investigator knock out the gene in the first place? One mechanism by which this could be accomplished was provided by results of further analysis of the first *E. coli-Streptococcus* shuttle vector described earlier in this chapter. Attempts were made to decrease the size of the shuttle plasmid pVA838 by digesting it with restriction endonucleases for which there were few sites. After digestion, the resultant fragments were religated and used to transform *E. coli* and *S. gordonii* with selection for the appropriate resistance phenotype. One product of these experiments was pVA891, which was isolated from an erythromycin-resistant *E. coli* transformant but had lost the ability to replicate in streptococci. The region of pVA838 mediating replication in streptococci was not present on the religated fragment, but because the *erm* gene had been retained, selection in streptococci was still possible. If fragments of streptococcal DNA internal to genes of interest were cloned into pVA891, in *E. coli*, the resultant recombinant plasmid could be isolated from *E. coli* and used to transform a strain of *Streptococcus*. Erythromycin-resistant streptococcal transformants could be obtained if the plasmid was rescued via integration into the transformant chromosome, due to homology between the cloned gene fragment and the intact gene in the streptococcal chromosome. Thus, pVA891 was the first of many streptococcal "suicide" or "integration" vectors to be described. Such a vector cannot survive by replication when introduced into a streptococcal strain, but if DNA with homology to chromosomal DNA has been cloned onto it, the entire plasmid will become integrated into the transformed host chromosome at the site of homology. The plasmid DNA will now be replicated as part of the chromosome, and the gene of interest will be inactivated due to insertion duplication of just an internal fragment of it. This same approach can be applied to virtually any oral bacterial species that is transformable, due either to the ability to achieve a natural state of competence or via artificial means such as electroporation, as long as the integration vector encodes a resistance gene that is expressed in that species. Numerous integration vectors with a variety of resistance markers have been described. Two or more such vectors may be used in the same bacterial species to construct a strain with multiple gene knockouts.

Very often it is not advantageous to examine gene functions when they are expressed on a plasmid vector, possibly because the vector is structurally unstable in the host species of interest, or because the plasmid is rapidly lost in the absence of antibiotic selection, and such selection may interfere with or alter the phenotype(s) expressed by the cloned gene. In other instances, the expression of multiple copies of the cloned gene, as is the case when the gene is encoded on a plasmid vector, may not provide an accurate picture of its true physiological function in the cell when present in a single copy on the host chromosome. And, in some cases, overexpression of a gene may be toxic to the bacterial cell. Several genetic systems have been devised by which a cloned gene can be integrated into a bacterial host chromosome so as to examine the effects of a single copy expression of that gene. One such system is of particular interest because it provides a mechanism by which a cloned fragment of DNA can be transferred to, and integrated into, the chromosome of either a transformable or non-transformable streptococcal species, and it is applicable to DNA that may or may not share homology with the chromosome of the target bacterial species. The system is composed of a specialized integration vector and one or more transformable streptococcal strains in which the vector can integrate into the chromosome. The integration vector pDP36 consists of pVA891 flanked by DNA from a conjugative element, Ω6001, which is similar to the conjugative transposon, Tn916. The construction of pDP36 resulted in a 1.1-kb deletion of Ω6001 DNA that caused a deletion of its tetM gene. Virtually any DNA, with or without homology to the target host species, can be ligated to pDP36 and cloned in E. coli by selection for resistance to chloramphenicol, which is encoded on the pVA891 plasmid. Subsequently, the resultant recombinant plasmid can be isolated from E. coli and transferred to a naturally transformable streptococcal species, e.g., S. gordonii that carries Ω6001 in its chromosome. Since pDP36 cannot replicate in a streptococcal host, the only way that it, or a recombinant DNA molecule derived from it, will survive in such a host is to integrate into the new host chromosome, due to the extensive homology on either side of pVA891 to Ω6001. Transformants are selected in the presence of erythromycin, resistance to which is also encoded by pVA891. Such transformants will also be susceptible to tetracycline, due to the replacement of a large segment of Ω6001, including its functional tetM gene, with the portion of this element containing the inactivated tetM gene. The function(s) encoded by the DNA cloned into pDP36 in E. coli can now be studied in the S. gordonii transformant, in which they are present in this host's chromosome in single copy. Also because of the integration of the recombinant pDP36 molecule into Ω6001, it has now become an integral part of a conjugative element that can be transferred to nontransformable streptococcal strains via conjugation. Thus, the pDP36 recombinant DNA system could theoretically be used to clone virtually any bacterial gene and to subsequently study, and utilize for various purposes, its expression by any species of Streptococcus.

Variations of the concept described above were used to clone a Streptococcus pyogenes gene, emm6.1, into the pVA891 portion of such an integration vector. The cloned gene, emm6.1, encodes the surface-expressed protein, M6, transcriptionally fused to a constitutively expressed S. gordonii promoter. The recombinant vector was then used to transform S. gordonii, and in transformants the expression of M6 on the S. gordonii cell surface was demonstrated. This concept has been developed even further by showing that cloned gene products expressed on the surface by S. gordonii could be used to elicit the production of specific antibodies by animals colonized by the recombinant S. gordonii strains. In one instance, a gene encoding the E7 protein of a human papillomavirus was cloned as a translational fusion with the constitutively expressed M6 protein. This recombinant plasmid was then used to transform S. gordonii, and it became integrated into the chromosome. The resultant recombinant strain was shown to make the viral E7 protein, and because it was made as a fusion protein with M6, it was transported to and expressed on the surface of the S. gordonii cells. Such a strain was then used to inoculate mice, and was shown to colonize the mice as readily as the original wild-type S. gordonii strain. The recombinant strains, however, were shown to induce a systemic immune response by the mice, and their sera were shown to contain immunoglobulin G antibodies specific for the viral protein. Thus, it was demonstrated that recombinant S. gordonii strains, expressing foreign proteins on their surface, could potentially be used for the production of vaccines against viral pathogens.

Another integration vector, pBGK, specifically constructed for the study of *S. mutans* promoters, was designed to overcome a number of problems often faced in the cloning and analysis of streptococcal genes. The vector consisted of the *E. coli* plasmid, pBR322, flanked by sequences of the nonessential *S. mutans* gene, *gtfA*, and a kanamycin resistance element, ΩKm, just upstream of a cloning site containing the recognition sequences of several restriction endonucleases. DNA cloned into this vector, following transformation of *S. mutans*, would be integrated into the chromosome via a double crossover event due to the flanking *gtfA* sequences. Originally, the integration vector had contained the *E. coli* cloning vector, pUC19, but it was found that when *S. mutans* promoters were cloned into it, the recombinant molecules would suffer deletions of various sizes in the *gtfA* regions. This may have been due to high copy number of pUC19 and/or to the toxicity of products made in such a high copy number. Thus, pUC19 was replaced with the lower copy number plasmid, pBR322. The ΩKm element, which expressed resistance to kanamycin in both *E. coli* and *S. mutans*, was included just upstream of the cloning site because it is flanked by transcriptional terminators, as well as translational terminators in all six reading frames, which would serve to prevent any potential readthrough from the promoter of the operon that controls expression of *gtfA*. Such expression through *gtfA* DNA might complicate interpretations of results of studies on the intended promoter(s). The utility of pBGK has been demonstrated by cloning the promoter of the *S. mutans* gene, *fruA*, encoding fructan hydrolase, fused to a promoterless *cat* gene. After integration of the recombinant plasmid into the *S. mutans gtf* gene, the influence of different carbohydrates on the expression of the *fruA* promoter could be followed by measuring the expression of the reporter gene, *cat*.

Integrative vectors have been described for oral bacterial genera other than *Streptococcus*, and very likely will be constructed for a variety of uses in virtually any species that can be transformed, either by natural transformation or by some artificial means, such as electroporation. The only absolutely required feature of any integration vector is the presence of DNA with sufficient homology to the intended host's chromosome to facilitate integration.

Genes of bacterial species that are naturally transformable, such as many of the oral streptococcal species, can be manipulated without a requirement for vectors of any kind. Linear double-stranded DNA can be used to transform such species, and transforming molecules of virtually any composition can be constructed by a method referred to as fusion PCR. For instance, if one wished to delete a gene designated gene B completely, in the order ABC on the host chromosome, then it would only be necessary to construct an amplicon composed of an antibiotic resistance gene, e.g., gene X, flanked on one side by DNA from gene A and on the other side by DNA from gene C. If such an amplicon was used to transform a strain containing gene B, followed by selection on a medium containing the antibiotic to which resistance is encoded by gene X, then transformants would be selected in which gene B has been displaced by gene X, due to a double crossover event based on the homology between genes A and C in the amplicon and the host chromosome. In fusion PCR, the transforming amplicon composed of genes AXC is constructed as follows. Pairs of oligonucleotide primers would be designed such that for the first pair, one would consist of perhaps the first 20 bases at the 5' end of gene A, for synthesis of the 5' to 3' strand of gene A, and the second would contain 10 or so bases from the 5' end of gene X and 10 or so from the 3' end of gene A for synthesis of the 3' to 5' strand of gene A, such that the amplicon synthesized would consist of the 3' end of approximately 1,000 bp of gene A DNA with about 10 bp of homology to the 5' end of gene X. Oligonucleotide primers for the synthesis of gene X would be designed so that the 5' end of the gene amplicon would have approximately 10 bp of homology to the 3' end of gene A and the 3' end of it would have approximately 10 bp of homology to the 5' end of gene C. The gene C amplicon would contain approximately 1,000 bp of the 5' end of the gene with approximately 10 bp at its 5' end of the 3' end of gene X. Because of the overlapping homologies, the amplicon comprising the 3' end of gene A and the gene X amplicon would be combined and used as a template for synthesis of a gene AX amplicon (similar to the PCR processes described in Fig. 7). This AX gene fragment can subsequently be used as a template, along with the gene C amplicon, for the synthesis of the final gene AXC amplicon using a similar approach. This would then be used as the transforming DNA for the isolation of a transformant in which gene B has been deleted and replaced with the antibiotic resistance-encoding gene X. This fusion PCR approach can be employed for the synthesis of transforming amplicons encoding virtually any combinations of DNA segments from the same source or different bacterial sources. If gene B is essential to the host species, or part of an operon in which essential downstream genes are not expressed as a result of the chromosomal insertion, then its deletion would not be possible by transformation with the AXB gene amplicon, as described above. Approaches to address these situations would also use fusion PCR to generate DNA fragments possessing the essential genes and their promoters, or other functional promoters, for insertion elsewhere in nonessential regions of the chromosome. Once a functional essential gene is inserted elsewhere, one would then show that the allele could now be deleted from its original chromosomal site by the insertion of the AXB amplicon.

TRANSPOSON MUTAGENESIS

The identification and analysis of genes that encode a variety of phenotypic traits have been aided by application of transposons to the random insertional mutagenesis of bacterial genomes. When a transposon inserts into a bacterial genome, if the site of insertion is within a structural gene, a defective gene product (protein) will be made, if any product at all is synthesized. The phenotypic trait(s) imparted by that gene product (or an operon, if the interrupted gene is followed by other genes within the operon, and the insertion resulted in polar effects) can be identified by comparing the properties of the isogenic mutant to its wild-type parent strain. A variety of transposons have been employed in the random mutagenesis of oral bacterial genomes, followed by studies of the phenotypes affected. One of the most useful transposons for insertional mutagenesis has been the conjugative transposon, Tn*916*. The use of Tn*916* for this purpose was prompted by observations that it, or closely related conjugative elements, had either been shown to transfer to a variety of oral bacterial species or was present in tetracycline-resistant isolates of these species from the oral cavity. The presence of these elements has been reported in such oral streptococcal species as *S. mutans, S. sanguis, S. mitis,* and *S. oralis,* as well as gram-negative species such as *F. nucleatum.* Selection for the transfer of Tn*916* via conjugation involves the use of media selective for recipient strains that have become resistant to tetracycline, followed by screening of the resistant isolates for alterations in detectable phenotypes. The site of transposon integration can be detected by the cloning, from the mutant strain, of Tn*916*-associated DNA carrying the *tet*M gene and flanking chromosomal DNA. Among the oral streptococci, Tn*916* has been used in the identification and study of genes encoding intergeneric coaggregation in a strain of *S. gordonii,* a fibronectin-binding protein in *S. sanguis,* and the ability to produce rods, exhibit aciduricity, and accumulate intracellular polysaccharides by strains of *S. mutans.*

Tn*916* was also employed for insertional mutagenesis of *A. actinomycetemcomitans,* but the transposon was not transferred by conjugation, but rather by electrotransformation. The plasmid, pAM120, into which Tn*916* had been cloned, was isolated from *E. coli* and used to transform the Y4 strain of *A. actinomycetemcomitans* by electroporation, followed by selection for resistance to tetracycline. Since pAM120 cannot replicate in *A. actinomycetemcomitans,* bacterial cells were able to become resistant to tetracycline only if the *tet*M-encoding Tn*916* inserted into the new host chromosome via transposition. The results of Southern hybridization experiments showed that Tn*916* had inserted at a variety of chromosomal locations among several tetracycline-resistant Y4 transformants examined. Several tetracycline-resistant isolates were subsequently shown to be defective in the production of the capsule-like serotype b-specific antigen, SPA, due to the insertion of the transposon into the corresponding gene.

Transposons other than Tn*916* have been employed for the insertional mutagenesis of oral streptococcal species. One small transposon, Tn*4001,* a 4.5-kb erythromycin resistance-encoding element first isolated from *Staphylococcus aureus,* was transferred to *S. gordonii* on the recombinant *E. coli* plasmid pα. The transposon was shown to insert randomly into the *S. gordonii* chromosome, and its usefulness for insertional mutagenesis was demonstrated by the isolation of transformants defective in the utilization of lactose. Tn*4001* was also shown to undergo transposition in a strain of *S. mutans.*

The methods of transposon insertional mutagenesis described above are dependent on transposition, a low-frequency event, immediately following the introduction of the transposon to the recipient cell via conjugation or following transformation with a suicide plasmid, both transfer methods also low-frequency events. Thus, the number of mutant isolates obtainable from each transfer experiment is generally quite low. Frequencies of mutant isolation can be increased dramatically by the construction of a transposon delivery plasmid that is temperature sensitive for replication. One such plasmid, designated pTV1-OK, consists of (i) a mutant

L. lactis plasmid, *repAts*-pWV01, able to replicate in numerous gram-positive and gram-negative species at temperatures around 30°C, but unable to replicate if the temperature of incubation is shifted to 40 to 45°C; (ii) the enterococcal transposon Tn*917*, which encodes resistance to erythromycin and can be induced to transpose at a higher than normal frequency in the presence of subinhibitory concentrations of erythromycin; and (iii) *aph3A*, a gene encoding resistance to high levels of kanamycin in both gram-positive and gram-negative species. pTV1-OK is introduced into the bacterial strain of interest by transformation, followed by selection for resistance to kanamycin. The plasmid is distributed to all cells in a culture if propagated at a temperature permissive for its replication. If the culture is also incubated in the presence of subinhibitory concentrations of erythromycin, then transposition of Tn*917* will be induced, with many copies of it inserting into various sites on the host chromosome. If such a culture is diluted and then incubated at a temperature nonpermissive for replication, the plasmid will be lost as the cells divide. Subsequent culture with a concentration of erythromycin selective for the transposon causes colonies to appear that have lost pTV1-OK but contain Tn*917* in their chromosomes. Evidence for the loss of pTV1-OK is demonstrated by showing that the erythromycin-resistant isolates have become susceptible to kanamycin. This transposon delivery vector has been used to interrupt, identify, and study a variety of genes involved in the metabolism of *S. mutans* as well as a number of genes whose expression is regulated by different environmental conditions.

Two transposons originally described in strains of *Bacteroides fragilis*, Tn*4351* and Tn*4400*, have been used for the transposon insertional mutagenesis of *P. gingivalis*. Tn*4351* is delivered on the plasmid R751::*Ω4 to strains of *P. gingivalis* from *E. coli* by conjugation. R751 is a broad-host-range conjugative plasmid that can transfer to, but cannot replicate in, *P. gingivalis*, whereas R751::*Ω4 is R751 containing a partial tandem duplication of Tn*4351*. Theoretically, the only way Tn*4351* can survive in *P. gingivalis* following transfer on R751::*Ω4 is via transposition to the *P. gingivalis* chromosome, which can be selected for in the presence of erythromycin, as resistance to this antibiotic is encoded by the transposon. However, in at least one strain of *P. gingivalis*, among the majority of mutants obtained, plasmid R751 had accompanied Tn*4351* into the chromosome via cointegration, rather than a simple transposition event that would have resulted in the insertion of Tn*4351* only. Although the mutations that were caused by a cointegration event were stable, the presence of the large plasmid (53 kb), in addition to the transposon, at the site of insertion made it more difficult to characterize the interrupted gene. The second *B. fragilis* transposon, Tn*4400*, is transferred to *P. gingivalis* strains on the delivery vehicle, pYT646B, which, in addition to Tn*4400*, consists of the *E. coli* plasmid, pBR322, and *oriT* from RK2, which facilitates transfer from *E. coli* to *P. gingivalis* by the mobilizing plasmid, RK231. Integration of the transposon is confirmed by selection for tetracycline resistance encoded by the transposon-mediated, anaerobically expressed *tetQ* gene.

Integration or suicide vectors enable targeted mutagenesis of genes of interest. In contrast, transposons enable mutagenesis at undefined sites, so mutants that display the loss of a phenotype of interest can be characterized to determine which genetic loci contribute to that phenotype. The use of transposons could then be considered to be phenotypically targeted, as opposed to the use of integration vectors, which are genetically targeted. With the wealth of genome sequence data available, genetically targeted mutagenesis is facilitated by knowledge of the sequence and organization of genes predicted by their DNA sequence to be of interest. However, it is significant that often more than a third of the genes in an annotated genome are unassigned in function. This highlights the need for phenotypically targeted mutagenesis, which provides a powerful approach to delineate novel genes contributing to a phenotype.

KEY POINTS

Investigations of the ability of strains of a few species of oral streptococci to achieve a natural state of competence for genetic transformation were being conducted in the early 1960s. However, the true origin of the genetics and molecular biology of the oral microbiota can be traced to the isolation of plasmid DNA from a strain of *S. mutans* in 1973, followed shortly thereafter by demonstration of the transfer of plasmids between oral streptococci.

DNA can be acquired by bacterial cells through either vertical or horizontal (lateral) transmission. In vertical transmission there is transfer of a copy of the parental DNA to daughter cells upon cell division. In horizontal transmission there is acquisition of foreign DNA. The known mechanisms responsible for horizontal gene transfer are transformation, the uptake of naked DNA by competent recipient cells; conjugation, the transfer of DNA through cell-cell contact; and transduction, the introduction of DNA into a bacterial cell by bacteriophages containing either random (generalized transduction) or specific (specialized transduction) pieces of DNA from the previous host of the phage.

The development of competence (the ability to uptake DNA by transformation) in streptococci can involve quorum sensing with small peptide signaling molecules that induce phosphorylation-dependent signaling cascades. In some gram-negative organisms, there is specificity of DNA uptake with the presence of USS being required. Regulation of competence in gram-negative organisms can occur by catabolite repression.

Plasmids are extrachromosomally replicating genetic elements. Most plasmids are present in their host cells as double-stranded, covalently closed, circular DNA molecules. Plasmids must encode the elements required for autonomous replication, including an origin of replication and contiguous gene(s) encoding replication proteins and other controlling elements. Some native plasmids encode genes that confer resistance to antibiotics. Other phenotypes that may be encoded by plasmids include virulence traits, metabolic capabilities, and the production of bacteriocins. Plasmids may be either conjugative or mobilizable. Conjugative plasmids possess all the genes necessary for conjugative transfer. Mobilizable plasmids require genes encoding conjugative functions to be provided by another plasmid or the chromosome. Circular plasmids replicate by theta and RC mechanisms.

Transposons are discrete nonreplicative segments of DNA capable of inserting into, and being replicated as part of, a bacterial replicon such as a chromosome, plasmid, or bacteriophage genome. They may also move from one site in a DNA molecule to another. Insertion of a transposon into DNA is mediated by insertion sequence elements, which are located at the ends of transposons and encode the enzyme transposase, which catalyzes the insertion events.

Transposon insertion is usually random, i.e., it may occur at virtually any site on a DNA molecule, independent of extensive homology. Thus, transposons can be used for random mutagenesis where screening for a phenotypic property is possible. Some transposons can be transferred by conjugation.

A bacterial mutant in which only a defined gene has been altered is termed an isogenic mutant, and this will lead to a change or loss of function specific to that gene. Restoration of the gene and/or its expression, referred to as complementation of the mutant, should restore function.

A common approach to generating isogenic mutants is to use a vector that does not replicate in the bacterium of interest (a suicide vector) but into which has been cloned DNA homologous to a region of the targeted gene as well as a resistance determinant that provides a marker for selection. A single recombination (or crossover) event will result in integration of the entire plasmid and disruption of the gene. A mutation in a gene can also be created by a double recombination event between two identical DNA regions of the plasmid (constructed to flank the selection marker) and the chromosome, resulting in an allelic replacement, essentially a swapping of a portion of the gene with the selection marker. A similar double recombination event can also be used to create a deletion mutation, a loss of a region of a gene without introduction of a selection marker. Phenotypic analyses are used to evaluate the effect of the gene disruption. In all cases it is important to assess any effects on genes downstream of the target gene.

Shuttle vectors that replicate in both *E. coli* and another species facilitate cloning (in *E. coli*) and transfer of genetic material into the species of interest. These vectors can be used to generate double

(continues)

KEY POINTS

(Continued from previous page)
recombination mutants or to provide an intact copy of a gene for complementation. Restoration of gene function by complementation ensures that the phenotypic effect observed was due to inactivation of the gene, not to a polar effect on a downstream gene or other unintended mutation.

The application of genetic and molecular biological tools to the study of oral microbiology has been expanded to such oral bacterial genera as *Actinobacillus, Porphyromonas, Actinomyces, Prevotella, Fusobacterium,* and *Treponema.* The inclusion of genetic and molecular tools in the analysis of additional oral microbial species and genera will, as with the above-mentioned genera, likely be made possible by the discovery of naturally occurring plasmids in some species or the identification of plasmids from related species that can replicate in others;

the development and optimization of genetic transfer systems for each species; and the use of plasmids that cannot replicate in these species, i.e., integration or suicide vectors, as well as a variety of transposons, for the construction of isogenic mutants by insertional mutagenesis. The pace of such studies is, and will be, hastened by the availability of the total genomic sequence of an ever-increasing number of oral bacterial species. Such sequences provide important information as to which genes of a species are present and likely to contribute to its role in the oral environment or, in some instances, its ability to cause disease. With the availability of genetic and molecular tools, it is, or will be, possible to confirm a function predicted by the sequence of a gene, to examine environmental conditions that regulate its expression, or to elucidate the function in each species of the 30 to 40% of genes whose function cannot be predicted by sequence alone.

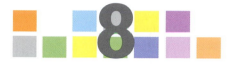

Applied Molecular Biology and the Oral Microbes

HANSEL M. FLETCHER, ANN PROGULSKE-FOX, AND JEFFREY D. HILLMAN

INTRODUCTION

Technological breakthroughs in the 1970s, collectively referred to as recombinant DNA technology, provided significant impetus for studies that should lead ultimately to a basic understanding of the biological processes of oral microbes. While standard biochemical, physiological, and classical genetic approaches had provided insights into the biology of several oral microbes, little was known regarding the basis of their virulence or even their ability to colonize a host until the advent of molecular genetics as a research tool. These advances also led to the development of molecular diagnostic protocols for the rapid identification of oral microbes.

Since the initial cloning of the first gene from a streptococcus in the late 1970s, significant progress has been made in the characterization of several genes from many streptococcal species, as well as other oral microbes including *Porphyromonas gingivalis*, *Actinobacillus actinomycetemcomitans*, *Treponema denticola*, *Actinomyces naeslundii*, and *Prevotella intermedia*. Furthermore, the nucleotide sequences of the entire genomes of several of these organisms have been determined. The postgenomic era with its developing technology now allows genome comparison of different strains and facilitates the identification of candidates for virulence genes, vaccine and antimicrobial targets, and diagnostics.

In this chapter, we describe the various recombinant DNA techniques that have been applied to the study of oral microbes. The continued progress and success of these technologies will bring many pragmatic benefits, particularly in therapeutics for oral and related systemic infections.

INVESTIGATING GENE EXPRESSION: GENETIC APPROACHES

DNA Cloning

The elucidation of the genetic code, and of the structure of DNA and its role as the genetic material, made it clear that to unravel the secrets of biological processes would require an ability to propagate specific DNA segments and determine their sequences. A first step in this process is the cloning of a gene into a vector that can be propagated in bacterial or viral host cells (Fig. 1). This step takes advantage of several types of enzymes that can act on and alter DNA, and in some instances, RNA. Important among these enzymes are restriction endonucleases that catalyze site-specific cleavage of DNA, often leaving complementary single-stranded ends; ligases, which permanently join DNA fragments via the formation of covalent bonds; reverse transcriptase, which can generate a DNA fragment from an RNA template; and a variety of DNA polymerases, which catalyze the synthesis of complementary DNA strands from single-stranded templates. As a first step in the cloning of a gene, purified genomic DNA from an organism is digested with a restriction endonuclease to produce specific fragments. The numbers and sizes of fragments produced will depend on the numbers and locations of sites along the

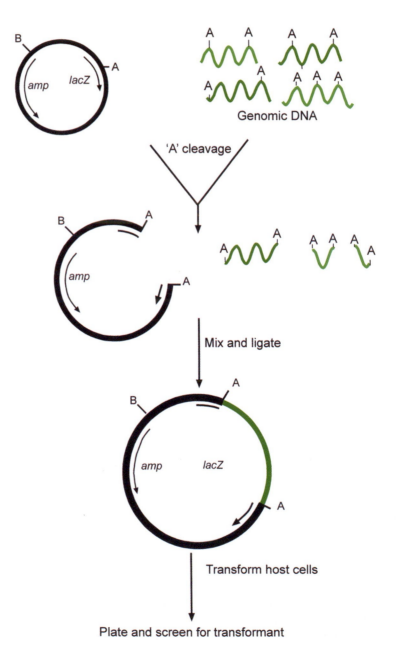

FIGURE I General method for cloning a DNA fragment onto a plasmid vector. Double-stranded plasmid vector and genomic DNA are purified separately and each is digested with the same or a compatible restriction endonuclease. The digested DNAs are mixed together and the complementary ends are ligated (covalent bonds are formed) by phage T4 DNA ligase. The ligated recombinant molecules are used to transform a host cell. The plasmid vector contains an origin of replication and an antibiotic resistance marker, thus selection of transformants that have received the vector will be resistant to the antibiotic, whereas cells that are not transformed will not survive on antibiotic-containing medium. In the transformants, the plasmid can replicate independently of the host chromosome and these cells can then be screened for a predicted phenotype imparted by a gene or genes that were inserted into the vector. Vector DNA with no inserts, or with miscellaneous inserted genomic DNA, will not impart the desired phenotype. See text for other methods for screening for specific cloned DNA.

genomic DNA molecules that are recognition sites for the enzyme used. The vector DNA, in which there is generally only a single site, is also digested with the same or a compatible enzyme. Depending on the type of restriction enzymes used, fragments may be generated with "sticky" (or complementary) ends that may have a 5' or 3' single-stranded overhang with 1 to 5 base pairs exposed. The digested fragments, under the appropriate conditions, and due to the complementary ends on each, can adhere to each other by hydrogen bonding. Fragments from the host genome may adhere to each other, and two or more digested vector molecules may also ad-here to each other. However, in many instances a single fragment of chromosomal DNA will adhere to a single digested vector molecule. In the presence of DNA ligase from the *Escherichia coli* bacteriophage T4, the ends of the combined fragments are covalently linked, thus producing new recombinations of DNA molecules (hence "recombinant DNA"). When the DNA molecules have been digested with an enzyme that produces complementary single-stranded ends, the ligated junctions of the recombinant molecules will contain the original restriction sites, which facilitates the future isolation and purification of cloned fragments. Alternatively, blunt-ended fragments, which are without a single-stranded overhang, can be generated by specific restriction enzymes or by the "filling in" of the 5' single-stranded overhangs or digestion of 3' → 5' single-stranded overhangs with an enzyme such as phage T4 DNA polymerase (or S1 nuclease). These blunt-end fragments may also come together in solution, and can be joined by DNA ligase, albeit with a bit more difficulty than fragments with complementary ends, to generate new recombinant molecules that may or may not contain the original restriction site. The mixture of ligated recombinant molecules is introduced into a bacterial host strain by transformation. The plasmid vector contains an origin of replication that is functional in the host of choice and also encodes a gene that mediates resistance to an antibiotic. By spreading the transformation mixture onto an agar-based medium containing the antibiotic, cells that have received recombinant plasmids will be resistant to the antibiotic and grow on the nutrients in the medium. However, cells that have received just recombined genomic DNA, or no DNA at all, will not grow in the medium. Colonies of transformants that have received plasmid vector DNA, with or without cloned genomic DNA fragments, may be subsequently screened for the presence of the cloned gene of interest.

The most direct way of identifying a DNA fragment carrying the gene of interest is by detecting an expressible phenotype from the cloned gene that allows the recombinant clone to be differentiated from those without the fragment. One such example is the identification of protease genes from *P. gingivalis*. Screening of a genomic library of *P. gingivalis* chromosomal DNA constructed with an *E. coli* plasmid vector produced a colony that showed pronounced proteolytic zones on skim milk agar plates when incubated in an anaerobic environment. A limitation associated with this method is the inability of some of genes to have an expressible phenotype in *E. coli*. This limitation has been overcome in some instances by the construction and availability of shuttle vectors. Such vectors consist of at least two origins of replication, one for replication in *E. coli* and one that allows replication in the bacterial host of interest, and also contain an antibiotic resistance gene or genes that are expressed in both bacterial hosts. Thus, the actual cloning is performed in *E. coli*, which still remains the best host system for most cloning experiments, and then a library of recombinant DNA clones is purified from a culture of *E. coli* and used to transform the host of interest, in which the desired gene can be expressed.

Another approach for identifying the appropriate clone is based on detecting the gene product by using antibodies and Western blotting technology. This is particularly useful if the phenotypic expression of the gene in *E. coli* is affected by protein processing or if antibodies are already available to the gene of interest.

Clones carrying the desired DNA fragment may also be identified by methods that do not require expression. Identification of these fragments may be based on hybridization of previously cloned homologous genes from another source or by generation of an oligonucleotide synthetic probe based on the amino acid composition of the gene product of interest. With this approach, DNA from a cloned source is transferred onto a nitrocellulose filter membrane. The DNA is then denatured to single strands by alkali treatment. Since single strands of DNA are fixed to the surface of the filter, they will not reanneal with each other. They will, however, anneal to complementary DNA (the probe) if a solution containing DNA homologous to the filter-bound target DNA is added to the filter. The extent of the hybridization (annealing) to the probe will be directly related to the stringency of the hybridization conditions and the degree of homology between the probe and the target DNAs (see Fig. 2 for an illustration of hybridization). The probe used can be labeled with radioactive or chemiluminescent compounds for ease and enhancement of detection.

When a single recombinant molecule composed of a vector plus an inserted DNA fragment is introduced into an appropriate host cell, the cloned fragment is amplified along with the vector, usually producing large numbers of the recombinant DNA molecules. The cloning of a variety of genes from oral microorganisms has been accomplished with a wide range of cloning vectors and systems.

Another method of preparing genomic DNA for insertion into a vector is the amplification of specific genes from DNA by polymerase chain reaction (PCR) (see below). These fragments can be joined to a vector by ligase to generate a new recombinant molecule. A major advantage of this method is the ability to clone only the gene, or DNA fragment, of interest, to the exclusion of all other genomic DNA from the host of origin. Another advantage of this method is the ability to engineer into the DNA fragment to be cloned any restriction endonuclease site of choice.

PCR

The primary objectives of genetic cloning are to isolate and amplify genes or DNA fragments for functional analyses or further manipulations. PCR is a powerful tool for the amplification of specific DNA fragments from any DNA molecule in which they are present (Fig. 3). For PCR amplification, two oligonucleotide primers (typically 20 to 30 nucleotides in length) are added in vast excess compared to the DNA to be amplified. They hybridize to opposite strands of the DNA and are oriented with

A. DNA Isolation and digestion by endonuclease

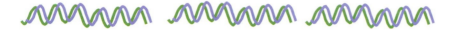

B. DNA gel electrophoresis

C. DNA transfer to filter membrane

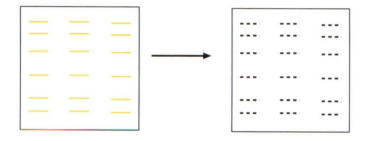

D. DNA hybridization

FIGURE 2 General method of Southern blot hybridization. (A) DNA is isolated and digested with a restriction endonuclease. The DNA fragments are separated by gel electrophoresis (B) and transferred and fixed to a filter (C). (D) The filter is hybridized with a probe that has been labeled either with a radioactive isotope or a reactive chemical. A signal detection procedure (e.g., autoradiography) reveals bands where the target DNA is complementary to the probe.

their 3′ ends facing each other to enable synthesis by the DNA polymerase (which catalyzes growth of new strands 5′ to 3′) as it extends across the segment of DNA between them. The first cycle of synthesis results in new strands of indeterminate length, which, like the parental strands, can hybridize to the primers upon denaturation and annealing. The second cycle of denaturation, annealing, and synthesis produces two single-stranded products that together compose a discrete double-stranded product that is exactly the length between the primer ends. Each strand of this discrete product is complementary to one of the two primers and can therefore participate as a template in subsequent cycles. The amount of this product doubles with every subsequent cycle of synthesis, denaturation, and annealing, accumulating exponentially so that

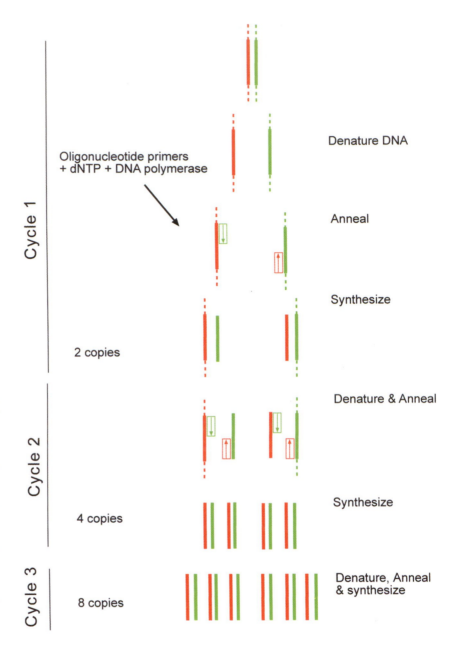

Cycle 1

Oligonucleotide primers
+ dNTP + DNA polymerase

Denature DNA

Anneal

Synthesize

2 copies

Cycle 2

Denature & Anneal

Synthesize

4 copies

Cycle 3

Denature, Anneal
& synthesize

8 copies

FIGURE 3 PCR. A solution containing the DNA in which the target sequence to be amplified is present is heated to a temperature that will allow it to denature. The solution is then cooled to a temperature that will permit renaturation, and a reaction mixture is added. This mixture contains the heat-stable DNA polymerase, the four nucleotides dATP, dGTP, dCTP, and dTTP, and a pair of short oligonucleotide primer sequences that are known to be complementary to base sequences on each strand at either end of the target sequence. The mixture is incubated for a time (minutes) and at a temperature that will allow annealing of the target sequence to the appropriate primer sequence, followed by the synthesis of complementary strands. This produces two copies of the target sequence. A cycle of heating for a few minutes to a temperature that permits denaturation, followed by cooling to a temperature that will permit reannealing and synthesis, is repeated several times (generally 30 to 40 cycles), giving rise to millions of copies of the target DNA in a few hours.

30 cycles can result in a 2^{28}-fold (270 millionfold) amplification of the discrete product. The PCR product can then be detected by electrophoresis on agarose gels, staining with a dye, such as ethidium bromide, that binds specifically to DNA, and visualization using ultraviolet light. Specific DNA fragments may also be detected by Southern hybridization (Fig. 2).

Since its initial development, PCR technology has been extended to numerous applications. For example, PCR products can be sequenced directly without the need for cloning. Because of the small quantity of template DNA required, in addition to the specificity in amplification that can be achieved by using unique oligonucleotide primers, PCR has been applied to the direct identification of oral microorganisms. Unique primers based on the nucleotide sequences of genes encoding a 16S rRNA subunit, which contains species-specific regions, are used in PCR to detect oral microorganisms without the need to culture those strains. This technique can also be used for the study of microbial communities, including unculturable species. Thus, PCR analysis of biological samples using oligonucleotide primers that recognize species-specific 16S rRNA sequences, in conjunction with other species-specific genes, has facilitated the identification of oral microorganisms including *Streptococcus* spp., *Porphyromonas* spp., *Actinobacillus*, *Treponema* spp., and *Actinomyces*. Direct amplification of 16S rRNA sequences by PCR from mixed culture biomasses followed by purification and sequencing has also allowed the analysis of complex communities. This technique has been applied to the microbiota associated with dentoalveolar abscesses, and a number of novel sequences that did not correspond to known, culturable organisms were identified. Novel taxa identified by phylogenetic analysis in this way are designated "phylotypes." Phylotypes related to *Bacteroides*, *Prevotella*, and oral asaccharolytic *Eubacterium* species were identified. While all three phylotypes were detected in periodontal sites, the phylotype related to oral asaccharolytic *Eubacterium* spp. was significantly associated with disease. Sequence data from unculturable organisms can be used to design specific PCR primers and DNA probes for rapid detection of the organisms in clinical specimens. These can then be used to determine the prevalence of the organisms in healthy and diseased tissues and, if specific associations are found, may provide useful markers of disease activity.

The development of rapid PCR-based molecular testing methods can be of major clinical significance, as the mixed microbiota associated with disease can be investigated in its entirety without the inherent biases associated with determinations of culturable organisms. Also, the ability to identify novel organisms associated with disease will improve our knowledge of the etiology of periodontal disease and lead to the discovery of additional marker organisms of value in disease diagnosis and treatment monitoring.

PCR has also been adopted for use with RNA templates for the production of cDNA using reverse transcriptase (RT). RT-PCR has been useful for gene regulation studies where the pattern of gene expression can be quantified by an approach referred to as real-time PCR.

INVESTIGATING GENE FUNCTION

Directed or site-specific mutagenesis is a powerful technique for dissecting the genetic basis of bacterial functions (e.g., the virulence of bacterial pathogens). Before the advent of recombinant DNA technology, chemical and physical methods were used to alter the phenotype of bacterial strains. However, these techniques lacked specificity in that mutations produced could occur anywhere on the bacterial genome and were not confined solely to the gene of interest. Thus, new phenotypes could have been the result of mutations in one or more genes, making analysis difficult. The development of intergeneric shuttle plasmids and efficient DNA transfer systems has provided the tools necessary to assess the molecular mechanism(s) of gene expression of several oral microorganisms.

Directed mutagenesis can involve insertion-duplication mutagenesis, allelic exchange, or transposon mutagenesis. For insertion-duplication mutagenesis, plasmids are used to construct specific isogenic mutants using available cloned DNA gene sequences. The type of plasmid used, called a "suicide vector," usually contains an *E. coli* origin of replication, which permits replication in *E. coli* but not the species under study, and antibiotic resistance markers that are expressed in *E. coli* as well as the bacterial species of interest. An internal subcistronic fragment of the gene of interest is cloned onto the vector in *E. coli*. The recombinant plasmid is propagated in and isolated from *E. coli*. The plasmid DNA is then used to transform the strain of interest, followed by selection for the appropriate antibiotic resistance phenotype. Because the plasmid is unable to replicate in the strain of interest, the resulting antibiotic resistant transformant cells must be those in which the vector has become integrated into the genome, thus producing a mutation at the site of insertion. This is accomplished by a reciprocal recombination event between the plasmid and chromosome involving the cloned subcistronic DNA fragments. The resulting insertion mutation splits the gene of interest. Because this method will give rise to duplication during the recombination event, it is critical that the subcistronic DNA fragment be internal to the gene of interest. A limitation of insertion-duplication mutagenesis is the need for selective pressure, i.e., growth in the presence of antibiotic, in order to maintain the integrated plasmid.

Allelic exchange mutagenesis (Fig. 4) is another technique that uses cloned gene sequences to generate a specific isogenic mutant. Construction of such mutants requires the exchange of gene alleles either between strains, such as from a plasmid into the appropriate chromosomal position, or from the chromosome onto plasmids. The ability to replace the wild-type chromosomal copy of a gene with a mutated derivative of the gene that has been constructed in vitro using a cloned copy of the gene allows the phenotype of the mutation to be studied under a defined set of in vitro or in vivo conditions, with the mutation present in a single copy at its normal or specific chromosomal location. Several widely used allelic exchange systems have been developed for gram-negative and gram-positive oral bacteria. Nearly all constructs used in these systems rely on the positive selection of an antibiotic-resistance gene (e.g., erythromycin or *erm*) that is also used to interrupt and mutate the target gene. Insertion of the antibiotic resistance marker must be within the coding sequence of the gene. When replacement constructs are linearized, the drug resistance gene is flanked by two regions of homology to the target gene. Selection of the cells using the appropriate antibiotic eliminates the great majority of cells that have not stably incorporated the construct. Antibiotic-resistant transformants are those mutants that have a defective gene as a result of additive integration (two double crossovers). The net effect is that the defective version of the gene replaces the wild-type copy, creating a gene-specific mutant strain. Unlike insertion-duplication mutagenesis, allelic exchange mutagenesis is stably maintained even in the absence of selective pressure.

Another useful technique for generating isogenic mutants without a need for first cloning the gene of interest is transposon mutagenesis. This involves the insertion of a transposable element into the host chromosome, giving rise to specific insertion mutations. Although some

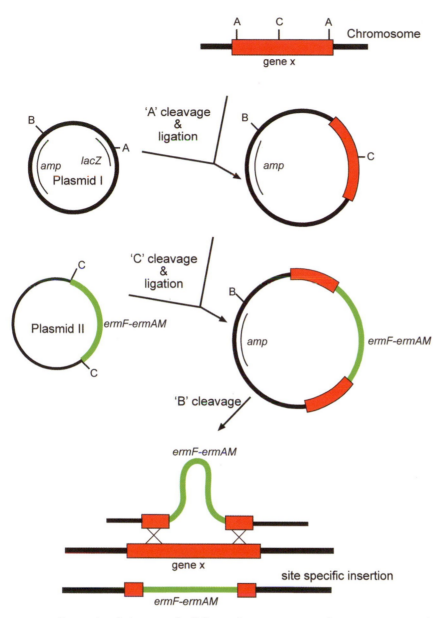

FIGURE 4 Example of the use of allelic exchange mutagenesis to construct a site-specific mutant. The chromosome of the organism under study and *E. coli* plasmid vector I are digested with restriction endonuclease A. This liberates numerous chromosomal fragments, one from each copy of the chromosome that encodes gene *x*. Alternatively, a chromosomal fragment containing only gene *x* can also be amplified from the chromosomal DNA by PCR. Insertion and ligation of DNA fragments into the cleaved site of plasmid vector I inactivate the *lacZ* gene. Plasmids containing fragment inserts are selected by screening for ampicillin-resistant transformants of *E. coli* that form white colonies on solid medium containing X-Gal. Recombinant plasmids that have been identified as those encoding gene *x* and plasmid vector II are digested with restriction endonuclease C. This enzyme is chosen because it either cleaves within gene *x* or results in the excision of a segment of gene *x*, which allows the insertion of an *erm* cassette (encoding erythromycin resistance) from plasmid vector II. Plasmids with the insertionally inactivated gene *x* are selected by screening for erythromycin-resistant colonies. This plasmid is then introduced (usually by electrotransformation or by natural transformation, depending on species and strain) into the original wild-type host cell. The inactivated gene shares homology with the host cell chromosome via the sequences of gene *x* that flank the *erm* gene. Thus the functional allele of the host is exchanged for the inactivated allele by homologous recombination. Successful integration of the inactivated gene into the host chromosome is monitored by acquisition of erythromycin resistance and loss of the phenotype encoded by the gene.

transposable elements may have "hot spots" or specific sites of insertion, many can insert into target DNA largely randomly during transposition. These elements usually contain an antibiotic resistance marker that facilitates direct selection. An added advantage of transposon mutagenesis is the ability to identify the inactivated gene based on the nucleotide sequence flanking the transposon. For example, genes involved in biofilm formation of *Streptococcus gordonii* strain Challis were characterized by screening isogenic mutants generated by Tn*916* transposon mutagenesis for defective biofilm formation. By using inverse PCR and DNA sequencing of the region flanking the transposon in these mutants, it was shown that genes required for biofilm formation include, among others, those that are involved in signal transduction, peptidoglycan biosynthesis, and adhesion. These functions are associated with quorum sensing, osmo-adaptation, and adhesion in oral streptococci. Transposons can also be modified to facilitate rapid cloning of the inactivated gene. This is observed in a mutagenesis system for *P. gingivalis* based on Tn*4400'*, a modified version of the *Bacteroides* transposon Tn*4400*. This transposon contains a pBR322 replicon and a beta-lactamase gene; thus, the cloning of disrupted genomic DNAs from a transposon insertion is easily accomplished after ligation of genomic fragments and transformation into *E. coli*.

A caveat associated with gene inactivation by any of the above methods is the possibility that these insertions can affect the expression of downstream gene sequences that can make interpretation difficult. To overcome this potential problem, the expression of downstream genes can be monitored by RT-PCR or Northern blot analysis if DNA sequences are available. In addition, the mutation can be complemented by introducing a replicative plasmid containing a wild-type copy of the mutated gene into the mutant. This should then restore the wild-type phenotpye if no polar effects are generated by the mutation. Further, additional mutagenesis on downstream sequences and evaluating the effect, if any, of such mutation would be required.

UNDERSTANDING GENE REGULATION

The regulation of a gene, e.g., induction or repression, in response to environmental signals can shed light on its function. For example, genes that encode iron-scavenging proteins are often up-regulated in response to low iron concentrations. The activities of most bacterial gene products are generally difficult to assay or detect. Thus, surrogate genes, referred to as "reporter genes," that encode well-studied and easily assayed enzymes are often used in regulation studies. Thus, to assess the effects of environmental signals on the expression of a gene of interest, a construct is designed such that a reporter gene is incorporated immediately downstream (and at times as a replacement) of the gene of interest. The result is a transcriptional fusion in which the regulatory region of the gene of interest now controls the expression of either both the original gene of interest and the reporter gene, or the reporter gene only. This type of fusion is easily created by cloning a promoterless reporter gene downstream of the promoter-operator of the gene of interest. One of the more common reporter genes used to study gene regulation in oral microorganisms is *lacZ*, which encodes β-galactosidase, an enzyme that hydrolyzes the disaccharide lactose to glucose and galactose. Another commonly used reporter gene is *cat*, which encodes chloramphenicol acetyltransferase, an enzyme that inactivates the antibiotic chloramphenicol via the addition of an acetyl group to the molecule. The reporter is particularly useful because the activity of the enzyme can be measured directly or by determining the MIC of chloramphenicol in the strain in which it is expressed, because it is one of the very few antibiotics for which the MIC is directly correlated with the level of expression of the encoding gene, i.e., enzyme copy number. Other useful reporter genes include *galK*, a gene whose product, galactokinase, phosphorylates galactose, an activity that can be measured by a radioactive assay using galactose and radiolabled phosphorous as substrates. Other reporters that can be used include *xa*, a gene encoding a bifunctional xylosidase/arabinosidase enzyme easily assayed by using β-nitrophenol derivatives as substrates, and a gene (*gfp*) encoding the green fluorescent protein, both fluorescent reporters, and bacterial luciferase (*luxAB*), a chemiluminescent reporter. The activities of fluorescent and chemiluminescent proteins can be detected visually and can also be quantitated with specialized instruments, such as fluorimeters.

A transcriptional fusion can be carried on a plasmid vector or can be inserted into the chromosome of the organism. However, in most cases, it is more desirable for the transcriptional fusion to be inserted in the chromosome via the insertion-duplication method (see above). This is important when it is necessary to maintain the gene dosage (a single copy on the chromosome, as opposed to multiple copies of a recombinant plasmid, i.e., plasmids that exist in anywhere from a couple to as many as 200 copies per chromosome equivalent) or when no stable vector is available for the organism of interest. In a transcriptional fusion, the RNA polymerase starts transcription from the promoter-operator region of the gene of interest. The fusion is expressed only under environmental conditions where the gene of interest is normally expressed. In *P. gingivalis*, use of a superoxide dismutase (*sod*)::*lacZ* fusion confirmed that SOD expression is maximal during the mid-exponential phase of growth and is influenced by oxygen, temperature, and pH. In this example, the β-galactosidase was readily detected using the chromogenic substrate indoyl-galactoside (X-Gal), which turns blue when the galactosyl bond is cleaved by the enzyme.

The identification of unknown genes regulated by similar environmental stimuli can be accomplished with a transposon-based strategy. Transposons having a selectable antibiotic resistance marker can be engineered to also carry the promoterless *lacZ* gene. Selection of antibiotic-resistant isogenic mutants will generate a library of clones in which the transposon is inserted randomly into the chromosome of the bacteria. The screening of the clones for the desired regulation of the *lacZ* reporter gene will facilitate the identification of those clones in which the transposon would have placed *lacZ* downstream of a promoter that is responsive to the environmental signal of interest. Once a clone is obtained, the nucleotide sequence flanking the transposon can be readily determined and will provide valuable information about the original gene(s) regulated by that promoter. In this manner Tn*917*-*lacZ* mutagenesis of *Streptococcus mutans* has been used successfully to identify environmentally regulated genes. In this case Tn*917*-*lacZ* mutants were isolated that expressed β-galactosidase activity under growth conditions of glucose limitation, acidic pH, 35 mM NaCl, and elevated (42°C) temperature. Further characterization of one of the mutants with increased β-galactosidase activity under glucose limitation revealed maximal activity in batch culture in stationary phase after glucose depletion. The β-galactosidase was also found to be repressed threefold in medium containing (excess) glucose relative to measured activity from cells suspended in the same medium containing no glucose. Sequence analysis of the region harboring the transposon revealed that the *lacZ* fusion occurred near the 3′ end of a gene encoding a homolog of an ATP-binding protein from a family of gram-positive bacterial ABC transporters.

Although multiple approaches for the global analysis of genes and gene function are available for certain organisms, their adaptation for use in oral microorganisms is limited. For example, reporter genes that can be used to detect expression in vivo, such as those encoding luciferase and green fluorescent protein, will need to be adapted for use in *P. gingivalis*. Approaches for detection of gene expression in novel environments can involve the use of several techniques including in vivo expression technology (IVET), signature-tagged mutagenesis, and differential display. IVET has been adapted for use in *P. gingivalis*. The IVET vector for *P. gingivalis* (pPGIVET) is a 9.3-kb self-transmissible suicide plasmid containing a cloning site upstream of two tandem promoterless reporter genes that encode tetracycline resistance *[tetA(Q)2]* and galactokinase (*galK*). Heterodiploids of *P. gingivalis* 381 in which the reporter genes were under the control of either the *hagB* or *hagC* promoter indicated that these genes are expressed during the infectious process in the mouse abscess model. This was the first direct evidence to support expression of two putative virulence factors in a host environment and further suggests that pPGIVET may be used to isolate *P. gingivalis* host-induced genes.

IVIAT: a Method To Identify Microbial Genes Expressed Specifically during Human Infections

Bacterial infections are complex, dynamic processes that evolve constantly within the host. In many instances, virulence gene expression is modulated in response to the changing environment encountered at the site of infection. Pioneering technologies such as IVET, signature-tagged mutagenesis, and differential fluorescence induction were designed to identify genes specifically expressed in vivo. All of these methods depend on a reasonable assumption; genes that are specifically induced during in vivo growth are likely to be important to the pathogenic process. These technologies all depend on the use of animal models of infection. However, animal models are not available for many pathogens and, in those cases for which an animal model is available, it might not closely approximate the human condition. In vivo induced antigen technology (IVIAT) identifies in vivo expressed genes but does not rely on animal models. Instead, it identifies genes expressed during an actual human infection. IVIAT uses sera from patients with the infection or disease of interest to probe for genes specifically expressed in vivo. IVIAT was initially developed to study the oral pathogen *A. actinomycetemcomitans* and is currently being used to study a number of other pathogens including bacteria, yeasts, and parasites. A general overview of the IVIAT scheme is presented in Fig. 5. IVIAT avoids the use of animal models by using

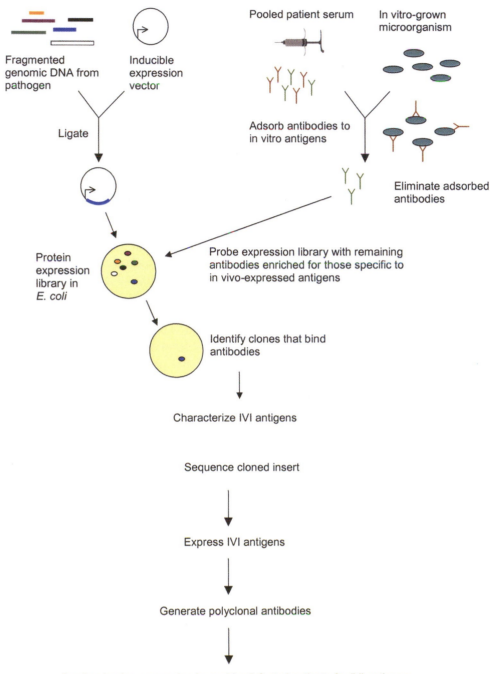

FIGURE 5 IVIAT. Sera from patients who have experienced an infection caused by the pathogen under study are pooled and exhaustively adsorbed with cells of the pathogen grown in vitro, leaving antibodies against antigens that are expressed only in vivo (top right). An expression library of the pathogen's DNA is generated in a suitable host (top left) and clones are probed with the adsorbed serum. Reactive clones, which are producing antigens that are expressed during a natural infection but not during in vitro cultivation, are purified and their cloned DNA sequenced. Genes are identified in this fashion as encoding IVI antigens. These antigens are purified and used to verify that the IVI antigen is expressed by the pathogen during an infectious process. This can be done with fluorescent-labeled antibodies raised against the purified IVI antigen to probe biological samples taken from infected patients.

serum from patients who have experienced disease caused by the pathogen of interest. The use of pooled sera allows the identification of the widest possible array of antigens produced during different stages of infection and, when appropriate, from patients infected via different routes. Reactive clones contain a DNA fragment from the pathogen that encodes an in vivo induced (IVI) antigen.

A particularly noteworthy feature of IVIAT is the potential it has in subacute and chronic infections such as periodontal diseases for defining a timeline for antigen production by the pathogen. Once one or more IVI antigens have been identified with the IVIAT scheme, sera of individual patients can be probed for reactive antibodies to each antigen. Provided that a detailed medical/dental history is available for these patients, the pattern of reactivity for each IVI antigen can then be correlated to the stage of infection (early, middle, or late) for each individual patient. The staging of individual sera can provide relevant information on the pathogenesis of the microorganism and on the host response to the infection.

IVIAT has been applied using sera from patients with well-characterized periodontal disease to screen the entire genomes of both *A. actinomycetemcomitans* and *P. gingivalis*. Hundreds of genes were confirmed as positive and sequenced. Sequence analysis revealed homologies to known virulence factors of these and other bacterial pathogens, to known genes in other organisms, and to hypothetical genes or genes of unknown function. Genes in the latter group are particularly interesting because they could well represent entirely novel virulence factors. Identification of IVI genes could lead to the discovery of new targets or pathways important for the development of antimicrobials, provide a logical basis for designing diagnostic tests, and suggest new targets for vaccine strategies.

GENOMICS: APPROACHES AND CHALLENGES

Genomics is the study of all genes, including their functions and regulatory elements, present in the genomes of organisms. The genome of an organism consists of its chromosomes and any extrachromosomal elements that may be present. With the advent of whole-genome sequencing, a new revolution in the search for an understanding of host-bacterium interactions began. Determination of the nucleotide base sequence of an organism's complete genome is a major goal of genomics, and was made possible by recent advances in DNA-sequencing automation and informatics. The completed genome sequences of eubacterial organisms are available for analysis through the World Wide Web (www.tigr.org); the anticipation is that many more genomes will be sequenced in the next few years. This includes the genome sequences of 13 oral microorganisms that are either completed or nearly completed (see chapter 7, Table 1).

Knowledge of the contiguous DNA sequence of a bacterium's chromosome provides important insights into its genetic makeup. This facilitates the identification of candidate virulence genes, and vaccine and antimicrobial targets, and can lead to the development of new diagnostic tools. Interpretation of completed genome sequences is accomplished by first identifying the predicted protein coding sequences or open reading frames (ORFs). While an ORF is identified as any stretch of codons that does not include a chain termination triplet, only a subset of all the ORFs present in the genomic sequence actually encode proteins. This prediction is based on the detection of regulatory sequences including a ribosomal binding site. In addition, many untranslated RNAs (mainly tRNA and rRNA genes) are identified and annotated. Various other features may be part of the annotation, including elements of the predicted protein structure, such as secondary structure motifs, which may help in the identification of function, and membrane spanning regions, which would suggest an association with the cell surface.

The mining of genomic sequences for genes that encode virulence factors and other functions of interest may be conducted by several approaches. The comparison of predicted coding sequences to sequences in databases (e.g., GenBank) with the BLAST program identifies matches to known genes. Typically, approximately 20% of the predicted ORFs in a genome do not match any other ORFs in GenBank, whereas another 10 to 70% match genes of unknown function, often discovered in other genome projects. Other databases, such as BLOCKS (a database of conserved regions of protein families obtained from multiply aligned sequences), provide information on different motifs within a protein. Hits in databases such as these are based on much smaller conserved regions of DNA and do not require extensive similarity elsewhere in the sequence, as may be the case with whole-gene matches. Other sequence-based clues as to function may also be unearthed in this type of analysis. For example, tandem repeats of sequences are often found in or near certain virulence genes, and motifs commonly associated with binding sites for regulators, such as inverted repeats, can sometimes be identified in regions of a genome that control genes involved in pathogenesis or known virulence traits.

In all of the completed genome sequences, a high proportion of genes with no assigned function have been identified. These genes classified as FUN (function unknown) range from 10 to 70% of the genome. Consistent with these observations, FUN genes for the sequenced genomes of oral microorganisms also fall within this range. Because the assignments of ORFs are based on homology searches of previous databases of known gene sequences, one caveat of the annotation process is the potential misassignment of some ORFs due to misassignment of the previous homologs. Thus, physiological characterization of gene products is necessary to verify function.

TRANSCRIPTOMICS AND PROTEOMICS

Transcriptomics

Elucidation of changes in gene expression associated with biological processes is central to assessing function. Because a gene is usually transcribed only when and where the function of its product is required, determining the environmental conditions under which a gene is expressed allows inferences about its function. Although several independent rapid methods for differential gene expression (including expressed sequence tag sequencing, subtractive cloning, differential display, and serial analysis of gene expression) may enable functional annotation of sequenced genomes, DNA microarray hybridization appears to be the most advantageous due to its simplicity, comprehensiveness, data consistency, and high throughput. First described in 1995, microarray experiments are based on the principle that labeled nucleic acid molecules in solution hybridize, with high sensitivity and specificity, to complementary sequences immobilized on a solid substrate, thus facilitating parallel quantitative measurement of many different sequences in a complex mixture.

Microarrays are usually made by deposition of spots of DNA sequence on a solid support such as a coated glass surface. The DNA spots that are homologous to regions of each ORF in the genome are obtained by PCR amplification using ORF-specific oligonucleotides. Analysis using homology-searching algorithms before oligonucleotide design is important in order to choose regions of genes that will not cross-hybridize with other regions of the genome. After a simple purification step, PCR fragments can be deposited on a coated glass surface by a robotic arrayer. The flatness of the glass surface makes it possible to array molecules in a parallel fashion, to miniaturize the procedure, and to allow the use of fluorescent dyes for detection. There is no diffusion of the applied material into the support, thus allowing reading of the slides by laser scanning microscopy.

For measuring relative gene expression, RNA is prepared from two or more culture samples to be compared, each having been propagated under a different environmental condition or for a different amount of time. Labeled cDNA is prepared by reverse transcription, incorporating different fluorescent cyanine dyes for each sample (e.g., Cy3 [green] or Cy5 [red]). The two labeled cDNA mixtures are combined and hybridized to the microarray, and the slide is scanned. With the use of image analysis software, signal intensities are determined for each dye at each element of the array, and the logarithm of the ratio of Cy5 intensity to Cy3 intensity is calculated. Cluster analysis of the data set can identify coregulated genes, which can become important in such instances as identifying sets of virulence genes. Because many virulence-associated genes are coordinately and tightly regulated, clustering gene expression profiles across a number of environmental conditions that can mimic infection, and precisely monitoring their coregulation, can reveal subtleties of regulation that may lead to the identification of virulence genes or groups of genes that are similarly regulated.

Microarray technology, which has only recently been used in a limited number of laboratories for the study of oral microorganisms, will likely become a standard tool for assessing environmental parameters that influence gene expression. Examples of genes that have been identified by this technology with *P. gingivalis* are those that are either up- or down-regulated in response to iron concentrations, genes regulated directly or indirectly by *luxS*, and genes that are regulated upon entry and invasion of host cells. Because microarrays cannot measure expression of genes that are absent from the reference strain, one limitation of the approach is their inability to identify genotypic differences between closely related strains that may be due to horizontal genetic transfer (as can occur with virulence factors). In addition, as with any method that quantifies transcription, posttranscriptional regulatory events, such as whether or not a message is translated, or the translational product is subsequently modified, cannot be detected. The large and comprehensive data sets that will be generated from microarray experiments require careful analysis. For example, as is demanded for candidate genes identified by any expression screening approach, a role in pathogenesis must be subsequently confirmed by mutation and assays of virulence.

Proteomics

Genes may be transcribed but not translated. Further, the number of mRNA copies may not necessarily reflect the number of functional protein molecules. Thus, insights into such factors as the relative abundance of a protein product, posttranslational modification, subcellular localization, turnover, and interaction with other proteins can only be monitored by analysis of the protein profile. A technology complementary to DNA microarrays for monitoring gene expression is proteomics, which is defined as the identification and quantitation of the complete set of proteins, both in space and time, that is synthesized under a given set of conditions.

There are two main approaches to proteomics: one is the expression model in which all proteins are analyzed, and the other is the cell map model in which only a selected set of proteins, like complexes, are studied. In the expression model, changes in the pattern of expression in response to different environmental conditions are observed quantitatively for a large number of proteins within a cell. This makes it possible to identify specific proteins that are expressed in response to specific conditions and also allows deductions as to entire regulatory networks by identifying proteins that may undergo coordinated changes of expression. One goal of the latter approach is to identify proteins that interact with and/or form complexes with other proteins. By documenting the physical interaction of proteins, the association of proteins in particular pathways can be deduced.

The analysis of genome-encoded proteins relies on the use of several technologies. One of the more commonly used techniques is two-dimensional gel electrophoresis. This technique, developed in the mid-1970s, provides higher resolution than one-dimensional sodium dodecyl sulfate-polyacrylamide gel electrophoresis analysis as it separates proteins both in terms of their isoelectric point and molecular weight. To establish the pH gradient, for separation on the basis of isoelectric point, two-dimensional polyacrylamide gel electrophoresis technology can use carrier ampholytes (amphoteric compounds) or immobilized pH gradients, which are an integral part of the polyacrylamide matrix. Quantitation of protein spots can be accomplished by the use of quantitative fluorescence. Radiolabeling in combination with scintillation counting can also be used to quantitate a small number of proteins. Methods of protein identification include immunoblotting, peptide sequencing following Edman degradation, determination of amino acid composition, matrix-assisted laser desorption/ionization mass spectrometry, and electrospray ionization. The last two methods, which rely on the comparison of peptide mass fingerprints, are fast and require only picomole amounts of proteins.

A more recent approach to protein separation that avoids two-dimensional gels altogether is multidimensional protein identification technology. In this system, proteins are separated by multiple high-pressure liquid chromatography runs and fed directly into a mass spectrometer for identification. With the increasing availability of complete genome sequences for oral and nonoral bacteria, global proteomics analyses are now possible.

KEY POINTS

Restriction endonucleases that cut DNA at specific stretches of bases, along with vectors such as plasmids that can be propagated, allow individual genes to be excised and recombined with vectors (cloned), thus facilitating their manipulation and study.

PCR is an iterative process of amplification of a stretch of DNA (such as a gene) using short oligonucelotides (primers) that bind to regions flanking the DNA of interest. PCR amplification of regions of DNA that are specific to individual organisms allows their detection in clinical samples without recourse to culture. RT PCR allows the detection and quantitation of RNA after the enzyme reverse transcriptase has been used to convert the RNA to cDNA

The activity of a gene (the amount of mRNA produced) can be measured by cloning the promoter region (the binding site for RNA polymerase) along with upstream regulatory sequences, next to a reporter gene, and returning this construct to the chromosome. The reporter gene generally encodes an enzyme for which substrate accumulation is easily measured. Bacterial strains containing such promoter-reporter constructs can be tested in animal models of disease, allowing the detection of genes that are activated in vivo.

Many bacteria, including important oral organisms, have had their genome sequenced and so their total genetic makeup is available. Thus, it is now possible to measure gene activity on a global, or whole-organism, scale using microarray technology. In a microarray, DNA sequence corresponding to every gene in a bacterium is deposited on a solid support such as a glass slide. mRNA from the organism under test conditions is then converted to cDNA and labeled with a fluorescent dye. The cDNA is hybridized (allowed to bind to matching sequences) to the target DNA on the array. After washing, the amount of fluorescent label remaining bound to the array for each target gene gives a measure of the amount of mRNA from that gene present in the test sample, which in turn reflects gene activity.

The availability of sequenced genomes has also driven the global analysis of proteins. An organism's total proteins can be separated by electrophoresis or by chromatography and identified by Edman degradation or by mass spectrometry. As in most cases the proteins are the effector molecules of the cell, the expressed proteome (total protein) provides a basis for understanding the physiology and pathogenicity of bacteria.

FURTHER READING

Maloy, S. R., J. Cronan, and D. Freifelder. 1994. *Microbial Genetics*, 2nd ed. Jones & Bartlett, Boston, Mass.

Salyers, A. A., and D. D. Whitt. 2001. *Bacterial Pathogenesis: a Molecular Approach*, 2nd ed. ASM Press, Washington, D.C.

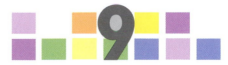

Population Genetics of Oral Bacteria

MOGENS KILIAN

INTRODUCTION

One of the results of the application of molecular genetics to bacteriology is recognition of an overwhelming genetic diversity within species of bacteria. It has become clear that bacterial species must be viewed as populations of individual strains that share basic housekeeping functions but otherwise may have very different properties. Analysis of the genetic structure of bacterial populations can elucidate the genetic mechanisms that cause this diversity. More importantly, population genetic analysis may identify particularly virulent variants within a species, thus providing a better background for the identification of important virulence factors. Such approaches may also yield a more detailed understanding of host-parasite relationships and may explain why temporal variations may occur in the prevalence of bacterial infections.

The goal of this chapter is to provide a brief overview of the molecular basis of bacterial population genetics and to demonstrate how the application of population genetic analysis to oral microbiology makes it possible to address many important questions about patterns of acquisition, transmission, and dynamics of the oral microbiota; whether particularly virulent forms of oral bacteria are responsible for oral diseases; and what the molecular mechanisms behind geographic and temporal variations in oral disease frequency and severity may be.

BACTERIAL SPECIES SHOW DIFFERENT PATTERNS OF EVOLUTION

Bacteria multiply by binary fission, a process that results in identical offspring. It was assumed previously that the major mechanism of genetic diversification is accumulation of point mutations in the bacterial genome. It is now clear, however, that recombinational replacements contribute significantly to diversification, but to different extents in different groups of bacteria. As a result, individual genera, species, and even subpopulations within species may display different population genetic structures.

Species in which accumulation of mutations is the dominant mechanism of genetic diversification consist of discrete phylogenetic lineages or clones. It has been estimated that the number of distinct evolutionary lineages within a given pathogenic species may range, at the global level, within a few hundred. Although members of individual clones are descendants of the same cell, they are not necessarily identical. Maynard Smith, a renowned population geneticist, defines a clone as "a set of genetically similar cells, recently derived from a common ancestor, without chromosomal recombination." What "recently" means in the evolutionary context is not clearly defined, but it may easily be thousands of years. The clonal population structure, which is the result of this evolutionary scenario, is characterized by linkage disequilibrium in the genome, i.e., particular alleles at individual gene loci cooccur (Fig. 1). For example, verotoxin production in *Escherichia coli* was for a long time associated with the serotypic trait O157:H7, the inability to ferment sorbitol, a particular DNA fingerprint pattern, and many other genotypic and phenotypic traits. As a practical matter, any of these properties could be used to trace bacteria with this particular virulence factor.

In most bacterial species interstrain homologous recombination or acquisition of new genes (horizontal transfer) by conjugation, transformation, or transduction is an additional, and often more important, source of genetic diversification. If recombination in a bacterial population is very frequent compared to the mutation rate, a panmictic population structure arises. This is characterized by a random (or nearly random) assortment of alleles and distinct phylogenetic lineages are no longer discernible. As a result, isolates with identical serotype, biotype, or other phenotypic trait are not necessarily genetically related. For example, genetically dissimilar isolates of *Neisseria meningitidis* or *Streptococcus pneumoniae* may express the same capsule serotype and yet show strikingly different pathogenic potential. Other examples of medically important species that show a panmictic population structure are gonococci and *Helicobacter pylori*. In practical terms, no single property will be able to identify a virulent phenotype in such bacteria unless that property is uniquely responsible for the pathogenic potential.

A bacterial population characterized by frequent recombination is constantly undergoing changes with new variants emerging and disappearing. This process may occasionally result in an explosive increase of a particularly successful variant, which may predominate for a time, possibly spread worldwide, and then eventually disappear as a result of erosion of its evolutionary success by recombination or resistance in the host population. A cross-sectional analysis may, mistakenly, interpret this as evidence of a clonal population structure, because repeated isolates from different geographic locations of one or more successful variants will

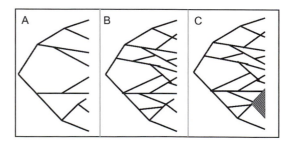

FIGURE 1 Three different genetic structures of bacterial populations: (A) clonal population structure; (B) panmictic population structure; and (C) epidemic population structure. The hatched area in panel C depicts a recently emerged, successfully spreading clone.

show the same combination of alleles. This evolutionary pattern, which accounts for the fluctuating prevalence of, for example, meningococcal meningitis, has been termed epidemic population structure. Another medically important species that shows this pattern is *Pseudomonas aeruginosa*.

It is not unusual that a single bacterial species includes subpopulations with different population structures. For example, serogroup A strains of *N. meningitidis* appear to have a largely clonal population structure, whereas the remaining part of this species is characterized by panmixia. Thus, the serogroup A population, which for unknown reasons has become genetically separated, may, in the long run, become a species distinct from *N. meningitidis* as it happened to the gonococcus many years ago when some genetic event(s) allowed it to take up a separate ecological niche.

LOCALIZED SEX IN BACTERIA

In most bacteria, the situation is more complex than described above. Different parts of a bacterial genome or even of a single gene may have a phylogenetic history different from that of the remaining genome. Thus, even in species that show a basically clonal population structure it is usual to find that genes encoding virulence factors or surface proteins reveal a mosaiclike structure as a result of local recombination. This localized process results in antigenic diversity of the encoded proteins, which confers ecological advantage under the selection pressure exerted by the immune system of the host.

Also complete virulence genes or whole "pathogenicity islands" may spread through a basically clonal population of bacteria by horizontal genetic transfer to confer the same virulence properties on otherwise evolutionarily distinct lineages. Pathogenicity islands are large genomic regions 10 to 200 kb in size that often have G+C content and codon usage that differ from those of the rest of the genome, suggestive of a "foreign" origin. Their location in the genome adjacent to highly conserved gene sequences facilitates their insertion in foreign genomes by homologous recombination. Pathogenicity islands usually contain multiple genes encoding adhesins, toxins, invasins, protein secretion systems, iron acquisition systems, and other proteins associated with virulence. The structure of the genes indicates that pathogenicity islands are generated through evolution by a multistep process. Similar mobile clusters of genes or genomic islands that enhance ecological fitness are also found in many nonpathogenic bacteria.

Other mobile genetic elements that may spread across evolutionary lineages and introduce new virulence-associated properties or antibiotic resistance are plasmids, bacteriophages, and conjugative transposons (see chapter 7).

As a result of such inserts, individual strains of bacterial species may show remarkable differences. For example, recent comparisons of the sequenced genomes of two strains of *E. coli* revealed that only 74% of the genes in an enteropathogenic strain of serotype O157 were found in another strain (K-12), in spite of a mean identity of more than 97% in those genes that were shared. Thus, bacterial genomes consist of a core of genes necessary for basic metabolism and survival and a flexible gene pool consisting of an assortment of strain-specific genetic information that may determine virulence or ecological success.

DIFFERENCES IN PATHOGENICITY OF STRAINS

Given the mentioned differences in genomes of closely related bacteria, it is not surprising that strains of a species may vary significantly in pathogenic potential. Even within strains of a subspecies or sero- or biotype that look identical when examined with traditional diagnostic tests, remarkable variations may occur. This difference explains the observation that the majority of cases of serious disease observed worldwide are often caused by a small proportion of the total number of extant clones. Even within a recognized bacterial pathogen like *Haemophilus influenzae* serotype b (Hib), there are distinct phylogenetic lineages within the basically clonal population that rarely, if ever, are associated with disease. Likewise, most of the genetic variants of meningococci that constantly emerge never cause disease but are found in healthy carriers, where they contribute to the induction of resistance to more virulent clones.

From bacteria that evolve without significant recombination, one may expect a relatively stable occurrence of infections over long periods, as long as there is no significant intervention from the environment. Conversely, in "pathogenic species" undergoing frequent recombination, either involving the entire genome or localized areas associated with virulence, clones with altered virulence will continuously emerge and disappear. Whereas evolution leading to new species ("macroevolution") is a very slow process (*E. coli* and *Salmonella* separated more than 100 million years ago!), generation of new variants with altered virulence or resistance to antibiotics may take only minutes or days ("microevolution"). These fluctuations in virulence explain temporal variations in the prevalence and severity of infections caused by some bacterial pathogens.

SPECIFIC HOST ADAPTATION OF BACTERIAL CLONES

There is convincing evidence in biology for the coevolution of parasites and their hosts and for the hypothesis that they have speciated in synchrony. A result of this close mutual adaptation is that many species of bacteria exclusively cause disease or colonize in one host species. The evolutionary process has included optimization of the bacterial genome, often leading to loss of metabolic versatility and, thereby, enhanced dependency on the host. Examples are found in the *Haemophilus-Actinobacillus-Pasteurella* group of bacteria (the family *Pasteurellaceae*), which include both pathogens and commensals associated with humans or various animal species. A closer look at the individual species in this group of bacteria reveals that they have developed strategies for iron acquisition and evasion of host defenses that work only in their respective hosts. Other known examples of strict host adaptation can be explained by specific interaction of adhesins of the bacteria with receptors uniquely present in their host.

Recent population genetic analyses of bacteria associated with humans suggest that this host adaptation may be even subtler in some species of bacteria. Comprehensive studies of some pathogens strictly associated with humans have noted significant differences in the occurrence of individual clones in different parts of the world. One well-studied example is the invasive pathogen *H. influenzae* type b. Before introduction of the Hib vaccine in most industrialized countries *H. influenzae* type b was an important cause of meningitis worldwide, though with markedly different prevalence of disease in different human populations. Analysis of disease isolates of *H. influenzae* serotype b revealed that different clones were responsible for disease in different populations, even within the same country. While single clones were responsible for disease in ethnically homogeneous countries, a variety of clones were isolates from patients in North America. A comprehensive look revealed that individual clones were distributed in the world in patterns resembling those of the very large population movements which occurred in the Middle Ages. Adaptation of individual clones of *H. influenzae* serotype b to hosts with a particular genetic constitution over many years of coevolution is an attractive hypothesis to explain this observation and is in accordance with occurrence of multiple clones in the ethnically heterogeneous North American population.

Likewise, population genetic analyses of the periodontal pathogen *Actinobacillus actinomycetemcomitans* (see below) and of *H. pylori* further emphasize that significant differences may occur between ethnic groups (and thus geographic locations). Moreover, different clones of *H. pylori* have been isolated from different ethnic groups of humans. Particular blood group determinants in the host serve as receptors for specific *H. pylori* adhesins required for efficient colonization.

The pattern of colonization, in which only hosts of a specific ethnicity or blood group are colonized, is not seen universally. For example, in the case of the pathogen *Bordetella pertussis*, the etiologic agent of whooping cough, and toxic shock syndrome-associated *Staphyloccus aureus*, a limited number of clones are known to have caused disease worldwide. Furthermore, metabolically versatile bacteria like *E. coli* and *P. aeruginosa* have multiple habitats.

POPULATION SIZES OF PATHOGENIC AND COMMENSAL BACTERIA

As mentioned above, most exogenous bacterial pathogens are represented worldwide by a relatively limited number of clones, although with frequently recombining bacteria it is necessary to operate with complexes of types to reach the same conclusion. The individual clones disseminate successfully in the human population and may cause disease in nonimmune individuals. Bacteria that form part of the commensal microbiota on mucosal membranes show a very different pattern. The population sizes are enormous as indicated by the observation that it is difficult to find two individuals who carry the same clone unless they belong to the same family or otherwise are in close contact. This indicates that the major mechanism of transmission of commensal bacteria is vertical (i.e., from parents to their children), whereas lateral transfer is limited and restricted to intimate contacts (Fig. 2). Constrained evolution and diversification of clones within families over millions of years may explain the

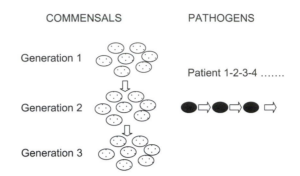

FIGURE 2 Different patterns of transmission and population sizes of commensal and pathogenic bacteria. Whereas commensals primarily spread from parents to their offspring (vertical transmission) and usually as a diversity of clones, pathogenic bacteria spread from patient to patient (horizontal transmission). Most pathogens consist of a limited number of clones.

immense number of distinct clones of commensal bacterial species, in contrast to pathogens, which spread horizontally from one individual to another. Furthermore, studies of the commensal bacteria in the oral cavity, pharynx, and gut demonstrate that multiple clones of some of the species often coexist in one individual.

ORAL BACTERIA SHOW VARYING DEGREES OF GENETIC DIVERSITY

The oral microbiota provides a remarkable example of biodiversity within a small habitat. Several hundred bacterial species have been isolated from the oral cavity and characterized in varying detail. However, recent analyses based on sequencing of 16S rRNA genes that may be amplified from dental plaque indicate that over half of the more than 700 species present are yet to be cultured and characterized. In addition to this complexity, application of sensitive DNA typing methods reveals considerable genetic diversity within species harbored by a single subject. This diversity makes it possible to disclose species-specific patterns of acquisition, population dynamics within the individual, and transmission between individuals.

It is clear that the degree of genetic diversity differs between species, although the available information is still incomplete due to methodological problems, and because only a limited part of the microbiota has been examined. Much of the actual diversity is likely to be missed in culture studies, which disclose only the predominant clones, even when selective isolation media are employed. Furthermore, results of such studies depend on the sampling technique, the number of isolates examined, and the resolving power of the typing method used. Extensive diversity has been demonstrated in populations of bacteria that are "true" commensals, i.e., *Streptococcus mitis*, *Actinomyces naeslundii*, *Fusobacterium nucleatum*, *Haemophilus parainfluenzae*, *Eikenella corrodens*, and some of the *Prevotella* species. In contrast, plaque populations of putative oral pathogens like *Porphyromonas gingivalis*, *A. actinomycetemcomitans*, and *Streptococcus mutans* (see chapters 11 and 12) usually consist of a single or a very limited number of genotypes at any one time.

Comparison of isolates of oral bacteria has demonstrated that the same genotypes of oral bacteria often are present in members of the same family, whereas unrelated individuals harbor distinct genotypes. In this respect, putative oral periodontal pathogens like *P. gingivalis* and *A. actinomycetemcomitans* resemble commensal bacteria rather than exogenous pathogens. As discussed below, the JP2 clone of *A. actinomycetemcomitans* constitutes a remarkable exception from this pattern. Members of this clone have been isolated from patients with juvenile periodontitis in virtually all continents of the world but restricted to individuals of northwest African descent.

THE ORAL MICROBIOTA IS A DYNAMIC POPULATION UNDERGOING CONSTANT CHANGES

It has long been recognized that the composition of the dental plaque microbiota is highly dependent on oral hygiene and dietary habits. In adults differences between individuals reflect differences in the proportions of individual species (and their detection by culture) rather than changes in their actual presence or absence. Thus, longitudinal studies of *A. actinomycetemcomitans* and *P. gingivalis* show that both species establish stable colonization in dental plaque of adults, although their proportions may change over time. However, recent studies in children using very sensitive detection by PCR show considerable instability. *A. actinomycetemcomitans* was detected in more than 50% of healthy children and *P. gingivalis* in more than 40%, but with random concordance between results obtained 1 to 3 years apart. Furthermore, in children who were colonized at both samplings different clones were present. Thus, in most children these two species colonize only transiently and a succession of colonizing clones may be observed during childhood.

S. mitis is one of the pioneers of the oral microbiota in infants. Within the first days of life several clones of this species may already be detected by culture studies. Throughout life a significant number of clones of this species inhabit the mucosa of the oral cavity and pharynx, but constant fluctuations occur in the relative proportions of the individual clones. While no clone remains detectable for more than 3 months in infants, more stability is present in adults.

S. mutans seems to be an exception to this pattern. This species colonizes the oral cavity predominantly during a brief "window of infectivity" after eruption of teeth. One or two clones of this species then seem to be stably present in dental plaque throughout life. In general, it is conceivable that clones colonizing dental plaque are more stable than clones colonizing mucosal surfaces in the oral cavity. The more stable colonization in adults may also be explained by more undisturbed microhabitats of dental plaque associated with the adult dentition.

Collectively, these studies emphasize the immense biodiversity of the oral microbiota and demonstrate the individuality of the microbiota in different subjects. The observed differences in population dynamics of oral bacteria raise important questions about mechanisms driving the fluctuations and how some bacteria are capable of coping with local selection pressures (including the mucosal immune system) whereas others are being rapidly eliminated.

TABLE 1 Strain-dependent differences in *P. gingivalis*

Virulence in animal infection models
Biological activities of cell wall lipopolysaccharide
Resistance to phagocytosis
Capsule production and capsule structure
Cytotoxic activity
Invasion of cells
Proteolytic activity
Expression and function of fimbriae
Expression of RagB protein
Autoaggregation
Glycosylation pattern of expressed glycoproteins

VIRULENCE DIFFERENCES WITHIN SPECIES OF ORAL BACTERIA?

From a disease perspective the individuality of dental plaques, particularly at the clonal level, has very significant implications. Individual genotypes of bacterial species present in dental plaques may have very different virulence properties. The putative periodontal pathogen *P. gingivalis* is an illustrative example. Studies of individual isolates of this species have revealed significant differences in virulence in experimental infection models in animals and in the expression of various properties that are likely to be of significance in the pathogenesis of periodontal disease (Table 1). Likewise, analysis of the complete genome of a pathogenic strain of *P. gingivalis* (W83) reveals numerous areas that resemble pathogenicity islands or "foreign" DNA by their significantly divergent G+C contents. Furthermore, the genome of strain W83 contains at least 96 complete or partial copies of insertion sequence (IS) elements that fall into 12 families. These IS elements may potentially inactivate genes and provide homology for intrachromosomal recombinations that may result in deletions and inversions (www.tigr.org). A recent comparison of the genomes of two strains with different pathogenic potential revealed numerous genes were highly divergent or absent in the type strain and confirmed that "hot spots" coincided with regions of lower G+C ratios (Fig. 3). Variably present proteins encoded by such regions included the putative virulence factor RagB, enzymes involved in capsular polysaccharide biosynthesis, and numerous proteins of yet unknown function.

Pioneering studies reported by DiRienzo and coworkers showed that among 12 genotypes detected by restriction fragment length polymorphism (RFLP) (see below) analysis of isolates of *A. actinomycetemcomitans*, one type was exclusively associated with periodontal disease whereas some others were exclusively associated with health. Furthermore, significant differences in the expression of leukotoxin, a toxin that kills human phagocytes (see chapter 12), have been demonstrated among *A. actinomycetemcomitans* strains (see below).

FIGURE 3 Distribution of divergent genes in the genome of strain W83 as compared to the type strain (ATCC 33277). (A) W83 genome and six-frame distribution of predicted genes. Dark blue, genes annotated with names or function; light blue, conserved hypothetical genes; gray, hypothetical genes and intergenic regions; red, tRNAs; yellow, rRNA. (B) GC distribution based on the G+C content of a 500-bp window and showing significantly divergent areas suggestive of recent acquisition by horizontal gene transfer. (C) Simulated heat map of the distribution of genes categorized from slightly (yellow) to highly (red) divergent between strains W83 and ATCC 33277. The black background indicates areas where genes are present in both genomes. Images were compiled with GenomeViewer software (http://www.oralgen.org). Reproduced with permission from T. Chen, Y. Hosogi, K. Nishikawa, K. Abbey, R. D. Fleischmann, J. Walling, and M. J. Duncan, *J. Bacteriol.* **186:**5473–5479, 2004.

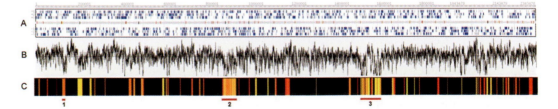

Experimental studies in animal models show striking differences in the cariogenic activity of human isolates of *S. mutans* and *Streptococcus sobrinus*, which are considered principal causes of dental caries (see chapter 11). However, it is notable that some isolates of the species *S. mitis*, which has been considered nonpathogenic, are as acidogenic and aciduric as these mutans group streptococci.

Studies of several other oral bacteria have revealed different allelic versions of genes encoding suspected virulence properties, but the functional significance of this genetic polymorphism has received only limited attention.

METHODS OF STRAIN DIFFERENTIATION AND SEARCH FOR VIRULENT CLONES

Application of DNA technology to the typing of microorganisms has resulted in numerous methods for strain differentiation. In contrast to traditional typing methods such as biotyping and serotyping, the discriminatory power of most of these DNA-based methods is very high. The choice of method depends primarily on the question that is being asked and on the genetic diversity within the population analyzed.

Single-locus typing targeted on a gene that shows significant polymorphism (e.g., genes encoding virulence properties or surface proteins under strong selection) usually has a high discriminatory power. The diversity may be demonstrated by nucleotide sequencing or by RFLP analysis using frequently cutting restriction enzymes and a labeled probe for demonstration of fragments. Ribotyping is a popular version of RFLP typing because a universal probe, e.g., from the *E. coli* rRNA operon, can be used for all bacterial species due to the conservation of parts of the rRNA gene. This fact may also be exploited to sequence or RFLP analyze the highly variable spacer region between 16S and 23S rRNA operons. In general, these techniques are suitable for short-term epidemiology, whereas in most cases they are inappropriate for global epidemiology because the high rates of evolution will obscure the overall genetic relationships between isolates. Furthermore, the plasticity of many bacterial genomes and the fact that some species are characterized by a random assortment of alleles at individual gene loci imply that studies focusing on single genes or limited parts of the bacterial genome, in most cases, will not provide an accurate picture of the overall phylogeny or genetic relationships within a bacterial population.

Methods that reveal the polymorphism in multiple random sections of the genome combine high discriminatory power with a more comprehensive view of the genome. The most commonly used methods are DNA fingerprinting achieved by restriction enzyme analysis or amplification of random DNA sequences by PCR. Restriction enzyme analysis is generally performed with frequently cutting restriction enzymes and separation of DNA fragments in agarose gels. Analysis of results obtained by this technique is often hampered by the complexity of the banding patterns, which makes it difficult to compare many strains. This problem may be overcome by pulsed-field gel electrophoresis, which allows separation of very large DNA fragments obtained by the use of rare-cutting restriction enzymes. An alternative restriction enzyme analysis method, which has been successfully applied to the typing of *A. actinomycetemcomitans*, is based on restriction fragment end labeling with a radioactive isotope. Separation of the fragments is performed in a polyacrylamide/urea sequencing gel and visualization is by autoradiography. With an appropriately chosen restriction enzyme this method produces very distinct patterns of fragments.

Amplification of random DNA segments with single primers of arbitrary nucleotide sequence is also used for genomic DNA fingerprinting. This technique is usually referred to as arbitrary primer PCR or random amplified primer DNA fingerprinting. Although this is a sensitive typing method, a number of experimental parameters have been found to influence the amplicon profiles, and the reproducibility of the technique has been questioned. A method that circumvents the inherent problems of the arbitrary method is rep-PCR, which targets repetitive DNA motifs. By detecting differences in copy number and chromosomal location of the repetitive element used as target, this method produces distinct and reproducible patterns.

The mentioned nontargeted multilocus methods are excellent for typing as they have high discriminatory power, but they do not provide a quantitative measure of genetic relatedness and are not suited for phylogenetic analysis. Thus, introduction of insertion sequences or recombination in part of the genome may blur the overall genetic relationships. Even more importantly, genome rearrangements, which are frequent events in some bacteria (e.g., *H. pylori*, *P. aeruginosa*, and *Salmonella typhi*) but do not necessarily affect their phenotype, may be mistaken as mutations at restriction sites. Finally, the methods are often too discriminatory to reveal overall relationships.

Population genetic analysis traditionally has been done by multilocus enzyme electrophoresis (MLEE), long a standard method in eukaryotic population genetics. In principle, this method maps the genetic polymorphism and relationships in a population of microorganisms by analysis of samples of the core genome. The targets are intracellular housekeeping enzymes in which mutations are assumed to be evolutionarily neutral as long as they do not affect function. A lysate of the bacterium is electrophoresed, usually in a starch gel, and the electrophoretic mobility of a number of metabolic enzymes is visualized by selectively staining for enzymatic activity. Different electrophoretic mobilities of the same enzyme in members of a population are equated with different allelic versions of the corresponding structural gene. A particular combination of electrophoretic mobilities defines an electrophoretic type, and cluster analysis of the data can be used to construct a tree. Provided that the population structure is basically clonal, the resulting tree will reflect the phylogeny of the population.

A further development of MLEE is multilocus sequence typing (MLST), which benefits by the fact that it has become feasible to amplify and sequence specific gene regions on a large scale. Instead of characterizing the housekeeping genes indirectly by comparing electrophoretic mobilities of the gene products, MLST characterizes the genes directly by nucleotide sequencing. The most important advantage of MLST over MLEE, and the many typing methods that compare DNA fragments on gels, is the unambiguity of nucleotide sequence data. In addition, results of MLST are electronically portable and can be directly compared between laboratories. The method was originally developed and validated by Spratt and coworkers in a study of *N. meningitidis* and subsequently has been applied to several other bacterial pathogens. The data of some of these studies are directly accessible on the Internet (http://mlst.net) where sequences can be directly compared.

Eventually, screening or even sequencing of entire bacterial genomes using pyrosequencing technology may become feasible for examination of populations of strains but will require powerful data analysis.

The crucial factor in any attempt to study the population genetic structure of bacteria is the sample. It must faithfully represent the population chosen for analysis and reflect the parameters under study, whether this is disease association or geographic or temporal variations. In contrast to many other infections in humans, studies of the etiology of oral diseases like periodontitis and caries pose significant problems due to the complexity of the microbiota. Isolation of a strain of *A. actinomycetemcomitans* or *P. gingivalis* or any other suspected pathogen from a patient with periodontal disease does not necessarily imply etiologic involvement. Conversely, an isolate from an apparently healthy subject is not necessarily nonpathogenic. The same problem applies to studies of dental caries etiology.

To approach the problem of identifying particularly virulent clones or subpopulations, clinical information on the isolates is compared with the clustering obtained by MLEE or MLST. If the bacterial population under study has a clonal population structure, this will usually disclose particular disease-associated clones or subpopulations if such occur. Conversely, in a population characterized by frequent recombination, pathogenic isolates may not cluster together but are characterized by distinct genes that encode virulence.

POPULATION GENETIC STRUCTURE OF ORAL BACTERIA

So far only two species of oral bacteria, *P. gingivalis* and *A. actinomycetemcomitans*, have been subjected to population genetic analyses. These studies utilized large collections of isolates that were both geographically and temporally diverse. Aimed at identifying particularly virulent subpopulations, all studies included isolates from healthy subjects as well as from patients with periodontitis.

Studies of *P. gingivalis* populations used MLEE, random amplified polymorphic DNA fingerprinting, and multilocus sequencing. All approaches demonstrate that virtually all isolates are genetically distinct and that isolates from cats, dogs, sheep, and New World monkeys belong to evolutionary lineages distinct from human isolates. In contrast, isolates from Old World monkeys are closely related to human isolates. In agreement with the conclusion that the population structure of *P. gingivalis* is panmictic, i.e., characterized by frequent recombination, there is no clear clustering within human isolates. Isolates for which pathogenicity has been demonstrated in animal models are randomly distributed across the population. These observations suggest that pathogenicity in *P. gingivalis* is associated with particular recombinant forms, presumably depending on genes in mobile chromosomal elements such as pathogenicity islands.

Screenings of comprehensive collections of isolates from clinically well-defined situations using microarray technology are required to identify specific combinations of genes that determine a virulent phenotype.

Studies of *A. actinomycetemcomitans* reveal a picture with both similarities and surprising differences from that observed for *P. gingivalis*. Cluster analysis of results obtained by MLEE and sequencing of selected gene loci demonstrate extensive genetic diversity as in *P. gingivalis*, with only few examples of isolates being identical. However, the population structure is clearly clonal with only limited evidence of genetic recombination. This conclusion is based on the observation that strains cluster according to serotype and that there is clear evidence of genetic linkage disequilibrium. In an analysis based almost entirely on isolates from Europeans, there was no evidence of single clonal types being responsible for multiple cases of periodontitis or systemic infections, nor was there evidence of disease-associated isolates clustering separately from isolates obtained from healthy individuals.

These observations are compatible with the conclusion that in the examined human populations both *P. gingivalis* and *A. actinomycetemcomitans* behave like commensals that spread among individuals primarily by vertical transmission. Thus, if etiologically involved in the pathogenesis of periodontal disease, they play the role of an opportunistic (endogenous) pathogen.

However, subsequent studies performed by Haubek and coworkers surprisingly revealed that a large number of isolates of *A. actinomycetemcomitans* from certain geographic regions belong to a single clone, i.e., the JP2 clone. The JP2 clone belongs to serotype b and differs from other strains of the species by significantly enhanced leukotoxic activity, by its hemolytic activity on horse blood agar, and by aberrant mechanisms of iron acquisition as a result of deleterious mutations in the gene encoding the hemoglobin-binding surface protein. The enhanced production of leukotoxin is due to a single deletion of 530 bp in the promoter region of the leukotoxin gene operon. Interestingly, in a Japanese isolate from juvenile periodontitis, similar enhanced activity was due to an insertion sequence interrupting the normal promoter of leukotoxin expression (Fig. 4).

The JP2 clone is strongly associated with juvenile, aggressive periodontitis in patients of northwest African descent living in the United States and in a variety of countries in South America and Europe. The clone is endemically present in Morocco, where it is associated with an unusually high prevalence of periodontal disease (15%) among adolescents (odds ratio, 29.4). It has also been detected in dental plaque from a group of Israeli children with an unusually high prevalence (38%) of early-onset periodontitis. Interestingly, other clones of *A. actinomycetemcomitans* showed no association with disease in the Moroccan population. Limited longitudinal observations confirmed the association of the JP2 clone with disease progression.

The characteristic epidemiology of the JP2 clone suggests that it originally arose in Africa and subsequently disseminated to most parts of the world, but still restricted to the original host population. Whether this restricted pattern of dissemination is due to adaptation of the JP2 clone to individuals of a particular genetic constitution or to predominantly vertical transmission is unknown. Its very strong association with early-

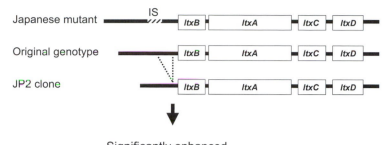

Significantly enhanced
leukotoxin production

FIGURE 4 The structure of the leukotoxin gene operon in *A. actinomycetemcomitans*. Two different genetic events have resulted in enhanced leukotoxin production in particular clones of *A. actinomycetemcomitans*. In a Japanese isolate an IS element has affected the normal promoter of the Ltx operon. In the JP2 clone associated with aggressive periodontitis in patients of northwest African descent, a 530-bp deletion interrupts the regular promoter.

onset aggressive periodontitis strongly supports its etiologic significance in this disease.

These findings emphasize that observations obtained in one geographic locality or in human populations consisting of individuals of a certain racial or ethnic background are not necessarily applicable worldwide. They further suggest that early-onset aggressive periodontitis may be a disease with dual etiology and epidemiology: In at least some persons of African descent disease is associated with a particular clone of *A. actinomycetemcomitans*, which has the epidemiological characteristics of an exogenous pathogen. The etiology in Caucasians is less clear. If etiologically involved, diverse *A. actinomycetemcomitans* clones may be acting as opportunistic pathogens. If this assumption is correct, it has important implications for treatment strategies. While eradication of the pathogenic clone with antibiotics or through vaccination may be relevant in the former situation, the most logical treatment in the latter situation would be to attempt to restore the natural balance in the commensal microbiota by hygienic measures.

KEY POINTS

Bacterial species can be viewed as populations of individual strains that share basic housekeeping functions but otherwise may have very different properties.

Genetic diversification can result from accumulation of point mutations in the bacterial genome or from recombinational replacements.

Species in which accumulation of mutations is the dominant mechanism of genetic diversification consist of discrete phylogenetic lineages or clones.

If recombination in a bacterial population is very frequent compared to the mutation rate, a panmictic population structure arises. This is

characterized by a random (or nearly random) assortment of alleles and the absence of distinct phylogenetic lineages. Hence, no single property will be able to identify a virulent phenotype in such bacteria unless that property is uniquely responsible for the pathogenic potential.

Different parts of a bacterial genome or even of a single gene may have a phylogenetic history different from that of the remaining genome. For example, surface proteins often demonstrate antigenic diversity as a result of local recombination. In addition, complete virulence genes or whole pathogenicity islands may spread through a basically clonal population of bacteria by horizontal genetic transfer to confer the same virulence properties on otherwise evolutionarily distinct lineages.   *(continues)*

KEY POINTS

(Continued from previous page)

Many bacteria appear to have coevolved with their hosts and have speciated in synchrony. A result of this close mutual adaptation is that many species of bacteria exclusively cause disease or colonize in one host species or even subgroups of that host species. The evolutionary process has included optimization of the bacterial genome, often leading to loss of metabolic versatility and, thereby, enhanced dependency on the host.

For bacteria that form part of the commensal microbiota on mucosal membranes, the major mechanism of transmission is vertical. Constrained evolution and diversification of clones within families over millions of years may explain the immense number of distinct clones of commensal bacterial species, in contrast to pathogens, which spread horizontally from one individual to another.

Molecular genetics has demonstrated a degree of biodiversity in the oral microbiota far exceeding earlier expectations and has provided new insight into the patterns of acquisition, transmission, and dynamics of oral bacteria. Combined with the recent realization that individual clones within bacterial species may have widely different properties, including widely differing virulence, this implies a remarkable degree of individuality of dental plaques. This new realization implies that previous attempts to identify etiologic agents of oral diseases by searching for associations between presence of particular cultivable bacteria and disease activity were too simplistic. Not all members of "pathogenic species" are likely to be virulent. Conversely, species considered nonpathogenic have been almost neglected, though there may be functionally important differences within such species. Even ubiquitous species, which are usually dismissed as lacking interest as potential pathogens, may include virulent subpopulations. Population genetic analysis of oral bacteria on a broad scale can reveal new insight into the genetic mechanisms of the genetic and phenotypic diversity that exists in the oral microbiota, and provide a better basis for our understanding of the etiology of oral diseases.

FURTHER READING

Maynard Smith, J. 1995. Do bacteria have population genetics?, p. 1–12. *In* S. Baumberg, J. P. W. Young, E. M. H. Wellington, and J. R. Saunders (ed.), *Population Genetics of Bacteria*. Cambridge University Press, Cambridge, United Kingdom.

Selander, R. K., and J. M. Musser. 1990. Population genetics of bacterial pathogenesis, p. 11–36. *In* B. H. Iglewski and V. L. Clark (ed.), *The Bacteria: a Treatise on Structure and Function*. Academic Press, New York, N.Y.

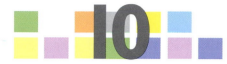

10

Oral Microbiology and the Immune Response

Michael F. Cole and Peter M. Lydyard

GENERAL PRINCIPLES

The oral cavity is the proximal part of both the alimentary and respiratory tracts. The mouth and nose are the principal portals of entry of infectious agents and allergens into the human body. Approximately two-thirds of all pathogens infect humans via these routes. The alimentary, respiratory, and genitourinary tracts, the conjunctiva, and the mammary glands are lined by glandular epithelia and are bathed by mucosal secretions. In the mouth the glandular (mucosal) secretion is saliva produced by the major paired parotid, submandibular, and sublingual salivary glands. In addition, the oral mucosa, with the exception of the midline region of the hard palate and the alveolar ridges, contains numerous minor salivary glands. In terms of immune protection, the oral cavity has much in common with the other mucosal surfaces of the body. However, the mouth is unique in that, in the dentate individual, there exist non-shedding surfaces, the crowns of the teeth, as well as shedding mucosal surfaces. The protrusion of the crown of the tooth through the oral mucosa results in a breach in the integrity of the mucosa with the formation of a cuff of keratinized squamous epithelium tightly apposed to the enamel surface. This cuff, the free gingiva, is lined with the sulcular epithelium that is continuous with the junctional epithelium that attaches the gingiva to the tooth surface. A space is thus formed between the tooth and the gingiva and is termed the gingival crevice (see Fig. 1 in chapter 3 and Fig. 5 in chapter 5). In health, gingival crevicular fluid (GCF), a tissue fluid-like transudate, flows from the gingival margin into the oral cavity. The flow of GCF serves to flush this area that is vulnerable to penetration by bacteria and their products. If dental plaque is allowed to accumulate at the gingiva margin, an acute inflammatory response ensues in the junctional epithelium and underlying connective tissue. The flow of GCF increases, and its nature changes from a transudate to a plasmalike inflammatory exudate that carries components of the immune system to the site of plaque accumulation.

The combined mucosal surfaces of the body comprise a considerable area of some 400 m^2, to which the mouth contributes some 240 cm^2 that must be protected from invasion by infectious agents and penetration by

201

toxins and allergens. It is not surprising, then, that a highly sophisticated and complementary host defense system has evolved in mammals to protect these surfaces. It should be realized that the mucosal surfaces are "open systems" unlike the vasculature and lymphatics (reticuloendothelial system), which are closed systems of tubes. All mucosal surfaces of the body are continuously flushed by secretions from closely associated exocrine glands, such as the salivary glands in the mouth. Persistence of microorganisms in the mouth requires, therefore, that they must attach to mucosal and dental surfaces or else multiply in the fluid phase, that is, saliva, at a rate exceeding the salivary flow or dilution rate.

In health, a state of dynamic equilibrium exists between the endogenous oral microbiota and host antimicrobial factors in the immunologically intact host. It should be appreciated that the principal oral diseases, dental caries (chapter 11) and periodontal disease (chapter 12), are the result of ecological imbalance between the components of the resident microbiota and the host immune response. For example, in the case of dental caries the frequent consumption of fermentable carbohydrate, particularly sucrose, provides a selective advantage to highly acidogenic and aciduric bacteria such as lactobacilli and, particularly, mutans streptococci. On the tooth surface these bacteria invest themselves in an adhesive, diffusion-limiting extracellular polysaccharide matrix synthesized from dietary sugars by glucosyltransferases and other enzymes to contribute to the biofilm known as dental plaque. If microcolonies of mutans streptococci are located in the biofilm close to the enamel surface, then the copious amounts of lactic acid produced by fermentation can result in enamel dissolution.

For purposes of discussion it is convenient to divide host defenses in the mouth and at other body surfaces into three levels or lines of defense. The first line of defense is a component of innate immunity, an evolutionarily primitive but, nonetheless, highly effective system. Innate immunity is nonspecific and does not require, nor is it intrinsically affected by, prior contact with the infectious agent. Thus, the innate immune system is in a continual state of readiness and can act rapidly to limit the infectious challenge. The initial strategy of innate immunity is immune exclusion. In the mouth, innate immunity acts to prevent a breach in the integrity of the barrier oral mucosa and enamel surface by attempting to combat infectious agents in saliva before they can attach to oral surfaces and by enhancing clearance of, or inactivating, agents that manage to adhere to these surfaces.

The second line of defense, also a component of innate immunity, comprises the inflammatory response (reticuloendothelial system), which serves to localize the infectious agent at the site of mucosal penetration if the first line of defense fails. The principal cellular elements of inflammation are phagocytic cells such as neutrophils (polymorphonuclear leukocytes), macrophages, and eosinophils; cells that release inflammatory mediators such as mast cells, basophils, and eosinophils; and natural killer cells. The inflammatory response utilizes a wide variety of pattern-recognition receptors that act in solution or on the cell surface of phagocytic cells. These receptors are able to differentiate molecular arrays displayed by infectious agents, termed pathogen-associated molecular patterns (PAMPs), from self. The inflammatory response acts as a link between innate immunity and adaptive immunity because it is able to function nonspecifically, but its activity is potentiated by the secreted products of B and T lymphocytes and by the classical pathway of the complement system. Moreover, many of the soluble mediators utilized by the first line of defense in mucosal secretions are also localized in the lysosomes of phagocytic cells and exhibit the same antimicrobial functions in the phagolysosome as they do in external secretions. A more complete discussion of inflammation can be found in chapter 2.

The third line of defense, acquired specific immunity, principally mediated by secretory immunoglobulin A (S-IgA) on mucosal surfaces, IgG and IgM from GCF, and effector T lymphocytes, is called into action in the event that the first and second lines of defense are unable to combat the pathogen. Acquired immunity, whether humoral or cellular, is adaptive and exhibits memory. Initial contact with the infectious agent or foreign molecule primes the immune system and it may be 7 to 10 days before specific antibodies or activated T lymphocytes are available to combat the infectious agent. However, this initial contact results in the development of memory cells that are able to initiate a secondary response that is more rapid, specific, and of greater magnitude. It is important to realize that, while convenient for purposes of discussion, the division of host defenses into first, second, and third lines is artificial, and in practice, there is extensive cooperation and overlap between components of each of the lines of host defense and they function as a fully integrated system.

INTRODUCTION

Immunologic defense in the mouth is mediated by a complex system of cells and molecules. Cells involved in host defense in the oral cavity include the mucosal barrier epithelium and phagocytes, lymphocytes, and other leukocytes involved in inflammation and adaptive immunity. Molecules involved in oral immunity include antibodies and nonimmunoglobulin proteins, glycoproteins, and lipoproteins that are derived from GCF, as well as from saliva. Salivary antibody in the healthy human mouth is predominantly S-IgA, although secretory IgM may be found in patients with selective IgA deficiency. GCF containing IgG, IgA, and IgM derived from plasma and synthesized locally in inflamed gingivae also contributes to the salivary antibody pool. The nonimmunoglobulin proteins include mucins (mucinous glycoproteins), lysozyme, lactoferrin, peroxidases, and a variety of other proteins with antimicrobial activity that are synthesized locally by salivary glands, the oral epithelium, and inflammatory cells in the gingival crevice/pocket or are derived from plasma. In the normal, healthy individual specific antibodies function in concert with these nonimmune host defense factors to maintain homeostasis in the oral cavity. A schematic representation of immune defense in the oral cavity is shown in Fig. 1.

There are several aspects of host defense in the oral cavity that are important to consider. It should be realized that many of the salivary molecules are multifunctional and have overlapping activities. Furthermore, some salivary molecules are able to form both homotypic and heterotypic complexes (Table 1). It is possible that such complexes have functions

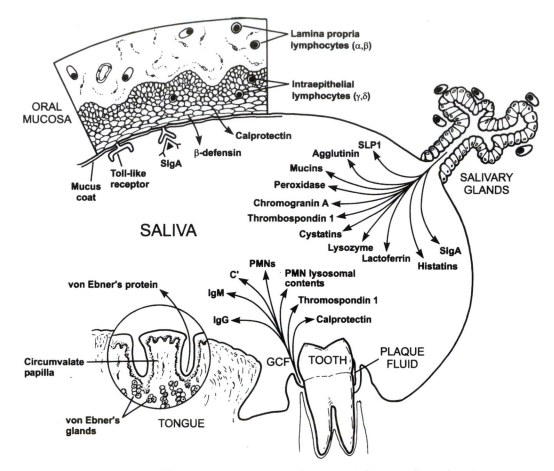

FIGURE 1 Schematic representation of immune defenses in the oral cavity.

additional to the individual molecules and/or that these complexes may exhibit synergistic activity (Table 2). In addition, the effector functions and properties of many of the immune factors may be different when they are adsorbed onto the mucosal, tooth, or microorganism surface compared to when they are in solution in saliva. This results from the fact that the proteins may undergo conformational changes when they become bound to surfaces that expose or create new epitopes or receptors. Additionally, immune factors in saliva may be modified by the action of bacteria-derived or host cell-derived proteases and/or glycosidases. Such modifications may abrogate their activity or, alternatively, reveal new activities of the molecule.

INNATE HOST DEFENSE

Oral Surfaces

THE MUCOSAL BARRIER

Because mucosal surfaces are required to serve a variety of functions, such as digestion, absorption, and gas exchange, they are thinner and more flexible than the keratinized, thick, and relatively impermeable skin. In the oral cavity only the free and attached gingiva, the hard palate,

TABLE 1 Heterotypic association

Mucin with S-IgA, lysozyme, cystatins, β-defensin

S-IgA with lactoferrin, agglutinin, agglutinin with lactoferrin

TABLE 2 Potential additive/synergistic interactions

S-IgA with lactoferrin

S-IgA with salivary peroxidase

Lysozyme with lactoferrin

Lysozyme with salivary peroxidase

Lactoferrin with salivary peroxidase

and part of the dorsum of the tongue are keratinized because these surfaces are subject to the abrasive forces of mastication. The remainder of the mouth is covered with nonkeratinized stratified squamous epithelium. While the keratinization of the skin and some areas of the oral mucosa aids in resistance to penetration by microorganisms and their products, the nonkeratinized oral mucosa is not defenseless and protects itself in a number of ways. The oral epithelium, in common with other epithelia and cells of the immune system, expresses Toll-like receptors. Toll-like receptors are signaling pattern-recognition receptors that recognize repeating patterns of molecules that are conserved among pathogenic microorganisms. These molecular arrays have been termed PAMPs and are not found on host cells. Examples of PAMPs are lipoteichoic acids of gram-positive bacteria, lipopolysaccharides of gram-negative bacteria, peptidoglycan, flagellin, pilin, and DNA of bacteria, fungal mannans, and double-stranded RNA of viruses. Currently 10 Toll-like receptors have been identified that are capable of engaging specific PAMPs (Table 3). Toll-like receptor engagement with a PAMP signals the epithelial cell to produce cytokines, chemokines, and peptide antibiotics known as β-defensins. Furthermore, epithelial cells also release nitric oxide and eicosanoids and express major histocompatibility complex (MHC) class II and nonclassical MHC class I molecules.

DEFENSINS

Defensins are a class of small (3- to 6-kDa) cationic peptides containing three to four disulfide bonds. They can be divided into α- and β-defensins based on the specific pattern of cysteine spacing and disulfide bonding. The β-defensin HBD-1 is the principal defensin produced by human epithelial cells. It is thought that defensins adopt multimeric anular complexes in bacterial membranes that are rich in negatively charged phospholipids. This leads to the formation of pores, which, in turn, increases the permeability of the membrane to solutes and leads, ultimately, to the disruption of the membrane. The lower phospholipid content of the cell membrane of higher eukaryotes, such as humans, provides protection from collateral damage by the defensin peptides. The mechanism of formation of a ring structure traversing the cell membrane by cationic peptides is similar to that of the membrane attack complex of the complement cascade (see chapter 2). β-Defensins are expressed in the duct cells

TABLE 3 Toll-like receptors (TLR) capable of engaging PAMPs

TLR	PAMP
TLR1	May associate with and regulate TLR2 response
TLR2	Lipoarabinomannan, peptidoglycan, mannan
TLR3	Viral double-stranded RNA
TLR4	Lipopolysaccharide, lipoteichoic acid
TLR5	Flagellin
TLR6	Lipopolysaccharide
TLR7	Small antiviral compounds
TLR8	Unknown
TLR9	Unmethylated CpG islands of bacterial DNA
TLR10	Possibly lipopolysaccharide

of salivary glands and have been detected in saliva. Defensins are active at micromolar concentrations against bacteria, fungi, and enveloped viruses in vitro. It is also possible that defensins have functions in addition to their direct microbicidal activity. β-Defensins induce the activation and degranulation of mast cells, thus releasing histamine and prostaglandin D_2 that are chemotactic for neutrophils. In this manner defensins function much like chemokines and may up-regulate inflammatory defenses. β-Defensins also appear to be chemotactic for immature dendritic cells and memory T cells, and in this manner, they may facilitate the initiation of adaptive antimicrobial humoral and cellular immune responses.

CALPROTECTIN

Calprotectin, another antimicrobial protein produced by nonkeratinized epithelia, is a calcium- and zinc-chelating protein. Calprotectin exerts antibacterial and antifungal activity by virtue of its ability to bind zinc and deprive microorganisms of this necessary ion. High concentrations of calprotectin also are found in the cytoplasm of neutrophils, monocytes, and macrophages. Therefore, inflammatory exudates, such as GCF, also may contain high concentrations of calprotectin, from where it can reach saliva.

ADHERENT MUCIN LAYER

Mucins are glycoproteins that exist in a number of glycoforms. Two major types of mucin, termed MG1 (MUC5B) and MG2 (MUC7), are found in the oral cavity. MG1 is a high-molecular-weight mucin that consists of many covalently linked monomeric protein subunits that contain heavily glycosylated domains interposed with those that are much less heavily glycosylated. In contrast, MG2 mucin is a low-molecular-weight molecule consisting of a single glycoprotein chain in which the carbohydrate side chains consist largely of sialylated di- and trisaccharides only. MG2 can be found in the adherent mucus coat and in the acquired pellicle on tooth surfaces. However, the viscoelastic gel-like properties of MG1, resulting from the large amount of carbohydrate, the large molecular mass of the molecule, and its threadlike structure, render it uniquely suitable for coating mucosal surfaces. All intraoral surfaces are covered by a thin film of mucus less than 0.1 mm thick that hydrates and lubricates the mucosa. The mucus coat forms a sticky, slippery gel that is selectively permeable and contains lipids, proteins, and ions. Lipids are localized on the surface and are distributed throughout the mucus coat. Immediately apposed to the surface epithelium is the glycocalyx consisting of short mucin fibers anchored to the cell membrane and forming a dense glycoprotein layer. The surface lipid layer and the glycocalyx contribute significantly to the selective permeability of the mucous layer, allowing transit of nutrients and waste products, but not bacteria and toxins. The lipids, together with the mucin saccharides, also serve as free-radical scavengers. Mucin is secreted continuously by the submandibular, sublingual, and minor salivary glands and then shed or partly digested by the commensal microbiota. The mucous layer is effective in trapping and blocking the penetration of particulates and small molecules. Entrapment in the mucous layer allows prolonged exposure to host antimicrobial substances including antibodies, such as S-IgA, which are held in the mucus by numerous short-lived, low-affinity bonds with the mucin fibers. The composition, rate of secretion, and shedding of mucus can change significantly and rapidly, depending on the diet and the variety of pathogenic and commensal microorganisms and toxic substances encountered on the mucosal surface. The life of mucus at the epithelial surface is short, and it can be replaced within minutes to hours. Movements of the lips, cheeks, and tongue promote the flow of mucus across the oral surfaces.

DESQUAMATION

Desquamation is an underappreciated, but essential, component of innate host defense. The mucosal and skin epithelium is continuously desquamating, and the rate of desquamation has been shown to be related to the microbial burden. The importance of desquamation in limiting microbial colonization readily can be appreciated by comparing the low numbers of bacteria observed in Gram-stained smears of buccal epithelial cells with the masses of bacteria observed in smears of dental plaque biofilm formed on tooth surfaces that do not shed.

EPITHELIAL ANTIBODY RECEPTORS

Receptors for secretory component (SC), a glycoprotein that is covalently linked to S-IgA polymers, are present on buccal epithelial cells. Thus, microorganisms captured by the tethered antibody are removed with the cells shed from the epithelium.

ACQUIRED ENAMEL PELLICLE

Just as the mucosal surfaces of the mouth are covered by a mucus coat, the dental surfaces are covered by an acellular organic film termed the acquired enamel pellicle. Within minutes salivary proteins and proteins from GCF and from oral bacteria are selectively adsorbed to clean enamel and other dental surfaces, such as exposed root surfaces and restorations. Pellicle formation is complete within less than 2 h but appears to undergo a maturation or stabilizing process that may require several days. Furthermore, there may be turnover of pellicle components over time. Interestingly, the acquired pellicle is not simply adsorbed onto the surface of enamel but appears to penetrate the subsurface. On self-cleansing enamel surfaces the acquired pellicle is between 30 and 100 nm thick. The major components of pellicle include proline-rich proteins, cystatins, lysozyme, S-IgA, MG1 mucin, lactoferrin, statherin, and amylase derived from saliva; IgG, IgM, and the complement component C3 from GCF; and the streptococcal enzyme glucosyltransferase. The principal functions of the acquired pellicle appear to be the protection of enamel surfaces from tooth-tooth and tooth-mucosa friction and from demineralization induced by bacterial acids and acidic foods. These functions are consistent with the presence in pellicle of lubricating molecules, such as MG1 mucin, and molecules that mediate remineralization, such as proline-rich proteins, statherin, and cystatins. In apparent contrast to its protective remineralization function, the acquired pellicle serves as the substratum for the initial adherence of the pioneer bacteria that initiate dental plaque formation, and dental plaque is a prerequisite for dental caries and periodontal inflammation. Oral bacteria begin to attach to the acquired pellicle within a few hours of its formation, despite the presence of several innate antimicrobial factors, along with S-IgA, IgG, and possibly IgM antibodies. In fact, these immune molecules appear to act as ligands for bacterial attachment. This apparent contradiction may be reconciled by considering the acquired pellicle as a gatekeeper facilitating selective attachment of harmless oral bacteria while inhibiting those with potential to damage the enamel. However, some potentially pathogenic oral bacteria, such as *Streptococcus mutans*, produce extracellular glucosyltransferases that have a high affinity for the enamel surface and are incorporated into the pellicle. These enzymes synthesize adhesive glucan polymers from sucrose in situ that assist the adherence of *S. mutans* via glucan-binding proteins. Normally, *S. mutans* does not have a high affinity for pellicle and cannot compete effectively with pioneer streptococci for sites on the tooth surface. Therefore, this mechanism, which is mediated by sucrose and enhances the adhesion of *S. mutans* to the tooth, could be seen as one that disturbs those normal ecological processes that lead to healthy teeth and, instead, promotes disease.

COMMENSAL ORAL MICROBIOTA

An intact endogenous microbiota is an important component of the innate host defense system at mucosal surfaces and functions in a number of ways. Commensal bacteria compete for nutrients and receptors with exogenous microorganisms.

Endogenous bacteria also produce antagonists, such as bacteriocins, that inhibit susceptible extrinsic bacteria. In addition, immunostimulatory components of the endogenous microbiota, such as lipopolysaccharide, maintain a low but constant expression of MHC class II molecules on macrophages and other accessory cells and stimulate the production of cross-protective antibodies. The importance of the endogenous microbiota can be appreciated in patients who have been treated with oral broad-spectrum antibiotics. In these patients susceptible bacteria in the endogenous microbiota are suppressed, allowing the emergence or colonization of resistant bacteria and fungi, such as *Candida albicans*, that are usually excluded from, or held in check within, the mouth by the normal commensal microbiota.

Fluid Phase: Saliva

About 0.5 to 1.5 liters of saliva is secreted into the mouth each day by the paired, parotid, submandibular, and sublingual major salivary glands and by numerous minor salivary glands distributed throughout the oral mucosa. The submandibular salivary glands contribute about 65%, the parotid salivary glands about 23%, the sublingual salivary glands about 4%, and the minor salivary glands about 8% to whole-mouth saliva, although these proportions change with different types and conditions of stimulation. An adequate flow of saliva is essential to the integrity of the hard and soft oral tissues. The deleterious effects of reduced salivary flow are readily observed in subjects who have received radiotherapy to the head and neck that has compromised the function of the salivary glands as well as in persons taking the many prescription drugs that reduce salivary flow. Saliva is a hypotonic, aqueous fluid that has about the same osmolarity as plasma. The average pH of whole saliva is 6.7, but salivary pH may vary by about 1 pH unit on either side of this value. Saliva contains both inorganic and organic components. The electrolytes bicarbonate, chloride, potassium, and sodium are the principal inorganic components in saliva. The total protein concentration in whole saliva is low, about 2 to 3 g/liter, and includes the digestive enzyme amylase, the lubricant mucous glycoproteins, acidic proline-rich and tyrosine-rich (statherin) proteins involved in the stabilization of calcium and phosphate in saliva, and a number of nonspecific and specific humoral host defense factors that function to protect the mucosal and dental surfaces. These defense factors are discussed in the following sections and their concentrations in whole saliva are shown in Table 4.

MUCINS

In addition to the mucus coat, MG1 and MG2 mucins are present in saliva. Because of low viscoelastic properties, MG2 functions principally in the salivary phase. Here it plays an important role in the aggregation

TABLE 4 Origin and features of humoral defense factors

Analyte[a]	Whole saliva[b]	Parotid gland	Submandibular/ sublingual glands	Minor glands	Von Ebner glands	Epithelium	GCF
Volume (liters/day)	1.0 (0.5–1.5)						
Flow rate (ml/min)	1.3 (0.2–3.0)						
pH	6.7 (5.6–7.9)						
Total protein (mg/ml)	2.3 (0.2–7.5)						
β-Defensin 1	N/A[c]	Yes	Yes	Yes	No	Yes	Yes
Mucin MG1	233 (SD, ±146[d])	No	Yes	Yes	No	No	No
Mucin MG2	133 (SD, ±116)	No	Yes	Yes	No	No	No
Agglutinin	N/A	Yes	Yes	Yes	No	No	No
S-IgA	299 (65–928)	Yes	Yes	Yes	No	No	No
IgG	21 (8–35)	No	No	No	No	Yes	Yes
IgM	4 (2–10)	No	No	No	No	Yes	Yes
Complement C′3	5 (3.0–8.0)	No	No	No	No	No	Yes
Peroxidase (immunochemical)	7.5 (0.5–40)	Yes	Yes	Yes	No	No	Yes
Peroxidase (activity, mU/ml)	1.0 (0.3–2.2)	Yes	Yes	Yes	No	No	Yes
SCN (mM)	0.9 (0.2–2.6)	Yes	Yes	Yes	No	No	Yes
HOSCN/OSCN (mM)	38.5 (0–113)	Yes	No	No	No	No	Yes
Lysozyme (immunochemical)	69.1 (14.4–159)	Yes	Yes	Yes	No	No	Yes
Lysozyme (activity)	14.1 (4.2–31)	Yes	Yes	Yes	No	No	Yes
Lactoferrin	3.5 (0.9–115)	Yes	Yes	Yes	No	No	Yes
Cystatins (total)	50.5 (17.9–125)	Yes	Yes	Yes	No	Yes (uncertain)	Yes (uncertain)
Histatins (total)	33 (14–47)	Yes	Yes	Yes	No	No	No
Von Ebner gland protein (VEGh)	N/A	No	No	No	Yes	No	No
TSP1	4.1 (1.1–12.8)	No	Yes	Unknown	No	No	Yes
Calprotectin	1.9 (0.5–5.7)	No	No	No	No	Yes	Yes
SLPI	1.2 (0.9–1.7)	Yes	Yes	Yes	No	No	Yes
Chromogranin A (ng/ml)	3.4 (no range)	No	Yes	No	No	No	No

[a]Grams per milliliter unless otherwise noted.

[b]Mean and range.

[c]N/A, data not available.

[d]SD, standard deviation.

and clearance of oral microorganisms. MG2 is effective in aggregating bacteria via lectinlike interactions between saccharides on the glycan chains of the mucin molecule and protein receptors on the bacterial surface. For example, submandibular and sublingual gland saliva aggregates some species of oral streptococci via sialic acid on the mucin glycan side chains. However, it is likely that many different sugars are involved in aggregating different genera and species of oral bacteria. In saliva the aggregation of bacteria by mucins is a highly effective clearance mechanism; however, when the mucins are coating the mucosa (see discussion on MG1 above), such interactions may potentially aid in the attachment and retention of these bacteria.

AGGLUTININ

Closely related to MG2, salivary agglutinin is a highly glycosylated protein that has the ability to agglutinate a wide range of oral bacteria. Both MG2 and salivary agglutinin are very sticky molecules that tend to complex with other salivary proteins such as S-IgA and lactoferrin. Salivary agglutinin is identical to gp340, a member of the scavenger receptor cysteine-rich superfamily.

VON EBNER GLAND PROTEIN

Von Ebner gland protein is a cysteine protease inhibitor that is secreted into saliva by the Von Ebner glands located at the base of the circumvalate and foliate papillae on the dorsum of the tongue. This multifunctional protein may scavenge peroxidation products, and also, it possesses nuclease activity that may be antiviral.

HISTATINS

Histatins are small multifunctional histidine-rich basic or neutral polypeptides, 7 to 38 amino acids in length. They display a number of functions including regulation of calcium phosphate crystal growth, neutralization of toxic molecules, chelation, and protease and cytokine inhibition. They also exert potent fungicidal and bactericidal activities and are able to inhibit intergeneric bacterial aggregation and bacterially mediated hemagglutination. At least 12 distinct histatin polypeptides are found in saliva. Histatin 1, a 38-amino-acid polypeptide, and histatin 3 (32 amino acids) are encoded by two distinct genes, and the other members of the family are generated by truncations and/or proteolysis of these two molecules. Histatin 5 is the N-terminal 24 amino acids of histatin 3. The three major histatins (1, 3, and 5) are secreted predominantly in parotid and submandibular saliva and account for some 80% of total histatin protein in whole saliva. It is unclear how histatins exert their microbicidal effect. It is possible that they alter membrane permeability by generating ion channels as do other cationic proteins. It has been suggested that the antifungal activity of histatin 5 results from its ability to bind to yeast membrane proteins and release cellular ATP that activates fungal ATP receptors. However, other microbicidal mechanisms cannot be excluded.

CYSTATINS

Cystatins are a superfamily of proteins that inhibit cysteine proteinases. Since many invasive microorganisms utilize cysteine proteases during their infectious life cycle, inhibitors of these proteases are considered to be important host defense factors. In addition, it seems most likely that cystatins play a role in regulating inflammation both by inhibiting host cell proteolytic activity and by up-regulating cytokines, both of which serve to maintain the integrity of the barrier epithelium. On the basis of structure and function differences, cystatins can be divided into three families. Family 1 cystatins are found intracellularly, and family 3 cystatins are high-molecular-weight kininogens. Cystatins S, SA, SN, C, and D belong to family 2 and are secreted into saliva. Cystatins S, SA, SN, and D appear to be restricted to saliva whereas cystatin C has been found in all external secretions so far examined. Salivary cystatins in saliva consist of at least nine isoforms encompassing acidic, neutral, and basic molecules. The cystatins are larger molecules than the histatins, with molecular mass of approximately 14 kDa, and are mainly secreted by the submandibular and sublingual salivary glands.

SECRETORY LEUKOCYTE PROTEASE INHIBITOR

Secretory leukocyte protease inhibitor (SLPI) is a small (12-kDa), cationic, acid-stable, nonglycosylated protein produced by serous acinar cells and epithelial cells, and it is a normal component of saliva and other mucosal secretions. SLPI is a serine protease inhibitor, and its proposed function is the protection of the mucosal epithelium from elastase and cathepsin B that are secreted by neutrophils in response to infectious agents. However, SLPI also exhibits bactericidal, fungicidal, and human immunodeficiency virus type 1 (HIV-1) antiviral activity. Indeed, SLPI has been shown to inhibit the infectivity of HIV-1 at salivary concentrations in vitro. SLPI is composed of two highly homologous domains. Interestingly, the carboxy-terminal domain contains the protease inhibitory site, whereas the amino-terminal domain is responsible for the majority of the antimicrobial activity, but the intact molecule is required for antiviral activity. SLPI appears to exert its antiviral activity at the level of the target cell. SPLI is without effect on the binding of HIV-1 to the target cell but appears to impede viral entry and/or uncoating. The mechanism(s) by which SLPI exerts microbicidal activity remain to be determined.

THROMBOSPONDIN

Thrombospondin 1 (TSP1) is a high-molecular-weight trimeric extracellular matrix glycoprotein that is secreted by the submandibular and sublingual salivary glands. TSP1 has been shown to inhibit HIV-1 infection of peripheral blood mononuclear cells and transformed T and promonocyte cell lines in vitro at concentrations found in whole saliva. The mechanism of action of TSP1 appears to be its ability to bind sites on the C2 and C3 regions of gp120 that are important in binding HIV-1 to CD4.

CHROMOGRANIN A

Chromogranin A is a salivary protein, the N-terminal 76-amino-acid peptide of which, termed vasostatin-1, exerts antibacterial and antifungal activity.

LYSOZYME

Lysozyme is a 14.6-kDa basic protein that is present in all major body fluids and is found at high concentrations in saliva, lacrimal fluid, and nasal and bronchial secretions. Lysozyme in whole saliva is derived from the salivary glands and GCF. Lysozyme exerts a bactericidal effect by several mechanisms. Functioning as a muramidase, lysozyme acts on the β(1-4) bond between *N*-acetylmuramic acid and *N*-acetylglucosamine present in the peptidoglycan of the bacterial cell wall. Disruption of the integrity of the cell wall leads to osmotic breakage of the cell membrane and death of the cell. Also, lysozyme may lyse bacteria by activating autolysins in the bacterial wall. In addition, lysozyme has been shown to be bactericidal in the absence of lysis. However, few species of commensal oral bacteria are susceptible to lysozyme under in vitro conditions except following an increase in pH to greater than 10.5 or the addition of salts or detergents. Therefore, lysozyme may be bacteriolytic only in environments that flux in pH and ionic strength, such as dental plaque. In addition to bactericidal and bacteriolytic activities, lysozyme effectively aggregates microorganisms and may act to inhibit their adherence to mucosal and tooth surfaces. Synergistic interactions between lysozyme and other nonspecific host factors, such as lactoferrin and the salivary peroxidase system, as well as with S-IgA have been demonstrated in vitro.

PEROXIDASES

Peroxidases are found in many, if not all, mucosal secretions. In whole saliva, peroxidase activity is composed of peroxidases synthesized by the salivary glands as well as myeloperoxidase from neutrophils and eosinophil peroxidase contributed by GCF. Salivary peroxidase catalyzes the peroxidation of thiocyanate (SCN^-) and the halides Br^- and I^-, by hydrogen peroxide, leading to the formation of, among other products, hypothiocyanite ($OSCN^-$). The SCN^- ion is a normal constituent of ductal and whole saliva as well as GCF and plaque fluid, while H_2O_2 is produced by the aerobic metabolism of glucose by several genera of commensal oral bacteria. $OSCN^-$ can inhibit the growth and acid production of a variety of oral microorganisms including streptococci, lactobacilli, and fungi by oxidizing bacterial enzymes in the glycolytic pathway that contain sensitive thiol groups. At acid pH, $OSCN^-$ becomes protonated to form hypothiocyanous acid (HOSCN), which, because it is uncharged, can rapidly pass through the cell wall and cytoplasmic membrane to the cytosol. Microbial inhibition results from interference of the NADH-NADPH balance of the cell, which is essential for glycolysis via the pentose shunt or via the NAP^+ dependent glyceraldehyde 3-phosphate dehydrogenase. Proteins in the cell membrane, as well as in the cytosol, also may be affected. Hydrogen peroxide is very toxic to eukaryotic cells and the reduction of H_2O_2 to H_2O by salivary peroxidase is considered to be important in protecting the oral mucosa. Salivary peroxidase retains activity when adsorbed to hydroxyapatite and can function effectively at the enamel-plaque interface. Contact between the enzyme and bacteria may, however, not be necessary because $OSCN^-$ diffuses readily. There is evidence of synergistic interactions between salivary peroxidase and lysozyme, lactoferrin, and S-IgA.

LACTOFERRIN

Lactoferrin is a multifunctional iron-binding glycoprotein (molecular mass, 78 kDa) that is synthesized by glandular epithelial cells and neutrophils. Lactoferrin is found in saliva and most of the other major secretions that bathe human mucosal surfaces. Lactoferrin exists in three forms, iron-free (apolactoferrin), ferric lactoferrin (one of two iron-binding sites occupied), and saturated lactoferrin (both iron-binding sites occupied). Iron binding requires the coordinate binding of bicarbonate. Because lactoferrin retards the growth of bacteria and fungi in vitro, it may play a role in the mucosal host defense. The antimicrobial action of lactoferrin in external secretions and of the closely related glycoprotein, transferrin, in plasma has been attributed to the ability of these glycoproteins to bind iron and render this essential nutrient unavailable to invading microorganisms. Lactoferrin has been shown to be bacteriostatic for a wide variety of bacteria and fungi by virtue of iron deprivation. However, lactoferrin is also directly bactericidal for many microorganisms and, although this effect depends on the ability of lactoferrin to bind iron, it is not reversed by the addition of iron. Lactoferrin binds tightly to the gram-positive and gram-negative envelope, and it may be able to perturb the organization of the cytoplasmic membrane, perhaps by lipid peroxidation. In addition to the antimicrobial activity of apolactoferrin, its hydrolysis by pepsin yields a 25-amino-acid residue cationic peptide referred to as lactoferricin. This peptide lacks glycosylation and the ability to bind iron but exerts potent antimicrobial activity against gram-positive and gram-negative bacteria and fungi. The mechanism of action is unclear, but lactoferricin may activate cell wall autolysins and/or cause a depolarization of bacterial cytoplasmic membranes. Lactoferrin forms a complex with S-IgA stabilized by disulfide bonds, and S-IgA antibody and perhaps complement may be required for the antimicrobial action of lactoferrin on certain microorganisms.

ROLE OF S-IgA IN INNATE IMMUNITY

The antigen-binding domains of certain S-IgA antibodies in saliva are encoded by germ line VH genes or by mutated VH genes in which the mutations are neutral, suggesting that antigen-induced selection has occurred. These S-IgA antibodies are polyreactive and are capable of binding a wide range of bacterial and host antigens (autoantibodies). It is proposed that these polyreactive S-IgA antibodies provide plurispecific mucosal protection prior to the induction of an acquired specific S-IgA immune response. This has led to the hypothesis that two different immune systems may function at the mucosal surface. One is a primitive system consisting of T-independent, self-renewing B cells, termed B1 or CD5 B cells, producing polyreactive S-IgA antibodies to commensal bacteria, food, and host tissue antigens. The other is a T-dependent system in the secondary lymphoid tissues at mucosal surfaces where IgA B cells undergo somatic hypermutation and produce monospecific antibody.

ROLE OF γδ T CELLS IN INNATE IMMUNITY

Within the epithelium is a population of intraepithelial lymphocytes (IELs), many of which bear the γδ T-cell receptor (TCR). γδ T cells express a very limited diversity of their TCR so that they can respond to antigens without the need for clonal expansion. γδ T cells do not appear to recognize antigen as peptides presented by MHC molecules, but directly in a manner analogous to the paratopes of antibody molecules. The functions of IELs are not completely understood, but they appear to recognize antigens expressed by epithelial cells that become infected or stressed. γδ T cells may play a role in maintaining epithelial integrity by secreting growth factors and removing epithelial cells that become injured or infected.

Acquired Specific Immunity in the Mouth

In humans and other mammals the mucosal surfaces of the body, including those of the oral cavity, are protected by a dedicated immune system termed the mucosal immune system. The mouth and the nose are the principal portals of entry for the majority of exogenous pathogenic microorganisms that infect humans. These mucosal surfaces are not sterile; they are colonized by stable complex communities of microorganisms referred to as commensal or resident microbiotas. These communities have coevolved with humans and, for the most part, exist in a homeostatic relationship with their hosts. Since the commensal microbiota is largely beneficial to the host, it would seem that the mucosal immune system must somehow differentiate between potentially harmful exogenous microorganisms and the endogenous microbiota. The mechanisms by which this is accomplished are not fully understood, but it appears that commensal bacteria induce a self-limiting humoral mucosal immune response.

Humoral mucosal immunity in the mouth is mediated principally by S-IgA. However, the gingival crevice and, possibly, the gingival one-third of the crowns of the teeth are protected by GCF that contains IgG, IgM, and IgA derived from plasma and produced locally by plasma cells in the gingivae. In contrast to IgA in plasma that is almost entirely monomeric and produced by plasma cells in the bone marrow, S-IgA is a polymeric immunoglobulin whose basic functional unit is a dimer, although tetramers are common. Covalently linked to the immunoglobulin polymers are two additional chains, SC and joining (J) chain. J chain is a product of the plasma cell and is required for the binding of IgA polymers to the SC, there being a single J chain in each polymer. SC is a glycoprotein that is a proteolytic fragment of the polymeric immunoglobulin receptor (pIgR). The pIgR is an integral membrane receptor that is found on the basolateral surface of epithelial cells lining mucous membranes and exocrine glands, such as salivary gland acini, that serves to transport J-chain-containing polymers into the external secretion. S-IgA is synthesized locally by plasma cells apposed to the mucosal epithelium and glandular acini. It is noteworthy that more IgA (plasma and secretory) is synthesized daily than the other four immunoglobulin isotypes combined.

There are two subclasses of IgA, IgA1 and IgA2. In addition, there are two allotypes of IgA2, A2m(1) and A2m(2). IgA2 lacks a sequence of 13 amino acids and five O-linked oligosaccharides that are present in the hinge region of IgA1. The deletion of this peptide from the hinge region of IgA2 renders it resistant to IgA1 proteases that are produced by certain mucosal pathogenic bacteria and commensal oral bacteria. In plasma almost all of the IgA is of subclass 1, whereas in mucosal secretions, such as saliva, there are approximately equal proportions of the two subclasses. Functionally, IgA1 antibodies appear to be directed largely against protein antigens, whereas IgA2 antibodies seem to recognize polysaccharides. Plasma IgA and mucosal IgA also differ in their rates of maturation. IgA in plasma does not reach adult levels until adolescence, whereas S-IgA reaches maturity in childhood. This difference reflects not only the different origins of plasma and mucosal IgA, but more importantly that the mucosal immune system is in contact with the outside world immediately after birth and stimulated by myriad foreign immunogens.

To function effectively at the mucosal surface, S-IgA must resist bacteria- and host-derived degradative enzymes. This is accomplished in several ways. Protection of the susceptible hinge region is afforded by SC and by glycosylation of this area of the heavy chain and, in IgA2, by the truncation of the heavy chain as described above. The IgA1 proteases cleave postproline bonds in a duplicated octapeptide region of the hinge region of IgA1 that is absent in IgA2. The resistance of IgA2 to proteolysis by IgA1 proteases may explain why there is a greater proportion of IgA2 in external secretions than in plasma.

Although defense of mucosal surfaces has been an important function of adaptive immunity since its evolution, the importance of S-IgA in the protection of mucosal surfaces of humans is enigmatic. IgA is a late evolving immunoglobulin isotype present in mammals and birds only. Furthermore, mammals make a significant commitment to the synthesis of IgA equal to the sum of the other four immunoglobulin isotypes. Teleologically, it would be expected that IgA must serve an important function in mammalian mucosal host defense and, accordingly, that humans with a selective- deficiency of IgA would be highly susceptible to mucosal infections. However, humans with selective IgA deficiency largely are asymptomatic, and the finding of their IgA deficiency frequently is incidental. An explanation to account for this observation is that there is considerable redundancy in host defense at mucosal surfaces and that many persons with selective IgA deficiency compensate by transporting IgM into external secretions in place of S-IgA. IgM also is a J-chain-containing polymeric immunoglobulin that can bind the pIgR.

It may be instructive to differentiate the potential influence that S-IgA exerts on the largely beneficial commensal microbiota and innocuous agents from that which it may exert on external pathogenic microorganisms. Overall, the role of S-IgA at mucosal surfaces is best described as one of immune exclusion. As maintaining the integrity of the epithelial barrier is of paramount importance in host protection at mucosal surfaces, S-IgA does not activate the complement system. As complement activation results in the generation of peptide mediators of inflammation such as C5a, C3a, and C4a, which could lead to disruption of the epithelial barrier, S-IgA is thus considered to be an anti-inflammatory immunoglobulin. The major functions of S-IgA are thought to be the prevention of microbial adherence to, and antigen penetration across, mucosal surfaces and neutralization of viruses, toxins, and enzymes. To this end, as has been mentioned earlier, receptors for SC that can immobilize S-IgA on the mucosal surface are present on oral epithelial cells. S-IgA can render bacteria mucophilic and reduce their negative surface charge and hydrophobicity. Furthermore, S-IgA binds to mucins. All of these functions serve to promote the clearance of microorganisms and other antigenic materials from mucosal surfaces.

S-IgA antibodies reactive with a variety of oral bacteria can be detected in saliva, and bacteria in saliva are coated with S-IgA. S-IgA is among the first glycoproteins to adsorb to naked enamel and it is a constituent of the acquired enamel pellicle. Pellicle-adsorbed S-IgA retains antibody activity. High concentrations of IgA are also found in the fluid phase of dental plaque, termed plaque fluid (see later). Studies conducted in vitro indicate that S-IgA can inhibit the attachment of bacteria and fungi to buccal epithelial cells and inhibit, but also, paradoxically, promote, bacterial sorption to hydroxyapatite (the base mineral of enamel). Clearly, as a polymeric immunoglobulin, S-IgA is very effective in agglutinating microorganisms via its multiple antigen-binding domains, but there is also evidence that the oligosaccharide side chains at the hinge region of the heavy chain may participate in lectin-receptor interactions with microorganisms. Whether the binding of S-IgA to a microorganism promotes or inhibits attachment to the mucosal or tooth surface may well depend on where S-IgA encounters the microbe. If the interaction occurs in saliva, then, likely, the outcome is clearance. However, if S-IgA is bound in the acquired pellicle, then the immunoglobulin may aid in attachment of the microbe to the tooth surface. Along similar lines, while salivary S-IgA appears capable of inhibiting the activity of certain microbial enzymes, it may enhance the activity of the glucosyltransferases of cariogenic streptococci.

There appear to be several mechanisms by which S-IgA can neutralize viruses. By binding to the virus particle, S-IgA can block the ability of the virus to attach to its cellular receptor. Even at antibody concentrations too low to inhibit attachment, S-IgA still may be able to inhibit penetration and/or viral replication. In addition, during transcytosis of J-chain-containing polymers of IgA through epithelial cells via binding to the pIgR, S-IgA exhibiting antiviral specificity can neutralize virus particles within the cell. However, this may be a two-edged sword because it has been shown that the pIgR and Fcα receptors, present on neutrophils, monocytes/macrophages, and eosinophils, can facilitate the uptake of certain viruses that are coated with S-IgA antibodies.

S-IgA is believed to limit the absorption of antigens through the mucosal epithelium. It is conceivable that antigens that penetrate the mucosa could be captured by polymeric IgA in the submucosa and returned to the mucosal surface via binding to the pIgR and trancytosis of the immune complex as described above.

MUCOSAL LYMPHOCYTES

Immunogens entering the mouth interact with lymphocytes in the mucosal-associated lymphoid tissues. These include oropharyngeal lymphoid tissues that are part of Waldeyer's ring and, if the antigen is swallowed and survives the acidity of the stomach, the Peyer's patches in the small intestine. Activated lymphocytes that have contacted antigen leave the mucosa lymphoid tissues via the efferent lymphatics and enter the circulation through the thoracic duct. These circulating lymphocytes home to epithelia and extravasate into the lamina propria and/or the intraepithelial compartment above the basement membrane. Most of the information about T-cell populations that are located in the mucous membranes has come from studies of the small and large bowel, but it is clear that the proportions of different T-cell phenotypes vary not only in different areas of the alimentary canal but also in other mucosae. T cells in the lamina propria appear to be resting memory cells awaiting reexposure to antigen. About two-thirds are $CD4^+$ and almost all express the $\alpha\beta$ TCR. They exhibit a low capacity to proliferate but a high capacity to produce cytokines. Perhaps because of the need to tightly regulate activation in the mucosae where there is an abundance of antigen, lamina propria $CD4^+$ T cells require an accessory CD2 signaling pathway for their activation. $CD8^+$ T cells expressing the $\alpha\beta$ TCR make up the balance of the T cells in the lamina propria where they serve to protect against intracellular parasites.

IELs are T cells located between the epithelial cells above the basement membrane. They are retained in this location because they express the integrin $\alpha_E\beta_7$, which binds to E-cadherin that is expressed on the basolateral surface of epithelial cells. IELs may be as frequent as one for every four to six epithelial cells. Phenotypically, IELs are much more heterogeneous than the T cells found in the lamina propria. For example, in the human small intestine as many as one-third of the T cells bear the $\alpha\beta$ TCR, and the majority of T cells are $CD8^+$ and many express both CD4 and CD8. The CD8 receptor is unusual in that it is an α chain homodimer instead of the usual $\alpha\beta$ heterodimer. The $\gamma\delta$ and $\alpha\beta$ TCR expressed by IELs exhibit limited V gene usage. As discussed, $\gamma\delta$ T cells do not appear to recognize antigen as peptides presented by MHC class I or II molecules, but directly in a manner analogous to the paratopes of an antibody molecule binding its epitope. Atypical MHC molecules expressed by injured epithelial cells appear to be among the targets of intraepithelial $\gamma\delta$ T cells. The functions of IELs are not completely understood but appear to include surveillance of the mucosa for microbial pathogens; maintenance of epithelial integrity by secreting growth factors, such as keratinocyte growth factor; the removal of epithelial cells that become injured or infected; and possibly, regulation of IgA responses.

In the oral cavity B cells are located in the lamina propria and, particularly, intimately associated with the acini of the major and minor salivary glands, where the vast majority are committed to the synthesis of IgA. For example, almost 90% of immunocytes in the parotid and submandibular salivary glands produce IgA, with the balance producing IgM or IgG. In histologic sections of parotid and submandibular salivary glands as many as 50 to 100 IgA-producing immunocytes may be observed in each square millimeter of the section.

GINGIVAL CREVICULAR FLUID

The function of GCF is to flush the vulnerable gingival crevice free of microorganisms, their products, and other noxious substances. The marginal gingivae are highly vascularized, being supplied with blood from both the periodontal ligament and the oral mucosa. There is a repeating pattern of capillary units, each unit consisting of a precapillary arteriole, arterial and venous capillaries, and a postcapillary venule. In gingival health, GCF is a tissue fluidlike transudate that enters the gingival crevice via intercellular spaces that exist between the cells of the junctional and sulcular epithelia. Gingival inflammation results in an increase in permeability of this extensive capillary network that directly underlies the junctional and sulcular epithelia. This leads to both an increase in the flow of GCF and a change in its composition to that of a plasmalike inflammatory exudate rich in immunoglobulins and inflammatory cells. It has been shown that in 15 min, as much as 40 µl of GCF can be collected from the upper anterior teeth of subjects with severe gingivitis, and it has been estimated that 2 to 3 ml of GCF flows into the mouth daily. Considering that the concentrations of IgG, IgA, and IgM in plasma are in the order of 10, 3, and 3 mg/ml, respectively, this would mean that some 20 to 30 mg of IgG and 6 to 9 mg each of IgA and IgM enter the mouth during a 24 h period. However, little of this immunoglobulin may retain functional integrity (see below). In addition to IgG, IgA, and IgM, the gingival sulcus also is the major site of entry of leukocytes into the mouth and the vast majority (95%) are neutrophils, with small percentages of monocytes (3%) and lymphocytes (2%). There are about three times as many B cells as T cells in gingival washings from healthy gingivae. About 10^5 neutrophils per milliliter can be obtained from gingival washings from an individual with healthy gingiva, and this number triples in subjects with gingivitis. Neutrophils retain their phagocytic functions both in the gingival crevice and in dental plaque.

DENTAL PLAQUE FLUID

Recent studies of intact natural human smooth surface dental plaque biofilms studied using confocal laser scanning microscopy have shown the plaque biofilm to have an open, extended structure with the biomass forming discrete structures. Overall, the architecture of the plaque biofilm is a heterogeneous distribution of cells, extracellular matrix, and fluid-filled channels, some of which extend from the enamel surface to the plaque-saliva interface. The aqueous phase circulating through the channels in the dental plaque biofilm is termed plaque fluid, and it comprises about one-third the volume of dental plaque. Dental plaque fluid is at the interface between saliva, enamel, cementum, GCF, and the junctional epithelium and it is here that innate and specific host defense factors likely exert their protective effects against dental caries and periodontal disease. Comparisons of the inorganic and organic components of plaque fluid, saliva, and GCF show that plaque fluid is a separate entity and not simply a mixture of saliva and GCF although it contains elements of both. Plaque fluid contains significantly greater concentrations of total IgA, IgG, IgM, the complement component C′3, lactoferrin, lysozyme, and peroxidase than does whole saliva (Table 5). These factors are present not only in plaque fluid but also bound to the biomass and can be eluted from it by using low pH buffers. However, examination of the structural integrity of host defense factors in plaque fluid reveals that, within a few days of dental plaque formation, they are extensively degraded by bacterial and host proteases.

IMMUNE REGULATION OF THE COMMENSAL ORAL MICROBIOTA

The question of whether S-IgA antibodies play a role in regulating commensal bacteria in the mouth is important because the two principal bacterial diseases in the oral cavity, dental caries and periodontal disease, are caused by members of the endogenous microbiota. Although saliva contains a complex, integrated secretory immune system, it is clear that many bacteria are capable of colonizing the various mucosal and dentate sur-

TABLE 5 Components of plaque fluid

Analyte	Plaque fluid, mean (range) (μg/ml)	Low-pH eluate, mean (range (μg/ml)
IgA (total)	2,096 (740–3,900)	100 (52–125)
IgG	594 (130–1,170)	30 (12–62)
IgM	64 (20–155)	18 (13–31)
Lactoferrin	283 (110–380)	91.0 (50–180)
Lysozyme	282.2 (90–450)	No data
Peroxidase	19.8 (2.2–52)	No data
C'3	85.0 (4–135)	28.0 (10–54)

faces of the mouth and can be found as constant components of the communities that establish there. In fact, it is the colonization of the mucosal surfaces by commensal bacteria immediately postpartum that drives the development of the adaptive immune system. The immune system of the infant either cannot exclude colonizing bacteria, with the survival of the strains being dependent on their physiology, or it is selective, eliminating those nonoral bacteria that attempt to colonize. It seems then that autochthonous oral bacteria are unaffected by, are not subjected to, or are able to avoid secretory immunity. That having been said, the absence of certain types of bacteria from the mouth may reflect effective suppression by immunological mechanisms, although one practical effect of an indigenous microbiota is the tendency to exclude newly introduced bacteria. It has been proposed that the control of bacterial populations constituting the commensal intestinal microbiota results from a combination of bacterial antagonism and immune mechanisms, and a similar situation likely pertains in the mouth.

IMMUNOLOGICAL CONTROL OF CARIOGENIC STREPTOCOCCI AND DENTAL CARIES

The identification of the viridans group streptococcus S. *mutans* as a principal etiologic agent of dental caries in humans stimulated research to determine whether there is natural immunological defense against this bacterium and, if so, whether it can be potentiated by active immunization. Immunity to oral bacteria can be mediated by the secretory immune system via S-IgA antibodies in saliva or by systemic immunity via IgG and IgM in GCF. The relative importance of mucosal versus systemic immunity depends, to a large extent, on whether one considers dental caries to be a mucosal infection.

NATURAL IMMUNITY

Numerous attempts have been made to correlate the levels of salivary IgA antibodies or serum IgG and IgM antibodies reactive with S. *mutans* or its antigens with either resistance or susceptibility to dental caries in cross-sectional studies. Such studies are complex because a correlation between current levels of immunoglobulins or antibodies with numbers of caries lesions may not exist. This is because a caries lesion is the manifestation of a process that may have begun months or years previously and even may be inactive at the time of sampling. Furthermore, such is the degree of cross-reactivity between different oral bacteria and between oral and intestinal bacteria that, unless a species-specific antigen is used for assay, the specificity of antibodies cannot be determined with any certainty. Consequently, a variety of studies have reported both direct and inverse relationships between dental caries and S-IgA and/or S-IgA antibody, in ductal secretions and/or whole mouth saliva. Thus the situation remains unclear.

SELECTIVE IgA DEFICIENCY

If salivary S-IgA antibodies are able to regulate oral bacteria, it would be expected that subjects with selective IgA immunodeficiency would exhibit increased susceptibility to dental caries and harbor *S. mutans* with greater frequency and numbers than immunologically intact individuals. However, while some studies report this to be the case, others have found no association between immunodeficiency and dental caries or, for that fact, periodontal disease. Indeed, some studies have found that patients with immune dysfunction have a lower caries experience than their immunocompetent counterparts.

ACTIVE IMMUNITY

The most direct evidence for a role of local S-IgA and/or systemically derived IgG/IgM antibodies in the regulation of the oral microbiota has come from the results of studies conducted in animals, principally rodents and primates, that have been immunized with antigens from, or whole cells of, *S. mutans* by routes designed to induce the preferred type of antibody response and then challenged with the immunizing strain.

Immunization of rodents

In general, rodents immunized by both mucosal and parenteral routes harbor fewer *S. mutans* bacteria, less dental plaque, and less dental caries than sham-immunized controls. However, there are several potential limitations of studies conducted in rodents. The first lies in the ecological relationship between *S. mutans* and the rodent host. *S. mutans* is not a normal inhabitant of the rodent oral microbiota, although *Streptococcus rattus*, a closely related species, has been isolated from wild rats. As has been discussed previously, it is evident that a host responds differently to its endogenous bacteria than it does to exogenous bacteria. In addition, many of the experiments have been conducted in germfree rodents that have been mono-associated with mutans streptococci and, thus, lack an intact oral microbiota. Second, rats become increasingly resistant to dental caries after 24 to 26 days of age. Typically, immunization is begun at weaning that occurs at 19 to 21 days of age, and the animals are not challenged with the cariogenic bacterium until several weeks later, when the animals are already highly resistant to dental caries. In fact, susceptibility to smooth surface caries decreases by 90% by the time rats are 30 days of age. Third, the experimental design of rodent studies has uniformly lacked a group of animals receiving an established cariostatic agent, such as fluoride, to serve as a positive control against which any effect of immunization can be compared. Last, often the experiments have utilized group sizes that are too small to provide statistical power and the methods used to score caries are not always clear. Because of these limitations, it is difficult to determine the significance of rodent data and to extrapolate the results of rodent studies to human beings.

Immunization of nonhuman primates

Nonhuman primates have been employed in immunization studies in an attempt to overcome the limitations of rodent models. Primates offer the many advantages of their close phylogenetic relationship with humans. Old World primates have a primary and secondary dentition comparable to that of human beings, and the composition of saliva, the oral microbiota, and the secretory immune system are quite similar. Importantly, nonhuman primates can be fed a human-type diet rich in fermentable carbohydrates. When infected with mutans streptococci, which are not part of their endogenous oral microbiota in the wild, and fed diets rich in sucrose, they develop caries lesions that are indistinguishable from those observed in humans. However, the use of nonhuman primates is not without drawbacks. First, they are difficult to obtain and expensive to maintain, and caries takes many months to years to develop. Therefore, the use of primates has been limited and, invariably, the group sizes have been small and the statistical power has been weak in experiments in which they have been utilized.

PARENTERAL IMMUNIZATION

The ability to protect against dental caries by intravenous immunization with *S. mutans* was first demonstrated by W. H. Bowen in 1969. Since this initial pilot study, other researchers have confirmed these findings. Clearly, protection afforded by parenteral immunization is unlikely to be mediated by S-IgA since systemic immunization is generally ineffective in inducing mucosal immunity. It is probable, therefore, that in this experiment protection resulted from IgG antibodies, derived from plasma, entering the oral cavity via GCF.

Potential adverse effects of parenteral streptococcal vaccines

Although parenteral immunization with *S. mutans* clearly is able to protect rodents and, importantly, nonhuman primates against dental caries, there is concern about the parenteral immunization of humans with *S. mutans* because it is clear that infection of susceptible humans with certain M types of another streptococcal species, *Streptococcus pyogenes*, can result in the development of rheumatic fever and acute glomerulonephritis. These diseases are thought to be the consequence of the ability of certain M types of *S. pyogenes* to induce autoantibodies and autoreactive T cells in humans that recognize joints, the myocardium, valves, and myocardial sarcolemma of the heart, the intima of blood vessels, the skin, the kidney, and the brain. In addition to molecular mimicry, several antigens of *S. pyogenes* also function as superantigens. Superantigens bind nonspecifically to MHC class II molecules on macrophages and to $\alpha\beta$ domains on the TCR of CD4 T cells. The result of bridging MHC II and the TCR is the activation of subsets of T cells bearing particular $\alpha\beta$ domains, some of which may be autoreactive.

What evidence is there that parenteral immunization with *S. mutans* also could lead to the induction of tissue-reactive antibodies? It is known that rabbits immunized with *S. mutans* produce antibodies that react with human sarcolemma and skeletal muscle. More significantly, *S. mutans* is able to absorb heart-reactive antibodies from acute rheumatic fever sera. Clearly, these findings would preclude parenteral immunization with a whole-cell vaccine, or even a subunit vaccine, if the subunit immunogen contained epitopes shared with human tissues. While it may be possible to identify immunogens that do not contain epitopes shared with human tissues, the likelihood is low that a parenteral anticaries vaccine would be acceptable for human use.

MUCOSAL IMMUNIZATION

The drive to develop a mucosal vaccine has been fueled, not only by the perceived importance of salivary S-IgA in protection against dental caries as a "mucosal infection" but, to a large extent, by the belief that mucosal immunity could be induced in the complete absence of circulating antibodies that might be host tissue-reactive. Although early experiments suggested that the mucosal immune system was independent from the circulatory immune system, this is not the case and mucosal immunization does induce circulating antibodies. Therefore, any prospective immunogen proposed for a mucosal vaccine must meet the same criterion as a parenteral vaccine, that of lacking epitopes shared with human tissues.

In contrast to the ease with which salivary S-IgA antibodies can be induced in rodents by various routes of mucosal immunization, it has proved much more difficult to induce salivary S-IgA antibodies by mucosal routes in nonhuman primates such as the rhesus monkey, *Macaca mulatta*, and the crab-eating macaque, *Macaca fascicularis*. One local route of immunization in monkeys that has proven effective in stimulating *S. mutans*-specific S-IgA antibodies in saliva is the retrograde instillation of killed bacteria into the parotid glands via the ducts. Monkeys immunized in this manner have been shown to be able to suppress implantation of *Streptococcus sobrinus*. However, frequent immunization is required because the antibody response is short-lived. Furthermore, this route of immunization results in functional impairment of the salivary glands and the induction of circulating antibodies and, therefore, would not be suitable for use in humans. Peroral immunization, which has been so successful in inducing salivary S-IgA antibodies in rodents, has been relatively ineffective in inducing S-IgA antibodies in the saliva of nonhuman primates. This discrepancy may result from anatomical and physiological differences between nonhuman primates and rodents, and additionally in primates there may be a greater need for a replicating antigen, or repeated, high doses of a nonreplicating antigen to overcome the destructive acidity of the stomach and digestive enzymes as well as peristalsis. As a result, researchers have employed other mucosal routes of immunization, such as intranasal immunization together with mucosal adjuvants, such as the B subunit of cholera toxin. However, S-IgA antibody induction in nonhuman primates remains unimpressive. Because of the difficulty in inducing salivary S-IgA antibodies, it has yet to be established that experimental dental caries can be prevented by mucosal immunization in experimental nonhuman primate models.

ACTIVE MUCOSAL IMMUNIZATION OF HUMANS

Almost all infants have S-IgA antibodies in saliva and IgG antibodies in blood that react with *S. mutans* prior to its colonization of the mouth. Thus, these antibodies are probably induced by other oral and/or enteric bacteria that share antigens with *S. mutans* or, perhaps, by cross-reacting food antigens. Clearly, in the majority of persons such antibodies are ineffective in preventing the colonization of *S. mutans*. Therefore, the purpose of a vaccine would be the extension of the specificity and avidity of salivary and/or circulating antibodies. Mucosal immunization with *S. mutans* cells or purified antigens such as glucosyltransferases, glucan-binding proteins, and fimbriae has been performed in humans. Intraoral, intranasal, and intragastric immunization routes have been employed in an attempt to stimulate IgA-inductive sites in the common mucosal immune system that would give rise to the appearance of specific S-IgA antibodies in saliva. Often liposomes have been used to deliver antigen to mucosal lymphoid tissues and to serve as an adjuvant. An alternative approach for antigen delivery to the mucosal immune system that has been considered is the utilization of commensal bacteria into which have been cloned genes that encode putative "virulence factors" of *S. mutans*. The rationale is to provide constant exposure of the cloned antigen to IgA-inductive sites of the mucosal immune system. As it is extremely difficult to introduce any bacterium into a climax community of commensal bacteria, this approach might be more fruitful in infants in whom the commensal oral microbiota still is in a state of development. Alternatively, attempts have been made to implant strains that may be at a selective advantage in the oral ecosystem because, for example, they produce a high level of antagonist, such as a bacteriocin.

Intractable problems with human subjects experiments include difficulties in obtaining a sufficient sample size, particularly in light of the large intersubject variation, and the lack of consistency in the means of statistical analyses of the data. Therefore, it remains to be determined whether specific salivary S-IgA antibodies can be effectively induced in the saliva of humans and, if so, whether these antibodies are capable of protecting against dental caries in humans.

PASSIVE IMMUNIZATION
Because of the concerns about the safety of actively immunizing humans with streptococci or streptococcal products, passive immunization has attracted considerable attention as a viable alternative. Attempts have been made to suppress or to reduce the repopulation of species of oral bacteria, particularly *S. mutans*, using antibodies delivered in drinking water, cows' milk, or other foodstuffs. The success of molecular biology in enabling the synthesis of properly folded, assembled, and fully glycosylated antibody molecules by plants, so-called "plantibodies," has made the economic, large-scale production and availability of antibodies of prescribed specificity a reality. Of course, antibodies utilized for passive immunization need not be S-IgA, nor need they be human in origin. Bovine milk IgG polyclonal antibodies, chicken egg yolk IgY antibodies, and mouse IgG monoclonal antibodies have all been utilized for passive immunization of animals and/or humans. In animal studies the antibody often has been included in the drinking water so that the antibody continuously bathes the oral tissues. In human studies, the antibody has been delivered less frequently by mouth rinse or by pipetting directly onto tooth surfaces. In some experiments that have sought to study the effect of passive immunization on recolonization of *S. mutans*, rinses and gels of the antimicrobial, chlorhexidine, have been employed to suppress this

bacterium to undetectable levels prior to beginning immunization. The use of chlorhexidine presents a confounding variable because this antimicrobial binds to the acquired pellicle and epithelium and has significant substantivity.

As might be expected, because of the greater frequency of antibody applications, the results of passive immunization experiments conducted in animals generally have been more impressive than those conducted in humans. Overall, the results of passive immunization studies conducted in humans, while mixed, have been promising in some cases. For example, following chlorhexidine treatment, passive immunizations with murine IgG monoclonal antibodies or with chimeric S-IgA antibodies six times over a period of 3 weeks were reported to suppress recolonization of *S. mutans* for 2 years. Since the duration of passively administered antibody in the mouth is, at most, a few days, the continued suppression of *S. mutans* after cessation of passive immunization was attributed to the ability of the initial antibody-mediated bacterial suppression to allow other oral bacteria to occupy the ecological niche of *S. mutans*, leading to its exclusion from the ecosystem. Passive immunization against commensal oral bacteria other than *S. mutans* also has been attempted in humans. *Actinomyces naeslundii* is a commensal bacterium that has been associated with caries lesions in dentine and exposed root surfaces. However, supervised twice-daily rinses with bovine milk containing IgG anti-*A. naeslundii* genospecies 1 and 2 antibodies for 4 days had no effect on the oral levels of these bacteria in comparison to rinsing with nonimmune milk or water. Therefore, it is as yet unclear whether passive immunization is a viable approach to dental caries prevention.

IMMUNOLOGY AND IMMUNOLOGICAL CONTROL OF PERIODONTAL DISEASES

The ability to develop a vaccine against periodontal diseases presupposes that the etiological agents of the various forms of the disease are identified, that it is clear which arm of adaptive immunity is the principal mediator of immune protection, and that suitable animal models exist in which to test candidate vaccines. Unfortunately, none of these is entirely the case. For localized aggressive periodontitis there is good evidence that *Actinobacillus actinomycetemcomitans* is the principal etiological agent, but an adequate animal model is lacking. For chronic adult periodontitis, there is neither a clearly identified etiologic agent nor an adequate animal model. From a bacteriologic perspective, chronic adult periodontitis is an endogenous infection that resembles mixed anaerobic infections elsewhere in the human body. These are complex polymicrobial infections that contain aerobes, along with facultative and obligate anaerobes. A characteristic of mixed anaerobic infections is that the microbial composition changes during the evolution of the infection and no single bacterium is considered to be the principal etiologic agent. Rather, pathogenicity results from synergism between the various microorganisms comprising the infection. That being said, *Bacteroides fragilis* is invariably associated with intra-abdominal infections even though it is a minor component of the gastrointestinal microbiota, and it is usually accompanied by fusobacteria. A similar situation may pertain in chronic adult periodontitis where a small cluster of species, such as *Porphyromonas gingivalis*, *Tannerella forsythia*, *Treponema denticola*, and perhaps several others, are consistently associated with sites of active disease. While it may not be possible to identify a single species as the etiologic agent, it is clear that the microbiota at diseased sites is different from that at healthy sites and at successfully treated periodontal sites. The initiating event or events that trigger the shift in the host-microbial balance from health toward disease remain unknown. However, localized deficits in neutrophil function may contribute to susceptibility, as may environmental factors such as tobacco smoking and stress, and systemic disease such as diabetes mellitus, and there is evidence of genetic predisposition. Although it is clear that certain bacteria are able to invade the periodontal epithelium, the vast majority of the biomass is found within the periodontal pocket attached to cementum as mineralized (subgingival calculus) or nonmineralized dental plaque, and the remaining bacteria are planktonic in GCF. Therefore, for the most part, the bacteria lie outside the reach of the humoral and cellular adaptive immune response. Accordingly, the periodontal lesion may be viewed as an example of "frustrated healing." In fact, gingival recession and alveolar bone loss could be viewed as host tissues retreating from the toxicity of the infectious front of the subgingival microbiota. Some periodontal bacteria such as *A. actinomycetemcomitans* produce cytotoxins that are capable of subverting the host immune response by killing neutrophils, monocytes, macrophages, and lymphocytes, while many others are masked from immune recognition by extracellular polysaccharide capsules or slime. In addition, many of the components and secreted products of the subgingival bacterial consortium are proinflammatory. Lipopolysaccharide, a component of the outer membrane of gram-negative bacteria, and peptidoglycan, the principal component of the gram-positive wall, are two potent inducers of inflammation. Added to these, many of the gram-negative, anaerobic rods that inhabit the periodontal pocket produce an array of hydrolytic enzymes that includes phospholipase, proteases, collagenase, fibrinolysin, neuraminidase, heparinase, and condroitin sulfatase, to name but a few, that are directly or indirectly tissue-damaging. Furthermore, many of these enzymes are able to degrade immunoglobulins. In addition, volatile and nonvolatile fatty acids, ammonia, and hydrogen sulfide, which are products of bacterial metabolism, also are capable of damaging host cells. The result of this assault is the recruitment of large numbers of neutrophils and other phagocytes into the nascent periodontal lesion by the release of chemokines from damaged cells in the periodontium and chemoattractant bacterial products. The attraction of neutrophils is aided by the activation of the alternate and lectin complement pathways generating the potent chemotactic factors C5a, C3a, and C4a. If there are naturally occurring antibodies in GCF reactive with the bacteria and their components, then the classical complement pathway also will be activated. In the process of engagement and phagocytosis of the subgingival bacteria, the phagocytes release a battery of cytokines and other inflammatory mediators. These include interleukin-1 (IL-1), IL-6, IL-8, IL-12, tumor necrosis factor-alpha, plasminogen activator, phospolipase, prostaglandins, leukotrienes, oxygen radicals, peroxides, and nitric oxide. In the nascent lesion where the bacteria are largely planktonic, neutrophils and macrophages, with the aid of Th1 T cells and an effective antibody response, may be successful in resolving or at least arresting the bacterial assault. However, biofilm formation largely places the subgingival bacteria outside the reach of the phagocytes so they cannot be eliminated, and the activation of, and the release of mediators and lysosomal contents from, the phagocytes causes considerable bystander damage to the periodontal tissues. Failing to achieve resolution or arrest of the lesion, the acute inflammatory response transitions into chronic inflammation with the replacement of neutrophils as the predominant cell type with T lymphocytes of the Th2 subset and finally plasma cells as the predominant cell type in the advanced lesion.

Since plasma cells dominate in the advanced periodontal lesion, the question can be asked as to whether antibodies are protective or whether they contribute to tissue damage. Low levels of IgG antibodies reactive with many oral bacteria, including those that have been associated with periodontitis, are present in the blood of almost all humans. It is clear that the majority of patients with periodontitis exhibit a humoral immune response reactive with members of their periodontal microbiota, which results in elevated levels of predominantly IgG, but also IgM, antibodies in GCF. Antibodies in GCF reactive with subgingival bacteria are derived both from the blood and increasingly from plasma cells in the inflamed periodontal tissues as the lesion progresses. However, it should be remembered that the absolute quantity of antibody may be far less important than the quality of its effector functions. There are four subclasses of IgG, and each has a different range of effector functions. IgG1 is the predominant IgG subclass and comprises about 70% of total IgG in the blood. IgG2, -3, and -4 comprise approximately 20, 8, and 2%, respectively. Of the four subclasses, IgG1 and IgG3 are most effective in fixing complement whereas IgG2 fixes complement poorly and IgG4 does not fix complement at all. IgG1 and IgG3 also bind more effectively to phagocytic cells and so are more efficient opsonins. In addition to the differences in effector functions of the IgG subclass antibodies, they may also exhibit different avidities. It is known that chronic infection and high antigen load, hallmarks of periodontitis, result in the production of low-avidity antibodies. A factor contributing to the production of low-avidity antibodies may be the polyclonal activation of B cells by lipopolysaccharide and muramyl dipeptide derived from the subgingival microbiota. Low-avidity antibodies have poor effector functions and tend to form immune complexes that promote inflammation. The finding of elevated levels of IgG4 antibodies in the GCF of patients with periodontitis is consistent with chronic immune stimulation. This supposition is supported by the finding that periodontal therapy consisting of scaling and root planing that removes the subgingival microbiota results in an increase in antibody titer and avidity. Whether these increases in titer and avidity result from the removal of the high antigen load represented by the subgingival microbiota or by the introduction of bacteria into the blood that stimulate peripheral lymphoid tissue is unclear. Thus, the induction of a highly avid and focused antibody response may be successful in eliminating or controlling the bacterial challenge, resulting in the resolution or at least the stabilization of the lesion, whereas chronic antigen stimulation and polyclonal B-cell activation may lead to the development of low-avidity, unfocused antibodies that are poorly protective and tissue-damaging.

Local dysregulation of immunity in the periodontium may also be promoted by components of the subgingival microbiota that function as superantigens and result in activation of, and the release of large amounts of cytokines from, subsets of T cells bearing particular αβ domains. Furthermore, the recognition of different PAMPs expressed by the subgingival microbiota by particular Toll-like receptors on macrophages and dendritic cells may result in the induction of different patterns of immune and inflammatory genes that may be polarized toward either a Th1 or Th2 response. It can be seen from the foregoing discussion that, in periodontal disease, the adaptive immune system is both protective and contributory to tissue destruction.

An examination of the results of experiments that have attempted to immunize against bacteria thought to be involved in the initiation and progression of the periodontal lesion might aid in clarifying the bacterial etiologic agent(s) as well as the role of humoral immunity. For the most part, the focus of immunization experiments has been on *P. gingivalis*, since this bacterium has come to be viewed as among the most important of several presumptive periodontal pathogens. Immunization experiments largely have been conducted in rodents while a few have employed nonhuman primates. It has been argued that the periodontium and the histology of the periodontal lesion are comparable in rats and humans despite the fact that the sulcular epithelium of the rat is keratinized and there is a predominance of neutrophils. However, all of the models involve infection with the presumptive periodontal pathogen and, in the case of rodents, almost always germfree animals have been employed. The relevance of such models to periodontitis in humans must be considered in light of the fact that human periodontitis is an endogenous polymicrobial infection rather than an exogenous monomicrobial infection as is the case in the experimental models. It is interesting in this regard that in neither rodents nor primates is it possible to establish *P. gingivalis* for more than a few weeks. However, despite these limitations, the data from studies in which rodents have been parenterally immunized with *P. gingivalis* cells or purified antigens prior to challenge with the bacterium suggest that immunized animals harbor fewer *P. gingivalis* organisms and exhibit less alveolar bone loss than controls.

The few primate studies conducted have been acute studies and have utilized ligation of the teeth with silk sutures to act as a reservoir for implanting high numbers of *P. gingivalis* organisms and/or as a mechanical irritant after parenteral immunization. The outcome variable in some studies has been colonization of *P. gingivalis* while others have also examined periodontal disease. The results have been equivocal due to small group sizes and large interanimal variability. Parenteral immunization with *P. gingivalis* appears to be able to reduce the numbers of this bacterium in some immunized animals and reduce alveolar bone loss when compared with controls. However, a reported collateral effect of immunological suppression of *P. gingivalis* was a significant overgrowth of other subgingival bacteria, such as *A. actinomycetemcomitans*, and enhanced progression of periodontal destruction. Thus, while parenteral immunization with presumptive periodontal pathogens is reasonably successful in inducing significant levels of IgG antibodies, there remains no clear evidence that such antibodies are able, consistently, to reduce the numbers of presumptive periodontal pathogens or, more importantly, protect against periodontal disease. Indeed, the suppression of one species in the periodontal microbiota, if it can be achieved, may allow the emergence of another and result in the exacerbation of the disease.

PROSPECTS FOR VACCINES AGAINST DENTAL CARIES AND PERIODONTAL DISEASES

Few would argue that, together with sanitation and public health, vaccination has made a significant impact on the reduction of infectious diseases that took place during the 20th century. Smallpox has been eradicated by an aggressive vaccination program, and there is the prospect that polio will follow in a very few years. An armamentarium of antibacterial and antiviral vaccines has been developed that protects against the principal causes of life-threatening infectious disease of humans. Despite the success of these vaccines, and perhaps because of it, there is increasing resistance by the general public to accept vaccination because of concerns about vaccine safety. With the incidence of infectious disease so low, there is concern that the adverse effects may outweigh the benefits. Initiated perhaps by the association of Guillain-Barré syndrome with the swine flu vaccine in 1976, and the frequent local and systemic adverse reactions including convulsions associated with the whole-cell pertussis vaccine, the real and imagined adverse effects of vaccines have grown to include arthritis, asthma, attention deficit disorder, autism, brain damage, cancer, chronic fatigue syndrome, diabetes, Gulf War syndrome, infantile spasms, inflammatory bowel disease, multiple sclerosis, and sudden infant death syndrome. Related to this, recent surveys show high numbers of parents refusing at least one recommended vaccine for their children. The reports of adverse effects have not been limited to parenteral vaccines. In July 1999, the Centers for Disease Control and Prevention recommended that health care providers and parents postpone use of the oral rhesus rotavirus tetravalent vaccine for children. This action was taken based on reports to the Vaccine Adverse Event Reporting System of intussusception among 15 infants who received the rotavirus vaccine. The manufacturer, in consultation with the Food and Drug Administration, voluntarily ceased further distribution of the vaccine. As a result of the increasing public concern about the safety and side effects of vaccines and the fear of litigation, the number of U.S. vaccine manufacturers continues to decline.

One of the tenets of vaccine development is that the disease should be serious enough to justify vaccination. It is a truism that no one has ever died from dental caries or periodontal disease (at least in their local manifestations), even though they are of major economic importance and frequently place a large health and financial burden on those least able to bear it. Furthermore, tooth brushing, the use of dental floss, and the application of sealants, fluoride, and antimicrobials in various forms can effectively control both diseases. Therefore, any vaccine designed to protect against these diseases would have to be completely safe. This criterion cannot be attained. Therefore, it is highly unlikely that a local or parenteral vaccine against dental caries and/or periodontal disease would be licensed for human use. Passive immunization may remain the single viable option.

KEY POINTS

Highly sophisticated and complementary host defense systems exist in the mouth.

The mucosal and dental surfaces of the mouth are continuously flushed by saliva produced by the major and minor salivary glands.

The cuff of free gingiva around the clinical crowns of the teeth permits the flow of GCF into the oral cavity, which serves to flush this vulnerable area.

In oral health, a state of dynamic equilibrium exists between the indigenous microbiota and host defense factors. The principal oral diseases, dental caries and periodontal disease, are the result of an ecological imbalance between members of the resident microbiota and host immunity.

There are three levels of defense mediated by innate and acquired specific immunity in the oral cavity. Innate immunity is nonspecific and does not require prior contact with the infectious agent, so it is in constant readiness and can act rapidly to limit the infectious challenge. Innate immunity comprises the mucosal and dental surface barriers, soluble antimicrobial factors in saliva and GCF, and the cells of the inflammatory response. This first line of defense combats infectious agents in saliva before they can adhere to oral surfaces or, if they adhere, enhances their clearance or inactivation.

The second line of defense is the inflammatory response that serves to localize infectious agents at the site of mucosal penetration if the first line of defense fails. The inflammatory response utilizes a wide variety of pattern-recognition receptors that act in solution or on the surface of phagocytic cells, principally neutrophils, macrophages, and eosinophils. Inflammation acts as a link between innate immunity and adaptive immunity because not only are the phagocytes able to function nonspecifically, but their activity is enhanced by the secreted products of B and T cells.

The third line of defense, acquired specific immunity, comprises S-IgA in saliva and IgG and IgM and effector T lymphocytes in the oral tissues. The role of S-IgA is immune exclusion at the mucosal surface. IgG and IgM antibodies are called into play in the event that microorganisms breach the mucosal barrier and cannot be successfully contained by phagocytes.

FURTHER READING

Challacombe, S. J., and P. J. Shirlaw. 1999. Immunity of diseases of the oral cavity, p. 1313–1338. *In* P. L. Ogra, J. Mestecky, M. E. Lamm, W. Strober, J. Bienenstock, and J. R. McGhee (ed.), *Mucosal Immunology*, 2nd ed. Academic Press, San Diego, Calif.

Cole, M. F. 1985. Influence of secretory immunoglobulin A on ecology of oral bacteria, p. 131–135. *In* S. E. Mergenhagen and B. Rosan (ed.), *Molecular Basis of Oral Microbial Adhesion*. American Society for Microbiology, Washington, D.C.

SECTION II ORAL DISEASES OF MICROBIAL ETIOLOGY

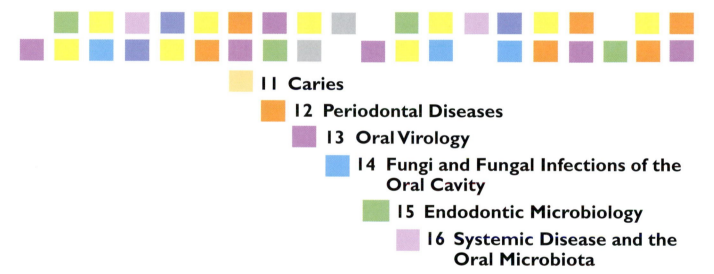

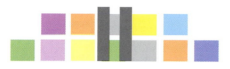

Caries

Robert G. Quivey, Jr.

OVERVIEW

Dental caries is a disease of human dentition characterized by loss of the mineralized surfaces of the tooth to the extent that the surfaces are permanently damaged and the underlying dentin is at risk or already damaged. The disease has been characterized as an ecological collision in the mouth, involving infectious bacteria and the ready availability of sugars in the diet, which the microbial population uses to produce destructive organic acids. If allowed to persist, the acidification brought about by bacteria results in permanent demineralization of the enamel.

The most heavily investigated etiologic agent of dental caries is *Streptococcus mutans*, a gram-positive coccus, though other bacteria including *Streptococcus sobrinus*, certain other acid-tolerant oral streptococci, *Lactobacillus* species, and, in some cases, strains of *Actinomyces* may be involved in human dental caries and have been shown to cause caries in animal models. The focus on *S. mutans* has come about because of its consistently high correlation with disease in epidemiological surveys of children and adults, its low abundance in the absence of disease, its demonstrated ability to grow at low pH values in vitro, and its ability to cause caries in animal models. The virulence factors of *S. mutans* are summarized in Table 1. Two key features of the physiology of *S. mutans* make it ideally adapted to cause dental caries. The first is that *S. mutans* readily metabolizes dietary sucrose to form insoluble polymers of glucose that aid in the persistent colonization of solid surfaces. The second feature is that *S. mutans* can survive at pH values that are toxic to most of the other bacterial species present in the mouth. Thus, the ability to adapt to acidic conditions is a key contributor to the pathogenic potential of *S. mutans*. The organism is also capable of utilizing a wide variety of sugars, which are rapidly metabolized to organic acids. In the presence of high levels of sugar, the predominant acid produced is lactic acid, which rapidly acidifies the environment around the bacterium. If bacteria are not physically removed from the tooth surface, plaque will accumulate as *S. mutans* grows, promoting accumulation and interaction of other bacteria, along with salivary proteins and food particles, with concomitant increase in acid production and retention.

TABLE 1 Virulence factors of *S. mutans*

Virulence attribute	Location	Function
SpaP (AgB, AgI/II, P1)	Surface, cell wall anchored	Adherence, binding to saliva-coated tooth surfaces and salivary agglutinin
Glucosyltransferases GtfB, -C, and -D	Secreted, often cell associated	Production of $\alpha 1,3/\alpha 1,6$-linked polymers of glucose from sucrose; important for adherence and biofilm accumulation
Glucan-binding proteins (GbpA, -B, and -C glucosyltransferases)	Surface, cell wall anchored	Binding of glucans produced by the glucosyltransferases; adherence to teeth, biofilm accumulation
Fructosyltransferase Ftf	Secreted, sometimes cell associated	Production of $\beta 2,1/\beta 2,6$-linked polymers of fructose from sucrose that can serve primarily as an extracellular reserve of carbohydrate; possibly implicated in adherence
Fructanase	Secreted and cell wall anchored	Hydrolysis of fructan polymers produced by Ftf; extends depth and duration of acidification
Dextranase	Secreted and sometimes cell associated	Endo-hydrolytic cleavage of $\alpha 1,6$-linked glucans; remodeling of glucan polymers to make them more water-insoluble and releases glucose from polymers that can be used to produce acids
Intracellular polysaccharides	Intracellular	Glycogen-like polymer of glucose used as a storage polysaccharide when exogenous sources are depleted; extends depth and duration of acidification
Phosphoenolpyruvate sugar:phosphotransferase (PTS)	Membrane/cytoplasm	Catalyzes high-affinity and high-capacity uptake of multiple different sugars; critical for growth and acid production
ATPase (F_1F_o ATPase or H^+-ATPase)	Membrane (F_o) and cytoplasm (F_1)	Large enzyme complex that uses ATP to pump protons from the cytoplasm; critical in acid tolerance
Acid tolerance and adaptation	Global, multifactorial	Allows organisms to acquire enhanced resistance and to grow more effectively at low pH

Caries is most often found in the industrialized nations, where sugar consumption is the highest. Not surprisingly, the organism has evolved to become a highly efficient sugar-processing engine, utilizing extracellular functions and intracellular metabolism to process the sugars that are common in diets. In particular, sucrose, the ordinary table sugar and the historical sweetener in cooking, is useful to the organism. In fact, results from early studies using human volunteers and animal models (see below) showed conclusively that irreversible colonization of the mouth occurred only in the presence of sucrose, and not in the presence of selected monosaccharides, like fructose or glucose. Some years later, after the advent of molecular techniques, the reasons for the sucrose dependence of attachment have become clearer.

As summarized in Fig. 1, *S. mutans* synthesizes and secretes four extracellular enzymes, three glucosyltransferases (Gtf) and a fructosyltransferase (Ftf), which function to split sucrose into glucose and fructose and, in the same action, form polymers of glucose (Gtfs) or fructose (Ftf). The glucosyltransferases are themselves diverse in that one of the enzymes, Gtf-I, acts to form insoluble glucans with a predominance of $\alpha(1\rightarrow3)$ linkages between the glucose monomers. The other enzymes, Gtf-S and Gtf-SI, function to produce glucans that are partly water soluble or insoluble, respectively. The Ftf product, a fructan polymer, is relatively water soluble. Of significant interest is the observation that the Gtf enzymes contain two domains, one of which possesses the glucan-synthesizing activity of the enzymes and the other functions as a glucan-binding domain. What makes this interesting from a biological standpoint is that *S. mutans* also synthesizes several additional extracellular glucan-binding proteins. Published reports have suggested that surface-binding of Gtf

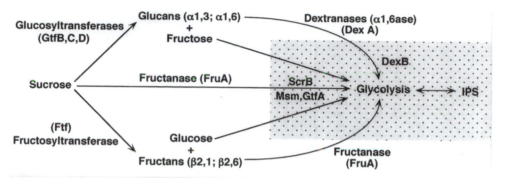

FIGURE I Metabolism of sucrose by *S. mutans*. The disaccharide sucrose can be converted to the polymers glucan or fructan by the enzymes glucosyltransferase (B, C, or D) or fructosyltransferase, respectively. Energy is provided by splitting of the glucose-fructose bond, and in both cases, monomers of the nonpolymerized monosaccharide (fructose or glucose) are produced. Fructanase can split sucrose or fructan and provide monosaccharides for glycolysis inside the bacterial cell. Similarly, dextranase can convert glucan into glucose for glycolysis. Intracellularly, glucose can also be polymerized into intracellular polysaccharide (IPS), which can be mobilized for glycolysis as necessary.

enzymes may result in a conformational change in the proteins, rendering them more highly active. In combination with data that show a disruption of normal biofilm development in mutant strains defective in glucan-binding protein synthesis, the conclusion is inescapable that glucan-binding is an important element of the *S. mutans* infectious process that facilitates the adherence and accumulation of the organisms on the tooth. Additional studies have shown enhanced binding of *S. mutans* to beads coated with saliva containing enzymatically active Gtf, revealing that the enzymes in free form may be able to synthesize binding sites on the tooth for the organisms to colonize. In summary, the picture that has emerged collectively from three decades of study is that *S. mutans* takes advantage of the presence of sucrose to bind irreversibly to surfaces through the ability to produce and adhere to glucans.

Caries itself is the dissolution of tooth enamel caused by the prolonged exposure to bacterially derived organic acids; the disease does not occur in the absence of bacteria. Tooth enamel is normally bathed in saliva, which at physiological pH levels is supersaturated with respect to calcium and phosphate, the primary minerals in enamel. If sugar is present in sufficient quantities in the diet, oral streptococci will preferentially produce and secrete lactic acid. The ionization constant of lactic acid (pK_a, 3.5) is below that of tooth enamel. When plaque pH values remain below a critical point, generally believed to be approximately 5.5, the balance between enamel remineralization and demineralization is disrupted and the caries process is initiated. With prolonged high levels of acid, mineral is dissolved and teeth can become permanently damaged (Fig. 2).

CARIES IN POPULATIONS

The incidence of caries in large populations has closely paralleled the industrialization of nations. As wealth has increased, so has sugar consumption in the form of foods and confections. In modern times, fluoridation of

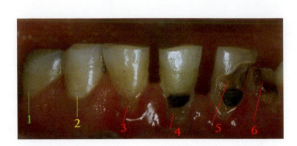

FIGURE 2 A patient presenting with caries in multiple stages. The stages of tooth decay are described as follows. (1) A tooth surface without caries. (2) A "white spot" lesion, which is not classified as a carious lesion but, rather, as incipient caries. (3) The tooth enamel has been penetrated; this lesion is referred to as a decayed surface. (4) A decayed tooth containing a restoration, or filling, in which the lesion has continued to expand. (5) Demineralization has proceeded, leading to and undermining the tooth. (6) Damage to the tooth has become severe enough to lead to a fracture. The image and legend were generously provided by Douglas Bratthall, Malmö University, Malmö, Sweden.

water systems, as well as the presence of fluoride in packaged foods and beverages, has greatly reduced the incidence of dental caries in the population of the industrialized countries. Nevertheless, reducing the risk of caries depends on behavior and access to dental care. It can be anticipated that though caries can be reduced by community water fluoridation, as not all communities in the United States have fluoridated water, there is still an abundance of caries in the nation. Moreover, access to health care is also unevenly distributed over the entire population. Indeed, this is borne out in the Surgeon General's report *Oral Health Care in America*, which summarizes a large number of studies and presents the most recent, comprehensive snapshot of the incidence of caries by age, racial/ethnic group, and economic circumstances. Caries was found to remain prevalent in groups with poor oral hygiene and limited access to health care. These general trends are likely to be applicable to other industrial countries.

The oral streptococci are now known to be transmitted primarily from mother to infant soon after the eruption of the deciduous teeth. The predictable result is that caries is found in all age groups in the United States, and it appears that virtually the entire population is infected to some extent with *S. mutans* and other caries pathogens. Despite the availability of fluoridated water, in 1997 slightly more than half of children between the ages of 5 and 9 had at least some caries experience, described as a decayed, missing, or filled tooth surface. By the mid-teenage years, the rate had increased to over 75% of the subjects and nearly 85% for persons over 18. The increase in the number of decayed, missing, or filled surfaces is not surprising given the accumulating nature of repaired tooth surfaces and the great abundance of carbohydrates in our society. The data point out that most individuals experience caries in their lifetimes. Moreover, nearly half the population over the age of 75 had at least one tooth exhibiting root caries, a number that will very likely increase as the overall population of Western nations increases. As might be expected, treatment of caries was roughly half as great among those living below the poverty line.

BACTERIAL ETIOLOGY OF DENTAL CARIES

Members of the genus *Streptococcus* are abundant in the oral cavity and include S. *mutans*, S. *sanguis*, S. *gordonii*, S. *sobrinus*, S. *salivarius*, S. *mitis*, and S. *anginosus*, among others. W. D. Miller, in the 1890s, published the parasitic germ theory of dental decay in which he articulated a cogent argument that acid-producing bacteria were the causative agent of dental disease. Moreover, he also cautioned that good dental hygiene with thorough removal of the organic matter was essential to prevent disease—a concept many years ahead of its time. The organism that presently enjoys the most attention with respect to dental caries, S. *mutans*, was first identified as an isolate from a human in 1924 by J. K. Clarke. The bacterium took its name from the different morphologies that it exhibited during growth on sugars. Later in that decade, S. *mutans* was identified in a high percentage of dental caries, suggesting a possible causal role in tooth decay. However, it was not until the late 1950s that Orland, Fitzgerald, and coworkers showed, using rats and hamsters, that strains of S. *mutans* could be used to inoculate germfree animals and that the infection would lead to the formation of dental caries.

In the late 1960s and early 1970s, Bratthall and coworkers showed that S. *mutans* itself was actually a group of organisms that could be distinguished on the basis of serology. Five serological groups were determined, and these were described as serotypes *a*, *b*, *c*, *d*, and *e*. Later work added two additional groups, *f* and *g*. The type most commonly associated with human disease has been the serotype *c* group. As technology advanced and came to include DNA-DNA reassociation kinetics, based on G+C content, Coykendall and colleagues proposed establishing four subgroups of S. *mutans*, which later became species in their own right: S. *mutans* (serotypes *c*, *e*, and *f*, genetic group I); S. *ratti* (sometimes called S. *rattus*) (serotype *b*, genetic group II); S. *sobrinus* (serotypes *d* and *g*, genetic group III); and S. *cricetus* (serotype *a*, genetic group IV).

The heterogeneity of mutans streptococci found in the human oral cavity is helpful to remember, in that the focus in caries research over the last 3 decades has been on S. *mutans*. While there is little doubt about the ability of S. *mutans* to cause dental caries in humans or animal models, there is relatively little understanding of the interplay of S. *mutans* with the many other organisms found in the oral cavity. Other commonly isolated bacteria from supragingival dental plaque include *Lactobacillus*, *Veillonella*, *Neisseria*, *Actinomyces*, and *Fusobacterium* species. Some of these, particularly lactobacilli and *Actinomyces* species, are potentially cariogenic in their own right.

WHERE DO CARIES OCCUR?

Supragingival Tooth Structures

Dental caries occurring on that component of teeth that can be easily seen is termed supragingival, or coronal, caries (see Figs. 1, 3, and 4 in chapter 3). Root surface caries, described in a following section, occurs on surfaces of the teeth that, in good health, are covered by the gums. The white, visible part of teeth is enamel, which covers the dentin, pulp, and cementum. Enamel is one of, if not the most, dense biologic tissues known. It is a mineralized tissue consisting, initially, of two proteins, amelogenin and enamelin, and protein-bound minerals, predominantly calcium, with phosphate, carbonate, and small quantities of many other minerals. As enamel is secreted, prisms of solid enamel are formed by the action of multiple cells called ameloblasts. Enamelin is elevated in aspartic and glutamic acid residues and is phosphorylated. Amelogenin, on the other hand, contains high levels of proline, histidine, glutamate, and leucine. As enamel develops, most of the amelogenin content is lost, whereas enamelin remains, bound in the crystal structure. The formation of enamel begins with the secretion of a product that contains relatively higher levels of water and protein, which is replaced over time with calcium, phosphate, and carbonate. The mineral content of enamel has been of great interest for many years, not only for the role of trace elements in the structure and function of enamel but also as reporter compounds for the effects of the environment on human development. Two important examples should be mentioned. The first is the element lead, which at high levels of exposure in women can lead to developmental disabilities in their children. Exposure to lead can also result in relatively softer enamel and a greater likelihood of dental caries formation. The second example is fluorine, which when present within the enamel leads to stronger crystal structures. This is a particular benefit of water fluoridation, in that saliva normally promotes remineralization of enamel, and in the presence of fluoride ion, the element can actually strengthen the tooth surface.

Dentin, the material directly under enamel, also contains a high mineral content, though much more closely related to bone, likely owing to its origins, as with bone, in mesodermal tissue. Dentin arises from the secretion of odontoblasts and contains approximately 20% protein made up of primarily type I collagen, along with phosphoproteins and proteoglycans. Cementum acts to join the teeth to their sockets, and like dentin, arises from mesoderm, with the result that the chemical composition is similar to that of dentin. The interior of the tooth is referred to as pulp, and in the case of rampant caries, pulp can be lost as well (Fig. 2).

Root Surface Caries

Root caries, as its name implies, is the formation of carious lesions on the surfaces of tooth roots. The disease is a significant oral health concern and one that is likely to become more problematic in the future, given that people are living longer than in the past and are retaining more of their natural teeth. As a result of aging or disease, the gums can begin to recede, resulting in the exposure of tooth roots. It has been estimated that approximately one-third of persons under the age of 60 have experienced root surface caries, and that the number climbs substantially with age; prevalence ranges as high as 60% and many patients present with multiple incipient and recurrent caries. As the roots lose their protective covering, in the form of the gum and the periodontal ligament, they become susceptible to bacterial infection and the subsequent accumulation of plaque. As it does in coronal caries, plaque on root surfaces presents the danger of concentrating metabolic acids on the enamel. Root surfaces are softer than enamel on the coronal portions of teeth, such that they are relatively more at risk for demineralization initiated by low pH environments. As erosion of the cementum progresses, the dentin also demineralizes, eventually leading to exposure of the dental pulp and loss of the pulp's collagenous matrix. The progression of root surface caries is paralleled by its discoloration (Fig. 2) and changes in the texture from hard to a softer or more leathery surface, and finally to a soft material as the pulp is exposed, weakening the entire structure and leading to the possibility of fractures in the tooth.

In bacteriological terms, the disease is very similar to coronal caries. Extensive research into the microbial etiology of root caries has resulted in a picture of predominance by aciduric bacteria. The bacterial etiology of root surface plaque historically has been somewhat troublesome to establish. Early studies had indicated the low abundance, or even absence, of streptococci and a far greater abundance of *Actinomyces* species. More recent reports have indicated abundant numbers of streptococci, with *S. mutans* and *S. sobrinus* being more prevalent than on healthy surfaces in the same subject. Moreover, levels of *Actinomyces* species are essentially equivalent on healthy and diseased sites in the same patient. Over time, therefore, the aciduric bacteria, mutans streptococci and *Lactobacillus* species, have emerged as the likely culprits that cause the disease we know as root caries. This is not to dismiss the possibility of other bacterial pathogens. As root caries progresses into the pulp, and the collagenous matrix is lost, it would be reasonable to consider the probability that proteolytic bacteria would also find a ready nutritional source in this advanced stage of disease.

ANIMAL MODELS IN CARIES RESEARCH

The use of animal models for caries was essential in showing that *S. mutans* is a causative agent of the disease and that the microbe is transmissible from one host to another. Fundamental studies by Orland and by Fitzgerald and Keyes, using rats and Syrian hamsters as models for caries, have led to decades of investigations into the pathogenesis of *S. mutans* in humans. The purpose of their research was not only to establish the bacterial etiology and transmissibility of dental caries but also to establish a coherent set of scoring procedures and language to standardize the methods by which research in caries formation could be conducted. The use of animal models has also provided a mechanism whereby modern molecular approaches could be used to investigate the impact of specific genes on bacterial pathogenesis. Moreover, the U.S. Food and Drug Administration promulgated a policy, in the late 1970s, that required demonstration of efficacy for oral therapeutic agents from two tests, the combination of an animal study plus an in vitro or in situ study. In practice, this has involved first showing efficacy of an agent in animal models; the second could be the demonstration of a reduction in solubility of hydroxyapatite caused by an active agent or demonstration of an increase of fluoride into enamel slabs. Importantly, to date, it has never been shown that agents successful in the rodent model are not also efficacious in humans under similar conditions. Experience has underscored not only the predictive ability of the animal model system but also emphasized its importance in the protection of humans until equally predictive in vitro models can be developed.

The use of animal models in caries experiments goes back to the 1920s, although far greater emphasis has been placed on attempts to standardize their use in recent times. The list of potential caries models has, in the past, included most available species of rodents along with larger animals, such as dogs, cats, horses, and pigs. However, nonrodent models are seldom used now, mainly because of issues of cost and susceptibility to caries. Primates, particularly macaques, have been used in many investigations related to caries vaccine work because of their similarity to humans, both in general physiology and in the organization of their dentition. However, the difficulty of working with macaques, the cost of maintaining them, and their availability have dramatically reduced their use in routine caries investigations.

The Rat Caries Model

Over the last 4 decades, the rat has been, by far, the most commonly employed caries model. The model has a number of important advantages. Their relatively modest size makes them considerably easier to maintain; however, their greatest advantage is that they will readily develop caries when fed a diet rich in carbohydrates. Use of the rat involves several important considerations, including the timing of infection, the diet and how it is presented to the animals, and the indigenous microbiota of the animals. Under optimal conditions, extensive carious lesions can be scored in less than 4 weeks. Moreover, it has been shown that caries formation can be greatly accelerated by preventing salivary gland secretions from reaching the mouth, usually by surgically removing the submandibular and sublingual glands of the animals and restricting flow through the parotid ducts.

Infection of Rodents for Caries Studies

Two types of experimental rat models are potentially available for use. In the gnotobiotic model, pups are delivered by cesarean section, raised in isolation, and fed sterilized food, thus preventing colonization by the normal, indigenous microbiota. The alternative used far more often is the specific pathogen-free animal model whereby the animals are screened, before their use in caries experiments, for the presence of human strains of oral microorganisms, especially *S. mutans*, and for the presence of other infectious agents, such as sialodacryoadenitis virus, which can compromise salivary gland function.

In Sprague-Dawley (albino) rats the first mandibular and maxillary molars usually erupt into the oral cavity around the 16th day of age. The second mandibular and maxillary molars erupt 1 or 2 days later, and by the 20th or 21st day, when rats are normally weaned, all three molars have erupted. In the experimental setting, the pups are usually infected around the time of weaning from their mothers, generally 17 to 21 days following their birth. The procedure involves dipping sterile cotton swabs into a bacterial suspension, and then using the swab to wipe the teeth of the animal. Difficulty in achieving a productive infection may arise when procedures are performed more than 27 or 28 days after birth. There appear to be at least two reasons for the need to infect the animals relatively quickly after weaning. The first is that the indigenous flora may block infection by virtue of sheer numbers; the second reason is that the density of the tooth enamel in rodents changes with age, thereby introducing another variable into the experimental design. Reintroduction of the infectious agent is often done in each of several successive days following the first infection; the purpose is to ensure infection. It is common to use genetically marked strains of bacteria, usually a resistance to a specific class of antibiotics, such that selective bacteriological media can be used to verify the success of swabbing.

The formation of dental caries is dependent on the availability of carbohydrates, and many foods have been examined for their ability to promote dental caries in rats, but typically rat model systems rely on sucrose in the diet. A number of commercially available dietary formulations have been used through the years; the emphasis was on relatively high-sucrose diets, at 56% (wt/vol), or diets with considerably less sugar, containing 5% (wt/vol) sucrose. The abundance of studies performed with both diets containing sugar at either level indicates that the sugar is in excess. Debate continues as to the usefulness of one type of diet over the other, but there is overwhelming agreement for the essential role of sugar in the formation of caries in model systems and in humans. Commercially prepared diets are available that contain appropriate mixtures of required nutrients and varying levels of carbohydrate.

Caries Scoring in Rats

A significant advantage of the rodent model for caries is the codified manner of scoring the disease, developed initially by Keyes and Fitzgerald and subsequently modified by Larson. The scoring system relies on the organization of the tooth surfaces into different zones and a numerical system assigned to score differences in severity of caries, as judged by penetration of a carious lesion from enamel into dentin. Examples of rat mandibles exhibiting caries, as compared to jaws prepared from rats fed a noncariogenic diet, are shown in Fig. 3.

Caries Models in the Future

Considerable effort has gone into the development of alternative models for caries, including artificial mouths and the use of prosthetic devices containing enamel slabs worn in the mouths of human volunteers. Artificial mouths will require some time to reach a reasonable facsimile of the human mouth. Intraoral devices, worn in human mouths, have the potential for delivering pertinent information, and some institutions are heavily investing in these devices. In these cases, the devices are slabs of enamel or other materials carried into the mouth on orthodontic brackets or similar mounting devices. The concept is to allow the devices to be bathed in normal saliva and for the subjects either to grow their normal microbiota on the device or to subject the device to a treatment schedule that includes the unaffected teeth, or additional considerations. The principal experimental issue with intraoral devices revolves around the device used to mount the slabs as the construction often introduces other variables or constraints into the experimental paradigm, which in turn may introduce differences in the observations as compared to normal tooth surfaces. It can be stated with certainty that exploration of intraoral devices, as a separate experimental tool, will continue for the foreseeable future.

Another model, albeit an alternative animal model to the rat, is the mouse. Mice have been used relatively infrequently in caries experiments,

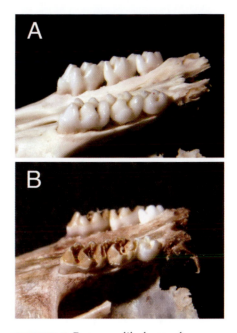

FIGURE 3 Rat mandibular molars prepared for caries scoring. (A) Jaws prepared from a rat fed a noncariogenic diet. (B) Jaws prepared from a rat fed a highly cariogenic diet. Reproduced with permission from W. H. Bowen and R. A. Lawrence, *Pediatrics* **116**:921–926, 2005, copyright 2005 by the American Academy of Pediatrics.

largely owing to their small sizes and their relatively more delicate association of molar teeth in the jaw. The advantage with mice is that the genetic stocks have become very well defined over the last 2 decades. As a result of mouse genomic sequencing, we have learned that mouse salivary protein genes are syntenic, that is, arranged in an identical fashion as human salivary protein genes, suggesting a high degree of conservation in form and function of salivary proteins between mice and humans. This fact alone could prove important in that loss of saliva is well known to lead to rampant caries in humans and rodents. Thus, the ability to manipulate salivary protein genes in rodents could be extremely useful for studies on the role of saliva in the balance between infection and protection of teeth. The procedures and tools established in the rat model are available for use with mice; the added advantage is the ability to genetically manipulate mice with a far greater degree of precision than is presently possible with rats. For these reasons, the mouse offers a potentially powerful system to examine the interplay of oral bacteria with host proteins and tissues.

IMMUNOLOGY OF DENTAL CARIES AND THE POSSIBILITY OF A CARIES VACCINE

The ubiquitous nature of *S. mutans* infection in the human population has been a driving force in the search for a successful vaccine to prevent dental caries. Although fluoridation of water supplies has been a dramatic public health success in reducing caries, its availability is not universal, even in the industrialized nations. As a result, research has continued vigorously in the pursuit of candidate target molecules that could be used as effective vaccine antigens.

The challenges faced in producing such a vaccine are formidable. A vaccine would have to be specific and efficacious, and it should have long-term positive effects with minimal negative side effects. Historically, successful vaccines generate systemic antibodies directed against a target, and they lead to the creation of memory cells that provide an anamnestic response, or memory, of the vaccination, leading to long-term resistance to the infectious agent.

The case of vaccinating against *S. mutans* is a particular challenge. It is found most abundantly on solid surfaces of the mouth, where the levels of systemic antibodies are quite low. Indeed, the largest proportion, by far, of immunoglobulin in saliva is in the secretory immunoglobulin A (sIgA) class. Moreover, no antigen identified to date represents an essential function that would either eliminate the ability of the organism to colonize the mouth or obviate its ability to cause dental caries. However, certain antigens have been identified, which are discussed below, whose elimination significantly reduces caries in rodent models. Moreover, exploration into the component pieces of vaccine strategies has contributed useful information that may ultimately lead to a vaccine for *S. mutans* and possibly other infectious agents that colonize wet surfaces of the human body. The following discussion is devoted to the current status of vaccine development and the challenges that exist.

What makes a caries vaccine problematic is that, to date, it is not known how to generate a truly long-term IgA response to antigens. Most published data from rodents and humans have indicated a period of elevated immunoglobulin levels for weeks or months, but not yet years. Many studies have been performed that show that sIgA levels directed against *S. mutans* in saliva (and other exocrine gland secretions) can be boosted repeatedly, but that the levels continue to fall off over weeks or months, requiring subsequent administration of a "booster" inoculation of antigen.

The other main issue is specificity, where two hurdles exist. The first is the certain identification of the causative organism, and the second is the identification of virulence factors whose elimination would lead to a decrease in disease. Here, far more information is currently available. As described above, *S. mutans* may not be the sole bacterial agent in dental plaque capable of surviving in the low pH environments required to initiate dental caries. However, an overwhelming body of evidence suggests that the organism is highly involved in the process. As a result, investigators with an interest in developing caries vaccines have focused on two key goals: the antigen(s) produced by *S. mutans* that would be reasonable vaccine candidate(s) and the mechanisms by which to stimulate a longer-lived immune response in the mouth. Both strategies have their roots in the concepts that the organism binds to tooth surfaces and then begins to grow, such that prevention of attachment would lead to a reduction in numbers and hence reduce the likelihood of disease.

Secretory IgA Is the Dominant Antibody in Saliva

Consideration of caries vaccines requires a brief discussion of the immune mechanisms available in the human mouth and the mouths of rodents, as most studies have been conducted in rats. In the case of humans, sIgA is by far the immunoglobulin in greatest abundance in the mouth. IgA is present in two subclasses, IgA1 and IgA2; the distinguishing feature between them is a glycosylated hinge region in IgA1 antibodies. Unfortunately, a number of mucosal pathogens produce and secrete an IgA1 protease, which cleaves the molecule, lowering its ability to agglutinate bacteria. Nevertheless, approximately 40% of the total salivary sIgA is of the A2 subtype. Secreted IgA is produced by all of the salivary glands, including a significant portion from the minor salivary glands in the lips, referred to as the labial glands, and the palatine glands in the roof of the mouth. Major production comes from the larger salivary glands, and earlier studies took advantage of the ability to stimulate antibody production by direct injections of antigen into lymphoid tissue near the salivary glands or directly into the salivary ducts (referred to as retrograde injections). The results of the direct injection approaches had the benefit of showing that levels of IgA could become elevated in saliva, a precondition for preventing colonization of the mouth by *S. mutans*, although these routes of immunization were less appealing and not practical for a large-scale immunization in humans. Many other ways have been explored to find alternative mechanisms by which the secretory immune system could be stimulated. Subsequent approaches have focused on methods to enhance stimulation of sIgA production and to refine the candidate antigens being used.

Studies involving tissue targeting of antigen via injections had shown that the nasal mucosa-associated lymphoid tissue of rodents might be a useful target for antibody production. Equivalent sites in the humans are the tonsils and the Waldeyer's ring, which have all of the anatomical structures associated with a healthy immune response. However, a key difference exists between the salivary immune repertoire of humans and rodents, and that is the availability of IgG in rodent saliva. Because the incisor teeth of rodents continually erupt, IgG makes its way into the oral cavity via exudates from the gingival crevices. It seems likely that the presence of IgG is of benefit in clearing microorganisms from the oral cavity of animals that gnaw on food and materials continuously. Thus, the effects of rodent vaccination, while an essential part of vaccine development, have to be interpreted in the context of saliva antibody composition, as well as the end-point data regarding efficacy against caries or other oral infectious diseases.

Vaccine Candidate Antigens and Delivery Systems

Early studies of immunization to dental caries were conducted using whole cells of *S. mutans*. Human volunteers swallowed boluses of killed streptococci, with the aim of increasing the abundance of salivary and serum levels of antibody to *S. mutans*. As most individuals infected with *S. mutans* already exhibit serum antibodies to the organism, the goal was to look for spikes in the production of antibodies to particular antigens, generally on the surface of the organisms, though antibodies to cytoplasmic proteins were often reported as well, consistent with reports regarding infection by other infectious bacteria. However, the finding that immunization could induce heart cross-reactive antibodies (see below) provided the impetus to explore more refined strategies with purified components. Fortunately, at about the same time, our knowledge regarding the molecular mechanisms of *S. mutans* colonization of the mouth was also beginning to evolve on the basis of molecular techniques. As a result, efforts have more recently been focused on proteins expressed on the surface of *S. mutans* or secreted by the organism. These efforts include the use of glucosyltransferases, glucan-binding protein, and antigen (Ag) I/II (SpaP) as candidate vaccine targets. The objective has been to prevent colonization of the mouth by reducing or eliminating the ability of the bacterium to get a foothold on the tooth surface.

In the case of AgI/II, the protein is known to bind salivary agglutinin, and likely binds salivary mucin, via a domain located in the N terminus of the molecule. As a vaccine candidate, the objective has been to interrupt the ability of the molecule to bind to salivary glycoproteins. This particular approach has had appeal because of the multifaceted role suggested for the molecule: blockade of early adherence mechanisms; inhibition of binding to early colonizers that have become coated with salivary molecules; and the possibility that the protein is involved in dentinal tubule invasion.

Work over the past decade has focused on the issue of prolonging antigen availability at sites of immune responses, that is, in the nasal mucosa-associated lymphoid tissue or at Peyer's patches in the gut, the gut-associated lymphoid tissue. Particulate materials such as alum powders combined with antigen or the incorporation of antigen into microspheres composed of poly-L-lactose have been used with at least partial success in raising sIgA levels. Initial efforts used intact molecules, such as glucosyltransferase or glucan-binding protein from *S. mutans*, in combination with particulates that were then introduced into rodent nasal tissue by spray or injection. Subsequent efforts have involved the use of peptide derivatives of Gtf and the AgI/II protein; the underlying assumption was that the peptides had innately higher abilities to function as epitopes. The approach also includes the notion that peptide constructs would be far easier to combine, using recombinant molecular techniques, to produce fusion peptides with biological adjuvants such as the cholera toxin B subunit or the detoxified *Escherichia coli* heat-labile toxin. Results from these studies have shown that molecules that act as adjuvants, such as the toxins, do improve the longevity of the IgA response to antigens from *S. mutans*, which is an important goal.

In addition to these approaches, the use of a living bacterium to deliver antigens has also been investigated. Attenuated strains of *Salmonella enterica* serovar Typhimurium have been created that take advantage of the organism's ability to infect the gut. Genetically engineered strains have been developed for seeding the gut-associated lymphoid tissue with organisms that continuously produce proteins of the target bacterial pathogen. Results from studies with a recombinant strain expressing a peptide-fusion of the salivary-binding region of *S. mutans* AgI/II coupled to the B subunit of cholera toxin have shown that nasal and gut administration of the vaccine strain induced the production of IgA in saliva. Moreover, the data indicated a reduction in recoverable *S. mutans*, indicating that the approach has potential. The challenge for implementing the use of such strains in the future is the requirement that the production strain must be able to produce the recombinant protein in a way that resembles the native production of the protein by the infectious agents themselves.

In summary, results from many studies support the principle that sIgA production in saliva can be boosted by a wide variety of approaches. These methods have generally led to reports of reductions of *S. mutans* numbers recovered from the animal hosts and incremental reductions in caries scores. The objective of future studies will clearly focus on reducing the frequency of boosters and on reducing caries scores to low levels. Because *S. mutans* infection is not lethal, the need for safety, efficacy, and cost-effectiveness for a caries vaccine will require significant improvements in longevity of IgA memory and the ability of antibodies to reduce caries incidence to a far greater degree than has been seen to date.

Cross-Reacting Antibodies to Streptococcal Antigens

An obvious component to caries vaccine work is information showing that any candidate vaccine is safe in humans. The original report by van de Rijn et al. showed that serum from rabbits immunized with strains representing the *a, b, c,* and *d* serotypes of the mutans group of oral streptococci reacted with human heart tissue. The observation quite naturally sparked many investigations into the nature of the antigenic reaction.

It was shown subsequently that the cross-reacting antibody could be removed by preadsorption using extracts of heart tissue and membranes from the group A streptococci, but, importantly, not from the media constituents used to grow the bacteria. These findings led to a number of studies designed to identify the antigens responsible for the cross-reactivity.

The focus of the work was primarily directed to the reasonable notion that epitopes on the surface of *S. mutans* were responsible for the cross-reactivity, much like what was established for M protein on the surface of group A streptococci. Moreover, the immunogenicity of the AgI/II cell wall protein was also well known, and that protein is highly conserved in oral streptococci. However, it was shown that the *S. mutans* heart cross-reactive antibody could not be adsorbed by purified AgI/II protein and that mutant strains defective in the production of AgI/II were capable of eliciting heart cross-reactive antibodies in rabbits, clearly indicating that other epitopes are involved. The issue then became one of elucidating other sources of antigenicity in *S. mutans* that would lead to the formation of antibodies directed against human heart tissue. The difficulty was that several possibilities existed: that the process of immunizing rabbits itself elicited the production of autoantibodies at low levels; that an unknown molecule on the surface of *S. mutans* elicited the cross-reactive antibodies, and the event could be a posttranslational modification of protein and, hence, not directly identifiable from genomic information; or that two or more surface molecules combined to yield an antigenic site. These concerns were somewhat mitigated by the well-established knowledge that anti-*S. mutans* serum antibody was readily identified in persons infected with *S. mutans* and that complications do not commonly arise from those antisera. Nevertheless, a number of studies were conducted to determine the origin of the heart-reactive antibodies. These studies included examination of whether bacteriologic media components, either themselves or bound to *S. mutans*, would contribute to the elicitation of heart antibodies. Molecules, presumably on the cell surfaces of *S. mutans,* that could drive strong antibody production in rabbits but did not result in human heart reactivity were identified as antigen A and antigen ID. Further characterization of these molecules has not been pursued, since use of selected highly purified targets does not appear to induce the adverse immune responses.

Probably the clearest insight has come from work with *S. ratti*, a species that is capable of eliciting the production of heart cross-reactive antibody in rabbits but does not encode an AgI/II protein. Membrane constituents from *S. ratti* were found to bind antibodies derived from rabbits that had been immunized with heart muscle. The converse was also true, in that antibodies to *S. ratti* membrane preparations recognized multiple antigens in preparations of heart tissue. These observations, taken together, support the idea that similar structures may exist in both heart tissues and streptococcal membranes. Conservation of the phenomenon among streptococcal species was established when it was shown that monoclonal antibodies to a 62-kDa protein of *Streptococcus pyogenes* could react with myosin, a muscle protein, and that the antibodies also reacted to proteins of similar mass in *S. mutans* and *S. ratti*.

At present, arguments have been made that the myosin-directed antibodies that cross-react with streptococcal membrane proteins are actually by-products of rabbit immunization. Indeed, higher levels of heart-reactive antibodies have not yet been identified in human antiserum in which antibodies to oral streptococcal antigens have been measured. This is not to say that these antibodies are nonexistent, but that they have not been found. What the data so far affirm is that material to be used as part of an immunizing vaccine has to be free of material that elicits antibody to host tissue.

APPLICATION OF MOLECULAR TECHNIQUES TO THE STUDY OF DENTAL CARIES

The contribution of molecular biology and its associated techniques in deciphering the mechanisms by which *S. mutans* causes disease is difficult to overemphasize. The application of nucleic acid-based technologies to the study of dental caries has included a number of exciting facets in modern biology and promises to involve the genomic and proteomic procedures that are being developed. Examples of how modern biology has contributed to oral microbiology, and vice versa, include not only the relatively standard DNA cloning approaches but also the ability to create precisely engineered mutations in the chromosome of *S. mutans*; the preparation of putative virulence proteins for biochemical study; the expression of virulence genes and, potentially, ameliorative gene products in heterologous hosts; and the use of strains of bacteria containing biochemical reporter molecules for detailing the expression of specific genes under defined conditions.

A discussion of the molecular approaches to *S. mutans* pathogenesis should be considered in the context that the fundamental concepts of *S. mutans* pathogenesis had been established well before the advent of DNA cloning in the mid-1970s. That is, it was known that the bacterium formed organic acids that were capable of initiating the dissolution of tooth enamel. It was also known that mutant strains of the microbe could be derived following chemical treatments and that these strains would be defective in various types of binding assays and, indeed, in caries model systems. Moreover, the role of sugar in the diet and its contribution to glucan formation by *S. mutans* were also well established. At the time of the introduction of cloning technology, scientists were using biochemical approaches to decipher the number, types, and mechanisms by which intracellular, extracellular, and cell wall-bound proteins promoted colonization by streptococci. Against this backdrop, the ability to separate a single gene from a bacterial genome came into play and revolutionized the way genetics, physiology, and biochemistry could be intertwined to study an organism's ability to cause disease.

Molecular Approaches to Adherence and Colonization by *S. mutans*

The application of recombinant DNA technology to the study of caries has no better exemplar than the wealth of research conducted on the enzymes produced by *S. mutans* that are involved in producing extracellular carbohydrate polymers. Virtually every approach currently in use has been successfully applied to the research into polysaccharide production, and for that reason, the following discussion focuses on how a variety of techniques were used to elucidate important information regarding the glucosyl- and fructosyltransferases. These techniques have also been applied to many other elements of streptococcal pathogenesis, but the first targets of molecular investigation were genes encoding the extracellular proteins involved with sugar polymer formation. Biochemical approaches had established that *S. mutans* appeared to produce multiple enzymes, the Gtf and Ftf, capable of forming glucan and fructan chains from sucrose, and other gene products that appeared to be involved in degrading the products. What was not understood at the time was how the *gtf* and *ftf* genes, or their protein products, were regulated by environmental conditions; how many genes there really were in a given strain; and how the proteins contributed to virulence. To address these issues, *gtf* genes were cloned from a number of oral streptococcal species. The efforts of many investigators led to the discovery that three genes in the chromosome of *S. mutans*-encoded Gtf enzymes. The ability to isolate the genes from *S. mutans*, in turn, facilitated the production of large quantities of highly purified enzyme. The picture that emerged in the mid-1980s was that each of the genes encoded a protein that had unique enzymatic characteristics, which were reflected in the type of glucan formed. Determination of the nucleic acid sequence of each of the genes also revealed the presence of shared domains between the enzymes. That is, the observation was made that glucosyltransferases contained repeated amino acid sequences in the carboxy-terminal portions of the proteins and conserved domains in the amino-terminal portion of the protein. Experiments were then conducted to define the role of each domain in the ability of Gtf enzymes to produce glucan. In these studies, portions of *gtf* genes were deleted and the shortened genes were used to produce their incrementally shorter proteins for use in reactions to measure the ability of the proteins to synthesize and bind to glucans. The data showed that glucosyltransferases contained two distinct domains. The first, present in the amino terminus of the protein, is responsible for glucan synthesis and contains an aspartic acid residue that is conserved, throughout nature, among proteins that either synthesize or degrade a wide variety of glucose-based polymers, including such things as cellulose, chitin, and the glucan present in dental plaque. The second domain, in the carboxyl terminus, consists of a set of repeating amino acid sequences that form a coil that accounts for the ability of the enzyme to bind to glucan, in essence, a glucan-binding domain. Subsequent studies have shown that oral streptococci produce distinct glucan-binding proteins domains highly similar to those in the Gtfs but lack the enzymatically active domains of the Gtf enzymes.

The availability of the *gtf* genes also permitted key experiments in bacterial virulence. Regions of DNA from many other bacterial species had been identified and characterized for their ability to encode antibiotic resistance genes. Fragments of DNA containing these resistance genes, referred to as resistance cassettes, were found to be useful as tools to create mutant strains of *S. mutans*. In the case of *gtf* biology, DNA restriction enzymes were used to cut the genes and antibiotic resistance cassettes were then inserted into these specific sites, the result being *gtf* genes that had been artificially interrupted by the presence of the antibiotic resistance gene. Genes that have been manipulated with these approaches can be introduced into the *S. mutans* chromosome by genetic transformation (see chapter 7). The power of this approach to the study of bacterial virulence is that DNA encoding proteins potentially involved in pathogenesis can be altered by the insertion of antibiotic resistance cassettes and returned to the chromosome of the source organism. Thus, it has been possible to select strains of *S. mutans* with disruptions in each of the three glucosyltransferases and to be confident that, unlike other mutagenesis strategies, no other changes were introduced into the organism. The strains were used to evaluate the effects of losing one or more of the enzymes in caries experiments with rats. In fact, a number of laboratories performed exactly these kinds of experiments with mutant strains of *S. mutans* defective in multiple *gtf* genes and the *ftf* gene. Results from those experiments showed convincingly that glucosyltransferases were extremely important for the ability of *S. mutans* to cause caries, especially on smooth surfaces of the teeth. In other words, the studies created a molecular basis for caries in humans: *S. mutans* produces glucosyltransferases, and when exposed to dietary sugars, the Gtf enzymes act to produce water-insoluble glucans that facilitate irreversible binding of the organism to teeth. In the absence of the Gtfs and Ftf, the ability of *S. mutans* to cause disease was greatly, although not wholly, diminished.

Clearly then, molecular approaches were essential to elucidating the role of the extracellular polymer-forming enzymes in the pathogenic potential of *S. mutans*. The story does not end there. Work has continued on Gtfs, as established virulence proteins, in at least two ways that also involve DNA technology. The important role of Gtfs in colonization of the oral cavity has suggested the possibility that blockade of the activity of these enzymes, either by chemical means or by immunological intervention, would reduce or prevent the formation of caries. To that extent, a wide variety of Gtf-derived peptides and genetically engineered Gtf proteins containing additional protein segments, such as the cholera toxin B subunit, have been investigated for their potential as caries vaccine candidates (see chapter 10). Corollary to the vaccine studies have been expression studies in which the question has been asked: when are *gtf* genes turned on? In studies of this nature, chimeric proteins, or fusion proteins, have been constructed consisting of two genes: reporter genes linked, in the chromosome, to the *gtf* genes. Initially, the reporter genes were antibiotic resistance genes, particularly the chloramphenicol acetyltransferase gene. The advantage to its use is that it allows the investigator to measure the enzymatic activity of chloramphenicol acetyltransferase, if the activity of the target gene is not measurable because of the nature of the genetic construction. As a result of studies of this type, we have learned that the glucosyltransferases are produced at higher levels during growth of the organism at low pH, a setting that also promotes the dissolution of enamel and the initiation of dental caries. More recent studies with gene fusion proteins have relied on the use of green fluorescent protein, or its variants, as the reporter portion of the molecule. The advantage of green fluorescent protein is that the molecule, as it name implies, is capable of fluorescence, and by monitoring light emission one can track when a gene of interest is turned on or off without using a biochemical assay. This kind of approach has been of benefit to studies with biofilm cultures, in that the biofilms need not be disturbed in order for an image to be collected with fluorescence microscopes equipped with digital cameras.

The study of glucosyltransferases and their role in caries exemplifies many of the techniques that are currently available to the interested oral microbiologist. However, molecular biology has not been restricted to those three genes. The production of intracellular storage polysaccharides;

the uptake of a wide variety of sugars through the phosphoenolpyruvate-dependent transport system; and the AgI/II surface protein have all been heavily investigated with recombinant DNA technology in ways similar to the studies of the glucosyltransferases. Many other genes, most recently those related to biofilm formation, have received considerable attention using the techniques that have been discussed. It should be anticipated that in the current era, with the availability of more oral bacterial genomes, these approaches, briefly touched on above, will be ever more utilized.

Characterization of Stress Responses and Their Role in Pathogenesis

After *S. mutans* colonizes the tooth surface, it has to multiply and survive a variety of stresses, including coping with the fluctuation in the availability of carbohydrate, the presence of oxygen and its metabolites, and the accumulation of organic acids as sugars are metabolized. It has been reasoned that understanding the nature of the response of oral bacteria to stress would give rise to information that could lead to novel therapeutic targets. That is, it might be possible to develop new antibiotics effective against *S. mutans* by elucidating the mechanisms by which the bacterium resists stress. Stress responses in bacteria are not readily visible, and their study has relied on the use of molecular approaches to identify genes, create mutant strains defective in a given stress-response gene product, and create gene fusions to report on the activity of a gene under defined growth conditions.

Attention has been given to a variety of stress responses: those based on known, generalized stress-response proteins in other bacteria, those based on possibly more specific mechanisms attributable to acid- or oxidative-stress genes, or those involved primarily with growth in biofilms. Well over 100 *S. mutans* proteins have been identified that are differentially expressed in response to growth at pH 5.0. Of those proteins, more than 61 are known to be involved with stress responses, including the proton-pumping ATPase; the molecular chaperones GroEL, DnaK, and trigger factor; and at least one member of the Clp protease family, which is responsible for turnover of damaged proteins. In addition to these response proteins, oral streptococci also attempt to ameliorate acidic conditions by raising their internal pH through ammonia-producing systems. These include a urease, present in some species of oral streptococci, that liberates ammonia and carbon dioxide from urea in saliva. Recent data have also indicated that ammonia liberation from salivary peptides and quaternary amine-carrying amino acids may be more broadly conserved than previously appreciated. Generally, ammonia is produced in oral streptococci by the arginine deiminase system, but recent reports have shown that *S. mutans*, previously thought to be devoid of such a mechanism, actually produces an agmantine deiminase system that is capable of releasing ammonia, presumably to protect the cell from acidification. The role of these various stress-response systems in pathogenesis is not yet entirely clear for many of the identified enzymes, and remains for future studies. Nevertheless, the observation that expression of over 100 proteins is affected by growth at low pH indicates the significant commitment to the acidic lifestyle made by *S. mutans* and further suggests the likehood that proteins unique to *S. mutans* will be uncovered. Seminal work has already been done showing that expression of an *S. salivarius*-derived urease in *S. mutans*, where it is not normally found, resulted in higher pH minima in cultures, indicating that not only was the *S. salivarius* urease expressed in *S. mutans*, but that it could function to keep the organism from acidifying the medium to levels seen in the wild type. From this example, it appears that additional useful observations will be made from investigations into the stress responses of *S. mutans*.

The Genomic and Postgenomic Eras of Caries Research in Oral Bacteria

The determination of the complete sequence of bacterial genomes has dramatically enhanced the capacity to evaluate the role of specific genes in the pathogenesis of *S. mutans*. Using the PCR technique to amplify copies of highly specific regions of the chromosome, it is now possible to rapidly isolate any single gene without prior knowledge of its function. Comparison of *S. mutans* sequences to other bacterial genome sequences, housed in multiple databases around the world, has indicated that roughly one-third of the genome is likely to encode proteins with no presently known function. Clearly, the challenge now is to determine how to use current information about the genes to understand their role in disease initiation by *S. mutans* and to establish methods to elucidate the roles of the unknown proteins encoded in the genome. The techniques that have been described above will continue to play dominant roles for the near term.

Presently, considerable attention is being paid to the use of cDNA microarray technology to identify genes that are turned on or turned off under particular environmental conditions (see chapter 8). In this approach, solid supports, typically glass microscope slides that have been highly polished and chemically treated, are spotted with gene fragments or oligonucleotides representing an entire bacterial genome, creating what are referred to as gene chips. Cultures of the bacterium are then grown under specific conditions and RNA is prepared from the cells. Treatment of RNA samples with the enzyme reverse transcriptase converts the RNA into what is referred to as cDNA, or copy DNA. The DNA can be chemically labeled by the addition of fluorescent dyes after which it is used to hybridize to the glass slides containing the gene chips. The amount of fluorescing material on each gene "spot" is indicative of the level of transcription for that particular gene under the given conditions. The technique offers the possibility of rapidly identifying genes that are important to the survival of cells by seeing how expression levels change in response to various stimuli, for example, low pH or antimicrobial compounds. For that reason, it is hoped that novel, species-specific genes will be found and that eventually new therapeutic agents directed against these proteins will be developed. This sort of technology is already gaining wide use in bacterial studies and is being applied to gene expression of *S. mutans*. Results from studies with other bacteria have already shown that most bacteria regulate many dozens of their genes in response to stress, quite a few of which belong to that category of proteins for which no known function has yet been established. While this is daunting for the present, the next generation of genomic chips will more likely be coated with bits of protein produced by a given organism, such that the goal will be to decipher which proteins interact with each other. It is thought that this approach will circumvent one of the critical problems with gene chips: that virulence proteins that are directly affected by environmental signals, rather than up- or down-regulated at the genetic level, will escape detection in microarray experiments. Although the number of proteins for which this is true cannot be known at present, it is a potentially important problem that protein chips may circumvent.

The elucidation of the genome of *S. mutans* and other oral microbes also promises to speed research directed at determining the interaction of one bacterium with another or with many others. Mixed microbial communities have been used previously with relative success in simply measuring survival of species grown at differing pH values, oxygen tensions, or carbohydrate concentrations. The way is now open to the use of reporter genes to report on the effects of growth in the presence of other bacteria or in the presence of host cells. Indeed, research of this nature has already begun in a small number of laboratories, the results of which have the likelihood of leading oral microbiology into the next layer of endeavor: the behavior of microbial communities such as those found in dental plaque.

KEY POINTS

Caries is a physicochemical process whereby the mineralized tissues of the tooth become demineralized as a result of the metabolic activity of bacteria. Hence, caries requires a susceptible host, pathogenic bacteria, and a nutritional substrate for the bacteria.

Caries can occur on tooth smooth surfaces, pits and fissures, and roots. Untreated caries can extend into the dentin and pulp chamber.

Cariogenic bacteria include mutans streptococci, lactobacilli, and actinomycetes. Mutans streptococci include the predominant human pathogens *S. mutans* and *S. sobrinus*. Lactobacilli are often secondary invaders of established carious lesions that can accelerate demineralization. *Actinomyces* species are less commonly involved in caries but may be important in root caries where the cementum surface is less mineralized than enamel.

The physiologic process that leads to caries is the production by microbes of organic acids, including lactic acid, from dietary carbohydrates. The production of lactic acid requires the activity of the lactate dehydrogenase enzyme. The organic acids lower the pH at the tooth surface to the point where the substituted hydroxyapatite of enamel becomes soluble.

Cariogenic bacteria such as *S. mutans* are aciduric; that is, they can resist the adverse effects of the low pH that result from their metabolic activities. Mechanisms of acid resistance include pumping protons out of the cytoplasm, inducing of stress-response proteins, and raising pH through ammonia-producing systems.

S. mutans also utilizes dietary sucrose to produce polymers of glucan (built from monomers of glucose) and fructan (built from monomers of fructose) through the action of glucosyltransferases and a fructosyltransferase, respectively. Insoluble glucan polymers help attach the bacterial cells to the tooth surface. Glucan and fructan can also be used as a food reserve.

A vaccine against caries would require induction of sIgA in saliva and is problematical because of the difficulty in sustaining sIgA levels, and as some *S. mutans* surface proteins can induce antibodies that cross-react with human tissues.

FURTHER READING

Newbrun, E. 1989. *Cariology*, 3rd ed. Quintessence, Chicago, Ill.

U.S. Department of Health and Human Services. 2000. *Oral Health in America: a Report of the Surgeon General*. National Institute of Dental and Craniofacial Research, National Institutes of Health, Bethesda, Md.

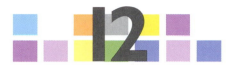

Periodontal Diseases

SUSAN KINDER HAAKE, DIANE HUTCHINS MEYER, PAULA M. FIVES-TAYLOR, AND HARVEY SCHENKEIN

General Concepts

Definitions

The Role of Plaque Bacteria in Periodontal Disease: Nonspecific, Specific, and Ecological Plaque Hypotheses

Suspected Pathogens in Periodontal Diseases

Virulence Traits of Suspected Periodontal Pathogens

P. gingivalis

A. actinomycetemcomitans

T. denticola

E. corrodens

F. nucleatum

P. intermedia

T. forsythia

Capnocytophaga spp.

Immunopathogenic Mechanisms of Tissue Destruction in Periodontitis

Pathogenesis of Gingivitis

Pathogenesis of Periodontitis

Bacterial Virulence and Evasion of the Immune System

Destruction of Periodontal Tissues by Immunopathologic Means

A Model for Periodontal Pathogenesis

Immune Cells and Bone Resorption

Use of Animal Models To Study Pathogenesis of Periodontitis

Genetic Factors That Influence Responses to Periodontal Infections

KEY POINTS

FURTHER READING

GENERAL CONCEPTS

Definitions

The term "periodontal disease" refers to a broad group of pathological alterations of the periodontal tissue. The common forms of the disease are known as gingivitis and periodontitis (Fig. 1) and represent one of the most widespread infectious diseases of humans. Plaque-induced gingivitis is the most frequently occurring gingival disease and is manifest as a reversible inflammation in the marginal periodontal tissues associated with dental plaque. The severity and duration of gingivitis can be modified by factors that modulate bacterium-host cell interactions, including systemic factors (e.g., endocrine changes associated with puberty, pregnancy, diabetes), medications, and malnutrition. A key feature of gingivitis is a lack of destruction of the periodontal attachment apparatus, although gingivitis may be found at sites with prior attachment loss.

Periodontitis is an inflammation-based infection of the supporting structures of the teeth characterized by progressive destruction of the periodontal ligament and alveolar bone that may result in tooth loss. Periodontitis is caused by bacteria or groups of bacteria found within the dental plaque biofilm (see discussion below). The two distinct forms of periodontitis that occur in otherwise healthy individuals are chronic and aggressive periodontitis, and these conditions have been the focus of most investigations of pathogenesis. A third form of the disease occurs in individuals with systemic conditions, most commonly genetic or hematological disorders (e.g., leukemia and neutropenia) that profoundly compromise the host response to bacterial infection.

Chronic periodontitis is the most common form of periodontitis. It is found predominantly in adults but may occur in children. One key diagnostic feature is that the severity of disease is consistent with local factors of plaque and calculus (a hard deposit of calcified plaque that forms on the tooth or root surface). A second key diagnostic feature is a slow to moderate progression of tissue destruction, although short periods of rapid progression may occur. Disease progression and severity may be accentuated by systemic conditions such as diabetes or environmental

253

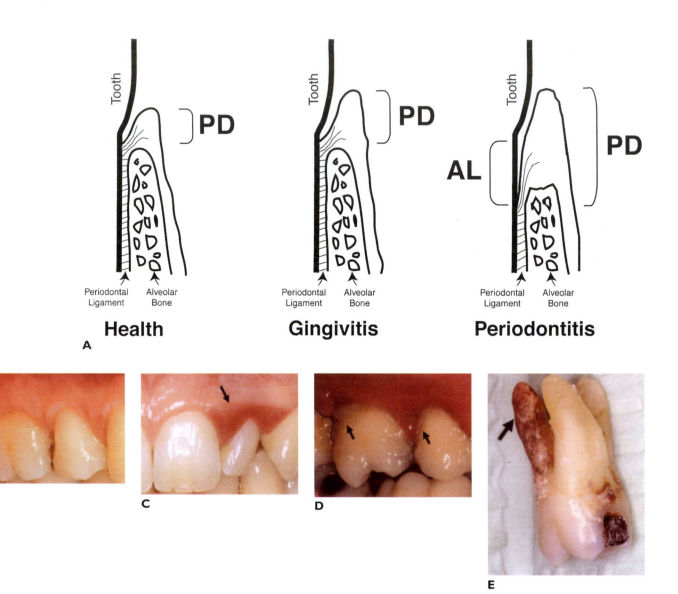

FIGURE I Periodontal diseases. (A) Schematic representation of health, gingivitis, and periodontitis. The periodontal pocket depth (PD) is increased in gingivitis due to tissue swelling associated with inflammation. In periodontitis the PD is further increased due to the loss of the tissue attachment to the root of the tooth (AL, attachment loss). Periodontitis is further characterized by loss of supporting alveolar bone. (B) Health. Note the lack of evidence of inflammation in the tissues. (C) Gingivitis. Pronounced inflammation is present in the gingival tissues (arrow), evident by the red coloration and swelling present. (D) Periodontitis. Tissue inflammation is evident by the redness and swelling present and is associated with local plaque and calculus (arrows). (E) Extracted molar from patient in panel D. Note the presence of calculus on the distal root (arrow) that extends to the apex of the root.

factors such as smoking. The plaque microbiota associated with chronic periodontitis is variable, as discussed below.

Aggressive periodontitis is distinguished from chronic periodontitis by three primary factors: the severity of disease is not consistent with the occurrence of the local factors of plaque and calculus, the progression of tissue destruction is rapid, and there is often a familial pattern of occurrence, suggesting genetic factors play a significant role in disease susceptibility. The lesions of aggressive periodontitis are most commonly associated with the gram-negative pathogen *Actinobacillus actinomycetemcomitans*. Individuals with aggressive periodontitis commonly demonstrate abnormalities in polymorphonuclear leukocyte (PMN) function or hyperresponsive macrophages that produce increased amounts of the mediators involved in tissue destruction, such as prostaglandins and interleukin-1β. Aggressive periodontitis is further classified into two forms: localized (previously termed localized juvenile periodontitis) and generalized. Localized aggressive periodontitis (LAP) has an onset at the time of puberty and typically involves the incisors and first molars, and afflicted individuals demonstrate a strong antibody response to the infecting bacteria. Generalized aggressive periodontitis is usually found in individuals under 30 years of age and involves at least three teeth other than incisors and first molars, and afflicted individuals typically display a poor serum antibody response to the infecting bacteria.

In patients with underlying disease there can be invasion of organisms, particularly spirochetes, into the tissue, resulting in necrotizing periodontal diseases. This painful condition often occurs in individuals experiencing high levels of stress, and indeed was termed trench mouth among soldiers during World War I. Another result of tissue invasion by periodontal bacteria is the formation of periodontal abscesses. A variety of gram-positive and gram-negative organisms participate in abscess formation. Often the patients are immunocompromised such as diabetics.

The Role of Plaque Bacteria in Periodontal Disease: Nonspecific, Specific, and Ecological Plaque Hypotheses

Advances in our understanding of the microbial ecology of dental plaque biofilms and their interaction with host tissues have led to several transitions in the conceptual framework through which periodontal diseases are viewed. In the mid-20th century the prevailing concept of the etiology of periodontitis was that it was caused by dental plaque as a whole, accumulating over time on the teeth. This concept was supported by epidemiologic studies that correlated periodontitis with age and the amount of plaque present, as well as studies of the natural history of periodontitis that described a slow progressive course of the disease process. This concept, called the nonspecific plaque hypothesis, assumed that all plaque bacteria were equally capable of causing disease. Disease onset and progression were thought to result from the increase in plaque beyond a threshold level at which the host defenses were no longer able to neutralize the plaque bacteria and their toxic products.

Several factors led to a transition away from the nonspecific plaque hypothesis. Many individuals with considerable amounts of plaque, calculus, and gingivitis never develop destructive periodontal disease. In addition, the pattern of disease evident in individuals with periodontitis reveals advanced lesions adjacent to sites that are largely unaffected. These observations do not support the concept that all plaque bacteria are equally pathogenic. In the latter part of the 20th century, major advances were made in techniques to culture and characterize plaque bacteria, resulting in taxonomic refinements and characterization of new plaque species. Distinct differences in the composition of plaque at sites

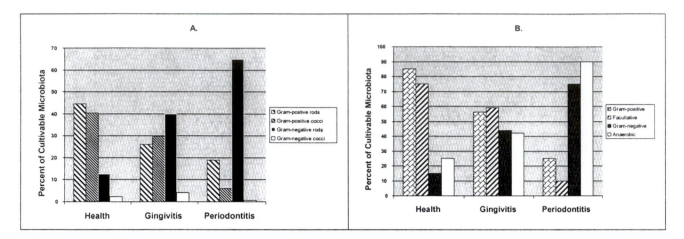

FIGURE 2 Cultivable subgingival bacteria in periodontal health and disease. (A) Analyses of bacteria by morphological groupings demonstrate increases in gram-negative rod-shaped bacteria in gingivitis and periodontitis as compared to health, with corresponding decreases in gram-positive species. (B) Gram-positive facultative species predominate in health sites while gram-negative anaerobic species predominate in periodontitis sites. Sites with gingivitis demonstrated a more balanced distribution of these bacterial groupings.

TABLE I Bacterial species implicated as pathogens in periodontitis

Gram-negative anaerobic species

Porphyromonas gingivalis

Tannerella forsythia

Fusobacterium nucleatum

Prevotella intermedia, P. nigrescens

Campylobacter rectus

Treponema denticola and other oral spirochetes

Gram-negative facultative species

Actinobacillus actinomycetemcomitans

Eikenella corrodens

Gram-positive anaerobic species

Eubacterium nodatum

Peptostreptococcus micros

Streptococcus intermedius

of health and disease were described, providing the foundation for recognition of the specificity in the etiology of periodontitis. The specific plaque hypothesis, defined in the mid-1970s, maintains that the pathogenicity of plaque depends on the presence of, or relative increase in, specific microorganisms. An underlying tenet of the specific plaque hypothesis is that plaque bacteria are not all equally pathogenic, and thus specific bacteria in plaque are responsible for the changes that lead to destructive periodontitis. Acceptance of the specific plaque hypothesis was furthered by the recognition of *A. actinomycetemcomitans* as the predominant pathogen in LAP.

Considerable effort in the later part of the 20th century focused on association studies designed to identify periodontal pathogens by examining the composition of plaque associated with health and varying states of periodontal disease. The findings support the view that of the more than 500 bacterial species found in plaque, destructive periodontal diseases are associated with a relatively small subset of bacteria that are suspected pathogens in the disease process. Clear distinctions in the proportions of specific bacterial species are evident in states of health, gingivitis, and periodontitis (Fig. 2). Bacterial species implicated as pathogens in periodontal diseases (Table 1) are predominantly gram-negative and anaerobic species. Recognized pathogens are also found in health, although at lower levels and with less frequency than evident in disease states. Colonization by the putative pathogen *Porphyromonas gingivalis* occurs early in life, and this organism can be detected in over a third of all children under 18 years of age (Fig. 3). Similar results have been documented for *A. actinomycetemcomitans* and other suspected pathogens. That these microorganisms are present early in life and at healthy sites

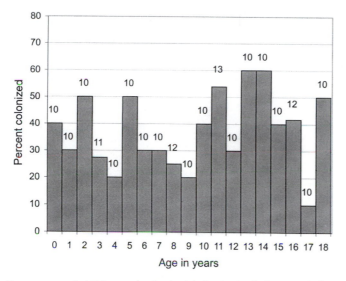

FIGURE 3 Percentage of children colonized with *P. gingivalis* by age. Colonization of a substantial number of subjects with *P. gingivalis* was evident regardless of the age. The total number of subjects investigated was 198, and the number at the top of each bar indicates the number of subjects in whom *P. gingivalis* was detected for that age group.

begs the question of how they increase in proportion in the subgingival microbiota and come to predominate in disease.

Studies of mixed bacterial populations in vitro under conditions mimicking those found in vivo have begun to investigate microbial shifts in plaque. Based on the influence of environmental parameters on the ecology of plaque biofilms, the ecological plaque hypothesis has been proposed as an alternative to the specific plaque hypothesis. The ecological plaque hypothesis maintains that the microbiota undergoes a transition from a commensal to a pathogenic relationship with the host due to factors that trigger a shift in the proportions of resident microorganisms. For example, alterations in gingival crevicular fluid (GCF) flow and pH may result in the enrichment of pathogenic species in the subgingival region. The ecological plaque hypothesis is consistent with the specific plaque hypothesis in recognizing that plaque microorganisms vary in their pathogenic potential. However, the ecological plaque hypothesis focuses on understanding the ecological perturbations that result in the enrichment or emergence of pathogenic species. It further emphasizes the mixed microbiota within which any individual species functions, as it is unlikely that any one species is responsible for the complex processes leading to the inflammation and tissue destruction evident in periodontal diseases. Ecological studies based on the detection of 40 different species in over 13,000 plaque samples have defined five major bacterial "complexes," each consisting of bacterial species that are found in association with one another in the plaque environment (Fig. 4). The "red complex," which includes *P. gingivalis*, *Tannerella forsythia* (*Bacteroides forsythus*), and *Treponema denticola*, was found to be associated with increased pocket depth and bleeding on probing. The biological basis underlying the individual microbial complexes may involve essential metabolic or signaling interactions between bacterial species or the common emergence of the

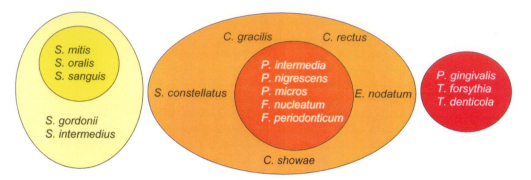

FIGURE 4 Schematic illustration of microbial complexes detected in dental plaque. The organization of complexes and their relationships to one another were based on analyses for 40 microorganisms in 13,261 plaque samples. The complexes identified by each color group include species that tend to be detected together in subgingival plaque. The potential for pathogenicity is highest in the red group and lowest in the yellow group.

bacterial species under specific environmental conditions. The ecological plaque hypothesis additionally accommodates contributions from variations in the virulence of bacterial strains that could also influence host factors that lead to altered environmental conditions. For example, a strain of *A. actinomycetemcomitans* that produces high levels of a toxin (e.g., leukotoxin) may alter the environment by the destructive effects of the toxin on host cells and the release of mediators from the host cells that may influence the plaque composition. Similarly, differences in the host response to plaque bacteria may contribute to environmental alterations. For example, individuals with "hyperresponsive" tissue cells may produce greater amounts of mediators involved in tissue destruction. Another example of the host response variability relates to differences in the immune response in the production of antibody to specific bacteria, which may be important in preventing the progression of periodontitis.

Hypotheses regarding the bacterial etiology of destructive periodontal diseases provide a framework for understanding pathogenesis as well as strategies that may be of benefit in preventing or treating disease. Much of our current therapy is based on the nonspecific plaque hypothesis, with the strategy of overall plaque reduction to prevent disease or disease progression. The specific plaque hypothesis reoriented research efforts toward identifying individuals at risk for disease on the basis of the identification of specific bacteria and the development of strategies that target pathogenic species. Similarly, the ecological plaque hypothesis refocused investigations on ecological aspects of plaque biofilms and the host environment that may define new preventive and therapeutic strategies. Currently, treatment strategies aimed at both modulating the bacterial composition of plaque and modulating the host response to the bacterial challenge are in clinical use.

Suspected Pathogens in Periodontal Diseases

Considerable research over the past few decades has centered on identifying periodontal pathogens. The classic criteria for identifying a pathogenic microorganism, known as Koch's postulates, have been difficult to apply to periodontal diseases. Key reasons for this difficulty include the inability to culture microorganisms that are associated with disease (e.g., spirochetes [see discussion below]), the presence of suspected pathogens in healthy individuals, difficulties in identifying and culturing sites with actively progressing disease, and the lack of good animal model systems for the study of periodontitis. An alternative set of criteria for determining periodontal pathogens consists of the following:

1. Association with disease based on increased numbers of the pathogen at sites of disease;
2. Elimination or decreased numbers of the pathogen at treated sites that demonstrate a return to clinical health;
3. Evidence of a host response to the pathogen based on humoral or cellular immunity;
4. Pathogenic potential of the pathogen as demonstrated in animal model systems; and
5. Possession of virulence factors with the potential to contribute to periodontal tissue destruction.

According to these criteria, two periodontal microorganisms, *A. actinomycetemcomitans* and *P. gingivalis*, are considered as likely primary pathogens in periodontitis (Table 2). A relatively small number of additional bacteria are also suspected pathogens (Table 1). This section focuses on aspects of the association, elimination, and host response criteria for suspected pathogens. Virulence determinants of these pathogens and animal models used to assess their virulence are discussed in detail in later sections of this chapter. It should be pointed out, however, that advances in nucleic acid-based identification of noncultivable bacteria are reshaping

TABLE 2 Criteria implicating *A. actinomycetemcomitans* and *P. gingivalis* as pathogens in periodontal diseases

Category of criteria	A. actinomycetemcomitans	P. gingivalis
Association	Increased in number in LAP and some chronic periodontitis lesions. Detected within host tissues at sites of LAP lesions	Increased in number in periodontitis lesions
Elimination	Suppressed or undetectable in successfully treated lesions. Detectable in recurrent lesions	Suppressed or undetectable in successfully treated lesions. Detectable in recurrent lesions
Host response	Increased serum and crevicular fluid antibody levels in subjects with LAP	Increased serum and crevicular fluid levels in subjects with periodontitis
Animal studies	Pathogenic potential demonstrated in rodent models of periodontitis	Pathogenic potential demonstrated in rodent and nonhuman primate models of periodontitis
Virulence factors	Host tissue cell adherence and invasion, elaboration of leukotoxin, collagenase, endotoxin (LPS), CDT, fibroblast-inhibiting factor, bone resorption-inducing factor	Host tissue cell adherence and invasion, elaboration of proteases, collagenase, fibrinolysin, phospholipase A, phosphatases, endotoxin (LPS), and tissue-toxic metabolic by-products (hydrogen sulfide, ammonia, fatty acids)

our understanding of the composition of the periodontal microbiota. Some of these newly identified organisms may also be pathogens.

A. actinomycetemcomitans is a facultatively anaerobic nonmotile gram-negative rod, and evidence suggests that this species plays a primary etiological role in LAP. Subjects with LAP typically demonstrate *A. actinomycetemcomitans* at sites of periodontal lesions and have substantially elevated levels of antibody to *A. actinomycetemcomitans* in serum and GCF. Clinically successful treatment of LAP correlates with reduction or a loss of detection of *A. actinomycetemcomitans*, whereas unsuccessful clinical outcomes are associated with a lack of reduction. Antibody levels to *A. actinomycetemcomitans* and detection of the bacterium correlate with active periodontal breakdown in subjects with LAP. In some cases of LAP *A. actinomycetemcomitans* is not detected, but other periodontal pathogens present may be responsible for the periodontal destruction evident (see discussion below).

Some forms of chronic periodontitis are also found to be associated with *A. actinomycetemcomitans*, although the bacterium is isolated less frequently and at lower levels than in LAP. In addition, while successful treatment of chronic periodontitis is associated with decreased numbers of *A. actinomycetemcomitans*, the microorganism appears to persist in detectable numbers in treated lesions. *A. actinomycetemcomitans* is also found in periodontally healthy individuals and sites, but much less frequently and in much smaller numbers than in diseased sites. Phenotypic variation among strains of *A. actinomycetemcomitans* is evident and may account for differences in pathogenesis. Five distinct serotypes of *A. actinomycetemcomitans* (serotypes a to e) have been identified, with serotype b being the most commonly associated with diseased sites. In addition, colonization by strains producing high levels of a leukotoxin (see discussion of virulence factors below) has been associated with the onset and occurrence of LAP.

P. gingivalis is a gram-negative, anaerobic, nonmotile rod. Of the suspected periodontal pathogens, *P. gingivalis* has been most consistently and strongly associated with chronic periodontitis. This species is markedly increased in prevalence and proportions in diseased as compared to healthy sites and in sites demonstrating recent disease progression. Detection of *P. gingivalis* is indicative of increased risk for future disease progression, and successful clinical treatment of chronic periodontitis correlates with decreased levels. The host response to *P. gingivalis* is evident in increased serum antibody titers in subjects with periodontitis. In addition, *P. gingivalis* is one of the more common periodontal pathogens, other than *A. actinomycetemcomitans*, that is associated with LAP.

It is noteworthy that with sensitive PCR-based assays *P. gingivalis* is found in up to 25% of healthy sites. Variability in strains of *P. gingivalis* based on DNA sequence analyses has been detected, and specific subpopulations are more strongly associated with human disease. *P. gingivalis* possesses numerous properties that may contribute to its virulence, including the elaboration of proteases capable of degrading effectors of the immune response and a wide range of host tissue molecules of importance in periodontal support of the teeth (see discussion of virulence factors below).

The oral spirochetes are a group of gram-negative, anaerobic, spiral-shaped, and highly motile microorganisms. Spirochetes have been associated with periodontitis but historically have proved difficult to study due to the inability to cultivate many of these organisms in the laboratory and to distinguish among different species in clinical samples. Studies of oral spirochetes through molecular approaches indicate that around three-quarters of the oral spirochetal species in the genus *Treponema* have not been cultivated. Microscopic observations indicate that spirochetal microorganisms are associated with periodontitis and sites with recent bone loss and that spirochetes are detected within host tissues in LAP and advanced chronic periodontitis. Spirochete numbers are correlated with the severity of chronic and aggressive forms of periodontitis, and their levels are diminished with clinical treatment. Similar to other suspected pathogens, spirochetes are found at low levels in healthy periodontal sites. Two species that have been associated with periodontitis are *T. denticola* and *Treponema lecithinolyticum*.

Numerous other oral species have been implicated as pathogens in periodontal diseases (Table 1). Of the remaining species, the gram-negative anaerobe *T. forsythia* (*T. forsythensis* or *B. forsythus*) has been most closely associated with periodontitis. *T. forsythia* is found in higher levels in chronic periodontitis as compared to healthy sites, and decreases in the levels of this species correlate with a favorable therapeutic response. Detection of *T. forsythia* has also been found to be predictive of future destruction of the periodontal tissues. *Prevotella intermedia*, *Prevotella nigrescens*, *Fusobacterium nucleatum*, *Eikenella corrodens*, and *Campylobacter rectus* are all gram-negative species that are found in higher levels in periodontitis as compared to gingivitis and periodontal health. *P. intermedia* is also increased significantly in a form of gingivitis known as pregnancy gingivitis, and this may relate to an increase in environmental steroid hormones that stimulate the growth of this species. Whereas the predominant bacterial species associated with periodontitis are gram-negative, several gram-positive species have also been implicated in association studies, including *Peptostreptococcus micros*, *Streptococcus intermedius*, and *Eubacterium nodatum*. Recent studies have also demonstrated an association between herpesviruses (Epstein-Barr virus 1 and human cytomegalovirus) and chronic periodontitis, and the presence of these viruses in the subgingival region is associated with high levels of putative pathogens including *P. gingivalis*, *T. denticola*, and *T. forsythia*. The potential role of viruses in periodontal pathogenesis remains to be determined.

VIRULENCE TRAITS OF SUSPECTED PERIODONTAL PATHOGENS

The virulence of periodontal pathogens is complex and multifactorial. Often times activities with directly opposing functions can be demonstrated, especially with regard to modulation of innate immune response factors. However, these kinds of properties are consistent with the ecological plaque hypothesis whereby the organisms can be present in both health and disease and different environmental conditions can induce differing phenotypic properties of the bacteria. In this section the major potential virulence factors are summarized. Unfortunately, a unified theory that integrates all these factors into ecology in health and disease is lacking; however, models of disease based on bacterial and host factors are presented in the following section.

P. gingivalis

MOLECULES AND ORGANELLES

Proteases

P. gingivalis elaborates myriad proteases with assorted specificities. The main function of these enzymes is to provide peptides for growth, but because of their ability to degrade host proteins, they can also disrupt host defenses and many are thus believed to be key virulence determinants. The variety of names used to describe these enzymes, as well as the numbers of different strains used and incomplete biochemical characterization, has resulted in much confusion in the literature. However, the confusion surrounding these proteases is gradually abating due to the sequencing of the *P. gingivalis* genome together with the development of a meaningful gene classification scheme. In that regard, and to aid the reader, we will use genes and gene products to identify these enzymes whenever possible.

The best characterized *P. gingivalis* proteases are the R and K gingipains, arginine- and lysine-specific cysteine proteases. Three genes encode these proteinases: *rgpA* encodes the Arg-x-specific proteinase RgpA, which has adhesin/hemagglutinin domains (*hag* sequence domains); *rgpB* encodes the Arg-x-specific proteinase RgpB; and *kgp* encodes the Lys-x-specific proteinase Kgp, which has adhesin/hemagglutinin domains (*hag* sequence domains). Another group of *P. gingivalis* cysteine proteinases is made up of gene products of *prtT*, a streptopain-related protease and periodontain, an enzyme that cleaves and inactivates α1-proteinase inhibitor. The *prtT* gene also has a C-terminal region encoding hemagglutinin activity that is different from that of the *hag* sequences of the gingipains. Another protease gene, *tpr*, encodes Pz-peptidase, a papain-related enzyme. Evidence suggests that this enzyme is surface-associated and has broad activity. Although it does not act on native collagen, it hydrolyzes gelatin and Pz-peptide, which has led to the suggestion that it may play a role in late stages of collagen degradation. Other proteinases include aminopeptidases, an endothelin-coverting enzymelike endopeptidase, and prolyl dipeptidyl peptidase IV. In addition to providing peptides for nutrition, proteinases have a spectrum of biological activities of potential relevance to the disease process (Table 3).

Hemagglutinins

Bacterial binding to receptors on host cells with subsequent colonization may be mediated by surface-associated hemagglutinins. Thus, for a number of bacterial species, including *P. gingivalis*, these proteins are known virulence factors. *P. gingivalis* hemagglutinin activities include those associated with fimbriae, cell surface lipopolysaccharide (LPS) and lipid, hemagglutinin domains of proteases, and specialized hemagglutinin molecules such as HagA, HagB, and HagC. HagA is a large protein of over 230 kDa containing four contiguous direct 440- to 456-amino-acid residue repeat blocks. The *hag* sequences found in the *rgpA* and *kgp* genes

TABLE 3 Functions of *P. gingivalis* proteinases

Impairment of tissue integrity	Perturbation of host defenses	Bacterial function
Degradation of extracellular matrix proteins: fibronectin, laminin	Degradation of immunoglobulins	Release of hemin and iron from host proteins
Hydrolysis of collagens I, III, IV, and V	Inactivation or activation of complement components	Exposure of host and bacterial cryptitopes
Degradation of fibrinogen	Destruction of cytokines and chemokines	Posttranslational processing of proteases, fimbrillin, and outer membrane proteins
Inactivation of tissue and plasma proteinase inhibitors	Cleavage of leukocyte surface receptors	Involvement in intracellular invasion
Activation of matrix metalloproteinases	Degradation of antimicrobial peptides	
Activation of the kallikrein-kinin cascade		

that encode two of the gingipain proteases described above are nearly identical to the direct repeats found in *hagA*. In HagA, each repeat block may represent a functional hemagglutinin domain. The *hagB* and *hagC* genes are at distinct chromosomal loci, although the HagB and C proteins (~40 kDa) are very similar. These adhesins mediate the binding of *P. gingivalis* to host cells, e.g., epithelial cells, as well as to erythrocytes. However, surface-associated proteases may also participate in the binding.

It has become evident that the genetic and functional factors of *P. gingivalis* adhesion, hemagglutination, fimbriation, and proteolysis are tightly linked. This complex process is likely of great importance to *P. gingivalis*, both to fulfill its nutritional and growth requirements (e.g., peptides, iron) and for virulence.

LPS

Analysis of the chemical composition of LPS from a number of different *P. gingivalis* strains shows that in contrast to enterobacterial LPS, *P. gingivalis* LPS appears to have little or no heptose in its LPS core. Furthermore, the LPS fatty acids are branched and longer than those of the *enterobacteriaceae*. The biological properties of *P. gingivalis* LPS are clearly different from those of enteric LPS; a major difference is the relative lack of endotoxicity of *P. gingivalis* LPS. The differences in the biological properties likely reflect differences in their chemical structure that are in turn a reflection of their specific pathogenic roles.

Fimbriae

Peritrichous fimbriae adorn the surface of *P. gingivalis*. Two distinct types of fimbriae are visible by electron microscopy; other genetically distinct structures may also exist. The major fimbrial type, which varies in length from 0.3 to 3.0 μm and in width from 3 to 5 nm, is composed of ~45-kDa fimbrillin (FimA) subunits. These long *P. gingivalis* fimbriae share homology with fimbrial subunits from other species. One minor fimbrial type is shorter than the major type and is composed of a 67-kDa protein.

In vitro evidence strongly suggests a potential role for fimbriae in adherence, colonization, and periodontal destruction. A number of in vivo studies document the importance of fimbriae in the infection process. For example, preimmunization of rats with purified fimbriae (FimA) protects against *P. gingivalis*-induced bone destruction. Furthermore, in the same model, bone destruction is averted following infection with a mutant strain lacking the long fimbriae. Taken together, these studies provide strong evidence that fimbriae are *P. gingivalis* virulence determinants.

Outer membrane vesicles

Vesicles associated with the surfaces of gram-negative organisms result from evagination of the outer membrane. Thus, vesicle components include those associated with the outer membrane (for *P. gingivalis* proteases, LPS, and hemagglutinins) as well as entrapped periplasmic components. *P. gingivalis* vesicles mediate binding to red blood cells, other bacteria, and hydroxyapatite surfaces. More recently it has been shown that they possess marked platelet aggregation activity (see below). Furthermore, fimbriae are visible on the surfaces of *P. gingivalis* vesicles. It has been proposed that adhesive microvesicles can function as vehicles for the precise delivery of virulence factors, e.g., toxins and proteases; their small size enables them to access niches that whole cells could not enter.

Polysaccharide capsule

To date, six polysaccharide capsular serotypes have been described in *P. gingivalis*. Highly encapsulated strains exhibit reduced phagocytosis, and the capsule has thus been considered to be an important virulence factor. *P. gingivalis* capsular structures have also been correlated with pathogenicity in animal models. Differences in virulence within a capsular serotype occur, suggesting that the capsule plays a role in virulence but is not the only determinant for *P. gingivalis* virulence. Capsular polysaccharide on the *P. gingivalis* surface can mask LPS, thereby modulating its activity.

MECHANISMS
Adhesion, colonization, and dental plaque (biofilm) formation

Like all microorganisms, the first challenge *P. gingivalis* cells face in the oral cavity is the ability to adhere to a specific substrate. The oral cavity affords a number of different surfaces (teeth, precedent microorganisms and their metabolites, mucosa, extracellular matrix proteins, etc.) with which microbiota can interact. However, the surface of choice for *P. gingivalis* is developing plaque biofilm. A biofilm lifestyle protects organisms from environmental adversity; thus, by itself it should be considered a virulence determinant. In vitro studies have shown that *P. gingivalis* exhibits intergeneric coaggregation with many early oral plaque organisms, such as streptococci (*S. sanguis*, *S. gordonii*, *S. mitis*, *S. oralis*, and *S. cristatus*) and *Actinomyces naeslundii*. It can also coaggregate with later-colonizing plaque organisms, such as fusobacteria, an intermediary between the early and late colonizers, as well as with late colonizers per se (*T. denticola* and *T. forsythia*).

The major fimbriae are significant adhesion mediators of *P. gingivalis*. It has been shown that they affect adherence to oral epithelial cells, fibroblasts, and endothelial cells and to cell matrix components such as fibronectin and fibrinogen. Fimbriae also bind to other entities associated with the oral cavity, such as salivary components (proline-rich proteins and statherin), to saliva-coated hydroxyapatite, a tooth model, and to other oral bacteria (e.g., strepococcal and *Actinomyces* species). FimA per se is a participant in these binding activities, in contrast to fimbriae-mediated binding in many other gram-negative bacteria in which it is minor fimbrial components that mediate binding and major subunits that form the structural framework. Binding mediated by *P. gingivalis* major fimbriae is necessary for its colonization of the plaque biofilm. It has been shown that environmental cues can regulate *fimA*, the gene that encodes FimA. Evidence has also been presented that indicates that at least one plaque bacterium can also modulate *P. gingivalis fimA* expression. Contact of *Streptococcus cristatus* with *P. gingivalis* initiates a signaling mechanism that leads to the down-regulation of *P. gingivalis fimA* expression, preventing binding and subsequent biofilm formation. This suggests that the transition of plaque from commensally associated to pathogen-associated organisms can be modulated by the presence of *S. cristatus*, which is able to block the expression of *P. gingivalis fimA* and, in so doing, ward off its binding and incorporation into plaque biofilm and foster its elimination from the oral cavity. In contrast, a biofilm made up of towering microcolonies interspersed with fluid-filled channels forms following the adhesion of *P. gingivalis* to *S. gordonii* in vitro. Several specific adhesin-receptor pairs on the surfaces of both microorganisms, including both the major fimbriae of *P. gingivalis* and S. *gordonii* SspB, a multifunctional surface protein, are required for the formation of the mixed species biofilm.

Epithelial cell invasion

Periodontal disease requires interaction between bacteria of the plaque biofilm and the gingival tissues. *P. gingivalis* cells are found in vivo in gingival tissue, suggesting that the organism can pass through the epithelial barrier after colonizing this mucosal surface. *P. gingivalis* has the ability to invade epithelial cells and replicate in the intracellular environment. Invasion is driven by interaction between the major fimbriae of *P. gingivalis* and integrins on the surface of the epithelial cells. Activation of a signal transduction pathway by the occupied *P. gingivalis* receptor leads to cytoskeletal rearrangements that result in internalization of attached bacteria. Signaling involves fluxes in intracellular calcium ion concentrations and modulation of the eukaryotic mitogen-activated protein kinase pathways. The internalization process, a rapid event that is complete within minutes, results in the accumulation of large numbers of bacteria in the perinuclear region. *P. gingivalis* subversion of epithelial cell signaling can result in the inhibition of transcription and secretion of IL-8 by neutrophils. Furthermore, *P. gingivalis* can also antagonize IL-8 secretion after stimulation of gingival epithelial cells by commensal plaque organisms, a process that could clearly diminish the periodontal immune response. In addition to invasion within cells, *P. gingivalis* can also degrade components of the tight-junction (occludin), adherens junction (E-cadherin), and cell-extracellular matrix junction (β1-integrin) and thus facilitate intercellular invasion and intrusion deeper into the tissues.

Endothelial cell invasion

A relationship between periodontal disease and cardiovascular disease has been suggested (see chapter 16). Whereas oral bacteria are found predominantly in the mouth, the inflammation and bleeding associated with invasion of gingival connective tissue enable bacterial entry into circulating blood (i.e., dental bacteremia) and systemic locales where they may produce disease. Periodontopathogens, including *P. gingivalis*, have been shown to be associated with atherosclerotic plaques. Consistent with this, in vitro adherence to and invasion of human coronary artery and bovine aortic endothelial cells have been demonstrated. Invasion of endothelial cells by *P. gingivalis* likely involves an athrogenic process that stimulates both inflammatory cytokines and cell adhesion molecules, factors known to be involved in the pathogenesis of coronary heart disease and stroke. As with epithelial cell invasion, *P. gingivalis* major fimbriae are required for endothelial cell invasion. However, invasion is increased following treatment with amyloglucosidase to degrade the *P. gingivalis* polysaccharide capsule. Bacterial capsules are known to hinder the interaction of certain bacteria with both epithelial and endothelial cells. It has thus been postulated that the enzymatic treatment may be exposing additional adhesins. Once inside the endothelial cells, *P. gingivalis* evades the endocytic pathway to lysosomes by remaining in the autophagosome and blocking its maturation.

Proteolysis

It has been demonstrated that *P. gingivalis* proteolytic enzymes have the ability to degrade a variety of host proteins as well as the potential to disrupt host cell function (Table 3). They can degrade fibrinogen and plasma proteins; degrade or process cytokines, such as tumor necrosis factor alpha (TNF-α), interferon gamma (IFN-γ), IL-6, and IL-8; cleave or inactivate the phagocyte C5a receptor; and cause the release of neutrophil chemotactic activity from the C5 complement component. Thus, proteases are thought to play a role in interfering with the host cell inflammatory response. Furthermore, proteases can activate prothrombin, protein C, factor X, the kallikrein-kinin system, and neutrophils by means of cleavage of proteinase-activated receptor 2. It has also been shown recently that RgpA/B-mediated hydrolysis of CD14 on human gingival fibroblasts results in the down-regulation of LPS-induced IL-8 production.

Inflammatory response

P. gingivalis can both activate and suppress components of the host innate immune response. Whole cells and their components can induce the expression of a variety of cytokines and chemokines. *P. gingivalis*-stimulated PMNs, monocytes/macrophages, fibroblasts, and epithelial cells all elicit a cytokine response. Proinflammatory cytokines (IL-1β, TNF-α, IL-6, and IL-8) promote inflammation and stimulate bone and tissue destruction. However, *P. gingivalis* also induces anti-inflammatory cytokines (IL-1ra and IL-4), degrades existing cytokines, and antagonizes IL-8 production by epithelial cells.

P. gingivalis LPS does not stimulate endothelial cell expression of E-selectin and actually inhibits the LPS-stimulated expression of other bacteria. It is a poor activator of IL-1β and TNF-α in monocytes compared with *Escherichia coli*, and these cytokines are indirect activators of human selectin expression. Furthermore, in studies that involved a mouse model of early inflammation, induction of fibroblast-induced cytokine,

E- and P-selectins, and monocyte chemoattractant protein 1 by *P. gingivalis* LPS was poor compared to that of *E. coli* LPS.

Host cell Toll-like receptors recognize conserved patterns on bacteria and thus comprise part of the innate immune defense system capable of recognizing specific bacterial products, such as lipoproteins, peptidoglycan, DNA, and LPS. The interaction of Toll-like receptors with specific bacterial components initiates signals that exert control over the ensuing inflammatory response. Thus, Toll-like receptor signaling is a key factor in the innate immune response to pathogenic infection. It has been shown that the binding of *P. gingivalis* LPS to human gingival fibroblasts activates a number of second messenger systems. Furthermore, after LPS stimulation for 24 h, fibroblasts that express high levels of Toll-like receptor secrete much higher levels of IL-1 and IL-6 than those that express low Toll-like receptor levels. However, after LPS stimulation for more than 24 h, expression of Toll-like receptors on the fibroblast surface decreases, indicating that *P. gingivalis* LPS can modulate the immune response in the long term by down-regulating expression of Toll-like receptors.

P. gingivalis fimbriae and their peptide subunits induce the expression of inflammatory cytokines in mouse peritoneal macrophages and human gingival fibroblasts. They also induce IL-6 production, IL-6 mRNA gene expression, and tyrosine and serine/threonine phosphorylation of proteins in human peripheral blood mononuclear cells. These findings suggest a role for fimbriae in *P. gingivalis* host cell signaling. It has also been determined that fimbriae induce the expression of IL-1β and TNF-α genes in mouse peritoneal macrophages. The fimbrial receptor on the macrophages is β2-integrin, and it is believed that its β chain plays a key role in the signaling required for the fimbriae-induced gene expression. A significant IL-1β response is elicited in epithelial cells in conjunction with *P. gingivalis* adhesion and invasion. Interestingly, *P. gingivalis* invasion and infection of epithelial cells reduce IL-8 production and accumulation and intercellular adhesion molecule 1 (ICAM-1) expression and inhibit neutrophil migration through the epithelium. Thus, it appears that *P. gingivalis* uses a powerful combination of antagonistic strategies for down-regulation of ICAM-1 and IL-8 and thus disables one aspect of the host defense mechanisms.

Bone resorption, bone destruction, and bone formation inhibition

P. gingivalis can stimulate bone resorption, inhibit bone formation, and induce bone destruction. LPS and fimbrial and outer membrane constituents appear to play key roles in abrogation of the homeostatic relationship that occurs in health between bone deposition by osteoblasts and bone resorption by osteoclasts.

Activation of osteoclasts by *P. gingivalis* LPS causes the release of bone resorption mediators (IL-1β, prostaglandin E_2 [PGE2], and TNF-α) from fibroblasts, macrophages, and monocytes. Besides causing bone resorption, these mediators can also induce the production of host cell proteases that destroy both bone and connective tissue and inhibit the synthesis of collagen by osteoblasts.

The major fimbriae have been shown in vitro to stimulate bone cells to express both IL-1β and granulocyte-macrophage colony-stimulating factor and to induce fibroblasts, macrophages, and monocytes to produce bone resorption mediators (IL-1β and TNF-α).

A. actinomycetemcomitans

MOLECULES AND ORGANELLES

Leukotoxin

Leukotoxin is probably the most studied *A. actinomycetemcomitans* virulence factor. First described in 1979, this 116-kDa toxic protein was later shown to be produced by about half of the strains isolated from patients with LAP. A protective role for the antibodies to this toxin is suggested by studies that showed that attachment loss was less in patients with early-onset periodontitis with *A. actinomycetemcomitans* leukotoxin-reactive antibody than in patients who lacked the antibody. An association between leukotoxin and periodontitis is also suggested by the high levels of leukotoxin in *A. actinomycetemcomitans* strains isolated from patients with Papillon-Lefèvre syndrome, a keratoderma associated with severe periodontitis. Leukotoxin belongs to the RTX family of pore-forming hemolysins/leukotoxins expressed by a variety of pathogenic bacteria. The structural gene for leukotoxin (*ltxA*) is the second gene of an operon consisting of four genes, C, A, B, and D. Proteins encoded by *ltxB* and *ltxD* are involved with transportation of the toxin to the cell surface, whereas the *ltxC* gene product activates the toxin posttranslationally.

Leukotoxin is both species specific (human and primate) and cell specific. It binds only to monocytes, neutrophils, and a subset of lymphocytes, and forms pores in the membranes of these cells. Death can result from the leukotoxin-induced pores interfering with osmotic homeostasis capabilities or through an apoptotic effect. In addition, leukotoxin actually triggers the release of enzymes from PMNs capable of degrading the molecule. However, protease inhibitors within serum can inhibit the proteolytic degradation; thus serum actually enhances leukotoxic activity.

Cytotoxins

Cytolethal distending toxin (CDT)/immunosuppressive factor (ISF). CDT is a bacterial heat-labile holotoxin whose biological activities include eukaryotic cell distention and cell cycle arrest, actin rearrangement, and apoptosis; however, the activity elicited depends on the cell type under investigation. ISF produced by *A. actinomycetemcomitans* is a member of the family of Cdts encoded by the *cdtB* gene; CdtB protein and ISF are essentially equivalent entities. Three genes, *cdtA*, *cdtB*, and *cdtC*, encode three polypeptides, CdtA, CdtB, and CdtC (27, 29, and 20 kDa, respectively). The functions and the functional relationship(s) of the three proteins have not been clearly defined. However, it is known that CdtB is a type I deoxyribonuclease. *A. actinomycetemcomitans* CDT has been shown to cause G2 cell cycle arrest in CHO and HeLa cells and in the B-cell hybridoma cell line and lymphocytes. CHO cells were used to show that *A. actinomycetemcomitans* CdtA anchors the toxin to the cell surface, whereas CdtB and CdtC are responsible for the toxicity. Cdt can stimulate a specific network of cytokines in peripheral blood mononuclear cells; it was shown to cause the production of IL-1β, IL-6, IL-8, and IFN-γ, but not of IL-12, TNF-α, or granulocyte-macrophage colony-stimulating factor. The inhibition of proliferation and cytokine induction both likely contribute to the pathogenesis of *A. actinomycetemcomitans*. Leukotoxin and Cdt can also induce apoptosis in human immune cells, which would disrupt immune surveillance.

LPS

The high-molecular-mass O polysaccharide component of *A. actinomycetemcomitans* LPS harbors the *A. actinomycetemcomitans* immunodominant antigen. It is known that *A. actinomycetemcomitans* LPS causes bone resorption, platelet aggregation, and skin necrosis. *A. actinomycetemcomitans* LPS has also been shown to bind strongly to hemoglobin, a source of iron for its growth. In addition, *A. actinomycetemcomitans* LPS can activate macrophages. At low concentrations it stimulates macrophages to produce IL-1α, IL-1β, and TNF, cytokines that are involved in tissue inflammation and bone resorption. At higher doses LPS stimulates the production of both proinflammatory and anti-inflammatory cytokines in whole blood. It has been proposed that the ratio of the production of the two types of cytokines may affect the outcome of periodontal diseases.

Fc-binding proteins

The binding of antibody to specific receptors on PMNs is mediated by the Fc region of the antibody molecule. Bacterial Fc receptors (immunoglobulin [Ig]-binding proteins) are proteins associated with, or released from, the cell surface that can bind to the Fc region of Igs. These proteins can thus compete with PMNs for binding to the Fc region and in so doing inhibit phagocytosis. Fc-binding activity is associated with a member of the OmpA family of gram-negative heat-modifiable membrane proteins and with surface capsular material. Since Fc receptors are also believed to play a role in complement activation, the *A. actinomycetemcomitans* Fc-binding protein(s) would inhibit both of these important host defense functions.

Membranous vesicles

Vesicles (blebs) are a prominent feature of the surface of *A. actinomycetemcomitans*. These structures either remain attached to the cell surface or bud off from it. Large numbers of vesicles are released into the external environment. Vesicles associated with *A. actinomycetemcomitans* grown on agar are thick fibrils with knob-like ends. Highly leukotoxic *A. actinomycetemcomitans* strains have an abundance of vesicles, whereas low- or nonleukotoxic strains have few or no vesicles. In addition to leukotoxin, *A. actinomycetemcomitans* vesicles also possess LPS with endotoxin activity, bone resorption activity, and actinobacillin, a bacteriocin. *A. actinomycetemcomitans* vesicles must also contain adhesins as the addition of vesicles to weakly adherent or nonadherent strains significantly increases the ability of those strains to attach to epithelial cells. The observation that *A. actinomycetemcomitans* vesicles exhibit adhesiveness prompted the hypothesis that vesicles can also function as delivery vehicles for *A. actinomycetemcomitans* toxic materials.

Extracellular amorphous material

The surfaces of certain *A. actinomycetemcomitans* are associated with an extracellular amorphous material (ExAmMat), which actually embeds adjacent cells in a matrix. It has been determined that ExAmMat is proteinaceous, most likely a glycoprotein, with both bone resorbing activity and adhesive properties. Moreover, when *A. actinomycetemcomitans* strains that normally adhere weakly to epithelial cells are suspended in ExAmMat, they adhere tightly, a phenomenon termed conveyed adhesion.

Fimbriae

A. actinomycetemcomitans fimbriae are peritrichous, may be ~2 μm in length and 5 nm in diameter, and frequently occur in bundles. Freshly isolated strains are fimbriated, but in vitro subculture results in organisms that, in general, lack or have few fimbriae. *A. actinomycetemcomitans* adhesiveness to epithelial cells and to both hydroxyapatite and saliva-coated hydroxyapatite is associated with colonial variation and fimbriation. Fimbriae contain a 54-kDa fimbrial subunit (fimbrial associated protein) that is involved in adherence. An additional 6.5-kDa protein, Flp, can also be present, and this exhibits some amino acid sequence similarity to type IV pilin. Clearly there is a correlation between *A. actinomycetemcomitans* fimbriation and adhesion; however, nonfimbriated *A. actinomycetemcomitans* also exhibits adhesive properties, indicating that nonfimbrial components also function in adhesion.

MECHANISMS

Adhesion

A. actinomycetemcomitans adhesion to the gingival crevice epithelium is likely a key step in its colonization and in the subsequent tissue destruction associated with periodontal disease. Adhesion of *A. actinomycetemcomitans* to the tooth surface is also important and is more efficient in fimbriated strains. Unlike many later colonizers, *A. actinomycetemcomitans* has few coaggregation partners and coadhesion has only been demonstrated with *F. nucleatum*.

Nonspecific adhesion. Certain strains, especially fresh clinical isolates, generate tenacious biofilms on solid surfaces, such as plastic, glass, and hydroxyapatite. This nonspecific adherence requires the *tad* locus, a cluster of seven genes (*tad*ABCDEFG) associated with the formation of long fibrils and bundled pili. This formation of strongly adherent biofilms could be an early step in *A. actinomycetemcomitans* colonization of the tooth surface.

Specific adhesion to epithelial cells. Most *A. actinomycetemcomitans* strains that have been tested to date adhere to epithelial cells strongly. Cell surface entities that mediate adherence include fimbriae, ExAmMat, and vesicles. However, *A. actinomycetemcomitans* strains that express the smooth colonial phenotype bind strongly to epithelial cells, yet they bear little or no fimbriae. This indicates the presence of adhesins on *A. actinomycetemcomitans* that are not associated with fimbriae. A surface-associated protein determined to be an autotransporter has been shown to be involved in *A. actinomycetemcomitans* adhesion to epithelial cells. The adhesin, termed Aae for adhesion to epithelial cells, is encoded by a gene (*aae*) that is homologous to autotransporter genes of *Haemophilus influenzae* and *Neisseria* species. Thus, the adhesion of *A. actinomycetemcomitans* to epithelial cells is multifactorial with several adhesins and mechanisms playing a role.

Adhesion to extracellular matrix proteins. The extracellular matrix is a complex network of proteins and polysaccharides that surrounds the cellular components of connective tissues. Collagen is the major protein component of the extracellular matrix. Collagen types I, II, III, V, and XI (fiber-forming types) are predominant in connective tissue, whereas type IV, which differs structurally from the others, is a major component of basement membranes. Fibronectin and laminin, noncollagenous glycosylated proteins, are also found in connective tissue and basement membranes. *A. actinomycetemcomitans* binds to immobilized collagen types I, II, III, and V, but not to type IV collagen. Binding to collagen types I, II, III, and V does not occur with soluble collagen, suggesting that a specific conformation of the fibrillar collagens is required for binding. *A. actinomycetemcomitans* outer membrane proteins are essential for the binding to fibrillar collagen. *A. actinomycetemcomitans* also binds to fibronectin, but not to the plasma protein fibrinogen. Binding, therefore, is highly specific. The binding of *A. actinomycetemcomitans* to the insoluble form of proteins that are major structural components of the extracellular matrix may aid the organism in its spread and colonization of both oral and extraoral connective tissues.

Invasion of epithelial cells

Early clinical studies showed that *A. actinomycetemcomitans* can penetrate the gingival epithelium. These in vivo studies revealed that *A. actinomycetemcomitans* occurs in very specific intracellular locations and exhibits a very specific penetration pattern. In vitro studies have demonstrated that *A. actinomycetemcomitans* can also invade epithelial cells. Invasion is a dynamic, complex process that involves attachment to the host cell with initiation of *A. actinomycetemcomitans* uptake in a host-derived membrane-bound vacuole from which it quickly escapes and enters the cytoplasm.

Intracellularly, *A. actinomycetemcomitans* is not quiescent. A short time after escape from the vacuole into the cytoplasm, it transits through the cell to neighboring cells via bacteria-induced protrusions that appear to be extensions of the host cell membrane. Bacteria can be seen within these protrusions by scanning, transmission, and fluorescent microscopy. Microtubules are strongly implicated in the intra- and intercellular spread of *A. actinomycetemcomitans*. Internalized *A. actinomycetemcomitans* interacts with host cell microtubules. In vitro studies show that *A. actinomycetemcomitans* localizes exclusively with the plus-ends of microtubules of taxol-induced microtubule asters, indicating a specific *A. actinomycetemcomitans*-microtubule interaction.

On the basis of these in vitro observations, it is proposed that invasion of epithelial cells and the dynamic process of inter- and intracellular spread are the means by which *A. actinomycetemcomitans* spreads to the gingival connective tissue and initiates the destruction associated with periodontal disease.

Colony phase variation

A. actinomycetemcomitans produces three distinct colonial morphologies on solid medium. Upon primary isolation from the gingiva, it typically forms a rough colony phenotype. These are small (~0.5 to 1 mm in diameter), translucent, rough-surfaced circular colonies with irregular edges that pit the agar. They have a distinctive internal star-shaped or crossed-cigar morphology from which the genus name of the organism is derived. In liquid medium, the rough colony phenotype cells form aggregates on the vessel walls, thereby leaving the medium clear. Repeated subculture on agar yields two types of colonial variants; one is smooth-surfaced and transparent, the other is smooth-surfaced and opaque. The transparent smooth-surfaced variants appear to be an intermediate between the transparent rough-surfaced and opaque smooth-surfaced types. In contrast to the rough-to-smooth variant transition, which in general occurs rapidly soon after isolation during in vitro culture, a smooth-to-rough variant transition, which appears to be associated with nutritional factors, occurs only rarely in vitro.

Bacterial colonial variation is indicative of the differential expression of cell surface components. It has been determined that *A. actinomycetemcomitans* rough colony variants express 43- and 20-kDa outer membrane proteins, rough colony protein A and rough colony protein B, respectively, that are not expressed in smooth colony variants. The genes that encode these proteins have homology to genes known to encode fimbriae-associated proteins. In that regard, *A. actinomycetemcomitans* rough colony variants are heavily fimbriated, whereas smooth colony variants have few or no fimbriae associated with their surface. Although the role of the phenotypic variation is not known, it has been proposed that it may play some role in the episodic nature of periodontitis.

Interference with host defense mechanisms

Similar to other periodontopathogens, *A. actinomycetemcomitans* elaborates factors that can modulate and suppress host defense mechanisms. The host's first line of defense against invading bacteria is phagocyte recruitment (chemotaxis) to the region. A number of steps are involved in this process: binding of chemotactic signaling factors, upregulation of adhesion receptors, binding to the endothelium, and movement of phagocytes to the underlying tissues. This is a major host defense mechanism that represents a significant challenge to invading organisms. Thus, the ability to disrupt chemotaxis promotes survival of the organism. *A. actinomycetemcomitans* can inhibit PMN chemotaxis, and the capsularlike serotype-specific polysaccharide antigen can resist phagocytosis and killing by PMNs. PMNs can also kill bacteria by fusing the phagosome-containing intracellular bacteria with lysosomes from which they acquire potent antibacterial agents. Bacteria able to inhibit the fusion or ward off the antibactericidal action are protected. *A. actinomycetemcomitans* can inhibit the production by PMNs of some of these compounds and it is resistant to others. A heat-stable protein in *A. actinomycetemcomitans* inhibits the production of hydrogen peroxide by

PMNs, and many strains are intrinsically resistant to high concentrations of hydrogen peroxide. Furthermore, *A. actinomycetemcomitans* is resistant to a number of defensins, cationic peptides that occur in neutrophils.

In addition to phagocytosis and killing, leukocytes and monocytes/macrophages also release biologically active agents, such as cytokines and oxidizing agents. Components of *A. actinomycetemcomitans* that can induce or enhance the synthesis of cytokines by monocytes include LPS, ISF, serotype-specific polysaccharide antigen, and a 65-kDa antigen. This modulatory activity likely interferes with host immune homeostasis and contributes to the initiation and progression of disease.

Bone resorption

Periodontal disease is associated with loss of alveolar bone, the structure supporting the tooth. *A. actinomycetemcomitans* can cause bone resorption through at least three different effectors: a surface-associated material (SAM), LPS, and a proteolysis-sensitive factor in microvesicles. The active component of SAM is the molecular chaperone (heat shock protein), GroEL. This chaperone seems to act directly with osteoclasts, the major bone-resorbing cell population. SAM can also exert an antiproliferative effect on osteoblastlike cells. The mechanism of action of SAM is distinctly different from that of LPS. *A. actinomycetemcomitans* LPS causes the release of calcium from fetal long bones. Dexamethasone completely inhibits LPS-induced bone resorption activity by a mechanism that likely involves prostaglandin and IL-1. In contrast, GroEL bone resorption activity is not inhibited by IL-1 receptor antagonist protein.

Apoptosis

Leukotoxin-mediated killing of promyelocytic HL-60 cells involves the induction of apoptosis through the activation of caspases. Induction of apoptosis by leukotoxin also involves the mitochondrial apoptosis pathway. Removal of acute inflammatory cells by apoptosis may play an essential role in the pathogenesis of diseases mediated by *A. actinomycetemcomitans*.

T. denticola

MOLECULES

Major outer membrane protein

The major outer membrane protein (Msp) of *T. denticola* is a 53-kDa adhesin with pore-forming activity that mediates attachment to a variety of matrix and cell surface molecules such as fibronectin, laminin, and fibrinogen. Besides functioning as a porin and adhesin, Msp exhibits cytotoxic effects on epithelial cells and erythrocytes, most likely through its pore-forming activity.

Proteinases

In close association with Msp in the outer membrane are the 95-kDa chymotrypsinlike proteinase complex (CTLP), also termed dentilisin, and PrtP, which is composed of the 72-kDa PrtP protein along with 40- and 30-kDa proteins. This prolyl phenylalanine-specific protease complex has broad substrate specificity, which includes bioactive peptides. The gene encoding the complex, *prcA*, produces a 70-kDa product (PrcA), which is cleaved by PrtP to generate the two smaller 40- and 30-kDa proteins, now termed PrcA1 and PrcA2. It is proposed that the cleavage may be a requirement for either formation or stability of outer membrane complexes. This protein complex contributes to cell attachment, tissue destruction, and tissue invasion. *T. denticola* possesses a variety of other proteolytic enzymes that can degrade structural components of the periodontal tissue and bioactive host molecules.

Hemin- and lactoferrin-binding proteins

At least two hemin-binding activities are exhibited by *T. denticola*. One of these is associated with phospholipase C. It has been proposed that these hemin-binding proteins are components of a unique pathway for iron acquisition. Proteins that can bind lactoferrin also have been identified in *T. denticola*, and the organism can utilize salivary lactoferrin through 17- and 43-kDa receptors expressed on the surface of the outer membrane.

MECHANISMS

Motility and chemotaxis

Spirochete motility is a key virulence factor, as motility mutants fail to infect their host. Locomotive ability enables maneuvering in viscous fluids, and like other spirochetes, locomotion of oral spirochetes is viscosity-dependent. The gingival crevice is a highly viscous environment, and motility may permit these organisms to translocate to the tissues. Spirochete chemotaxis is likely also involved in tissue penetration and infiltration.

Hemagglutination and hemolytic activity

T. denticola organisms can agglutinate and lyse red blood cells. The hemagglutinating activity is growth phase related and depends on a 45-kDa hemolysin that is homologous to aminotransferases and binds to a D-glucosaminelike-containing component. Dentilisin can also cause hemolysis of erythrocytes.

Adhesion

Fibroblasts. Attachment of *T. denticola* to human gingival fibroblasts occurs under both aerobic and anaerobic conditions; it appears to be lectin-mediated via a galactose- and mannose-containing receptor on the fibroblast.

Extracellular matrix. Most strains of *T. denticola* adhere to extracellular proteins. The organism binds to basement membrane proteins, such as fibronectin, laminin, and type I and type IV collagen, as well as to fibrinogen and gelatin. Binding to laminin is most tenacious. Specific mechanisms that involve protein-SH groups and/or carbohydrate residues are used for each protein type. Laminin, fibronectin, and fibrinogen bind to Msp, the 53-kDa major surface protein of *T. denticola*. The purified outer membrane-associated CTLP can hydrolyze IgA, IgG, fibrinogen, α_1-antitrypsin, gelatin, laminin, serum albumin, and transferrin. It also binds to hyaluronan, a polysaccharide that is found in the stratified squamous epithelium of the oral mucosa.

Epithelial cells. *T. denticola* can bind to epithelial cells and potentiate cytopathic processes. Dentilisin (CTLP) is believed to be involved in the adherence. The adherence mechanism involves the interaction of dentilisin with Msp, the 53-kDa major outer membrane protein. It is believed that Msp becomes integrated into the host cell plasma membrane where it is involved in the transport of certain bacterial surface components into the host cell. Dentilisin is also cytotoxic, causing epithelial cell membrane blebbing and inhibiting adhesion and locomotion of migrating cells.

Endothelial cells. *T. denticola* can adhere to endothelial cells; binding occurs both at the cells tips and at various places along their lengths and frequently involves host cell microvilli.

Coaggregation. *T. denticola* coaggregates with both *P. gingivalis* and *Fusobacterium* species. These interactions could play a role in the formation of dental plaque as well as provide nutritional components required by the organisms.

Invasion
Tissue invasion. In an abscess model using both normal conditions and those which mimic neutrophil dysfunction, *T. denticola* causes persistent, deep tissue lesions. Other oral treponemes also produce such lesions; however, formation of the lesions is not associated with chymotrypsin-like protease activity.

Cellular invasion. Although intracellular invasion by *T. denticola* is not thought to occur, the organism can penetrate epithelial and endothelial tissue monolayers with tight junctions.

Proteolytic activity
Dentilisin/PrtP/CTLP can disrupt cell-cell junctions and impair the barrier function of epithelial monolayers. In the murine virulence model, lesions produced by protease-deficient mutant cells are smaller than those produced by wild-type cells, and these mutants can no longer disrupt epithelial cell junctions.

Immunosuppressive activity
Human lymphocyte proliferative responses to antigens and mitogens have been shown to be suppressed by *T. denticola* lysates. This is a monocyte-dependent phenomenon which has no effect on lymphocyte viability. It has also been shown that a lipoprotein fraction from *T. denticola* can modulate the oxygen-dependent and -independent defense mechanisms used by human PMNs.

E. corrodens

E. corrodens is a human pathogen associated with periodontal disease, as well as with extraoral infections, but a causal role has not been clearly established, and factors that may contribute to its pathogenicity and virulence are not well studied.

MOLECULES AND ORGANELLES

Type IV pili

The *E. corrodens* surface exhibits type IV pili that are associated with phase variation. Piliated variants form small corroding (pit-forming) colonies on agar; nonpiliated variants form large, noncorroding colonies. The piliation-associated phase variation of *E. corrodens* resembles that of the pathogenic species *Neisseria gonorrhoeae* and *Moraxella bovis*.

Slime layer: exopolysaccharide

E. corrodens has a slime layer, a coating of bacterial surface-associated exopolysaccharide that may inhibit phagocytosis. Purified slime extract also exhibits immune suppression.

LPS

E. corrodens LPS demonstrates hemagglutinating activity, which could possibly play a role in adhesion to epithelial cells. It has also been shown to induce bone resorption in organ culture.

Outer membrane proteins

E. corrodens outer membrane proteins induce a number of cytotoxic effects on host cells and represent potential virulence factors. The principal outer membrane protein (POMP) has an apparent mass of 33 to 42 kDa. Although its function is unknown, it may be a porin. POMP at low doses induces the release of lysosome enzymes from macrophages, whereas at high doses it is cytotoxic. In addition, POMP affects macrophage phagocytosis, induces platelet aggregation, and consumes complement activity.

MECHANISMS

Adhesion

E. corrodens adheres to a variety of host cells, including epithelial cells, macrophages, and erythrocytes. Adhesion to all of these cells is mediated by an N-acetyl-D-galactosamine-specific lectinlike substance (EcLS). The identity of EcLS is not known, but a porinlike protein is one of its components. *E. corrodens* in vitro coaggregates with certain strains of *Actinomyces viscosus* and *Streptococcus sanguis*. Coaggregation appears to be mediated by EcLS. Studies suggest that EcLS is not the only adhesin present on the surface of *E. corrodens*. To date there is no evidence to suggest that *E. corrodens* invades epithelial cells.

Induction of proinflammatory cytokines

Human epithelial cells exposed to *E. corrodens* whole cells or supernatants secrete inflammatory mediators (IL-6, IL-8, and PGE2). The *E. corrodens* components that induce this effect are small (<10-kDa), soluble molecules. Induction of expression of inflammatory cytokines by epithelial cells may initiate and perpetuate inflammation during chronic infection.

Growth inhibition

A protein, designated P80/lysine decarboxylase, isolated and purified from cell-free saline-soluble extracts of *E. corrodens* and from dental plaque, causes growth inhibition of epithelial cells by depleting lysine from cell culture medium via conversion to cadaverine.

F. nucleatum

MOLECULES AND ORGANELLES

Toxins

An important potential virulence determinant of *F. nucleatum* is the production of toxic metabolites, which can stop host cell proliferation or kill cells (e.g., fibroblasts). Butyrate, proprionate, and ammonium ions produced by *F. nucleatum* can inhibit proliferation of human gingival fibroblasts and are important toxic components of dental plaque extracts.

MECHANISMS

Coaggregation

Fusobacteria, which are among the most commonly occurring species in the human gingival crevice, are highly promiscuous intergeneric coaggregation partners. Because of their ability to coaggregate with so many other strains and species of oral bacteria, they may play a key role in the development of plaque by serving as an anchor for some of the more fastidious, gram-negative late colonizers. Coaggregation is often associated with protein adhesins on the outer membrane.

Adhesion

Extracellular matrix. *F. nucleatum* binds strongly to fibronectin, a large glycoprotein, which in addition to its role in the extracellular matrix, is also found in saliva and plasma. It has also been shown that *F. nucleatum* binds to type IV collagen and to basement membranelike matrices in vitro.

Host cells. *F. nucleatum* can adhere to PMNs, macrophages, lymphocytes, HeLa cells, fibroblasts, both periodontal ligament and gingival fibroblasts, and buccal epithelial cells. Fusobacterial adherence to host cells is mediated by more than one mechanism. For example, adherence to lymphocytes and erythrocytes is mediated by a lectinlike mechanism that is inhibited by galactosides. On the other hand, *F. nucleatum* agglutination of erythrocytes is inhibited by L-arginine, but not by N-acetyl-galactosamine. Recently it has been determined that *F. nucleatum* can invade human gingival epithelial cells. Invasion is accompanied by the secretion of high levels of the proinflammatory cytokine IL-8 from the epithelial cells.

P. intermedia

MOLECULES AND ORGANELLES

Fimbriae

P. intermedia can express four different types of fimbriae that are classified exclusively on the basis of diameter. The type and extent of fimbriation vary among strains; some appear to have only one type, whereas others have at least some of all types, and still others are not fimbriated.

Hydrolases

A number of hydrolytic activities are associated with *P. intermedia*, including proteolytic, e.g., an IgG-degrading protease, and an IgA1 protease. Nucleolytic, lipolytic, and saccharolytic activities are also associated with *P. intermedia*. The individual activities vary markedly among strains. Whereas none of these activities are well characterized, some or all could play an important role in the *P. intermedia* infection process.

Hemolysin and hemagglutinin

P. intermedia outer membrane and surface-associated vesicles possess a heat-labile hemolytic activity. The activity appears to be associated with a multicomponent hemolysin with at least two functionally distinct forms of hemolytic activity.

P. intermedia strains can exhibit hemagglutinating activity. Two types of hemagglutinating activity have been demonstrated. One type is heat labile and may represent a major constituent of fimbriae; the other is heat resistant and LPS-like.

MECHANISMS

Coaggregation

Intergeneric coaggregation of *P. intermedia* appears to be highly specific. Certain strains participate in coaggregation with certain *Actinomyces* species, but not with others. Distinct *P. intermedia* molecules mediate the interaction with each *Actinomyces* species, i.e., the molecules are species specific. Either a protein or glycoprotein associated with the *P. intermedia* surface mediates the coaggregation.

Adhesion

Epithelial cells. *P. intermedia* can adhere to buccal epithelial cells. As with avidity in hemagglutination, strains vary considerably. Strains possessing only type C fimbriae demonstrate the highest affinity binding to buccal epithelial cells.

Host proteins. *P. intermedia* can bind to type I collagen, which could enable the organism to attach to and colonize the extracellular matrix. It also binds to fibrinogen, laminin, and IgG. In addition, binding to and degradation of lactoferrin, a molecule that inhibits the adhesion of *P. intermedia* to epithelial cells and fibroblasts, foster adherence and colonization.

Invasion of epithelial cells

P. intermedia is found in the oral epithelium and connective tissue of rats following infection with the organism. Invasion of epithelial cells by *P. intermedia* has also been reported and may require the presence of type C fimbriae.

Induction of inflammatory lymphokines

P. intermedia LPS and surface components can induce expression of inflammatory lymphokines, e.g., IL-1, IL-6, and IL-8. IL-1β causes bone resorption; IL-8 is a chemokine for PMNs; and IL-6 is a proinflammatory cytokine that causes T- and B-lymphocyte proliferation. Recently, a non-LPS glycoprotein fraction derived from *P. intermedia* was shown to increase the release of IL-8, granulocyte colony-stimulating factor, granulocyte-macrophage colony-stimulating factor, and ICAM-1 from human gingival epithelial cells. Furthermore, certain strains of *P. intermedia* can activate Vβ-specific CD4$^+$ T cells. These inflammatory mechanisms likely contribute to the pathogenesis of periodontal disease.

T. forsythia

The fastidious nature of *T. forsythia* has provided a cultivation challenge to researchers. Thus, this periodontopathogen has not been well studied, and only a few putative virulence factors have been identified to date.

MOLECULES

Hydrolases

T. forsythia produces a trypsinlike protease, an arginine-specific cysteine protease, and a sialidase. The cysteine protease also has hemolytic activity and is present in membrane fractions, indicating that it may be involved in the acquisition of iron from erythrocytes.

MECHANISMS

Coaggregation

T. forsythia exhibits coaggregation with *P. gingivalis*. The binding, which is inhibited by serum, involves protein-protein interactions. Coaggregation also occurs with the commensal plaque organism *S. cristatus*.

Adhesion

BspA, a *T. forsythia* surface antigen with a leucine-rich repeat region, is involved in binding to both fibronectin and fibrinogen. *T. forsythia* can also bind to red blood cells, fibroblasts, and leukocytes.

Capnocytophaga spp.

To date, *Capnocytophaga* spp. associated with dental plaque include *C. gingivalis*, *C. ochracea*, *C. sputigena*, *C. granulosa*, and *C. haemolytica*.

MOLECULES

Hydrolases

A trypsinlike protease has been described for *C. gingivalis*. In addition, *Capnocytophaga* spp. have been reported to express elastase- and chymotrypsinlike proteases.

An aminopeptidase with broad specificity against artificial substrates has been purified from *C. gingivalis*, and a serine dipeptidyl peptidase has been detected in all strains of *Capnocytophaga* spp. tested.

Capnocytophaga spp. secrete also proteases, which cleave the hinge region of IgA1 to produce intact Fab and Fc fragments.

IMMUNOPATHOGENIC MECHANISMS OF TISSUE DESTRUCTION IN PERIODONTITIS

Pathogenesis deals with the mode of origin or development of disease. Immunopathogenic mechanisms are those processes that lead to disease due to engagement of the immune system. The concept that the immune system may cause tissue destruction in periodontitis does not necessarily exclude the likelihood that bacteria may also directly cause tissue damage due to virulence factors such as toxins, enzymes, or other noxious substances. It is likely that tissue destruction in periodontal diseases is due to a combination of such factors that may play roles at different stages of disease.

An early noteworthy contribution to our concepts of immunopathogenesis came from the studies of Page and Schroeder, who described in detail the histology of the developing periodontal lesion. They organized their description of periodontal lesions into four stages that demonstrate characteristic pathologic changes to the tissues and concomitant appearance of cell types known to participate in immune responses. These stages were termed the initial lesion, the early lesion, the established lesion, and the advanced lesion, and they are described in more detail below.

Pathogenesis of Gingivitis

Chronic gingivitis is characterized by gingival redness, edema, bleeding, changes in tissue contour, loss of tissue adaptation to the teeth, and increased flow of an inflammatory exudate termed GCF. Development of chronic gingivitis is clearly dependent on the presence and accumulation of plaque bacteria, which can promote pathologic processes mediated by the immune system. The initial lesion is histologically an acute inflammatory response characterized by vascular changes, collagen degradation, alterations in the appearance of epithelial cells, and infiltration of the tissues by neutrophils. Since bacteria themselves are not found within these tissues, it is surmised that these alterations are likely due to chemotactic attraction of neutrophils by bacterial constituents and direct vasodilatory effects of bacterial products, as well as by activation of host immune systems such as the complement and kinin systems, and arachidonic acid pathways. A hallmark of the early lesion is the appearance of a lymphoid cell infiltrate dominated by T lymphocytes, with increased loss of collagen and further changes in the epithelium that portend the migration of the epithelium down the root surface. The number of B lymphocytes increases during this stage of disease, leading to the established lesion, which is dominated by B lymphocytes, plasma cells, and mononuclear phagocytes, while large numbers of neutrophils infiltrate the epithelium.

The chronic inflammatory infiltrate and vascular alterations seen in early and established gingivitis lesions, and the observed tissue changes including collagen destruction and epithelial proliferation, are consistent with a variety of host immunopathological mechanisms. Although direct evidence for the specific mechanisms involved is lacking, it is likely that bacterial products are interacting with mononuclear phagocytes and fibroblasts to recruit and activate the local immune system and cytokine pathways that have all the elements necessary to provoke the observed tissue changes. Cytokines responsible for the recruitment, differentiation, and growth of lymphocytes and monocytes are likely to mediate the progression of the lesion from a T-cell to a B-cell-predominated lesion, whereas chemotactic factors from the bacteria themselves or from host-derived systems such as complement and arachidonic acid pathways recruit neutrophils to defend against the bacterial insult. Remarkably, the damage to the gingival tissues due to gingivitis can be substantially reversed by removal of dental plaque bacteria from the tooth surface.

Pathogenesis of Periodontitis

The clinical hallmark of periodontitis is the destruction of the connective tissue attachment to the root surface and resorption of bone, with concomitant migration of the epithelial attachment toward the apex of the tooth. The histopathology of this stage of disease, termed the advanced lesion, shares many of the characteristics of the established lesion of gingivitis. Thus, the tissue is predominated by plasma cells, there is further loss of connective tissue elements, and in addition, there is osteoclastic bone loss.

Despite the histopathologic similarities between the established lesion of gingivitis and the advanced lesion in which there is "loss of attachment" of connective tissue elements to the tooth, there is little evidence indicating that the advanced lesion is the inevitable consequence of progression from the established lesion. Indeed, the established lesion may persist for many years in some patients without indication of clinical progression. Current thinking is that individual susceptibility to periodontitis in otherwise healthy individuals is likely to be due to a combination of patient-specific risk factors that include specific behaviors such as smoking, as well as hereditary factors. Genetic factors influencing immunopathogenesis are discussed later in this chapter.

NEUTROPHILS AND ANTIBODIES

A persistent characteristic of the histology of gingivitis and periodontitis is the presence of neutrophils, creating a barrier along the junctional epithelium and within the gingival crevice or periodontal pocket. The histological appearance of gingivitis and periodontitis lesions implicates neutrophils as the "first line of defense" against dental plaque microorganisms. This role for neutrophils in host defense is emphasized by the observation that a number of rare conditions in which neutrophil function is compromised are characterized clinically by early and severe periodontitis. Severe periodontitis, as well as other extraoral infections, is a frequent finding in young children suffering from chronic neutropenia, cyclic neutropenia, and leukocyte adhesion deficiency. These rare conditions teach us that properly functioning neutrophils are crucial for periodontal health and that profound defects in their function lead to a breakdown in the barriers against plaque bacteria.

More subtle defects in neutrophils also exist, and some of these are also associated with early and rapid periodontal tissue destruction. The most studied of these is aggressive periodontitis, which is characterized by severe and rapidly progressing disease that usually starts at puberty or in early adulthood. It has been known for many years that a significant proportion of patients with localized aggressive periodontitis have aberrant neutrophil function most frequently observed as defective chemotaxis. Interestingly, the chemotactic defect is not complete or profound but rather is partial, that is, the neutrophils can respond to chemical chemotactic gradients but respond more slowly and with fewer cells than those from a healthy individual. Remarkably, these patients have no other obvious health problems; their defective chemotactic function may be only manifested as aggressive periodontitis.

Though the absence of neutrophils or some defects in their function can lead to increased disease, the presence of these cells in periodontal lesions may also be destructive to the periodontium. The fundamental activities of neutrophils include synthesis and release of a variety of biologically active substances associated with periodontal pathology. That the interaction of bacteria with neutrophils can damage cellular components of the periodontium, including endothelial cells, keratinocytes, and fibroblasts, is well established. It is likely that under the challenge faced by the periodontal tissues, wherein a large biofilm mass harboring a variety of pathogenic bacteria encounters many neutrophils filling the periodontal pocket and lining the junctional epithelium, the release of constitutive enzymes and the synthesis and release of metabolites such as prostaglandins are likely. Such neutrophil-derived factors would give rise to tissue-damaging enzymes and bone resorption factors.

Antibodies specifically reactive with periodontal pathogens are commonly found in sera and GCF from patients with periodontitis. For example, both systemic and locally produced antibodies reactive with *P. gingivalis* are commonly found in patients with chronic periodontitis, whereas high levels of antibodies reactive with *A. actinomycetemcomitans* are found in patients with aggressive periodontitis. Such antibodies are usually considered to be protective in the sense that they promote phagocytosis in vitro, and high concentrations in serum are usually associated with decreased disease severity. On the other hand, it is obvious that the defensive posture of neutrophils at the junctional epithelium is not entirely effective and that bacteria or specific antigens coated with antibodies are likely enhancing the release of hydrolytic enzymes, oxidative metabolites, and prostanoids into the surrounding tissues.

Bacterial Virulence and Evasion of the Immune System

A comprehensive description of bacterial virulence factors appears earlier in this chapter. However, it is worthwhile to summarize and emphasize some of the characteristics of oral bacterial virulence that impact the immunopathogenesis of periodontal diseases.

The destruction of periodontal tissues may be viewed as a consequence of the ability of virulent oral pathogens to both incite destructive immune responses and to impair the host immune systems that would otherwise protect against bacterial infection. One of the conceptually simple strategies for bacteria to accomplish this is by simply numerically overwhelming the immune system by exercising characteristics that promote their growth and accumulation in the biofilm. Thus, as described above, the ability of *P. gingivalis* to induce inflammation and bleeding and then utilize its hemagglutinins and proteases to lyse erythrocytes and extract needed nutrients from their environment would be highly beneficial to the organism. By promoting its own growth, overwhelming the protective barrier provided by neutrophils, and inducing production and release of tissue-damaging substances, the organism enhances its ability to produce disease.

However, more subtle mechanisms have been developed by some oral bacteria that subvert the protective function of the immune system. Consider the fact that *P. gingivalis* produces proteases that not only provide peptides needed for its propagation, but that these proteases also degrade serum antibacterial components (i.e., antibody molecules, complement proteins) and immune cell-derived peptides (e.g., cytokines) aimed at promoting antibacterial immune responses. Furthermore, these bacteria can hide from elements of the local gingival immune system by invading epithelial cells, and can escape into the systemic circulation by invading endothelial cells. While this is occurring, the bacteria can enhance pathologic immune responses as they release small packages (membrane vesicles) of proinflammatory virulence factors as well as soluble proteins, peptides, and lipids that can make their way into the tissues. It is the interaction of bacterial components, such as LPS and a variety of other antigens, with immune cells that is thought to be responsible for a great deal of the damage to the periodontal tissues.

A second instructive bacterial species is the periodontal pathogen *A. actinomycetemcomitans*, which has been associated with both periodontal and systemic diseases. *A. actinomycetemcomitans* has the special characteristic of being able to produce a protein (leukotoxin) that specifically is toxic to host immune cells such as neutrophils and monocytes. This characteristic of some strains of this organism is closely associated with the occurrence of LAP. Furthermore, strains of *A. actinomycetemcomitans* can produce factors that inhibit immune responses (ISF), thus further guaranteeing their survival. Additionally, *A. actinomycetemcomitans* invades epithelial and endothelial cells, which provide a protected environment, facilitate entry into the circulation, and offer a base from where it can seed other tissues.

Thus, evasion of elements of the immune system by periodontal pathogens permits their growth and accumulation to critical levels, setting the stage for the initiation of destructive disease processes in response to the infection.

Destruction of Periodontal Tissues by Immunopathologic Means

Various pathways that could explain the histopathological alterations to the periodontium in the advanced lesion described above have been cited. Recall that hallmark signs of periodontitis include destruction of the periodontal ligament, resorption of the alveolar bone, and the migration of the epithelial and collagenous attachment apparatus towards the apex of the tooth. The absence of evidence of overwhelming bacterial infiltration or invasion of these tissues implicates host mechanisms in at least a portion of their destruction. It is likely that a combination of host mechanisms may play roles in this process.

A Model for Periodontal Pathogenesis

INADEQUACY OF HOST DEFENSE IN THE GINGIVAL SULCUS

As bacterial plaques mature they become increasingly populated with gram-negative bacteria. The capacity of local defense mechanisms to resist virulent constituents of plaque bacteria may be breached due to overwhelming numbers of such bacteria and their numerous virulence mechanisms. Recall, for example, that *P. gingivalis* secretes proteolytic enzymes known to degrade host proteins including complement components and immunoglobulins. Thus, opsonization within the gingival crevice or periodontal pocket may be compromised. Furthermore, *A. actinomycetemcomitans* produces a leukotoxin that kills neutrophils and monocytes. These and other features of virulent bacterial plaques enhance the survival of pathogens in the biofilm and thus increase the likelihood of the exposure of their constituents to the underlying host tissues.

There is little doubt, based on direct observation and indirect measurements, that bacteria or their constituents and metabolic products access the underlying periodontium. The invasive capacity of some oral pathogens such as *P. gingivalis* and *A. actinomycetemcomitans* has been documented above, and these bacteria have been observed in the superficial layers of diseased periodontal tissues. Some species of virulent bacteria in plaque, including those "red complex" bacteria described earlier in this chapter, and/or their constituents, clearly have the ability to access the local (gingival) and the systemic immune systems. This capacity is reflected in detectable specific local and systemic immune responses, notably production of IgG antibodies. The specificity of these antibodies for bacterial antigens reflects the fact that virulence factors such as LPS are present in sufficient quantities and for sufficient time to access the constituents of the innate and adaptive immune systems.

INTERACTIONS WITH THE INNATE IMMUNE SYSTEM
A likely pathway utilized by gram-negative periodontal pathogens is via interaction with mononuclear phagocytes in the periodontium. Bacteria directly (via bacteria chemoattractive peptides) or indirectly (via induction of release of chemoattractant cytokines and prostanoids from host cells) attract additional leukocytes to sites of infection. Bacterial LPS interacts with monocytes/macrophages via CD14 and Toll-like receptors on macrophages and dendritic cells to induce production of cytokines and inflammatory mediators. The major cytokine pathways likely involve IL-1, due to its association with bone-destructive mechanisms and collagenolytic activities. This pathway is also implicated by data demonstrating genetically controlled hyperreactivity to LPS-stimulated IL-1 production in susceptible individuals (see below). Additionally, LPS interactions with monocytes/macrophages lead to the synthesis and secretion of prostanoids, notably PGE2, which is found at high concentrations in GCF from periodontal sites that are losing attachment. PGE2 is likely to be important in promoting bone resorption during periodontitis. This has been illustrated both in animal models and in human patients, where inhibition of PGE2 production by nonsteroidal anti-inflammatory drugs results in decreased loss of alveolar bone.

INTERACTIONS WITH THE ADAPTIVE IMMUNE SYSTEM
Although the generation of protective immune responses is known to be important in limiting destruction of periodontal tissues, such responses also are likely to participate in immunopathological reactions that can enhance disease.

As previously mentioned, early periodontal lesions are histologically characterized by the presence of T lymphocytes and macrophages, whereas established and advanced lesions contain larger numbers of B lymphocytes and plasma cells. This progression is likely controlled by cytokines. The production of cytokines, notably the types, their location, and quantity, is regulated by both individual host variation (both genetic and environmental) and the interaction of bacteria with host cells. Under specific conditions of environment, host characteristics, and the nature of the infection, the resulting cytokine production may orchestrate a protective immune response or, alternatively, a pathological or destructive response.

The early lesion of periodontal disease, which is clinical gingivitis, appears histologically to be consistent with expected outcomes of a T-helper 1 (Th1) response. Such a response entails stimulation of IL-12 production, which in turn induces IFN-γ production, leading to macrophage activation, increased phagocytic activity, and protective immunity. On the other hand, the established and advanced lesions, with clinical periodontitis, are histologically consistent with a Th2 response characterized by production of IL-4, IL-10, and IL-13, leading to antibody production. It is well known that periodontitis may persist and progress despite the presence of high concentrations of systemic and local (GCF) antibody. This implies not that such lesions have resolved but rather that there is continued inappropriate production of cytokines and overproduction of inflammatory cytokines such as IL-1.

Regulation of immune responses to periodontal pathogens and dysregulation of such responses leading to pathology have been studied for several years with inconclusive and sometimes conflicting results. Studies examining gingival tissue cells for cytokine production or mRNA expression, or studies examining interactions between bacteria and leukocytes, frequently demonstrate a mixture of Th1 and Th2 cytokines or a predominance of one over the other. Limitations of these studies relate not only to technical differences and varying sources of cellular material for study, but also to the difficulty in differentiating active from inactive disease lesions and different disease phenotypes from each other. The cumulative data to date appear to favor the association of the Th2 response with chronic periodontitis.

Th1-DEPENDENT ANTIBODY PRODUCTION IN AGGRESSIVE PERIODONTITIS

Immune responses to etiologic organisms in patients with aggressive periodontitis are characterized by extremely high levels of specific IgG2 antibodies reactive with bacterial carbohydrate antigens. Patients with LAP are further characterized by having elevated levels of serum IgG2 protein compared to other subject groups. IgG2 is a unique antibody subclass in the human repertoire in that its production is dependent on Th1 rather than Th2 cytokines. The reasons for this predominant systemic Th1 response in patients with aggressive periodontitis are not entirely clear. However, it is known that serum IgG2 levels are under genetic control. Thus, LAP may represent a periodontal patient group in which elevated Th1-dependent responses predominate due to genetic factors and the direction of the immune responses by the major pathogen towards production of Th1 cytokines.

Immune Cells and Bone Resorption

There are functional links between immune system cells and bone cells that could explain the bone loss seen in periodontitis infections. Factors essential to bone resorption and remodeling include the TNF-TNFR superfamily proteins RANK-L (receptor activator of NF-κB ligand), RANK, and the inhibitor protein osteoprotegrin (OPG). The receptor for RANK-L is RANK, which is found on osteoclast precursor cells. In bone, RANK-L is expressed in osteoblasts and can be up-regulated by various bone-regulating hormones as well as by IL-1, IL-6, IL-11, IL-17, TNF-α, and PGE2. Up-regulation of RANK-L induces osteoclast production and activation. Bone remodeling and bone loss are controlled by a balance between RANK-L/RANK and the RANK-L decoy receptor OPG.

It has been found that RANK-L is also expressed by T cells and can be up-regulated by antigen activation. Experiments have shown that activated T cells, which express RANK-L, can directly induce osteoclasts. In a variety of inflammatory and infectious diseases, it is thought that T cells expressing RANK-L participate in bone resorption. In diseases characterized by T-cell activation as well as production of inflammatory cytokines such as IL-1 and TNF-α, bone resorption can be enhanced via elevated RANK-L expression on T cells and induction of RANK-L on other cells in the lesion by inflammatory cytokines. In periodontitis, the presence of proinflammatory cytokines and activated T cells in the advanced lesion sets the stage for bone resorption via RANK/RANK-L interactions. RANK-L and OPG have been demonstrated in gingival epithelia and connective tissues, and bacteria such as *A. actinomycetemcomitans* can up-regulate RANK-L. Thus it is likely that the immune and inflammatory milieus of periodontitis lesions provide an environment for immunoregulation of bone resorption via RANK-L and its inhibitor OPG.

Use of Animal Models To Study Pathogenesis of Periodontitis

There are no animal model systems that entirely recapitulate the "natural history" and pathological characteristics of human periodontitis. Nevertheless, animal models have been successfully utilized to demonstrate aspects of bacterium-host interactions that could not be otherwise studied in human systems. Additionally, animal models have been used to study fundamental aspects of pathogenesis that provide clues as to which systems are worthy of further study in human disease. Some examples of these systems that are currently in favor, and how they have been utilized in recent years, are given below:

PRIMATES

Primate models of periodontitis are used by researchers because of the anatomical similarities of the dentition and periodontal structures to those of humans. In addition, the bacterial microbiota of some primates resembles that of humans with respect to the presence of major periodontal pathogens. Several species of primates have been shown to spontaneously develop periodontitis with age. The histopathology of both gingivitis and periodontitis in most species of primates is similar, but not identical, to that seen in human disease.

Most studies of pathogenesis attempt to examine events that accompany active loss of periodontal tissues. Therefore, periodontal lesions in animals with mature periodontal microbiota but minimal periodontitis are induced by tying silk ligatures or orthodontic elastics (with or without infection with bacteria) around the teeth. This procedure can result in rapid local plaque accumulation and periodontitis lesions after several weeks. The histology of these lesions appears to vary with primate species. In squirrel monkeys, for example, the primary inflammatory infiltrate in periodontitis lesions is composed of neutrophils and macrophages, while in cynomolgus monkeys the lesions contain lymphocytes and plasma cells. Thus, cynomolgus monkeys may be considered to be more appropriate for studying pathogenic mechanisms related to human periodontal diseases.

One of the more notable early observations linking immunopathologic reactions to periodontal pathology was that high concentrations of antibody specifically reactive with periodontal microorganisms are present in patients with periodontitis. This led to speculation that formation of local antigen-antibody complexes could contribute to periodontitis. Indeed, induction of a type II (Arthus-type) reaction in ovalbumin-sensitized primates by inoculation of the gingiva with this nonoral antigen was shown to lead to inflammation and alveolar bone resorption. This model appears to implicate Arthus-type reactions in pathogenesis, though this mechanism of tissue injury has not yet been readily demonstrable in human periodontitis.

Primate models are now utilized in studies of immunomodulation of periodontal infections, in particular, studies of vaccine efficacy. *Macaca fascicularis* has been shown to naturally harbor strains of *A. actinomycetemcomitans*, *P. gingivalis*, *T. forsythia*, *C. rectus*, *P. intermedia*, and *F. nucleatum*. Furthermore, this species produces a serum antibody response to *P. gingivalis*. Several approaches have been used to examine the feasibility of immunization against periodontitis. *M. fascicularis* immunized with killed *P. gingivalis* demonstrated protection against ligature-induced periodontitis. This occurred in spite of the fact that periodontitis in primates induced in this manner appears to be polymicrobial and could be a result of cross-reactivity between the LPS of periodontal pathogens. Alternatively, this result may be a reflection of a required role for *P. gingivalis* in the maintenance of the biofilm and support of its constituents. Promising results have also been obtained with cysteine proteases of *P. gingivalis* as immunogens in primates.

Experimental periodontitis in primates has also been useful to test hypotheses about the pathogenesis of periodontal bone loss. A notable example of this is the examination of the role of the inflammatory cytokine IL-1 in periodontal bone loss. Administration of soluble IL-1 receptor and TNF-α receptor locally in animals undergoing experimental periodontitis significantly reduces loss of connective tissue attachment and alveolar bone. Such studies confirm the central role of IL-1 and TNF in periodontal pathogenesis in this animal model and might also suggest modes of immunotherapy.

RODENT MODELS

Rodents are frequently utilized to study pathogenic mechanisms of periodontitis despite the major differences between rodent dentition and that of humans. The obvious economy of utilizing rodents as well as the availability of inbred strains and genetic variants provides advantages not available in studies utilizing primates.

Mice

Mice have been extensively utilized for many years to study pathogenic mechanisms in periodontitis. In a model system designed to examine the relative "tissue invasiveness" or "pathogenicity" of bacterial isolates, bacteria are injected subcutaneously into the backs of mouse strains. Strains of some organisms, in particular *P. gingivalis*, are particularly dramatic in this assay, wherein they can cause lesions ranging from localized ulcerations to disseminating dissecting lesions and death. This assay has been used to initially assess the pathogenicity of *P. gingivalis* strains, and has been further utilized to assess the efficacy of immunization with various antigens derived from *P. gingivalis*. In addition, mutant strains of periodontal pathogens lacking crucial virulence factors can be tested for their pathogenic potential.

A variation on this model entails the surgical implantation of a subcutaneous coil that becomes encased in a fibrous chamber after healing. Bacteria injected into the chamber are retained due to fibrous enclosure, but elements comprising the inflammatory and the immune response can be sampled from the site and analyzed. Thus, the nature of the local response to such infections can be determined.

It has been noted that the application by oral swab of certain bacterial pathogens, notably *P. gingivalis*, results in alveolar bone resorption in some mouse strains. This observation and the availability of inbred congenic strains with defined defects in genes coding for immunologic factors of importance in periodontal pathology have facilitated systematic studies of isolated genetic defects on periodontal infections. Additionally, the development of transgenic strains that under- or overexpress a variety of factors has also allowed studies leading to hypothesis development regarding human disease.

Mouse models of alveolar bone loss have been utilized to examine the efficacy of vaccines derived from a variety of bacterial antigens. Immunization with whole *P. gingivalis* cells or RgpA, but not RgpB, has been shown to provide protection against *P. gingivalis*-stimulated alveolar bone loss. IgG antibody reactive with *P. gingivalis* was induced by all three antigens. This result implicates RgpA, or its associated hemagglutinin, as a critical virulence determinant for bone loss in this model. Other antigens of *P. gingivalis* have also proved to be effective immunogens in preventing bone loss in mice. For example, immunization with capsular polysaccharide led to production of both IgG and IgM antibodies reactive with *P. gingivalis* and inhibited bone loss caused by oral administration of the organism.

Genetically defined mouse strains have proved useful in examining immune responses to oral bacteria and the role of various immune factors in periodontal bone loss. For example, in studies utilizing mouse strains differing by H-2 haplotype, it was observed that significantly differing cytokine profiles (reflecting the balance of Th1 versus Th2 cytokines) were observed following immunization with *P. gingivalis* antigens. Studies of this type indicate that there is genetic control over the response to periodontal organisms that may reflect the pathological pathways leading to disease. The results of studies using targeted gene knockout mice have provided further insight into potential pathogenic mechanisms in periodontitis, for example, mice without CD4$^+$ T-cell function, as well as those lacking IFN-γ and IL-6, fail to lose alveolar bone. Other studies have shown that polymorphic genes controlling IFN-γ production influence bone loss; mice producing high levels of IFN-γ are most susceptible to periodontitis. Such studies may reflect pathogenic mechanisms that could occur in patients with periodontitis.

Rats

An advantage of rats over mice in rodent models is that the teeth are large enough for the local induction of periodontal lesions by ligatures tied around the teeth. This allows induction of isolated periodontal lesions at particular sites in the oral cavity. Furthermore, in a variation of the basic model, gnotobiotic rats can be utilized in experiments that examine monoinfection of sites in the oral cavity with selected pathogens. Bacteria can be delivered via swab or can be impregnated into the ligature used to induce periodontal lesions.

As in the mouse model, studies have focused on the influences of immunization with various bacterial antigens on pathogen-induced alveolar bone loss. For example, it has been shown that immunization of rats challenged orally with *P. gingivalis* with whole bacteria or with gingipain proteases (RgpA and Kgp) resulted in significant protection against alveolar bone loss. Examples of other immunogens shown to provide protection against alveolar bone loss include the hemoglobin-binding HA2 domain and the 43-kDa major fimbrial protein of *P. gingivalis*. The induction of specific antibody against these antigens could act in various ways, by promoting opsonization or inhibiting bacterial colonization or nutrient acquisition.

Genetic Factors That Influence Responses to Periodontal Infections

ROLE OF GENETICS IN INFECTIOUS DISEASE SUSCEPTIBILITY

An individual's response to the presence of pathogens is a function of the nature and route of exposure to the pathogen and the host's susceptibility to the infection. Susceptibility to infection, in turn, is a function of previous exposures to the pathogen, host genetic variability that modifies responses to pathogens, and environmental exposures that also modify susceptibility. These factors are not necessarily additive to each other but rather interactive in nature. Genetic factors may influence the host's reactivity to both the pathogen and other environmental risk factors, and these factors in turn interact with each other in a complex manner.

In most cases, genetic susceptibility to infectious agents involves multiple genes rather than single major genes. In general, these diseases are multifactorial and have a complex genetic component. It becomes a challenge, therefore, to identify the relative contributions of a variety of factors that can lead to the manifestation of the disease. Understanding the role of such genes in susceptibility to infectious diseases is important for a variety of reasons. This information would elucidate the molecular pathways of immune regulation and chronic infectious diseases such as periodontitis. Understanding which genes are involved in pathogenesis and how they influence the course of infection would assist in the development of drugs and vaccines.

Studies of genetic susceptibility to periodontitis are currently in their early stages. Such studies are problematic for a number of reasons, not the least of which is a lack of clear and stable definitions of the several disease phenotypes. This problem arises from the heterogeneity of periodontal disorders with respect to diagnosis and clinical variability, the variety of pathogens that may induce disease states via differing pathogenic pathways, the inconsistent biological risk factors evident in patient populations, and the alterations of disease phenotype that may occur due to therapy, antibiotic usage, or dental hygiene practices.

ESTIMATION OF THE CONTRIBUTION OF GENES TO PERIODONTAL INFECTION

It is clear that there is a heritable component to risk of periodontal infection. The best data in this regard come from studies of chronic periodontitis in twins. If a disease has a genetic component, then the disease phenotypes of monozygous twin pairs (who share all their genes) must have higher concordance than that observed in dizygous twins. Variations in manifestation of periodontitis between identical twins must be due only to environmental factors. Twin studies indicate that there is less variability of clinical measures of periodontal disease in monozygous twin pairs than in dizygous twin pairs. Twin pairs are assumed to share environmental risk factors (they grew up in the same household), so the proportions of disease variation in monozygous and dizygous pairs are assumed to be about the same. Thus, the observed phenotypic difference in pairs of individuals who share all their genes and pairs who share only half their genes is thought to be due to hereditary factors. Estimates of the contribution of genes to the population variance in periodontal measures indicate that about 50% of such variance is due to genes.

Additional evidence for genetic risk for periodontitis is from family studies of individuals with aggressive periodontitis. Such studies verify that these rare diseases are familial and that the distribution of disease within family structures is consistent with heritable disease. Furthermore, a variety of uncommon inherited diseases characterized by aberrations of inflammatory and immunological function, such as leukocyte adhesion deficiency, chronic neutropenia, cyclic neutropenia, and other related syndromes, are characterized by early periodontal infection and loss of teeth at a young age.

GENETIC FACTORS ASSOCIATED WITH PERIODONTITIS

Studies of specific genetic risk factors for periodontitis are limited, but it is likely that there are multiple polymorphic genes that each can contribute to overall risk for periodontal attachment loss. In view of the paradigm for the pathogenesis of periodontitis presented above, risk factors related to inflammatory and immunological processes have been targeted for study in various populations. As shown in Table 4, genetic polymorphisms associated with cytokines such as IL-1, TNF-α, IL-10, and IL-4 have been found to be associated with risk for chronic or aggressive periodontitis.

Associations between IL-1 polymorphisms and periodontitis severity have been the most intensively studied of such genetic influences on disease. The IL-1 polymorphisms are functional in the sense that the alleles

TABLE 4 Genetic polymorphisms associated with periodontitis or periodontal health

Polymorphism	Gene	Disease association
IL-1A (+4,845) and IL-1B (+3,954)	IL-1 gene	Chronic periodontitis
TNF-α-308 allele 1	TNF-α gene	Chronic periodontitis
TNF-β Ncol, ET-1 gene, and ACE gene insertion/deletion polymorphism	Lymphotoxin alpha (TNF-β), endothelin-1 (ET-1), and angiotensin-converting enzyme (ACE) genes	Chronic periodontitis
FcγRIIIb-NA2 allotype	Fc receptor polymorphism	Chronic periodontitis
NAT2	N-acetyltransferase polymorphism	Chronic periodontitis
MMP-1 promoter polymorphism	Matrix metalloproteinase 1 gene	Chronic periodontitis
IL-1A (+4,845) and IL-1B (+3,954)	IL-1 gene	Aggressive periodontitis
IL-1RN	IL-1 receptor antagonist gene	Aggressive periodontitis (localized)
IL-4 promoter and intron polymorphisms	IL-4 gene	Aggressive periodontitis
FcγRIIIb-NA2 allele (and possibly FcγRIIIa-158F)	Fc receptor gene polymorphisms	Aggressive periodontitis (generalized)
Gc locus chromosome 4q	Unknown	Aggressive periodontitis (localized)
fMLP receptor	N-formyl peptide receptor polymorphisms	Aggressive periodontitis (localized)
VDR ApaI polymorphism	Vitamin D receptor polymorphism	Chronic and aggressive periodontitis (localized)
VDR gene TaqI polymorphism	Vitamin D receptor polymorphism	Aggressive periodontitis
HLA-A28 and HLA-B5	HLA haplotype	Periodontal health
FcγRIIIb-NA1	Fc receptor polymorphisms	Periodontal health

more commonly present in patients with chronic periodontitis have been shown to be associated with increased in vitro monocyte secretion of IL-1 in response to bacterial LPS. Due to the known pathogenic sequelae of IL-1 production, such as bone resorption, matrix metalloproteinase production, and prostaglandin E synthesis, the genetic associations found in these patients are reasonable. It has been observed, however, that the associations between published IL-1 polymorphisms and chronic periodontitis do not apply to some subject populations because of racial or geographic heterogeneity in the population prevalence of these alleles.

Interestingly, the associations observed between IL-1 polymorphic genes and aggressive periodontitis are with the alleles that would promote lower levels of IL-1, or otherwise no association at all has been detected. These findings also appear to be population-dependent, and also may indicate a difference in pathogenesis of chronic and aggressive periodontitis that could relate to the role of IL-1 in antibody production.

The related cytokine TNF-α has been found to be associated with increased severity of periodontitis in some studies, but other studies have failed to detect such a difference. This result exemplifies the general principle that different human populations as well as different clinical phenotypes may be found to have different associations with individual polymorphisms. Several investigators have examined IL-10 polymorphisms for associations with chronic or aggressive periodontitis. For the most part, these studies have not supported a role for the tested polymorphisms in periodontal pathogenesis.

Another set of polymorphisms showing associations with disease severity or recurrence are those in genes coding for leukocyte Fc receptors. Some functional polymorphisms in Fc are responsible for the affinity of association of immunoglobulin Fc to the Fc receptor, which in turn influences phagocytotic ability and therefore protective antibacterial responses. As shown in Table 4, FcγRIII receptor gene polymorphisms have been shown to be associated with periodontitis severity in Japanese populations. The polymorphic alleles coding for lower-affinity receptors are more commonly present in patients with more severe and more rapidly progressing disease.

A number of other genes of note have shown similar associations. Of particular interest are those controlling connective tissue metabolism or homeostasis. These include polymorphisms in the *VDR* gene (for the vitamin D receptor) and the *MMP-1* gene (for matrix metalloproteinase 1).

Relationships between genes in the major histocompatibility complex and periodontitis seem possible, especially in view of data indicating that destructive immune responses may explain the pathogenic mechanisms of attachment loss. There is evidence of an association of HLA class I and class II antigens with chronic periodontitis, aggressive periodontitis, or periodontal health. However, definitive relationships have not been found, mainly because most of these studies were carried out with small groups of subjects.

Finally, the interesting observation that genetic polymorphism in the *NAT2* gene (*N*-acetyltransferase), which controls the rate of acetylation and detoxification of substances in cigarette smoke (as well as other compounds), may be associated with periodontitis risk exemplifies the complex relationships that may exist between genes, the environment, and disease susceptibility. Cigarette smoking has been repeatedly shown to be a risk factor for periodontitis. In addition, patients who smoke have been shown to have a number of immunological dysfunctions, including defective PMN function and depressed immunoglobulin levels. Thus, in patients with an unfavorable *NAT2* genotype who smoke, one may hypothesize that this interaction would influence immunological and inflammatory responses to oral bacteria and predispose patients to increased disease severity.

■ KEY POINTS

Disease characteristics
Periodontal diseases are a broad group of pathological alterations of the periodontal tissue.

Gingivitis is a reversible inflammation in the marginal periodontal tissues associated with dental plaque.

Periodontitis is an inflammation-based infection of the supporting structures of the teeth characterized by progressive destruction of the periodontal ligament and alveolar bone that may result in tooth loss.

The two distinct forms of periodontitis that occur in otherwise healthy individuals are chronic periodontitis and aggressive periodontitis. Chronic periodontitis is the most common form of periodontitis

and occurs mainly in adults. The severity of disease is consistent with local factors of plaque and calculus. There is a slow to moderate progression of tissue destruction, although short periods of rapid progression may occur. Disease progression and severity may be accentuated by systemic conditions such as diabetes or environmental factors such as smoking. In aggressive periodontitis the progression of the disease is rapid, the severity of disease is not consistent with the occurrence of the local factors of plaque and calculus, and there is often a familial pattern of occurrence, suggesting genetic factors play a significant role in disease susceptibility. Individuals with aggressive periodontitis commonly demonstrate abnormalities in PMN function or hyperresponsive macrophages. Aggressive periodontitis is further classified into two forms: localized (previously termed

(continues)

KEY POINTS

(Continued from previous page) localized juvenile periodontitis) and generalized. LAP has an onset at puberty and typically involves the incisors and first molars. Generalized aggressive periodontitis is usually found in individuals under 30 years of age and involves at least three teeth other than incisors and first molars.

Current thinking on the etiology of periodontitis invokes the ecological plaque hypothesis that maintains that the microbiota of the gingival crevice undergoes a transition from a commensal to a pathogenic relationship with the host due to factors that trigger a shift in the proportions or pathogenic capability of resident microorganisms. Thus, the presence of sufficient numbers of potentially pathogenic organisms, or groups of these organisms, in combination with the absence of beneficial species and the existence of specific susceptibility factors in the host, is required for the initiation and progression of disease.

In chronic periodontitis potential pathogens are often gram-negative anaerobes, including *P. gingivalis*, *T. forsythia*, *T. denticola*, and *P. intermedia*. LAP is usually associated with *A. actinomycetemcomitans*.

Pathogenic mechanisms

The virulence of periodontal pathogens is complex and multifactorial. A number of pathogenic mechanisms have emerged as important:

1. **Colonization.** Periodontal bacteria adhere to epithelial cells in the gingival crevice and to other bacteria in subgingival plaque. Adhesins are often associated with fimbriae on the bacterial surfaces. Adhesion to sites outside the gingival crevice can be followed by translocation to the subgingival area by spreading proliferation or translocation of dislodged progeny. Spirochetes, which are motile by means of their axial filaments, can reach the gingival crevice and tissues via chemotactic attraction.

2. **Invasion.** *P. gingivalis* and *A. actinomycetemcomitans* can direct their uptake into the otherwise nonphagocytic gingival epithelial cells. An intracellular location protects the bacteria from the immune system and can result in modulation of production of immune effectors such as cytokines. Spirochetes and other organisms invade the gingival tissues, causing inflammation and tissue damage.

3. **Toxins.** *A. actinomycetemcomitans* produces a potent leukotoxin that kills human neutrophils and monocytes by causing pore formation in cell membranes and by inducing apoptosis. The leukotoxin can be packaged in membrane-derived vesicles that readily penetrate the tissues.

4. **Enzymes and toxic products.** *P. gingivalis* produces a number of proteolytic enzymes to provide peptides for nutrition. These proteases also degrade immune effector molecules, structural component of tissues, and iron- and hemin-sequestering molecules. Fatty acids produced by bacteria can inhibit cell division and neutrophil chemotaxis.

5. **Cell constituents.** LPS interacts with monocytes/macrophages via CD14 and Toll-like receptors on macrophages and dendritic cells to induce production of cytokines and inflammatory mediators such as IL-1. Additionally, LPS interactions with monocytes/macrophages lead to the synthesis and secretion of prostanoids, notably PGE2. These pathways can result in bone and collagen destruction. Capsule and other extracellular material can prevent phagocytosis.

6. **Resistance to neutrophil killing.** Some organisms can prevent fusion of lysosomes with the phagosome, others are resistant to killing by the toxic compounds of the neutrophils.

7. **Immunosuppressive factors.** *A. actinomycetemcomitans* produces an immunosuppressive factor or cytolethal distending toxin that inhibits critical functions of lymphoid cells such as cell division, along with antibody and cytokine production.

Host factors

Periodontal lesions can be categorized into four stages that demonstrate characteristic pathologic changes to the tissues and the appearance of cell types known to participate in immune responses.

The initial lesion is histologically an acute inflammatory response characterized by vascular changes, collagen degradation, alterations in the appearance of epithelial cells, and infiltration of the tissues by neutrophils. The early lesion is characterized by the appearance of a lymphoid cell infiltrate dominated by T lymphocytes, with increased loss of collagen and the migration of the epithelium down the root surface. This is consistent with expected outcomes of a Th1 response. The number of B lymphocytes increases during this stage of disease, leading to the established lesion, which is dominated by B lymphocytes, plasma cells, and mononuclear phagocytes, while large numbers of neutrophils infiltrate the epithelium. In periodontitis, the advanced lesion that occurs predominates with plasma cells. Further loss of connective tissue elements occurs, as does osteoclastic bone loss. The established and advanced lesions are consistent with a Th2 response.

Neutrophils create a barrier along the junctional epithelium and within the gingival crevice or periodontal pocket. Neutrophils are considered the first line of defense against dental plaque microorganisms. Indeed, a number of rare conditions in which neutrophil function is compromised are characterized clinically by early and severe periodontitis. More subtle defects in neutrophils also exist, and some of these are also associated with early and rapid periodontal tissue destruction. In contrast to their protective function, the encounter between neutrophils and bacteria within periodontal tissues can lead to release of toxic compounds that can damage cellular components of the periodontium.

Formation of immune complexes in the tissues may also contribute to tissue destruction.

In aggressive periodontitis there are high levels of specific IgG2 antibodies reactive with bacterial carbohydrate antigens. IgG2 production is dependent on Th1 rather than Th2 cytokines. Thus, LAP may represent a periodontal patient group in which elevated Th1-dependent responses predominate.

IL-1 and TNF appear to be important mediators of tissue destruction and bone resorption. Regulation of bone resorption also occurs through RANK-L and its inhibitor OPG.

Several genetic factors may influence susceptibility to periodontal infection. These include polymorphisms in genes that control neutrophil chemotaxis, IL-1 and TNF production, and the Fc receptor on phagocytic cells.

FURTHER READING

Loesche, W. J. 1976. Chemotherapy of dental plaque infections. *Oral Sci. Rev.* **9**:65.

Page, R. 1986. Gingivitis. *J. Clin. Periodontol.* **13**:345–359.

Schluger, S., R. Yudelis, R. C. Pages, and R. H. Johnson. 1990. *Periodontal Diseases,* 2nd ed. Lea and Febiger, Philadelphia, Pa.

Schou, S., P. Holmstrup, and K. S. Kornman. 1993. Non-human primates used in studies of periodontal disease pathogenesis: a review of the literature. *J. Periodontol.* **64**:497–508.

Weinberg, M. A., and M. Bral. 1999. Laboratory animal models in periodontology. *J. Clin. Periodontol.* **26**:335–340.

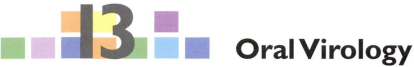

Oral Virology

Matti Sällberg

INTRODUCTION

What Is Oral Virology?

In a broad sense, oral virology could be defined as viruses present in the oral cavity. This does not, however, imply that all these viruses infect and replicate in the tissues of the oral cavity. Rather, many viruses are present in the oral cavity merely as a consequence of infection and replication elsewhere in the body, but reach the oral cavity through the circulatory system or other transport mechanisms. Thus, these viruses are directly or indirectly of interest to the dental profession. This is the definition of oral virology that is used in this chapter.

In this chapter the reader is introduced to the basic concepts of virology, such as the structure of viruses and the replication cycle of viruses, and to viruses that can be defined as being related to the field of oral virology. The chapter also covers the basics of how viruses are recognized by the immune system. This is very important, since in many viral diseases it is not the virus that directly causes the clinical symptoms. Instead, it is the immune system that when fighting the infection produces cytokines that cause fever and actively kill infected cells. Finally, the chapter discusses the basics of viral vaccines and modern antiviral therapies.

What Is a Virus?

One could say that a virus is the smallest form of life. This may, however, be debated, since viruses lack the ability to replicate in the absence of a host cell. The term virus, which in Latin means poison, reflects, to some degree of accuracy, the behavior of many viruses. For example, a virus can be transmitted through air on small droplets of water exhaled by an infected person. The mere touch of the skin by an infected person may, under certain circumstances, transmit the infection. Thus, it is not difficult to understand that viral infections throughout time have been considered as something that behaves like a poison. All viruses have some common basic characteristics, regardless of whether they infect prokaryotic or eukaryotic cells (Table 1). The components of the smallest viruses are a viral genome surrounded by a protein shell, termed capsid or nucleocapsid.

TABLE 1 Three basic characteristics common to all viruses

1. They lack their own metabolism.
2. They can replicate only inside a prokaryotic or eukaryotic cell.
3. They contain a genome and a surrounding protein shell that protects the genome from the environment, attaches to the cell to be infected, and determines the host range of the virus.

So, now we know the basic prerequisites for viruses. The question is, What does a virus look like? Viruses are small, ranging from 20 to about 300 nm in size. All viruses have their own genome. The genome has two basic functions. One is to code for all viral proteins and these sequences, or regions, are called the coding regions. The second is to interact with the machinery of the host cell, such as binding transcription factors or ribosomes. These genomic regions are called the noncoding, or untranslated, regions. The coding region of the viral genome encodes two types of viral proteins. The first type is called structural proteins, and by definition, they are the proteins found in the extracellular virus. Examples of structural proteins are nucleocapsid and envelope proteins. The second type of viral protein is called nonstructural proteins. These proteins are not present in the extracellular virus but can be found in the infected cell. Examples of viral nonstructural proteins are enzymes, such as DNA or RNA polymerases or proteases, and viral proteins that inhibit the host immune response. To summarize, the viral genome consists of coding regions that encode all viral proteins and noncoding regions that interact with the host cell machinery. The viral proteins are either structural proteins (present in the extracellular virus) or nonstructural proteins (only present in the infected cell).

The viral genome can be one of many different types such as composed of single-stranded RNA, double-stranded RNA, double-stranded DNA, and so on. To simplify the taxonomy of viruses, the two major groups of viral genomes are either RNA or DNA. Both RNA and DNA genomes can be divided into the subclasses listed in Table 2. Apart from these five subclasses, the viral genome can be linear, circular, or segmented. A segmented viral genome can be compared to the human genome in that it is composed of several chromosomes. An advantage of a segmented genome is that it can be large without risk of strand breakage. From a viral point of view, there are other advantages to a segmented genome. A classical example is the segmented RNA genome of the influenza A virus. We all know that the influenza A virus causes the respiratory disease, termed influenza, that appears every winter. However, in some years the impact of the influenza A virus epidemic takes global proportions, called pandemics.

How can influenza A virus cause such a massive spread of the infection when most individuals already have had one or more infections with the virus? The answer is directly related to the advantage of possessing a segmented genome. Influenza A virus has a very broad host range, meaning that a rather substantial number of animals can be infected by human influenza A virus. Many species, such as pigs, pigeons, and ducks, have their own species-specific influenza A virus. There are times when, for example, a duck cell is infected by both a human influenza A virus and a duck influenza A virus at the same time. If both viruses start to replicate, this will result in a number of human and duck influenza A virus gene segments in the same cell. These human and duck gene segments can, by recombination, or more correctly in this case reassortment of segments, be combined and be packaged into the same virus. Thus, the resulting virus will contain a new combination of human and duck influenza A virus genes. The virus now represents a new form of influenza A virus that is quite different from the influenza A viruses we will have previously encountered. Consequently, we lack complete protective immunity against

TABLE 2 Classes of viral genomes

Positive-sense single-standed RNA
Negative-sense single-stranded RNA
Double-stranded RNA
Single-stranded DNA
Double-stranded DNA

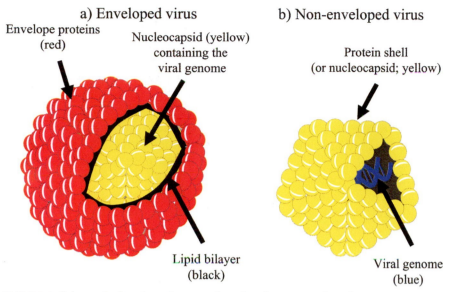

a) Enveloped virus

Envelope proteins (red)

Nucleocapsid (yellow) containing the viral genome

Lipid bilayer (black)

b) Non-enveloped virus

Protein shell (or nucleocapsid; yellow)

Viral genome (blue)

FIGURE I Schematic drawing of an enveloped and a nonenveloped virus.

this newly established strain. This allows a rapid and extensive spread of the virus throughout the human population. The molecular basis for this is, of course, that the virus has a segmented genome that allows for a recombination between human and animal influenza A virus genes. From this it can be deduced that the organization of the viral genome is an important factor determining the behavior of the virus.

All viruses have a shell that surrounds and protects the viral genome. However, depending on the virus type, more than one layer of shells may be present. Two major types of outer shells exist. The first is a protein shell composed of one or more proteins coded by the viral genome and is called the nucleocapsid, or capsid. The capsid can have two different structures, icosahedral or helical. An icosahedral capsid looks like the geometric solid called an icosahedron (Fig. 1). The helical capsid has the appearance of a helical wheel, much like when the histone proteins assemble our own DNA. Viruses that only have this type of shell are termed nonenveloped viruses (Fig. 1). The second type of outer shell is a lipid bilayer, derived from the infected cell, that surrounds the inner protein shell, the nucleocapsid. Within the lipid envelope, viral envelope proteins have been inserted. These types of viruses are termed enveloped viruses. Viruses with a helical capsid structure are always enveloped. However, viruses with icosahedral capsids can be either enveloped or nonenveloped. The schematic representation of these two groups of viruses is shown in Fig. 1.

THE VIRAL LIFE CYCLE

The life cycle of all viruses can be generalized to some common and basic steps. Of course, the exact life cycle of the different viruses varies extensively, but these general steps are relevant for most viruses. Let us consider an extracellular virus, also termed the virion, containing everything needed to transmit the viral infection. The first event that has to take place is binding to the surface of the cell to be infected. This event is called attachment (Fig. 2). Attachment is mediated through the interaction between the surface of the virus and a molecule, or receptor, present on the surface of the cell. The attachment event is an important factor in determining the host range of a virus. Cells that are not permissive to infection by a particular virus can often be made permissive by genetically introducing a surface receptor to which the virus can bind.

After attachment, the virus has to enter the cell. Depending on the structure of the virus, three mechanisms are most often used. First, if the virus has a lipid envelope, the lipid membrane of the cell can fuse with the lipid envelope of the virus. Thus, the two lipid membranes "melt" together and the viral capsid containing the viral genome is released in the cytoplasm (Fig. 3). Second and third, if the virus is a nonenveloped virus, i.e., does not have an outer lipid envelope, the virus entry into the cell is mediated by endocytosis or translocation (Fig. 3). These are the common ways for cells to take up macromolecular substances from the outside of the cell membrane. The virus will enter the endosome and be transported into the cell cytoplasm. Release of the virus from the endosome can occur in many different ways.

After the viral capsid enters the cell cytoplasm, the viral genome has to be released in order to perform the needed functions. This step is known as uncoating and describes the dissociation of the capsid and the release of the viral genome in the cell (Fig. 4). This step takes place in different compartments of the cell depending on the virus. Most DNA

FIGURE 2 The first steps in the viral life cycle.

Viral infection of a cell

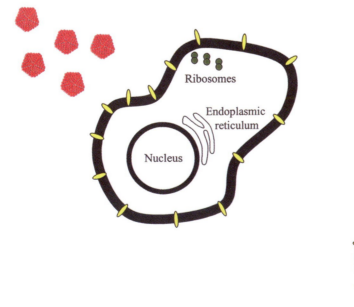

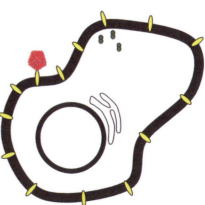

Attachment
The virus binds to a cellular membrane protein

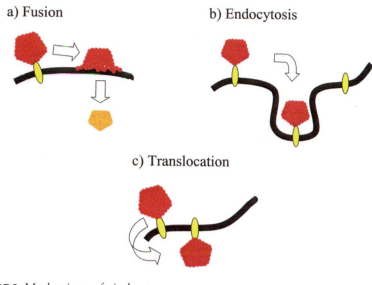

FIGURE 3 Mechanisms of viral entry.

FIGURE 4 Uncoating and release of the viral genome.

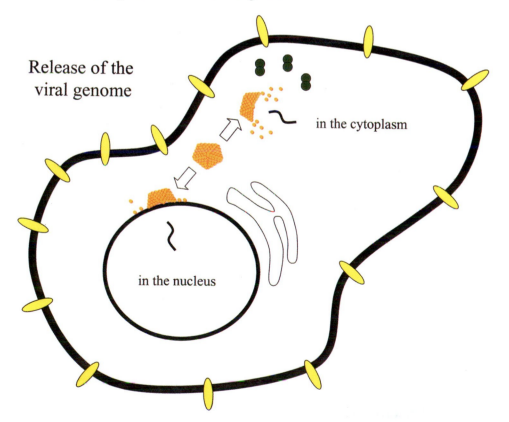

viruses, with few exceptions, replicate their genome in the cell nucleus. Thus, the capsid containing the viral genome is transported to the nuclear membrane, where the capsid dissociates and releases the viral genome into the cell nucleus (Fig. 4). In contrast, the replication of most RNA viruses takes place in the cytoplasm. Thus, the viral capsid disintegrates after entry into the cell cytoplasm where the viral genome is released.

The initial steps after uncoating of the viral genome are largely dependent on the virus. In general, two events can take place, either replication/transcription or translation of the viral genome. To better describe the next steps, two viruses are used as examples.

As previously mentioned, most RNA viruses replicate their genome in the cell cytoplasm. One such virus family is the *Flaviviridae*, to which hepatitis C virus (HCV), GB virus C (GBV-C), and tick-borne encephalitis virus belong. The genomes of the members of the *Flaviviridae* have some common features. All genomes are composed of one RNA strand approximately 10,000 bases long. The coding region of the genome, the part that encodes the viral proteins, is surrounded at both ends by important noncoding regulatory sequences. They all have an RNA strand with positive polarity, meaning that the RNA can directly interact with cellular tRNA, which is an essential step in regulation of this family of viruses. An internal ribosome entry site (IRES) is present in the 5′ noncoding region of the genome, which allows the RNA to bind ribosomes and be translated, and which is followed by the coding region that encodes all of the viral proteins. In addition, at the extreme 3′-end of the genome, a polyadenosine [poly(A) tail] stretch is often found. Thus, the basic structures of these viral genomes are very similar to those of cellular mRNAs and are therefore directly translated after entry into the cell cytoplasm. The ability to be immediately translated by the cellular machinery is essential for replication of the genome, since eukaryotic cells are unable to make new RNA copies from an RNA template. Let us take HCV as an example and look at what happens after the viral genome has been released in the cytoplasm.

After the HCV genome is released in the cytoplasm, the 5′-IRES directs the viral genome to ribosomes (Fig. 5). After binding, translation of the coding region is initiated and a large precursor polyprotein corresponding to the complete coding sequence is synthesized. The first part of the polyprotein, containing the viral structural proteins, is cleaved by host cell proteases, causing release of the individual viral proteins (Fig. 5). The remaining part of the polyprotein, containing the viral nonstructural proteins, is cleaved by a viral protease. This releases the viral RNA-dependent RNA polymerase required for the replication of the RNA genome. To summarize, the capsid containing the HCV genome disassembles in the cytoplasm, the viral genome is translated, and the individual proteins are released, and now replication of the RNA genome can take place (Fig. 6).

The second example is hepatitis B virus (HBV), a small enveloped virus with a circular partially double-stranded DNA genome and a member of the *Hepadnaviridae*. The capsid containing the DNA genome is transported to the nucleus, and the capsid dissociates at the nuclear membrane. The HBV DNA genome is released into the cell nucleus, and transcription of the genome is initiated (Fig. 7). The viral RNAs are transported to the

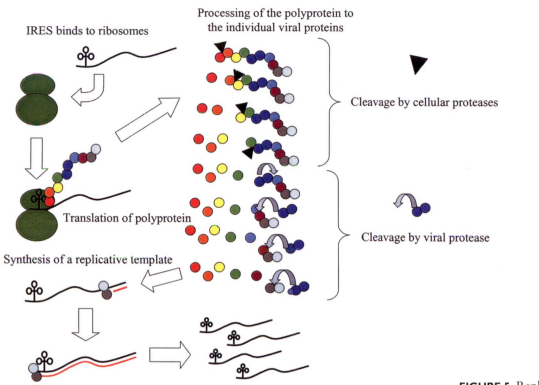

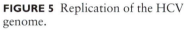

IRES binds to ribosomes

Processing of the polyprotein to the individual viral proteins

Cleavage by cellular proteases

Translation of polyprotein

Cleavage by viral protease

Synthesis of a replicative template

Synthesis of new genomes on the replicative template

FIGURE 5 Replication of the HCV genome.

FIGURE 6 Replication of a viral genome in the cytoplasm.

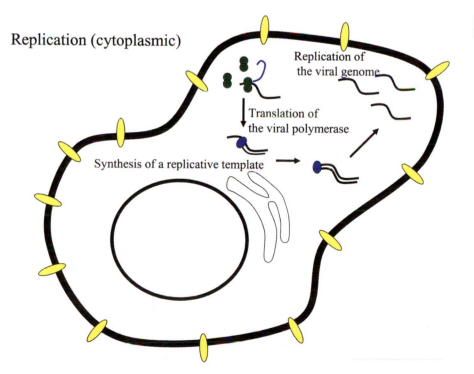

Replication (cytoplasmic)

Replication of the viral genome

Translation of the viral polymerase

Synthesis of a replicative template

Replication (nuclear)

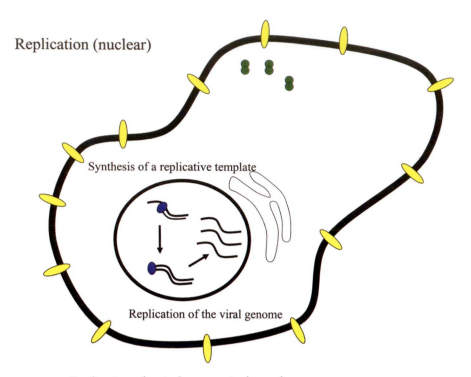

FIGURE 7 Replication of a viral genome in the nucleus.

cytoplasm for synthesis of viral proteins or retained in the nucleus to be used as the RNA pregenome. The genome is replicated from the RNA pregenome by use of the viral DNA polymerase. This forms a DNA-RNA hybrid genome that together with the viral polymerase is encapsidated into new viral capsids. Inside the capsid, the polymerase completes the final steps of the replication by replacing the RNA strand with a DNA strand to form the partially double-stranded DNA genome of HBV.

Before, after, or simultaneous with replication of the viral genome, synthesis of viral proteins occurs. Translation and protein processing are performed by the cellular machinery. Some viruses encode their own proteases that participate in the processing of the viral proteins. Transcription of viral DNA genomes is initiated by the binding of host cell transcription factors to the promoter sequences within the viral genome. The mRNA transcripts are transported from the nucleus into the cytoplasm followed by translation (Fig. 8). The viral proteins are transported to different cellular compartments using the same types of localization sequences as present in normal cellular proteins.

At this stage, all components needed to build new viral particles have been generated. The process of building the new viral particles is termed assembly (Fig. 9). The different viral proteins have specific characteristics. For example, the nucleocapsid proteins contain DNA- or RNA-binding domains by which the proteins assemble around the viral genome to form a mature nucleocapsid (Fig. 9). Viral envelope proteins contain membrane-binding domains, which target these proteins to cellular membranes. The envelope proteins form clusters within the cell membrane that attract the mature nucleocapsids or the precursors of the capsid proteins.

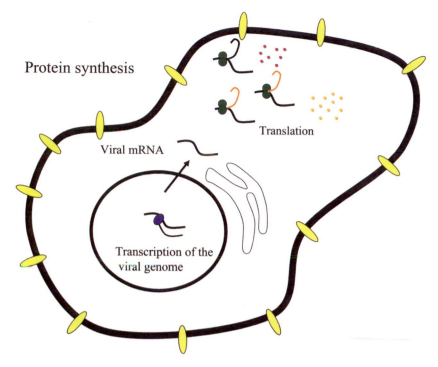

Protein synthesis

Translation

Viral mRNA

Transcription of the
viral genome

FIGURE 8 Synthesis of viral proteins.

FIGURE 9 Assembly of viral particles.

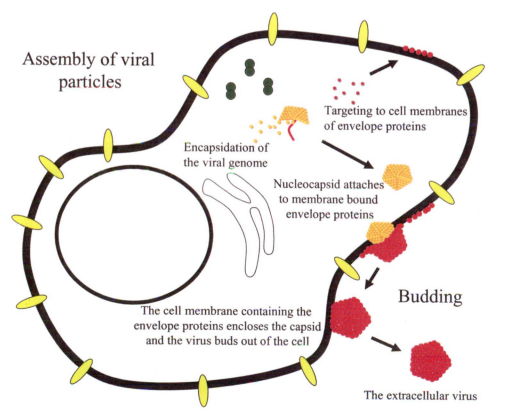

Assembly of viral
particles

Targeting to cell membranes
of envelope proteins

Encapsidation of
the viral genome

Nucleocapsid attaches
to membrane bound
envelope proteins

Budding

The cell membrane containing the
envelope proteins encloses the capsid
and the virus buds out of the cell

The extracellular virus

How does the virus leave the infected cell? There are two major pathways by which viruses leave cells, either by replicating and building new virus particles until the cell ruptures by lysis (lytic replication cycle) or by leaving the cell by nonlytic pathways (nonlytic replication cycle). Nonenveloped viruses often leave the infected cell through cell lysis, but this is not always the case. Some can leave the infected cell by exocytosis and the cell is not killed immediately.

Enveloped viruses leave the cell by a process termed budding. Budding is really the reverse form of entry by fusion described in Fig. 3a. This means that the viral nucleocapsid buds through a cellular membrane (usually the outer membrane but can be an intracellular membrane), allowing the viral nucleocapsid to be enclosed by a lipid envelope (Fig. 9). A high level of replication of an enveloped virus may eventually kill the cell, since the cell is not able to synthesize the membrane components rapidly enough to prevent cell shrinkage and death.

Once the virus leaves the cell and matures, the viral replication cycle is completed and new mature extracellular viruses, or virions, can now infect new cells.

VIRUS TAXONOMY

To better understand the relationships between organisms, humans have a tendency to arrange different life forms into groups where each group consists of similar or closely related life forms. This is also true for viruses. There are many ways by which viruses can be grouped into different families. Presently, the most important criteria to classify viruses are based on the structure and composition of the viral genome. As previously mentioned, there are five major classes of viral genomes; this is the first and most simple way to classify a virus. During the past 2 decades, techniques in molecular biology have been developed that have revolutionized our understanding of genes and genomes. Thus, as soon as a new virus is discovered, the first thing to do is to look at the viral genome. The sequence of the viral nucleic acids can tell us if it is similar to any known virus family. If so, we may rapidly understand the possible mechanisms of transmission and possible host range of the virus, based on what is already known about other members of the same family. The sequence of the virus also reveals the organization of the viral genome, i.e., which proteins the virus encodes, which regulatory elements are present, and so on. Thus, by characterizing the viral genome at the nucleotide sequence level, we can predict much about the properties of the virus without having to see or grow the virus. A simplified scheme for the taxonomy of human viruses is given in Fig. 10.

The identification of a viral genome can be problematic. To give an example of how challenging it can be to isolate a virus and how molecular technology can accelerate the process, the recently discovered GBV-C is discussed. In 1995 a group of scientists at Abbott Laboratories in Chicago, Ill., was successful in isolating a viral genome from a small monkey, a tamarin, which had been experimentally infected by human serum. The human serum derived from a surgeon with the initials G.B., who in the 1960s developed hepatitis due to an unknown agent. The serum from the surgeon had been used to inoculate nonhuman primates since the early 1970s, but no virus had been isolated. By 1995 a new technique called representational difference analysis had been developed. This technique can be described in the following simplified manner. Take a serum sample from a tamarin prior to any experimentation. Next, take another serum sample from the same tamarin after infection by the GB serum at the time point when symptoms of disease are present. Then isolate all genetic material present in the two serum samples. Serum does not normally contain genetic material, but if a virus is present in serum, that is a good source for genetic material. Then mix (hybridize) the genetic material from the samples before and after infection, and digest (destroy) all hybridized genetic material (i.e., present in both samples). Thus, any genetic material only present after infection of the tamarin, such as a virus, can be isolated and characterized. This is basically how two genomes, representing GB viruses A and B (GBV-A and GBV-B), were discovered. However, none of the viruses isolated from the tamarins could be found in human sera. The Abbott group therefore started searching for a third GB-related virus in humans using the sequence knowledge obtained from the tamarin viruses GBV-A and GBV-B. This search led to the discovery of GBV-C. By characterizing the GBV-C genome it was clear that it should belong to the *Flaviviridae* family, to which HCV, a known cause of viral hepatitis, belongs. In addition, the genome of GBV-C was often detected in patients with severe liver disease. Thus, the early data suggested that it was likely that GBV-C, like its close relative HCV, might also cause hepatitis.

However, microbes, including viruses, are present in all humans at varying degrees of frequency. Thus, there remained a chance that the genetic material originally isolated from an infected human may not be the genome of the virus that originally caused the symptoms of disease. Instead, the isolate may be a virus that is rather common to humans and that by chance was present in the infected human at the time of testing. It now appears that this is possibly what actually occurred in the case of GBV-C. The Abbott scientists in all discovered three GB viruses, GBV-A, GBV-B, and GBV-C. GBV-A and GBV-B have so far been found only in various monkey species, whereas GBV-C has been found in humans. However, after years of intensive research it does not seem that GBV-C causes any disease in humans. GBV-C most likely infects the human liver, but despite this, it seems rather harmless. These studies have resulted in the worldwide decision not to test for GBV-C at blood banks. We now know that around 3% of the population worldwide is infected by GBV-C. Thus, if GBV-C caused any major disease after blood transfusion, it would be evident by now.

In this particular example the genome of a new virus was discovered, but we still do not know whether it causes any disease. We now know that the first studies that showed that GBV-C was present in patients with hepatitis turned out to be an association without importance to the disease. Extensive research demonstrated that the reason for this association was that the virus was common to the general human population. Thus, anyone who received a lot of blood or blood products was, or actually still is, likely to become infected by GBV-C as a consequence of the therapy. Hence, the relation to hepatitis was accidental.

You could now call GBV-C a virus looking for a disease. The GBV story highlights how new viruses are often discovered today and contrasts with how

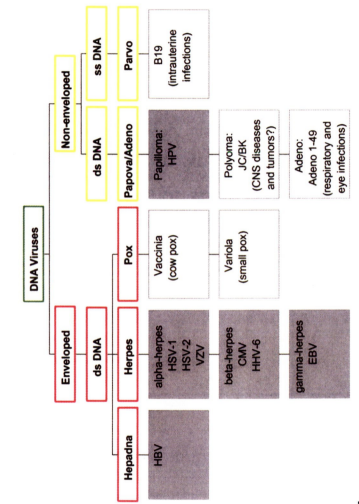

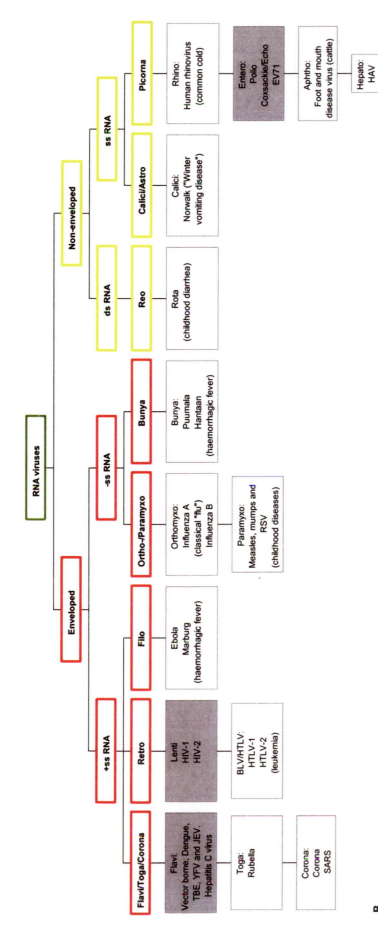

FIGURE 10 A simplified taxonomy of the most common and well-known human viruses. Viral families or genera that contain one or more viruses that can be related to oral virology are in gray boxes. (A) DNA viruses; (B) RNA viruses.

B

they have been discovered historically. A disease was first recognized, and then a virus could be identified from patients with the disease by trying to grow the virus in different cell lines. Then the viral genome could be characterized. A perfect example of this traditional way of discovering viruses is the discovery of human immunodeficiency virus type 1 (HIV-1), which is described later.

Other characteristics widely used in viral taxonomy are the basic shape and structure of the virus particle. As previously mentioned, some viruses have a lipid envelope and some do not. The basic structure of the nucleocapsid can be either icosahedral (Fig. 1b) or helical (spiral shaped). The appearance of the virus in electron microscopy allows morphological characterization of the size and shape of the virus particle.

Different viruses give different appearances (cytopathic effects) when grown in tissue culture. As described in the viral life cycle, the virus can leave the cell either by budding or by lysing the infected cell. Lysis of infected cells can be determined by using ordinary light microscopy to view the destruction of cells. Budding is not visible by means other than electron microscopy. However, some viruses cause syncytia (clusters of cells that melt together into a large cell) that are visible under light microscopy.

The array of different viral proteins can also be a useful taxonomic tool. They can be characterized biochemically with respect to their basic properties such as size, composition, and enzymatic functions. Some enzymes are only encoded by the genomes belonging to certain virus families. As an example, the enzyme reverse transcriptase (RT), which has the ability to transcribe DNA from an RNA template, is almost exclusively found among retroviruses. However, a polymerase with reverse transcriptase activity is also found among the *Hepadnaviridae*.

ORAL VIROLOGY: THE VIRUSES

The following text describes viruses with which dental professionals should be familiar. Some of these viruses can cause symptoms affecting tissues in the oral cavity. Others are present in the mouth following replication and release from other tissues and organs. The presence of such viruses in the oral cavity or in the circulation may result in an increased risk of infection for the staff involved in treating the patient. These two criteria make the following viruses relevant to a discussion of oral virology. Viruses that are not discussed in detail include those with a minor relation to pathologies in the oral cavity but with severe pathologies more relevant in the field of general medicine and others that occasionally cause symptoms related to the oral cavity, but that cause major symptoms elsewhere. Examples of these are viruses that cause many childhood infections such as measles, rubella, and mumps. These can be further explored in textbooks dedicated to virology.

VIRUSES THAT CAN CAUSE PATHOLOGIES IN THE ORAL CAVITY

Picornaviridae

One virus family commonly related to oral ulcerations is the *Picornaviridae* family, which contains over 70 viruses. A characteristic of the *Picornaviridae* is a single-stranded RNA genome of positive polarity consisting of around 10,000 bases. The viruses are small (25 nm), nonenveloped, and relatively resistant to environmental factors, and are easily transmitted from host to host by several routes. The most famous members of the *Picornaviridae* family are the polioviruses. Fortunately, due to mass vaccination schemes, we may be close to the eradication of the polioviruses. Picornaviruses cause a wide spectrum of diseases ranging from subclinical or mild respiratory disease, to myocarditis, encephalitis, or meningitis.

A good example of the *Picornaviridae* is hepatitis A virus (HAV), which does not cause any oral pathologies, in that it is highly contagious. During the acute disease, HAV is excreted in large amounts in the feces. Thus, in areas of the world where the purity of the drinking water is suboptimal, waterborne HAV is a widespread childhood disease.

Some picornaviruses have been related to pathologies in the oral mucosa. Hand-foot-and-mouth disease is caused by members of the *Enterovirus* genus, coxsackie A virus 16 and enterovirus 71. These viruses are transmitted by contact and cause blisters in the mouth (Fig. 11) and on the hands and feet of small children. This disease is, in general, harmless. However, there have been reports of hand-foot-and-mouth diseases caused by enterovirus 71 with neurological complications or a fatal outcome. When hand-foot-and-mouth disease is discussed, it is important to mention the similar infection, foot-and-mouth disease, seen in cattle. The latter disease is caused by a picornavirus named foot-and-mouth disease virus. This virus cannot infect humans, and thus the veterinary disease, although of great importance, is not the same as hand-foot-and-mouth disease seen in humans.

A rather common lesion or ulceration seen in the oral mucosa is the aphthous lesion. These lesions seem to recur at varying intervals in different subjects and can be painful. It has been proposed that there may be a relationship between aphthous lesions and picornaviruses. However, despite numerous attempts, there are only a few reports of picornaviruses actually being isolated from such lesions. Thus, a causal relationship between picornaviruses and aphthous lesions has not been established.

Human Herpesviruses

The family *Herpesviridae* contains eight known human pathogens. The first five discovered members were given names describing either the appearance in tissue culture or the names of the discoverers. Later, a new taxonomy was agreed on; in the new taxonomy, all new members were given the name human herpesvirus followed by a number based on the order of discovery.

CHARACTERISTICS OF THE *HERPESVIRIDAE* FAMILY

Herpesviruses are large viruses (150 to 200 nm) with large double-stranded DNA genomes. The genomes vary from 150 kb to around 220 kb in size. The genome is surrounded by an icosahedral nucleocapsid. Herpesviruses leave the infected cell by budding through a cellular membrane, whereupon the mature virion obtains an outer lipid envelope. The lipid envelope contains glycoproteins encoded by the genome and membrane proteins derived from the host cell. Subsequently, when the virus infects a new cell, it enters the cell by membrane fusion.

A feature of all members of the *Herpesviridae* is that they encode several enzymes that participate in nucleic acid metabolism. The best characterized of these enzymes is thymidine kinase. This enzyme can

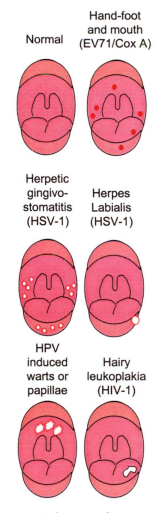

FIGURE 11 Schematic drawings of the clinical appearance of viral infections in the oral cavity (from top in each schematic: upper lips, palate, tongue, and lower lips). Red spots indicate ulcerations, and white spots with a red border indicate blisters.

phosphorylate nucleotides, resulting in incorporation into the genome. The discovery of viral thymidine kinase led to the development of a number of antiviral compounds that target this enzyme. The mechanism of action of these compounds is described later in the section on antiviral therapies.

HERPES SIMPLEX VIRUSES 1 AND 2 (HUMAN HERPESVIRUSES 1 AND 2)

Virology

Herpes simplex viruses 1 and 2 (HSV-1 and -2) are probably the most well-known human herpesviruses. The genomes are around 150 kb long. HSV-1 is a common virus, and about 50% of the population worldwide is infected. HSV-2 is less common and approximately 5% of the population worldwide is infected. The primary target cells for HSV-1 and -2 are epithelial cells. A feature common to all herpesviruses is the ability to establish latency. Latency means that the cell is infected, but for long periods the virus does not replicate. Latency mainly occurs at privileged sites, such as in nerve cells or neurons. Following infection of the primary target cell, one or more sensory neurons innervating the target cell area become infected. The virus is transported along the axon, and latency is established in the nerve cell nucleus. During latency, the genome is maintained episomally (separate from the chromosome) with a low level of transcription from the genome. The advantage of latency to the virus is that it effectively evades the host immune response. Reactivation of latent virus, often brought on by some sort of stress, is also the basis for the clinical appearance of the recurrent infection.

Epidemiology and clinical features

HSV-1 and HSV-2 infections have a worldwide distribution. HSV-1 is mainly transmitted in early childhood by contact with saliva from an infected person. If acquired later in life, viral transmission often occurs through kisses or contact with contaminated saliva or skin surfaces. The primary HSV-1 infection is often asymptomatic but can in some cases cause pharyngitis, tonsillitis, or herpetic gingivostomatitis. Stomatitis often appears as small white blisters or ulcerations that are present bilaterally in the epithelium of the oral mucosa (Fig. 11). The primary infections heal within 2 to 3 weeks. After the primary infection, HSV-1 is transported retrograde along the neural axons and lies latent in sensory nerve cells that innervate the oral cavity. These nerve cells often stem from one of the trigeminal ganglia and, subsequently, during reactivation the virus is transported along the axon and infects the epithelial cells present at the nerve end. Replication takes place in the local epithelial cells and a visible lesion always appears unilaterally at the same site (Fig. 11). Recurrences often appear two to four times per year. Before each episode, the patient can experience what are called prodromal symptoms, which include itching and discomfort at the involved area. When the blisters appear, they heal within a week. Thus, clinical symptoms of a primary HSV-1 infection can involve the whole oral cavity, whereas the clinical symptoms during a reactivated HSV-1 infection are unilateral. The mechanisms responsible for reactivation are not fully understood, although different factors have been associated with reactivation, such as exposure to UV light, other infections, or temporary immune suppression. HSV infections in the facial region can in rare cases cause paralysis of the facial nerve, called Bell's palsy.

HSV-2 is a sexually transmitted disease (STD), and symptoms occur around the genital tract. A primary HSV-2 infection presents as blisters filled with liquid in, on, or around the genital organs. Like symptoms of HSV-1, HSV-2 symptoms can recur. During recurrences, the viral infection is effectively transmitted. Because of changing sexual habits, oral HSV-2 infections are becoming more common.

Both HSV-1 and HSV-2 infections can cause severe complications such as encephalitis, which can be fatal. This is rare, however, and these complications occur mainly in patients with a suppressed immune system caused either by therapy (immune suppression after transplantation) or by another infection, such as HIV-1 infection.

The presence of HSV-1 or -2 is determined by detecting either the virus or viral genome in scrapings from blisters or lesions. The virus is detected either directly by immunohistochemistry or by first culturing the virus in cell lines. The viral genome can be detected in cells present in various body fluids or in other types of samples by PCR. Detection of specific immunoglobulin M (IgM) antibodies is sometimes used as a diagnostic tool. There is, however, a delay in the appearance of antibodies; hence direct detection of the virus or the genome is preferred. The infections can be treated with an antiviral compound, which is discussed in detail below.

VARICELLA-ZOSTER VIRUS (HUMAN HERPESVIRUS 3)

Virology

Varicella-zoster virus (VZV) is a close relative of HSV-1 and -2. The genome of VZV is around 120 kb long. Like all members of the *Herpesviridae*, VZV has an icosahedral capsid and a lipid envelope. VZV also latently infects sensory neurons. VZV is highly contagious and is transmitted through aerosols and by direct contact.

Epidemiology and clinical features

VZV causes a childhood disease that occurs worldwide. Primary VZV infection causes the disease known as varicella, or chicken pox. The incubation period lasts for 2 to 3 weeks, when the person is highly infectious. During the incubation period the virus first replicates in the regional lymph nodes of the throat, followed by infection and replication in the liver and spleen. Then a second viremia (virus particles in the bloodstream) spreads the virus to the skin and mucous membranes. The first symptoms to appear are flulike, with fever and respiratory tract involvement. During this period the infected person is highly contagious. A few days later, the typical cutaneous symptoms appear in the form of an exanthema that develops into blisters. The blisters develop during the first week and then slowly dry out. Clearance of the blisters is often accompanied by an irritating itch. The symptomatic period usually lasts for 1 to 2 weeks, during which latency of VZV in a spinal ganglion is established. Occasionally blisters in the oral mucosa are seen during the acute phase of the disease.

Reactivation of VZV is termed herpes zoster, or shingles. The reactivation, like that of HSV-1, is characterized by the appearance of blisters along the area innervated by one nerve, a dermatome, in which the virus has established a latent infection. The recurrences do not appear as often as for HSV, but the symptoms are more severe. A very painful zoster neuralgia can appear. The location is usually on the trunk but can also be oral or ocular.

VZV is often diagnosed clinically. However, as with HSV, the presence of VZV can be detected by immunohistochemistry, tissue culture, or PCR.

CYTOMEGALOVIRUS (HUMAN HERPESVIRUS 5) AND EPSTEIN-BARR VIRUS (HUMAN HERPESVIRUS 4)

Virology, epidemiology, and clinical features

Cytomegalovirus (CMV) causes a very common infection and around 70% of the world's population are asymptomatic silent carriers of this virus. Most immune-competent subjects who become infected with CMV have asymptomatic infections. If symptoms develop, they are often diffuse and flulike with subfebrile periods. However, a primary CMV infection during the early phase of pregnancy can lead to severe complications for the fetus. The major problem with CMV is reactivation in immune-suppressed patients, in whom the infection can be life-threatening. In transplant recipients and AIDS patients, CMV infection is closely monitored because of the immune suppression.

CMV productively infects several types of lymphocytes, and the reservoir for latent CMV infection seems to be macrophages. These cells are present in most secretions including saliva, and CMV infection can therefore be transmitted by several routes. This may be one reason why CMV has been related to various oral symptoms and diseases where a lymphocyte infiltrate is present. For example, CMV has been detected in periodontal pockets in patients with different forms of periodontitis. However, the CMV present in the periodontal pocket is most likely derived from infected lymphocytes, and there is no conclusive evidence that CMV plays a role in periodontitis. It has also been proposed that CMV can be an infrequent cause of oral mucosal lesions, mainly in patients with virally or chemically induced immune suppression. There are antiviral therapies today, such as ganciclovir, that can be used to treat CMV infection.

Epstein-Barr virus (EBV) is one of the few viruses that have a clear relationship to the development of cancer. Most people become infected with EBV early in childhood and do not develop any symptoms of the primary infection. A primary disease later in life is more likely to be symptomatic, with fever and swollen adenoid glands, also called infectious mononucleosis or kissing disease.

EBV infection is mainly transmitted by saliva but can also be transmitted via blood. The target cell for EBV is the B lymphocyte. In vitro, the transforming properties of EBV are evident, and EBV is widely used to immortalize B cells. Burkitt's lymphoma, which is mainly found in Africa, was the first oncological disease to be associated with EBV. Other oncological diseases with an association with EBV are nasopharyngeal cancer and certain types of lymphomas. No specific antiviral therapy has yet been developed for EBV infections.

Also of note is that EBV has been implicated in the etiology of periodontitis. However, since EBV effectively infects B cells and periodontitis is characterized by a lymphocyte infiltrate, this association may be accidental, and a direct cause-and-effect relationship may not exist.

HUMAN HERPESVIRUSES 6, 7, AND 8

Human herpesvirus 6 (HHV-6), HHV-7, and HHV-8 are three recently discovered human herpesviruses. HHV-6 seems to be a close relative of CMV. HHV-6 infection is very common, and the infection can be transmitted through saliva. HHV-6 causes an early childhood disease known as exanthema subitum, or the sixth disease. Most infections are, however, subclinical. Severe disease as a consequence of primary HHV-6 infection is rare.

HHV-7, which is related to HHV-6 and CMV, was identified in the early 1990s. No unequivocal causal relationship between HHV-7 and any severe human disease has been documented yet. The most common association with disease for HHV-7 seems to be febrile periods in childhood. It is also possible that HHV-7 can cause complications in transplant patients because of immune suppression. HHV-7 can be detected in saliva, and the target cells seem to be $CD4^+$ T cells.

HHV-8 has been found to be the possible cause of the oncological disease Kaposi's sarcoma, a tumor involving the blood vessels in the skin. Kaposi's sarcoma has mainly been observed in Africa and in AIDS patients. HHV-8 seems to be transmitted by saliva and sexually.

Human Papillomaviruses

VIROLOGY

Human papillomaviruses (HPV) are members of the family *Papovaviridae* and are named for their most common clinical symptoms, papillomas and warts. HPV has a double-stranded DNA genome and an icosahedral capsid (55 nm in diameter) and lacks a lipid envelope. There are more than 70 HPV types, some of which constitute the natural viral flora of the skin. The primary target cells for HPV are the epithelial cells in the dermis. HPV has also been associated with human cancer. Two HPV proteins have been found to have oncogenic properties in cell lines, since they are capable of independently transforming cells in vitro.

EPIDEMIOLOGY AND CLINICAL FEATURES

Many HPV types seem to be natural inhabitants of the skin, and have not been associated with any clinical symptoms. The common symptom caused by HPV is warts on the skin, or on the oral or genital mucosa. Most warts caused by HPV are harmless, but a few HPV types have been associated with development of cancer. In particular, HPV type 16 (HPV-16) and HPV-18 have been associated with invasive cervical cancer. HPV-16 has been detected in up to 50% of cervical cancers. However, infection by HPV-16 does not guarantee development of cancer, which complicates various screening measures to prevent development of cervical carcinoma. A seemingly effective HPV vaccine has been tested in humans.

The genital disease associated with HPV is called condyloma. Genital HPV infection is an STD where the primary infection occurs after the sexual debut. Genital HPV infection is most common in those who have many sexual partners. Diagnosis is generally performed by clinical inspection and cytology.

As previously mentioned, HPV can cause warts at many sites. In the oral cavity, some clinical symptoms have been associated with HPV (Fig. 11). Focal epithelial hyperplasia has been associated with HPV-13 and HPV-32, two HPV types that seem to be restricted to the oral cavity. Other forms of oral warts, such as condyloma acuminatum and verruca vulgaris, are associated with infections with genital types of HPV. HPV-16 and HPV-18 have been suggested to be associated with malignancies in the nasopharynx and the oral cavity. However, these correlations are not as clear as that of HPV with cervical carcinoma.

VIRUSES PRESENT IN THE ORAL CAVITY

The following text discusses viruses that are present in the oral cavity but do not, as far as we know, replicate in oral tissues. This is not always a clear distinction, and some of these viruses have been proposed to participate in pathologies found in the oral cavity. However, the major reasons for including these viruses here are that they are present in the oral cavity and that the diseases which they cause in other organs are often life-threatening. Thus, those in the dental profession should be familiar with these infections because the large number of patients treated and the types of procedures performed may increase the risk of becoming infected or transmitting the infection.

Hepatitis B Virus

VIROLOGY

HBV was discovered in the mid-1960s by Baruch S. Blumberg as he was looking for new coagulation factors. He noticed in an immune precipitation assay that a precipitate was formed between wells filled with sera from hemophiliacs and Australian aborigines. He designated this new antigen the Australia antigen. Further studies revealed that the presence of the Australia antigen was related to different forms of hepatitis, in particular to parenterally transmitted hepatitis, also known as "serum" hepatitis. Later on, the virus was observed by electron microscopy and the complete virus particle was named the Dane particle. During the 1970s it became clear that the Australia antigen was the envelope, or surface, protein of a virus that became known as the hepatitis B virus. In 1980 the complete genome of HBV was sequenced, revealing that HBV was the first member of a new family of viruses, the *Hepadnaviridae* (Latin *hepar*, liver; *dna*, DNA genome). The partially double-stranded genome is circular and approximately 3.2 kb long.

The virus has an icosahedral nucleocapsid consisting of 180 to 240 copies of a single protein, the hepatitis B core antigen (HBcAg). The mature capsid contains the partially double-stranded DNA genome and a DNA polymerase. The DNA polymerase of HBV has a unique property; it can synthesize a new DNA strand on an RNA template, thus having reverse transcriptase activity. This enzymatic activity is found only among the *Hepadnaviridae* and *Retroviridae* families.

The nucleocapsid is surrounded by a lipid bilayer into which the three viral envelope proteins have been inserted. These proteins are called the small (S), medium (M), and large (L) form of the hepatitis B surface antigen (HBsAg). The mature extracellular and infectious HBV virion thus contains the viral genome, HBcAg, the viral polymerase, and a lipid layer containing HBsAg.

The small genome is organized in an effective way. The genome encodes seven viral proteins (S-HBsAg, M-HBsAg, L-HBsAg, HBcAg, HBeAg, the polymerase, and the X protein). Theoretically, if only one reading frame within the genome were used, then the entire coding capacity would be approximately 1,070 amino acids. However, to increase the coding capacity the HBV genome has overlapping reading frames. This means that, for example, the same gene segment codes for more than one protein using two or three different reading frames. By this approach the coding capacity of the genome is drastically increased. As a consequence, a mutation at one nucleotide position may affect the sequence of more than one protein. This is most likely the basis for the genetic stability of the HBV genome.

HBV has a rather complicated replication cycle, and not all steps of the cycle are fully understood. In brief, one or more of the HBsAg proteins bind to an unknown receptor on the liver cell, or hepatocyte. The virus is then internalized by cellular endocytosis, the endosome and the viral envelope are disrupted, and the capsid is released in the cytoplasm. The capsid containing the genome disintegrates on the nuclear membrane, causing the genome and the polymerase to be released into the nucleus. The partially double-stranded DNA genome is then converted to a covalently closed circular DNA (cccDNA). Replication of the genome starts with the synthesis of large RNA transcripts from cccDNA. The transcripts are exported to the cytoplasm and used as templates for protein synthesis, except for one, which functions as the pregenome. The pregenome and the viral polymerase are encapsidated by HBcAg in the cytoplasm, and reverse transcription takes place within the capsid. This is distinct from the replication cycle of retroviruses where the reverse transcription occurs in the cell cytoplasm after dissociation of the viral capsid. The viral capsid becomes enveloped by budding through areas of the endoplasmic reticulum membrane containing HBsAg, and the mature virus is secreted into the bloodstream.

The HBV genome encodes five structural proteins, S-, M-, and L-HBsAg, HBcAg, and the polymerase. Two proteins, HBeAg and the X protein, are nonstructural proteins. The functions of these proteins are not fully understood. HBeAg is a protein that is secreted into the bloodstream during periods of high-level viral replication. It has been proposed that HBeAg can pass from the circulation of the infected mother across the placenta to the developing fetus. Thus, if HBeAg is present during the development of the neonatal immune system, HBeAg will be perceived as a self-protein. The child will, therefore, have a selective defect in the T-cell response to HBV. The HBx protein has been proposed to function as a regulator of host cell gene transcription by acting as a transactivator that can turn on various cellular genes.

The HBV genome, or more likely parts thereof, can be integrated into the host cell genome. HBV infection is correlated with the development of liver cancer, or hepatocellular carcinoma (HCC). The mechanisms of HCC development are not understood, but integrated HBV sequences are often found in cancerous tissues.

EPIDEMIOLOGY AND CLINICAL FEATURES
To understand HBV epidemiology, it is important to know the different phases of HBV infection. HBV can cause acute and chronic infections. HBV replication and virion secretion are very effective. During periods of high levels of replication the levels of HBV can reach 10^{10} to 10^{12} virus

particles per milliliter of blood. Under such circumstances 1 μl (10^{-6} liters) of blood contains 10,000 to 1,000,000 infectious virus particles; during this time the infected person is highly contagious. In acute HBV infection, a period of high-level HBV replication can last for up to 2 months but is generally much shorter. In chronic HBV infection, periods of high-level viral replication can last for more than 30 years. Consequently, the major sources for new infections are individuals with chronic HBV infection and high levels of viral replication. Keep in mind that despite the high levels of viral replication, these persons generally do not display any obvious clinical symptoms of the disease.

Age is the most important factor determining whether the outcome of the infection will be acute or chronic. A neonate infected by vertical transmission, meaning transmission from an infected mother to her infant at birth, has a 95% chance of developing a chronic HBV infection. In contrast, an adult with a normal immune system has a 5% chance of developing a chronic infection. Thus, the ability of HBV to establish a chronic infection is to a large extent determined by the maturity and the functionality of the immune system.

HBV has a global distribution and is transmitted through contact with contaminated blood or other human fluids (such as saliva and vaginal and seminal fluids), contaminated blood products, or contaminated medical devices. The prevalence of HBV infection varies greatly in different parts of the world. In developed countries such as those in Europe and North America (where vaccination is readily available), the prevalence of HBV infection in the general population ranges between 0.1 and 1%. In many parts of the world, including Africa, Asia, and South America, prevalence rates range between 1 and 15%. In certain areas of Asia, prevalence rates of up to 20% may occur. The main mode of transmission in Asia is vertical transmission, which, as previously explained, is the most effective means of establishing a chronic HBV infection.

In developed countries, HBV is transmitted mainly through sexual contact and through sharing of contaminated needles and syringes among intravenous drug users (IVDUs). Among IVDUs the incidence of HBV infection ranges from 20 to 50%, depending on the country.

HBV can cause a wide spectrum of clinical symptoms, with the most common being no symptoms at all (a subclinical or asymptomatic infection). The incubation period for acute HBV infection ranges from 2 to 6 months. Often the symptom debut can be pinpointed to a specific day. The classical symptom is icterus, a yellow tone of the skin or the sclera of the eyes, caused by the leakage of bilirubin from damaged liver cells to the circulation. Patients who develop chronic HBV infection generally do not display any symptoms within the first years of infection. Instead, they have a high risk of developing severe liver disease after 5 to 20 years. Such patients also have the highest risk for developing HCC. The clinical symptoms of HBV infection, which reflect the killing of infected hepatocytes, are not caused directly by the virus. Instead, these symptoms are caused by the host immune system trying desperately to kill all the virus-producing factories, i.e., infected hepatocytes.

Today the serological diagnosis of HBV infection is an excellent clinical tool. A single blood sample can be used to readily determine the phase of the infection, namely, acute, chronic replicating (i.e., highly

TABLE 3 Serological markers of HBV infection

Phase (infectivity under normal circumstances)	Marker detected in a serum sample				
	HBsAg	HBeAg/HBV DNA	IgM anti-HBc	IgG anti-HBc	IgG anti-HBs
Acute (highly infectious)	+++	+++	+++	+	+/−
Chronic, replicating (highly infectious)	+++	+++	−	+++	−
Chronic, nonreplicating (not infectious)	+++	−	−	+++	−
Past infection (not infectious)	−	−	−	++	++

infectious), chronic nonreplicating, or cleared (Table 3). The presence of HBsAg in serum always signals that the person is infected by HBV, but it does not indicate the phase of the infection or whether the patient is highly infectious. To determine infectivity, serum samples are tested for the presence of HBeAg or viral DNA. As none of these tests give a 100% reliable result, a better technique is to quantify the level of virus in the serum by quantitative PCR, unfortunately a very expensive technique. To know whether the infection is acute or chronic, the presence of IgM antibodies to HBcAg (IgM anti-HBc) is tested. If they are present, the patient has an acute HBV infection, and if the patient is an adult, the infection is likely to clear within a couple of months. Patients who have cleared HBV infections have no HBsAg in serum, but rather have IgG antibodies to HBsAg (anti-HBs) and anti-HBc. The markers described in Table 3 are those most widely used to diagnose HBV infections.

As a final remark, one could ask whether we ever can clear an HBV infection. The answer is, unfortunately, most likely not, as revealed by some interesting studies. For example, there are patients with serological evidence of cleared HBV infections from 20 years ago who for many years have had no HBsAg in serum. These patients became immune suppressed, and shortly thereafter the HBV infection was reactivated. In addition, similar types of patients who died from accidents had their livers transplanted to HBV-negative recipients. Within a couple of weeks to months after the transplantation, the recipients, who were put on aggressive immune suppressive therapy, developed an HBV infection. It is believed that the immune suppression allows small foci of HBV-infected cells in the transplanted liver to start replicating and spreading. Thus, it appears that once a person is HBV infected, he or she is always HBV infected.

Hepatitis D Virus

Hepatitis D virus (HDV), or hepatitis delta virus, is a satellite virus to HBV. This means that HDV cannot replicate in persons who are not infected by HBV. The reason for this is that HDV uses the envelope from HBV. Hence, HDV is a virus which is composed of the HDV genome and HDV-encoded capsid and the envelope derived from HBV. HDV is mainly spread among IVDUs. Infection by HDV is effectively prevented by HBV vaccination.

Hepatitis C Virus

VIROLOGY

HCV belongs to the *Flaviviridae* family. Thus, HCV is enveloped and has a single, positive-sense RNA strand as the genome. As described above, the HCV genome is targeted to ribosomes by the IRES and directly translated when released from the capsid. Following production of the viral RNA-dependent RNA polymerase, a negative RNA strand is synthesized, which is the template for the synthesis of new viral genomes. Apart from CD81, the cellular receptors for HCV, along with the mechanisms of viral entry and exit, are not known. Much of the life cycle of HCV is also unknown, since no tissue culture system for HCV was available until recently.

A key feature of HCV is the variability of the HCV genome. The molecular basis for this is that the viral RNA polymerase lacks proofreading ability. This means that any incorrect bases that were incorporated during genome synthesis are not removed. The effects of such mutations span the range from being lethal to being beneficial for the virus. If the mutations are beneficial, for example, helping the virus escape the immune system or antiviral compounds, they can be selected for in the next generation of viruses. Certain regions of the genome accumulate mutations. In particular, one of the two envelope proteins has regions that seem to allow a large set of different mutations. It is believed that the main reason for this localized variability is to allow the virus to escape the host immune response. In studies in chimpanzees, it has been shown that immunization with the envelope proteins from one strain does not protect against infection with another HCV strain. From this it is clear that vaccine development to prevent HCV infections will encounter the same problems of strain specificity as for HIV (discussed below).

Like HBV, HCV has a very high replication rate. This, in combination with the high genetic variability, means that a person infected by HCV carries not just a single variant of the virus, but multiple, closely related variants. These variants are termed quasispecies. Again, these viral variants aid in immune avoidance.

By comparing HCV strains from different parts of the world, at least six major variants have been described. The most common variant, genotype 1, accounts for around 50% of all HCV infections worldwide. There are some regional differences in the presence of the different genotypes. For example, genotypes 1, 2, and 3 are the dominating HCV variants in Europe and the United States, whereas genotype 4 is common in Egypt.

EPIDEMIOLOGY AND CLINICAL FEATURES

The incubation period for HCV ranges from 1 to 6 months. HCV shares many of the transmission routes used by HBV, such as contact with contaminated blood and blood products and contaminated medical devices. However, HCV is not transmitted effectively by either sexual or vertical transmission. The reason for this is not known but may be due to the fact that the levels of HCV in the circulation are around 1,000-fold lower than those for HBV. As a consequence, the levels of HCV in secretions outside the bloodstream are generally low. In contrast to HBV, HCV infection is not as dependent on the maturity of the immune system, since over 70% of those infected develop a chronic infection. One reason for this may relate to the extreme genetic variability of the HCV genome. Chronic HCV infection leads to an increased risk for developing HCC. Severe liver disease as a consequence of a chronic HCV infection is a slow process. It often takes more than 20 years from infection to develop a severe liver disease, although alcohol consumption can accelerate the process.

HCV has in fact been proposed to participate in various oral manifestations such as Sjögren's syndrome and lichen planus. Several reports have suggested that HCV genomes can be detected in various oral tissues such as salivary glands. However, these observations are far from conclusive.

HCV is effectively transmitted in hospital settings, such as wards where many patients are given intravenous injections, and where hygienic standards are suboptimal. Hence, HCV can be a nosocomial infection. Several reports have described outbreaks of HCV infections that can be due to the presence of a single HCV-infected patient in the ward. It is believed that HCV infections can be transmitted from patient to patient by hospital staff through the use of multidose vials. This is very important to remember within the dental profession and dental clinics in light of the extensive use and reuse of devices and materials. However, most epidemiological data suggest that HCV transmissions are rare at dental clinics in developed countries. Whether the same is true for developing nations is not known.

The prevalence of HCV infection in developed countries is generally less than 1%. In particular, the screening of blood donors at blood banks for antibodies to HCV has drastically reduced the frequency of transfusion-associated HCV infections. In developing countries, the prevalence of HCV can reach up to 5 to 10% of the general population. There are many reasons for this higher prevalence, including contribution by contaminated blood products and medical devices, suboptimal hygienic standards, and the practice of traditional medicine.

HCV infection is diagnosed by detecting HCV-specific antibodies and the viral RNA genome in a serum sample. There is no specific tool to distinguish acute from chronic infections. In contrast to HBV infection, it is highly likely that HCV infection can be cleared. The rather unstable RNA genome has no ability to integrate into the host cell genome, nor does there appear to be a latent phase. Thus, continuous replication is most likely needed to ensure survival of the virus, which also means that these cells will be recognized by the immune system.

Human Immunodeficiency Virus

VIROLOGY

HIV was discovered in the early 1980s after the observation that several young homosexual men died from what was called an acquired immunodeficiency syndrome (AIDS). The virus was isolated from peripheral blood and was found to grow rapidly in tissue culture using fresh T cells or T-cell lines. HIV-1 mainly infects cells expressing the CD4 cell surface marker, which is present on T helper (Th) cells, macrophages, dendritic cells, and certain types of neural glia cells.

HIV-1 and its close but less pathogenic relative found in West Africa, HIV-2, belong to the genus *Lentivirus* in the *Retroviridae* family. The characteristic feature of this family is that all viruses have the RT enzyme. The life cycle of HIV is rather complex but can be illustrated as follows. The virus binds to its receptor, the CD4 molecule, and to one of its co-receptors, CCR5 or CXCR4. After binding occurs, the viral envelope fuses with the cell membrane and releases the capsid containing two RNA strands and the RT enzyme. The key feature of retroviral infection is that the viral RNA genome has to be reverse transcribed to DNA and integrated into the host genome before replication of the viral genome. In the cell cytoplasm, the RT enzyme converts the RNA strands to double-stranded DNA, which is transported to the cell nucleus and integrated in the host genome. Following integration, replication and transcription of the viral genome occur. Thus, HIV-1 genome replication is then initiated and performed by the cellular machinery, such that all offspring from one integrated proviral genome are identical. New viral proteins are synthesized, and new viral particles are then formed.

An important aspect of the HIV-1 replication cycle is that the RT enzyme lacks proofreading capabilities. Thus, each time an HIV-1 RNA genome is reverse transcribed to DNA, one mutation is introduced. As is the case for HCV, these mutations can be beneficial for the virus and help HIV-1 escape the host immune system or acquire resistance to antiviral compounds. This is the molecular basis for the evolution of viral quasi-species.

The genetic variability of HIV-1 is one of the most problematic features to overcome, both for the immune system and in vaccine development. The high variability of HIV-1 will most likely prevent the development of a universal vaccine against HIV-1, at least with the techniques and strategies that are used today.

EPIDEMIOLOGY AND CLINICAL FEATURES

HIV-1 infection has now spread throughout the world. Mathematical calculations propose that the HIV-1 epidemic may have started in Africa around 1930. Changes in infrastructure and human habits and increased movement of people over great distances are most likely the reasons for the global spread of HIV-1 during the late 1970s and early 1980s. It is generally believed that HIV-1, originating from a chimpanzee virus or a similar ancestor, was introduced to humans from chimpanzees on several occasions throughout history. The earliest evidence for HIV-1 infection of a human has been found in samples derived in the 1950s.

HIV-1 infection is mainly an STD, but it is also effectively transmitted by contaminated blood and blood products and poorly sterilized medical instruments. Many types of medical procedures can transmit HIV-1 infection if the correct precautions are not taken.

There are several phases of HIV-1 infection (Fig. 12). Within 2 to 4 weeks of becoming HIV-1 infected, around 50% of patients develop a clinical syndrome called primary HIV-1 infection (PHI). The symptoms of PHI are often characterized by fever, rash, and swollen lymph nodes. These symptoms last for around 1 to 3 weeks. PHI is diagnosed by the presence of HIV-1 in peripheral blood simultaneous with absence of HIV-1-specific antibodies. If no laboratory testing is performed, PHI can easily be misdiagnosed as some more harmless infection such as mononucleosis. During PHI, a high rate of viral replication and a strong activation of the host immune response occur. Paradoxically, the activation of CD4$^+$ Th cells facilitates the establishment of HIV-1 infection, since HIV-1 replicates very effectively in activated CD4$^+$ T cells. During or after PHI, antibodies to HIV-1 develop and can be easily detected by laboratory tests.

PHI is followed by an asymptomatic phase of the infection that can last for many years, during which the virus continues to replicate at very low levels. A particular group of HIV-1-infected patients has been found

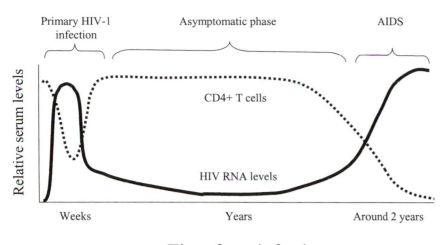

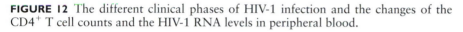

Time from infection

FIGURE 12 The different clinical phases of HIV-1 infection and the changes of the CD4$^+$ T cell counts and the HIV-1 RNA levels in peripheral blood.

to remain asymptomatic without treatment for up to 10 to 15 years, with a generally very low level of HIV-1 replication. These patients have been referred to as long-term asymptomatics, or long-term nonprogressors. The vast majority of HIV-1-infected patients eventually develop a gradually progressing immune deficiency. This can be monitored by laboratory tests that determine the number of CD4$^+$ T cells in the peripheral blood.

As the immune deficiency progresses, patients become susceptible to infections, particularly opportunistic infections (Fig. 12). In an opportunistic infection, the patient develops a symptomatic disease caused by a microbe present in the normal microbiota or by an exogenous organism that is usually nonpathogenic. In the presence of an intact immune system, these microbes are in general unable to cause disease. The onset of opportunistic lung infections such as *Pneumocystis carinii* pneumonia is one of the criteria for diagnosis of AIDS.

If HIV-1 infection is left untreated and allowed to develop into AIDS, it will inevitably lead to death. This rather dark perspective has now been radically changed by the introduction of effective antiviral compounds (discussed below).

As with all other conditions and infections that lead to suppression of immune function, HIV-induced immune deficiency also has oral manifestations. Studies have shown that HIV-1-infected patients with an asymptomatic disease and a functional immune system usually do not differ in their oral health status from uninfected individuals. However, as the immune deficiency progresses, symptoms in the oral cavity start to appear. The most common condition seen in AIDS patients is stomatitis caused by the fungus *Candida albicans*. In fact, oral candidiasis can be used diagnostically to discover otherwise asymptomatic HIV-1 infections.

Another condition associated with HIV-1 infection is necrotizing ulcerative gingivitis (NUG). The clinical appearance of NUG is characterized by swelling and necrosis of the smooth gingival epithelium surrounding the teeth. Early on, it was believed that NUG was caused directly by HIV-1. However, it is now well documented that NUG is a consequence of the severe immune deficiency. In fact, HIV-1-related NUG closely resembles the gingival necrosis seen in patients treated with immune suppressive drugs. NUG is effectively treated by an intense regimen of oral hygiene.

A condition which is almost exclusively seen in AIDS patients is hairy leukoplakia (HLP). The symptoms of HLP are represented by a white hyperplastic epithelium at the side of the tongue (Fig. 11). A substantial amount of data suggests that HLP is caused by EBV, although definite proof has yet to be provided. Importantly, the frequency of HLP seems to be reduced by effective antiviral therapy.

IMMUNE RESPONSES TO VIRUSES

Viruses and the Innate Immune System

INTRACELLULAR RESPONSES

Viruses are obligate intracellular parasites. The host has therefore developed intracellular defense mechanisms and specific cell types to fight the viral infection. Systems are present inside most human cell systems that react to a perceived assault. Such events are often referred to as danger signals, i.e., activating the response mechanisms of the cell. One such danger signal is the presence of double-stranded RNA, which is not normally found in cells. When an RNA virus infects a cell, double-stranded RNA is present during replication of the viral genome. The danger signal generated by double-stranded RNA leads to activation of interferons that in turn activate several antiviral pathways such as Toll-like receptor 3 (TLR3), RNA-dependent protein kinases (PKR), and oligoadenylate synthetase (OAS). Both PKR and OAS can directly interfere in different steps in the viral replication cycle to block the formation of new viral particles. Alternatively, the cascade of intracellular events can cause the cell to undergo programmed cell death, or apoptosis. Both pathways lead to the shutdown of the virus-producing factories. These intracellular antiviral systems are part of innate immunity.

EXTRACELLULAR RESPONSES

Several factors prevent infection by viruses. The most important is of course the first line of defense, i.e., intact skin and mucosal surfaces. If these barriers are broken, there are components of the innate immune system that initially combat most infections. Humoral components associated with innate immunity include various enzymes at mucosal surfaces, the complement system, and natural antibodies. Cell types most commonly associated with innate immunity are phagocytic cells such as macrophages, dendritic cells, and natural killer (NK) cells. The major role for macrophages and dendritic cells is as scavengers that engulf and degrade foreign substances. Through this mechanism they can also signal to cells in the adaptive immune system. The NK cell is of particular importance in the defense against viral infections. The NK-cell response to an infection is almost immediate and results in the release of several antiviral cytokines and cytotoxic substances. Such NK-cell activation most likely assists in the activation of the specific immune system. One well-characterized mechanism for the activation of NK cells is if the infecting virus blocks the surface presentation of major histocompatibility complex (MHC), or human leukocyte antigen (HLA), class I molecules. The

NK cell is actively inhibited by the presence of class I molecules, so if the virus somehow blocks the display of these molecules, the NK cell will be activated and kill that particular cell.

Viruses and the Adaptive Immune System

Three major cell types comprise the adaptive immune system: B cells, CD4$^+$ Th cells, and CD8$^+$ cytotoxic T cells (cytotoxic T lymphocytes [CTLs]). The function of B cells is to produce specific antibodies reactive against the invading virus. If these antibodies can block the attachment of the virus to its cellular receptor, or mediate uptake of the virus by macrophages or dendritic cells, they are called neutralizing antibodies. Thus, B cells and their associated antibodies are mainly restricted to acting directly on viruses or viral protein outside the cell. The production of neutralizing antibodies is most likely of key importance in the protection against viral infections. Thus, a major aim in vaccine development to protect against viral infections is to induce B cells to produce antibodies that can neutralize a particular virus. Most often such neutralizing antibodies are directed against surface-exposed regions of the extracellular virus, i.e., the structures that mediate binding to the cellular receptor. Another important role for B cells in the defense against viral infections is to act as antigen-presenting cells (APC). A B cell can, through its surface-bound immunoglobulins, bind a virus particle or a viral protein. The particle or protein is taken up by the B cell, degraded into short peptides, and presented on the surface using MHC/HLA class II molecules. These peptide-containing class II molecules are then recognized by specific Th cells, which thus become activated. Activated Th cells subsequently induce an antigen-presenting B cell to differentiate into a highly efficient antibody-producing cell, called the plasma cell.

T cells are key mediators of the defense against viral infections. The two types of T cells, Th cells and CTLs, are activated by two distinct, but similar, pathways. As described, the Th cell is activated by short peptides derived from viral proteins that are presented by MHC/HLA class II molecules on the surface of professional APCs such as B cells, macrophages, and different types of dendritic cells. The professional APC takes up the virus or the viral protein and degrades the protein(s) into peptides in the phagosome. These peptides, usually 10 to 15 amino acids long, contain target sequences by which they bind to the MHC/HLA class II molecules present in the phagosome. The peptide-MHC complex is then transported to the surface of the APC and thus becomes accessible to the Th cell. The T-cell receptor (TCR) of a Th cell specific for that particular viral peptide will recognize the peptide in the context of the MHC/HLA class II molecule on the surface of the APC. The TCR binds to the class II-bound peptide in a manner by which a number of surface molecules of the APC bind to surface molecules of the Th cell. This leads to activation signals in the Th cells whereby the Th cell becomes activated and starts to produce factors called cytokines. Some of these factors, such as interleukin-2, will induce cell division of the specific Th cell, leading to a clonal expansion, i.e., multiplication of that particular antiviral Th cell. Other factors, such as interferon-gamma, can directly activate PKR and OAS to start the antiviral cascades in the virus-infected cells nearby, thus blocking virus replication. The key role for Th cells is, however, to support the maturation and differentiation of specific B cells and CTLs. Some of the activated antiviral Th cells will differentiate into long-lived memory cells. These cells are partly responsible for the protection against reinfection with the same virus that is often seen. If the same virus is encountered a second time, let's say a few years later, the memory B and T cells are rapidly activated and will clear the infection before it establishes and begins to cause symptoms.

B cells and Th cells participate equally well in the immune response against bacterial and viral infections. In contrast, the activity of CTLs is exclusively directed against intracellular pathogens. After the virus has entered the cell, and replication and synthesis of viral proteins have started, another intracellular antiviral event takes place (Fig. 13). Most viral proteins synthesized in the infected cell are used to build new viral particles or perform important functions in the viral life cycle. However, some viral proteins are degraded within the proteosome into peptides, and shuttled by a peptide transporter system through the endoplasmic reticulum membrane, to associate with MHC/HLA class I molecules. Class I molecules containing viral peptides are transported to the surface of the infected cell where they can be recognized by specific CTLs. The TCR of the CTL will bind to the class I-peptide complex, which activates the CTL. After activation, one cytotoxic mechanism of CTL is the production of a protein complex known as the perforin complex, which punches a number of holes in the cell membrane of the infected cell. This leads to the killing of the virus-infected cell and thus to destruction of one of the viral factories.

FIGURE 13 Mechanism of recognition of a virus-infected cell by the MHC/HLA class I antigen-presenting pathway.

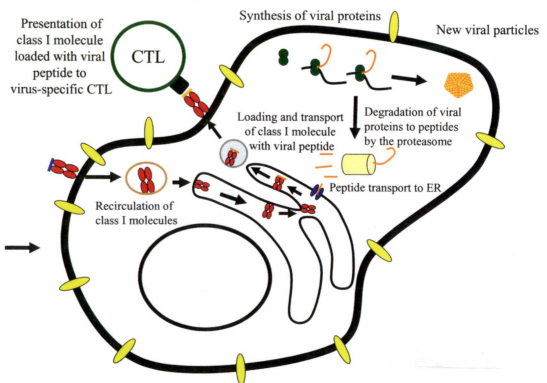

When all of these innate and adaptive immune system effectors are working perfectly, the infected host generally clears the viral infection. However, several viruses are able to establish chronic infections and remain in the host for extended periods. Exactly how viruses are able to establish chronic infections is largely unknown, but mechanisms that may be widely utilized have been identified. Strategies include blocking the activation of the host immune response or avoiding an activated immune response. The following text discusses three rather well-known strategies used by viruses to escape the host immune system.

1. Immune escape by inhibiting antigen presentation. The best-known example of inhibition of antigen presentation has been found among the *Herpesviridae*. For example, CMV produces four proteins called unique short region proteins that down-regulate the surface expression of MHC/HLA class I molecules on CMV-infected cells. Thus, no peptides representing the viral proteins produced by the infected cell are presented by class I molecules. Subsequently, there is no target for CTLs to recognize on the infected cell. One may ask, What about the NK cells that become activated by the absence of class I molecules? Correct, but CMV has a response to that and produces a homologue of HLA class I molecules that inhibits the activation of the NK cell. Thus, CMV effectively escapes the host immune system by blocking antigen presentation.

2. Immune escape by genetic variations in the viral genome. This is probably one of the better-known ways by which viruses escape the immune system. Both B and T cells specifically recognize viral proteins by recognizing regions of amino acid sequence (epitopes). Thus, if the virus accumulates mutations within the epitopes that are recognized by the B or T cells, the virus will be resistant to existing neutralizing antibodies and CTLs. Eventually new specific B cells or CTLs are generated to the new sequence, but at that time a different mutation may be introduced in the genome, so these cells are only antiviral for a short period. The best-known examples of viruses that use this strategy are HIV-1 and HCV.

3. Immune escape by using decoys or induction of immunological tolerance. The third way for viruses to avoid the host immune system is to produce viral proteins that keep the immune system busy or to produce proteins that reduce the activity of the antiviral immune response. A virus that actively pursues both these strategies is HBV. During HBV infection the infected hepatocytes produce and secrete into the circulation a large excess of HBsAg. These amounts are much more than needed for the synthesis of new viral particles. The excess HBsAg proteins serve two functions. First, they bind (or block) host antibodies directed against HBsAg, preventing these antibodies from neutralizing infectious virus. This is the decoy function of HBsAg. Second, the constant presence of high levels of HBsAg in the circulation leads to inactivation of HBsAg-specific T cells. This approach thus leads to the induction of an immune-tolerant state in the virus-specific T cells and they are unable to fight the infection.

As mentioned above, another HBV protein called HBeAg is also active in inhibiting the T-cell response to HBV. A proposed mode of action is that HBeAg passes through the placenta of the infected mother and enters the circulation of the fetus. If HBeAg is present during development of the fetal immune system, it is not recognized as a foreign antigen, so T cells specific for HBeAg are deleted, since they are regarded as reactive toward a self-protein. When the infant is infected by the mother's HBV strain at birth, a selective T-cell defect is present in the response to HBcAg and HBeAg (partly encoded by overlapping genes of the HBV genome). Thus, the newborn infant is unable to mount an effective immune response against HBV and the infant can become chronically infected. This is supported by the observation that newborns of mothers infected by a mutant variant of HBV that is unable to produce HBeAg more often develop a severe liver disease that leads to clearance of the infection. Thus, the function of HBeAg is to induce immunological tolerance to both HBeAg and HBcAg.

ANTIVIRAL VACCINES AND THERAPIES

The History of Viral Vaccines

The first recognized vaccine to be developed in the Western world was actually a viral vaccine. In the 1790s, Edward Jenner realized that women who milked cows (milkmaids) were resistant to infection with smallpox (variola). He noted a folk belief that the milkmaids often had blisters on their hands and developed a mild disease. He therefore concluded that these blisters might contain something that protected them from smallpox. He proceeded to isolate the liquid from the blisters from the women's hands and used it to inoculate a young boy. The boy was then exposed to smallpox and was found to be resistant to smallpox infection. This was the first step in the development of the smallpox vaccine.

The basis for the protection was that the milkmaids had been inoculated by a virus, closely related to smallpox virus, that is known as cowpox virus or vaccinia virus (*vacca* is Latin for cow). Vaccinia virus is able to infect human cells but causes only a mild disease. However, the replication of vaccinia virus in human cells leads to the activation of B and T cells that also react with the vaccinia virus proteins. Since vaccinia and variola viruses are closely related, the sequences of vaccinia and variola virus proteins are also quite similar. Consequently, most of the B and T cells that recognize vaccinia virus proteins also recognize the proteins from variola virus. Thus, a previous exposure to vaccinia virus primes an immune response that is then protective against variola virus. These findings started the human vaccine era as we know it today.

We have now, some 200 years later, been able to eradicate smallpox infections in humans by using the cowpox vaccine. How was this possible? Four very important criteria were fulfilled.

1. Humans were the only host for variola. If humans are the only reservoir for a virus, then vaccination of all humans will effectively eradicate the virus, since no other susceptible host is available.
2. Variola virus only caused acute infections. Variola virus caused an acute infection that led either to the death of the host or to a

complete clearance of the infection. Thus, when the infection was over, the host was either dead or resistant to reinfection. If a virus causes both acute and chronic infections, or there are asymptomatic carriers, then there will be reservoirs of infected hosts for a long time. If the vaccine is not 100% effective, then there will always be a small number of subjects who carry the virus.

3. The cowpox vaccine was effective, inexpensive, and easy to produce, allowing mass vaccination. The cowpox vaccine was quite easy to produce in large quantities and easy to administer. Almost everyone who received the vaccine developed an immune response that protected against infection with variola virus. Thus, those who were not effectively vaccinated could be infected by variola virus and either died or became immune to reinfection. This was the perfect setting to eradicate variola.

4. Smallpox virus has a stable genome. The smallpox virus genome does not vary. The genome does not differ substantially regardless of where in the world it is isolated. Thus, one single vaccine could be used globally to induce protective immune responses.

Smallpox was proclaimed eradicated by the World Health Organization in 1980, around 200 years after Jenner performed the first vaccination. Small amounts of the virus have been kept in well-guarded facilities in the United States and in the former Soviet Union. These stocks remain in case a new smallpox epidemic should occur. Whether we should destroy these virus stores has been widely debated. If the reservoir of smallpox virus were to fall into the wrong hands, this would constitute a serious threat of bioterrorism.

Antiviral Immunoglobulin Preparations and Vaccines

Viral infections can be prevented by either passive or active immunization. Passive immunization means the transfer or injection of immune components, in general immunoglobulins (antibodies) that in the host can protect against one or more infections. The disadvantage with passive immunization is that no immunological memory develops. Thus, if protection is to be maintained, the antibody supply needs to be restored by a new injection every 3 to 6 months. Today, immunoglobulin preparations are available for many diseases, including hepatitis A, hepatitis B, and rabies.

Active immunization introduces an inactivated form, or parts, of the virus so that the host actively develops immunity to the viral components. By this approach, an immunological memory is generated. This is the same approach used by Jenner, who coined the term vaccination, which was later used by Louis Pasteur (in honor of Jenner's work) to describe immunization against any infection.

Viral vaccines can be divided into different groups depending on how the vaccine is produced. The traditional way of making a viral vaccine is to use the whole viral particle of a nonpathogenic virus strain (attenuated vaccine) or to kill the pathogenic virus and use it as the vaccine (inactivated vaccine). Examples of attenuated whole virus vaccines are the smallpox vaccine (a nonpathogenic vaccinia virus strain), the orally administered attenuated poliovirus vaccine developed by Albert Sabin, and the combined measles, mumps, and rubella vaccine. Examples of inactivated whole virus vaccines are the injectable polio vaccine developed by Jonas Salk, the recent HAV vaccine, and the original plasma-derived HBV vaccine.

As shown in Table 4, there is great variability in the effectiveness of the different forms of vaccines in how they activate the host immune response. The most potent vaccines to date are the attenuated whole virus vaccines, as they allow a low level of viral replication. This means that the very potent danger signals are activated, which helps stimulate the immune response. In addition, since viral replication occurs, there is effective priming of CTLs. So, why are not all vaccines produced in this way? The answer is simple: either it is too dangerous (risk for disease) or it is not possible to accomplish. Reasons why it cannot be achieved include the inability to grow the virus in cell culture or to isolate sufficient amounts of the virus from infected individuals or animals. If the virus can be grown in different cell culture systems, but there is a risk that the attenuated virus may cause disease, the virus can be inactivated. This means that the virus present in the vaccine is unable to infect and replicate, in other words, is dead (assuming that a virus can be called a living organism in the first place). This is achieved by different chemical compounds, such as formalin, or by different forms of irradiation. Unfortunately, these types of vaccines do not prime as broad and long-lived immune responses as do the attenuated vaccines, although they are generally very safe.

Techniques developed during the past 20 years have enabled the production of vaccines by recombinant DNA technology. By this process, the gene for one or more viral proteins can be put into bacteria, which then produce large amounts of the viral protein. The protein is then purified and used as the vaccine. The first human vaccine produced in such a way was the HBV vaccine. The previous plasma-derived HBV vaccine was produced by purifying HBsAg (and virus particles) from blood plasma of HBV-infected individuals. The purified vaccine was then extensively inactivated. The plasma-derived HBV vaccine was highly effective, and no cases of hepatitis have ever resulted from vaccination. However, since human plasma may contain unknown, deleterious agents, such as prions, the possibility of a risk of transmitting other agents remained. Subsequently, a new vaccine was developed by using a recombinant protein.

Synthetic peptides have been used in several clinical trials, but no commercial human vaccine has yet been introduced. The major problem with peptides is that they are not always immunogenic in everyone due to immune system heterogeneity.

TABLE 4 Types of viral vaccines and the immune responses they prime

Vaccine type	Immune responses primed[a]		
	B cells (antibodies)	Th cells	CTLs
Whole virus, attenuated	+++	+++	+++
Whole virus, inactivated	++	++	−
Subcomponent	++	++	−
Peptides	+	+	+/−
Genetic vaccine	+	+	+++

[a]The effectiveness by which different cell populations are activated ranges from not at all (−) to highly activated (+++).

A new type of vaccine is a group called genetic vaccines. In a genetic vaccine, a viral gene is introduced into a modified bacterial plasmid or a modified apathogenic virus, for example, vaccinia virus, adenovirus, or Semliki Forest virus. The plasmid, or the viral vector, contains a eukaryotic promoter, which allows expression of the viral gene if the plasmid is introduced into a human cell. To explain the process, let us use plasmid DNA as an example. The plasmid DNA is purified and injected into the host to be vaccinated. Some of the plasmid is taken up by the host cells and is transported into the nucleus. In the nucleus, the eukaryotic promoter of the plasmid is activated, mRNA corresponding to the viral protein is produced, and viral proteins are generated in the cytoplasm of the cell. In this way, only the gene for the viral protein is injected and the host cells produce the viral protein themselves. This mimics the production of viral proteins during natural infection, and it has been found highly effective when priming of CTLs is desired. However, there are still many hurdles to overcome before DNA-based or other genetic vaccines become widely used.

Antiviral Compounds and Therapies

During the past 15 years, great progress has been made in the ability to treat viral infections. The major problem associated with the development of antiviral compounds is that the virus is an intracellular parasite and uses the host cell machinery for many steps in its life cycle. Thus, many compounds that are antiviral are also toxic for human cells. Despite this, several strategies have been used to block steps in the viral life cycle with compounds that have a higher specificity for viral enzymes. A classical example of an antiviral compound is the drug acyclovir, which is widely used to treat infections caused by HSV.

Acyclovir uses our knowledge about the HSV life cycle to act specifically against HSV. Acyclovir is what is known as a nucleoside analogue. It is very similar to thymidine, used in normal DNA synthesis, but lacks an active hydroxy group in the 3'-end of the molecule. However, to be selective for HSV-infected cells, the compound is nonphosphorylated and needs to undergo phosphorylation before it can be incorporated into the DNA strand (Fig. 14). Acyclovir is inefficiently phosphorylated by cellular kinases but is very effectively phosphorylated by the kinase (a thymidine kinase) encoded by HSV. When acyclovir is phosphorylated by HSV-thymidine kinase, acyclovir becomes incorporated into the viral genome. Since acyclovir lacks the 3'-OH group, no more bases can be added to the new DNA strand and the replication is terminated. This explains the specificity of acyclovir for HSV-infected cells, since these are the only cells that can activate the substance.

Since the development of acyclovir, several similar substances that are active against different viruses and different viral enzymes have been developed. In particular, the fight against HIV-1 has generated many new antiviral compounds and uses a wide range of targets. Examples of these are inhibitors of the RT enzyme, inhibitors of the viral protease, and inhibitors of viral fusion. The infections that today are effectively treated with different regimens of specific antiviral therapies are HIV-1, HBV, HCV, HSV, and CMV infections. Current therapy for HIV-1 infections consists of a combination of at least three compounds and is often

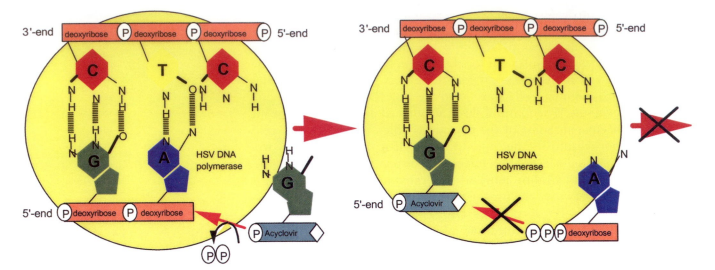

FIGURE 14 The mechanism of action of the antiviral compound acyclovir.

referred to as highly active antiretroviral therapy. These combinations usually contain one protease inhibitor and two or more RT inhibitors. The RT enzyme can be inhibited by two different approaches, nucleoside RT inhibitors and nonnucleoside RT inhibitors. Since these two types of RT inhibitors have different mechanisms of action, they often display synergistic effects. Unfortunately, there is enough plasticity in the viral genome to allow mutations within the viral target enzymes, which renders the virus resistant to one or all compounds. Viral variability is correlated with the number of replication cycles, since each replication generates mutations within the viral genome. It is therefore pivotal that the patient takes the different antiviral compounds at specific time points during the day, so that HIV-1 replication is continuously kept to a minimum. If the patient ignores this strict schedule, the virus can rapidly replicate, with development of resistant virus as a result. HIV-1 strains that are resistant to one or more antiviral compounds have now started to be spread in the Western world, where antiviral therapy for HIV-1 is common. Another problem is the ability of HIV-1 to maintain a latent infection in certain cell types, i.e., the virus does not replicate its genome until the cell is activated. It is thought that to eradicate HIV-1 present in one infected patient, an effective combination therapy would have to be maintained for several decades. This is, of course, almost impossible because the drugs cause rather severe side effects and the risk of developing resistant virus is high. The general aim at present is therefore to combine the antiviral compounds with some type of specific immune therapy such as vaccination. By this approach, it is believed that the antiviral compound will suppress the viral replication and that the vaccination will activate the T cells that can also kill latently infected cells. The paradox is, however, that the vaccine is designed to activate T cells, and HIV-1 replicates most efficiently in activated T cells.

Other ways to design antiviral therapies are to use different types of immune modulators, such as cytokines. The most widely used cytokine is alpha interferon (IFN-α). The mode of action of IFN-α is not fully understood and may differ from virus to virus. However, one major action is the activation of the PKR system. By this pathway viral RNA is degraded and the cell undergoes apoptosis. This is believed to be a major antiviral effect of IFN-α. There are most likely some additional antiviral effects exerted by IFN-α. For example, it has been shown that IFN-α effectively helps to activate the type of T cells that help to fight the viral infection. IFN-α is today often used to treat chronic infections caused by HBV and HCV. Around 50% of all those chronically infected by HCV can be cured by a combination therapy containing IFN-α.

Another compound for which the mechanism of action is even less well understood is ribavirin. Ribavirin is a nucleoside analogue. It has been shown that ribavirin therapy for chronic HCV infections does not have any effect on viral replication. However, when ribavirin is used in combination with IFN-α, the effect on viral replication is better than that of IFN-α alone. It has been suggested that ribavirin acts as an immune modulator or as a mutagen that forces the virus into an error catastrophe.

KEY POINTS

Viruses are obligate intracellular organisms, since they have no metabolism of their own.

All viruses currently known contain a viral genome surrounded by a protein shell. Some viruses may also have a lipid envelope surrounding the protein shell (nucleocapsid) that contains the viral genome. The viral genome comes in many shapes and sizes, ranging from around 2,000 bases up to around 200,000 bases. The viral genome can be composed of either RNA or DNA and can be linear or circular or consist of several chromosomes (segmented).

Viral genomes contain coding and noncoding regions. The coding regions encode all viral proteins and the noncoding regions interact with the cellular machinery.

The viral proteins are either structural proteins (present in the extracellular virus) or nonstructural proteins (only present in the infected cell).

The most widely used criteria for the classification of viruses are type of genome, presence or absence of a lipid envelope, and structure of the viral nucleocapsid (icosahedral or helical).

The viral life cycle can be summarized in the following steps: (i) attachment of the virus to the cell; (ii) entry of the virus into the cell by fusion, endocytosis, or translocation; (iii) uncoating, release of the viral genome; (iv) replication of the viral genome; (v) synthesis of viral proteins; (vi) assembly of new viral particles; and (vii) release of infectious virus by lysis of the cell or by nonlytic pathways.

The members of the *Herpesviridae* family are enveloped viruses with DNA genomes. The most important members of the *Herpesviridae* are HSV-1 (which causes the recurrent infection oral herpes); HSV-2 (which causes an STD); VZV (primary infection, chicken pox; recur-

rent infection, shingles); and CMV and EBV (which cause severe disease in immune-suppressed patients).

HPV is a DNA virus lacking a lipid envelope. HPV represents a group of viruses causing warts. HPV-16 and -18 have been associated with cervical carcinoma. HPV can cause oral warts, or papillomas.

HBV is an enveloped virus with a DNA genome. HBV is transmitted by contaminated blood and sexually. Infection is often asymptomatic for long periods, and HBV causes both acute and chronic infections. Chronic HBV infection increases the risk of developing liver cancer. The presence of HBsAg in serum signals ongoing infection. An effective vaccine is available.

HCV is an enveloped virus with an RNA genome. During each replication cycle new mutations are introduced into the HCV genome. HCV is transmitted by contaminated blood and blood products. HCV causes a chronic infection in >70% of all who become infected, and chronic infection increases the risk for developing liver cancer. Chronic HCV infection can be treated with IFN-α. No vaccine that can prevent HCV infection is available.

HIV-1 is a member of the *Retroviridae* family. HIV-1 is an enveloped virus that has an RNA genome and enzyme RT, which can synthesize DNA from an RNA template. The HIV-1 genome is integrated in the human genome as part of the viral replication cycle. HIV-1 infection can be asymptomatic for several years. HIV-1 infection is usually an STD and leads to the depletion of CD4$^+$ T cells. AIDS is a syndrome of opportunistic diseases which develops because of the immune deficiency caused by the HIV-1 infection. The mean survival of a patient who has developed AIDS and who is left untreated is 2 years. No effective vaccine is available to prevent HIV-1 infection, due in part to

(continues)

KEY POINTS

(Continued from previous page)
the high genetic variability of the viral genome. Effective combination antiviral therapies increase the life span of HIV-1-infected patients.

The most important cell types of the innate immune system in fighting viral infections are macrophages, dendritic cells, and NK cells.

The cells of the adaptive immune system that fight viral infections are B cells, Th cells, and CTLs. Antibodies from B cells can neutralize viruses when they bind to the surface of the virus particle. Th cells recognize viral peptides through the class II presenting pathway. CTLs recognize and kill virus-infected cells through viral peptides presented by the class I pathway. Viruses can escape the host immune system by inhibiting antigen presentation, changing their genome through mutations, producing decoys and inducing immunological tolerance, and immune dysregulation.

Jenner performed the first vaccination against smallpox in the 1790s. Smallpox could be eradicated because an efficient vaccine was readily available; humans were the only host; smallpox caused only acute infections that either resolved or killed the host, and thus, there were no reservoirs of the virus; and the virus was genetically stable.

Passive immunization (injection of antibodies) does not generate immunological memory. In contrast, active immunization generates immunological memory. Viral vaccines can be divided into attenuated whole virus, inactivated whole virus, subcomponent, peptide, and genetic vaccines.

Antiviral compounds can block or inhibit specific steps in the viral life cycle and act indirectly by activating or modulating the host immune system. The antiviral drug acyclovir is phosphorylated, i.e., activated, by a viral enzyme and is therefore only active in virus-infected cells. Future antiviral therapies will most likely be combination therapies consisting of several antiviral compounds.

FURTHER READING

Cann, A. J. (ed.). 2001. *Principles of Molecular Virology,* 3rd ed. Academic Press, San Diego, Calif.

Fields, B. N., et al. (ed.). 1996. *Fields Virology,* 3rd ed. Lippincott-Raven, Philadelphia, Pa.

Goldsby, R. A., T. J. Kindt, and B. A. Osborne. 2000. *Kuby Immunology,* 4th ed. W. H. Freeman and Company, New York, N.Y.

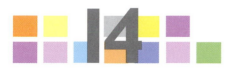

14

Fungi and Fungal Infections of the Oral Cavity

Richard D. Cannon and Norman A. Firth

INTRODUCTION

Fungi are normal, albeit minor, members of the oral microbial flora. The fungus that can be isolated most frequently from the human oral cavity is *Candida albicans*. This organism is a harmless commensal in approximately 20 to 40% of healthy individuals. Fungi can and do, however, cause oral mucosal diseases, particularly in immunocompromised individuals. The most common oral fungal infection is candidiasis, which has a variety of presentations, but several other fungi can cause oral lesions. There are fundamental structural and metabolic differences between fungi and other oral microorganisms, such as bacteria and viruses, and these differences affect the pathogenesis of the diseases they cause and the treatment of infected individuals. This chapter describes the biology and virulence of fungi, the major oral clinical conditions caused by fungi, and the treatment of people with oral fungal infections.

BIOLOGY

Fungi (singular: fungus) are a large group of microorganisms that constitute a kingdom within the domain *Eukarya*. As such, fungi are distinct from members of the animal and plant kingdoms and from *Bacteria* and *Archaea*. Fungi are ubiquitous microorganisms with important roles in the degradation of organic material, as food sources, and as key components in the baking and brewing industries. Of the approximately 100,000 recognized fungal species, only about 150 are pathogenic for humans, and of these, a handful cause oral and perioral lesions.

Fungi are vegetative organisms that do not synthesize chlorophyll, are nonmotile, and have a basic structure consisting of individual cells or chains of cylindrical cells (a hypha [plural: hyphae]), or both. Fungi are eukaryotic and share some structural and metabolic features of animal cells: they have DNA contained in a membrane-bound nucleus, possess organelles such as mitochondria and centrioles, and have 80S ribosomes (as opposed to the 70S ribosomes in bacteria). They also have features that distinguish them from animal cells: they almost always possess a rigid cell wall surrounding a plasma membrane that contains the sterol ergosterol rather than the cholesterol found in mammalian cell membranes. The cell walls of fungi are distinct from gram-positive or gram-negative bacterial cell walls. Fungal cell walls generally contain an outer amorphous layer of glycoproteins and inner layers, or enrichments, of polysaccharides such as glucans (polymers of glucose) and chitin (polymers of *N*-acetylglucosamine), which confer rigidity and determine cell morphology. *Cryptococcus neoformans* possesses a distinctive capsule composed predominantly of the polysaccharide glucuronoxylomannan. In filamentous fungi, growth is mostly limited to the hyphal tip; in yeast, there is general wall expansion over the entire surface during the cell growth cycle. The molecules on the outer surface of fungi are important as they are often involved in adherence and in interactions with the host defenses. The similarities and differences between fungi and mammalian cells, and between fungi and other microorganisms, are important for the development of specific antifungal drugs that are not toxic to humans and so will have fewer side effects.

Morphology

Fungal cells have a diameter of approximately 3 to 6 μm, and in general they are larger than bacteria and smaller than mammalian cells. Fungi have distinctive and varied cellular morphologies (Fig. 1). Those that exist predominantly in the unicellular state are usually ovoid and termed yeasts; examples are *C. albicans* and *C. neoformans*. Fungi that grow as hyphae are commonly called molds. Hyphae consist of chains of individual cylindrical cells, each containing a nucleus and divided from adjacent cells by walls called septa. The presence and structure of septa are important in the taxonomy of fungi. Fungal hyphae can branch and form a mycelial mat. Some fungi exist in more than one cellular morphological form and are termed dimorphic, or polymorphic, depending on the number of forms in which they grow. Dimorphic fungi include *Blastomyces dermatitidis*, *Paracoccidioides brasiliensis*, *Histoplasma capsulatum*, and *Sporothrix*

FIGURE 1 Growth morphologies of *C. albicans*.

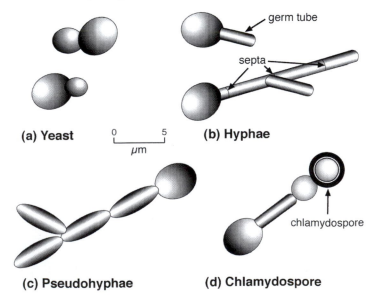

schenckii. C. albicans is often referred to as a dimorphic fungus, as it mostly exists in either the yeast or hyphal morphological form. Strictly speaking, however, it is polymorphic as it can also form sporelike chlamydospores on certain media, and grows as pseudohyphae, which differ from true hyphae in that they have constrictions at the septa and appear as chains of elongated yeast cells. Fungal dimorphism has been extensively studied, recently at the molecular genetic level, as it is believed to be involved in the pathogenesis of fungal diseases.

Macroscopically, yeast colonies on agar plates tend to be smooth with well-defined edges, whereas mold colonies are furry with individual hyphal threads visible at the edge of the colony. Mold colonies are sometimes pigmented toward the center (green, for example, for *Aspergillus* colonies) due to the maturation of spores.

Replication

Fungal replication can be either sexual or asexual, and some fungi can undertake both. Fungi that lack a known sexual state are classified in the phylum Deuteromycota (Fungi Imperfecti). *C. albicans* replicates asexually by budding. Although *C. albicans* possesses some genetic material homologous to that involved in sexual replication in the yeast *Saccharomyces cerevisiae,* there is currently no definitive evidence that *C. albicans* undergoes sexual reproduction in vivo. In the asexual replication of yeast, the mother cell produces a bud, which enlarges to form a daughter cell. The nucleus replicates by mitosis and migrates to the neck of the bud, and one replicated nucleus migrates into the daughter cell along with representative organelles. A cell wall septum is laid down at the neck between the mother and daughter cells and the cells separate, leaving a bud scar on the mother cell wall and a birth scar on the daughter cell.

Filamentous fungi can replicate asexually or sexually. Both types of replication can involve the production of spores; some asexual spores are termed conidia. Spores are often released from aerial fruiting bodies to be spread by air or water and are infectious agents. Sexual reproduction usually involves the fusion of either unicellular gametes or fusion of specialized hyphal elements.

PATHOGENESIS

Acquisition

Fungi are prevalent in the environment as well as being associated with humans and animals. Domestic animals are an important source of dermatophytic fungi such as *Microsporum canis,* which is associated with cats and dogs and can cause tinea corporis (ringworm) in humans. Other fungi are associated with birds; *C. neoformans,* for example, is carried by pigeons and can be disseminated through bird droppings. *C. neoformans* has also been associated in the environment with two species of eucalyptus trees, the distribution of which correlates with the occurrence of cryptococcosis caused by *C. neoformans* var. *gattii.* The fungus *Aspergillus* is commonly found in rotting vegetation but has also been isolated from some foods, including pepper and spices. Certain fungi are endemic in the environment in particular geographic areas. *H. capsulatum* is commonly found in North and South America, the Philippines, Indonesia, Turkey, Israel,

TABLE I Factors predisposing to oral candidiasis

Age: being very young or old
HIV infection
Mucosal trauma/irritation, including denture wearing
Drug therapy
Antibiotics
Corticosteroids (local or systemic)
Immunosuppressives
Cytotoxics
Malnutrition
Iron deficiency
Vitamin B$_{12}$ deficiency
Undiagnosed or poorly controlled diabetes mellitus
Leukemia
Agranulocytosis
Xerostomia
High-carbohydrate diet

Italy, Switzerland, Africa, Australia, and Asia. *P. brasiliensis* appears to be associated with subtropical forest areas with high annual rainfall.

Fungi can therefore be readily acquired by humans from the environment. The route of entry often depends on the nature of the infectious agent (spores, conidia, or yeast) and the nature of the environmental reservoir. It can be via the lungs for fungal spores, through the mouth for *Candida,* and by direct contact with the skin for dermatophytes. *C. albicans* has been isolated from primates, domesticated and other mammals, marsupials, and birds, but transmission to humans is usually from other colonized humans. In the clinical setting, transfer can occur via the hands of health care workers. Fungi can colonize the mouth and become a component of the oral microbiota. Filamentous fungi can rarely be cultured from the oral cavity, but yeast can be cultured from the saliva of approximately 40% of healthy individuals. The yeast most commonly isolated from saliva is *C. albicans*. Other yeasts that may be present include *Candida tropicalis, Candida dubliniensis, Candida glabrata, Candida parapsilosis,* and *Candida krusei*. Baker's yeast, *Saccharomyces cerevisiae,* can sometimes be isolated from the mouth, as can *Rhodotorula* species, which grow as distinctive red colonies on Sabouraud's agar. *C. dubliniensis,* which is phenotypically very similar to *C. albicans,* is a relatively recently described species found both in healthy individuals and individuals with human immunodeficiency virus (HIV) infection. *C. dubliniensis,* like *C. albicans,* forms germ tubes in serum and chlamydospores on cornmeal agar, but, unlike *C. albicans,* it cannot grow at the elevated temperature of 45°C. *C. dubliniensis* can be further distinguished from *C. albicans* by specific DNA probes or PCR amplification of specific DNA sequences. Yeast can colonize a variety of surfaces in the oral cavity and is often found associated with the dorsum of the tongue, the buccal (cheek) mucosa, and denture prostheses. *C. albicans* can also adhere to oral bacteria and salivary pellicles on oral surfaces, and has been detected in dental plaque. *C. albicans* is a harmless commensal in a significant proportion of the population, but if the host immune system is impaired, *C. albicans* can cause disease. A number of factors predispose humans to oral candidiasis (Table 1). Fungal colonization of the oral cavity can lead to colonization of the gastrointestinal (GI) tract, which can act as a reservoir for the infection of other body sites such as the vagina or for dissemination via the blood.

Virulence

Features associated with the growth and metabolism of fungi that cause damage to the host are termed virulence factors. Features that are not directly involved in host damage but are prerequisite for pathogenesis are termed virulence-associated factors. Such factors are involved in fungal adhesion, tissue damage and penetration, along with interaction with, and evasion of, the immune system.

Fungal adhesion is required for host colonization and usually involves cell surface adhesins that recognize and bind specific host receptor molecules. Adhesins are often glycoproteins, and the interaction with host receptors can be protein-protein or lectinlike (protein-carbohydrate). Tissue penetration is more easily achieved by fungi growing as hyphae as opposed to as yeast; thus the dimorphic transition from yeast to hyphal growth in *C. albicans* is proposed to be a virulence factor for that fungus. Fungi secrete hydrolytic enzymes, such as proteinases and phospholipases, which can cause tissue damage and facilitate tissue penetration. Proteinases can also destroy immunoglobulins and so help fungi evade innate and acquired host defenses. *C. albicans* possesses a family of secreted aspartic proteinases with at least 10 members (Sap1 through Sap10). Different Sap isozymes are secreted at different stages of *Candida* infections and are thought to be involved in nutrient acquisition, adhesion, tissue penetration, immune evasion, cell injury after phagocytosis, activation of the blood clotting cascade, and enhanced vascular permeability. *C. albicans* also secretes phospholipases and has at least eight genes with homology to lipases. The ability of some fungi to bind complement proteins is thought to enable them to avoid destruction by the immune system. The carbohydrate capsule of *C. neoformans* inhibits phagocytosis by macrophages and results in reduced killing by the immune system. Several fungi, including *C. neoformans* and *Aspergillus fumigatus*, produce the pigment melanin, which is associated with the cell wall. The *C. neoformans* melanin is thought to protect cells against oxidants and ultraviolet light and to interfere with cell-mediated immunity.

The identification of new fungal virulence factors and the elucidation of fungal pathogenesis may provide novel drug targets or alternative treatment strategies. The specific inhibition of fungal adhesion may, for example, prevent colonization, and hence preclude the initiation of disease. Drugs that inhibit proteinases may prevent the spread of fungal infections. The sequencing and annotation of the genomes of several pathogenic fungi, including *C. albicans*, *A. fumigatus*, and *C. neoformans*, are almost complete, and it is hoped that this information will help identify new drug targets. It is debatable, however, whether the inhibition of single virulence-associated factors would be sufficient to cure people with fungal infections.

HOST DEFENSES AGAINST FUNGAL INFECTION

Host defenses against fungal infections involve both nonspecific and specific defense mechanisms.

Nonspecific Defense Mechanisms

Natural, nonspecific defense mechanisms are in general very effective in preventing oral fungal infections. These innate defense mechanisms include the barrier function of intact mucosae, saliva flow, and antimicrobial components of saliva such as histatins, which are effective against *C. albicans*. Most oral surfaces are colonized by bacteria against which fungi have to compete for nutrients. Following fungal colonization of mucosae or invasion of tissues, a nonspecific inflammatory response is often elicited. Most fungi activate complement by the alternative pathway, become coated with C3 fragments, and attach to polymorphonuclear leukocytes, monocytes, and macrophages. The main leukocyte contributing to the containment and destruction of fungi is the neutrophil, but other components of the nonspecific response include eosinophils, basophils, platelets, and natural killer cells. Macrophages live longer than neutrophils and can persist at sites of infection. An early response to *H. capsulatum* infection is phagocytosis by macrophages, but the fungus can resist lysosomal killing.

Specific Defense Mechanisms

The specific immune response to fungal infections involves humoral and cell-mediated immunity. Antibodies are usually produced in response to fungi, and in the oral cavity the predominant immunoglobulin is secretory immunoglobulin A (IgA). The main function of secretory IgA is to agglutinate microorganisms and prevent them from adhering to oral surfaces. Although IgA responses to fungi can be detected, they are not always effective in preventing colonization. Cell-mediated immunity plays an important role in preventing several fungal infections of humans. Individuals with primary or acquired T-cell immunodeficiencies—AIDS patients, for example, who have depleted functional CD4$^+$ T cells—are very susceptible to deep-seated or superficial fungal infections such as aspergillosis or oropharyngeal candidiasis.

ANTIFUNGAL THERAPY

To treat people with oral fungal infections, it is often necessary to first grow and identify the fungus responsible for the clinical symptoms.

Growth and Identification of Fungi

Fungi can be cultured from clinical specimens on Sabouraud's agar. Methods for sampling oral sites include wiping with sterile swabs, using phosphate-buffered saline in oral rinses, and the plating of saliva samples. Antibiotics such as chloramphenicol and gentamicin can be included in the agar to inhibit the growth of bacteria from the samples. Inoculated agar plates are generally incubated aerobically at 30°C for 48 h. There are several methods for identifying fungi. Microscopic examination of clinical samples can be informative. Samples can be obtained by scraping mucosal surfaces with a wooden spatula, or tongue depressor, and transferring the material to a clean glass slide for wet-mount microscopy. Alternatively, a biopsy in which the sample is stained before microscopic examination may be indicated for some lesions (Table 2). This can reveal fungal cellular morphology: the presence of yeasts or hyphae, spores, conidia, or capsules and the size of these features (Fig. 2). Colony morphology of fungi is also distinctive. Fungal colonies can have a smooth surface or, for some molds, a furry appearance. The colony color, size, edge, elevation, and consistency are also informative. To identify fungi by growth features, specific agars may be required. Not all fungi, for example, will produce their characteristic spores on media used in primary culture from clinical specimens. Growth media containing various carbon and/or nitrogen sources can be used to determine fungal growth requirements and also determine fermentation patterns, which can distinguish species. Certain distinctive growth morphologies are used in the presumptive identification of fungi. *C. albicans*, for example, will produce characteristic hyphae if incubated in fetal calf, bovine, rabbit, or human serum for 3 h at 37°C. This is often referred to as the germ tube test, although this term is misleading as *C. albicans* does not germinate.

TABLE 2 Staining methods to visualize fungi in clinical samples

PAS
Potassium hydroxide (KOH)
Grocott-Gomori methenamine silver
Gridley's method
Calcofluor white

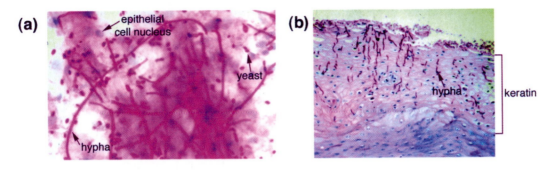

FIGURE 2 Histopathology of oral candidiasis. (a) Smear taken from pseudomembranous candidiasis lesion and stained with PAS; (b) Section of pseudomembranous candidiasis lesion stained with PAS.

Identification of fungi by growth characteristics is time-consuming, as it usually requires both primary and secondary culture on specific media, which may take several days. Some chromogenic agars containing antibiotics can be used to identify yeast directly from clinical samples as particular species grow on these agars as colonies with distinctive colors. The number of fungal species that can be reliably identified by this method is, however, limited.

Techniques have been developed to utilize the differences in the nucleic acid sequences of different fungal species in fungal identification. Hybridization of nucleic acids with labeled nucleic acid probes specific for a particular fungus can be used to detect that fungus in clinical samples. Usually there is amplification of the nucleic acid from the sample before hybridization. Alternatively, the ability to amplify a particular DNA sequence from a sample by using species-specific primers and PCR can be used to indicate the presence of a fungal species in the sample. These nucleic acid-based techniques can be relatively rapid and sensitive, but may have the problem of false positives due to nucleic acid contamination, and are presently carried out in laboratories rather than in the clinical setting.

Principles of Antifungal Chemotherapy

Once the fungus present in significant numbers in a clinical sample is identified, it is possible to devise a treatment plan involving the application of appropriate antifungal agents. Most effective antifungal drugs target features unique to the fungus and not present in mammalian cells. As fungi are eukaryotic, like their host, there are fewer potential specific drug targets than for bacteria. Most currently available antifungal drugs target membrane sterols (polyenes) and their biosynthesis (azoles) and nucleic acid replication (flucytosine [5FC]). Polyenes insert in fungal plasma membranes, associate with the sterol ergosterol, and form pores, which allow leakage of mono- and divalent ions and cytoplasmic components of low molecular mass. This leads to cell death and so polyenes are fungicidal. Polyene drugs have problems with host toxicity and are generally less soluble than the less toxic triazole drugs. Azoles such as imidazoles and the more recent triazole derivatives target fungal cytochrome

P$_{450}$ enzymes and inhibit sterol biosynthesis by preventing 14α-demethylation of lanosterol. 5FC is a pyrimidine analog that is taken up by fungal cells and deaminated to 5-fluorouracil, which causes aberrant RNA synthesis and inhibits DNA synthesis. 5FC is fungicidal, but certain fungi, including a proportion of *C. albicans* strains, are intrinsically resistant to 5FC. 5FC is usually administered in combination with other antifungals, such as amphotericin B (a polyene), in the treatment of patients with systemic cryptococcosis.

The cell walls of fungi contain components not present in mammalian cells that represent obvious antifungal targets. Inhibitors of chitin biosynthesis (nikkomycins) are available, but they are not effective against *C. albicans*. Glucan biosynthesis has proved difficult to target, but the echinocandin inhibitors caspofungin and micafungin are now available for intravenous use for esophageal candidiasis.

Fungal drug resistance has emerged as a problem in the treatment of certain patients. HIV-positive individuals and AIDS patients, for example, frequently suffer from oropharyngeal candidiasis, and long-term treatment with triazole antifungals such as fluconazole sometimes fails because of the presence of resistant *Candida* strains. *C. glabrata* and *C. krusei* appear to be intrinsically resistant to fluconazole (primary resistance), and fluconazole resistance in *C. albicans* can be induced by exposure to the drug (secondary resistance). The susceptibility of fungi to antifungal drugs can be determined by broth dilution or agar diffusion (Etest) methods. These techniques give a value (minimum growth inhibitory concentration) for the fungal susceptibility to the drug, and there is generally a correlation between the MIC value and clinical outcome of treatment with the drug. Drug resistance is most frequently seen with the azole and triazole antifungals. Fluconazole resistance in *C. albicans* can be due to overexpression of the drug target, mutations in the drug target, and most commonly for high-level resistance, overexpression of energy-dependent drug efflux pumps. Azole drugs are fungistatic and use of these drugs can contribute to the recurrence of oral fungal infections.

CLINICAL CONDITIONS

The most prevalent fungus in the oral cavity and the primary etiologic agent in oral candidiasis is the yeast *C. albicans*. The name of this fungus is interesting because both parts of the binomial mean white (*Candida* Latin adjective, white; *albicans* present participle of Latin verb *albico*, being white). The name therefore doubly reflects the growth characteristics of the fungus; it grows as creamy white colonies on Sabouraud's agar and it can also result in characteristic white lesions of the oral mucosae. In pseudomembranous and hyperplastic candidiasis there can be many small white lesions scattered over the mucosae, giving a speckled appearance. These speckled lesions could explain the common term for candidiasis, "thrush," which is thought to be derived from the Scandinavian word *torsk*, which is used for both the disease and the bird. Oral thrush has been recognized clinically for centuries, but the causative agent proved elusive. In his book *Epidemics*, Hippocrates in the 4th century B.C.E. described two cases of oral aphthae, which were probably thrush. The first reference to the word thrush is from the writings of Samuel

Pepys in 1665. In 1890, Zopf named the thrush fungus *Monilia albicans*, from which moniliasis, the early name for candidiasis, is derived. Although Berkhout proposed, in 1923, the genus *Candida* to accommodate *Monilia,* it was not until 1954 at the Eighth Botanical Congress in Paris that the generic name *Candida* was finally accepted.

   Candida infections are common in patients with T-cell-type deficiencies but are uncommon in patients with B-cell deficiencies. It has been postulated that susceptibility to oral mucosal *Candida* infections is related more to altered T-cell function than to defects in secretory immunity, whereas prevention of systemic infection is mediated by specific serum antibodies as well as oral epithelial effector cells (granulocytes and macrophages).

Candidiasis

In 1966 Lehner published a classification of oral *Candida* infections that was accepted for many years. Lehner's classification recognized two major subdivisions: acute (which included pseudomembranous and atrophic candidiasis) and chronic (including atrophic and hyperplastic candidiasis). The emergence of *Candida* infections in immunocompromised hosts such as HIV/AIDS patients and organ transplant recipients has resulted in several changes to the currently accepted classification. In particular, the simple temporal relationship is no longer considered valid as the pseudomembranous form can be long-lasting in the immunocompromised and other groups, for instance, long-term users of corticosteroid inhalers (asthmatics) in whom alterations in local immunity occur intraorally. Pseudomembranous candidiasis can therefore be considered to be acute or chronic. The term "atrophic" is a histopathological rather than clinical term; currently "erythematous" is favored as it describes the red nature of such lesions. This redness may be due to atrophy, but it may also be due to increased vascularity and inflammation. The clinical conditions angular cheilitis, denture stomatitis (chronic erythematous candidiasis), and median rhomboid glossitis may have a mixed bacterial and fungal etiology and therefore are considered to be *Candida*-associated lesions. The current classification of oral and perioral *Candida* infections is given in Table 3.

PSEUDOMEMBRANOUS CANDIDIASIS

Pseudomembranous candidiasis, colloquially known as thrush, most frequently affects infants, the elderly, and the terminally ill. It is uncommon

TABLE 3 Classification of *Candida* infections confined to oral and perioral tissues

Candida infection	Clinical presentation
Acute pseudomembranous	Multiple removable white plaques
Acute erythematous	Generalized redness of tissue
Chronic plaquelike/nodular	Fixed white plaques on commissures
Chronic erythematous	Generalized redness of tissue on fitting surface of upper denture
Chronic pseudomembranous	Multiple removable white plaques
Candida-associated angular cheilitis	Bilateral cracks, angles of mouth
Median rhomboid glossitis	Fixed red/white lesion, dorsum of tongue

but may be an indicator of an underlying serious medical condition such as diabetes, leukemia, other malignancy, or HIV/AIDS. In addition, drug therapy with corticosteroid inhalers (as a preventive measure for asthmatics) may be associated with the development of pseudomembranous candidiasis.

The clinical appearance is generally characteristic with the formation of nonadherent creamy white plaques, patches, or flecks that are easily wiped off with a blunt instrument such as a wooden spatula or a mouth mirror (Fig. 3a). Scraping may produce bleeding and generally reveals an erythematous mucosa. The commonly affected sites are the soft palate, oropharynx, tongue, buccal mucosa, and gingiva (gum). Generally pain is not a feature. When observed under a microscope, the plaques consist of a mesh of *Candida* hyphae, entangled with desquamated epithelial cells, fibrin, keratin, necrotic debris, and bacteria (Fig. 2). The clinical diagnosis can be confirmed by smears (stained with periodic acid-Schiff [PAS] stain), oral rinse, or culture. Smears are useful for a quick confirmation of diagnosis if hyphae are observed. Cultures are useful in determining which species is involved and to which antifungal agents the strain is susceptible. Biopsy is not necessary. Treatment is discussed below.

ERYTHEMATOUS CANDIDIASIS
Erythematous candidiasis may be acute or chronic depending on duration. The acute form has also been called acute atrophic candidiasis or

FIGURE 3 Oral candidiasis. (a) Pseudomembranous candidiasis lesions on the palate; (b) chronic erythematous candidiasis on the palatal mucosa of an edentulous, full-denture-wearing patient; (c) plaquelike/nodular candidiasis at the commissure of upper and lower lips (mucosal surfaces); (d) angular cheilitis at commissures of the mouth, involving skin.

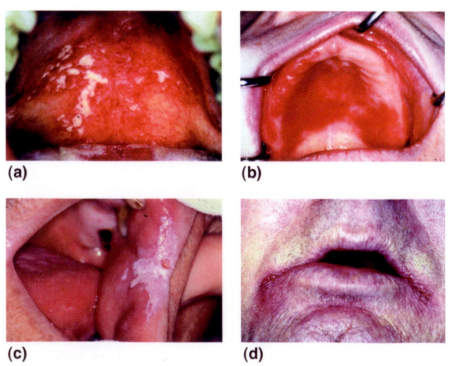

antibiotic sore mouth. As the latter term suggests, it is frequently associated with a preceding systemic course of broad-spectrum antibiotics or with topical antibiotic therapy. It may also be associated with the use of corticosteroid inhalers. This is the only form of candidiasis that is painful. The diagnosis can be confirmed by microscopic examination of smears or oral rinses, or by culture.

CHRONIC ERYTHEMATOUS CANDIDIASIS
Chronic erythematous candidiasis occurs on the palatal mucosa beneath full or partial maxillary dentures (Fig. 3b). There is a sharp demarcation between the affected and unaffected tissue. Occasionally the edentulous mandible may be involved. Usually patients are unaware of the condition. This form of candidiasis is more frequent among those who do not remove their dentures at night and wearers of old dentures. The diagnosis can be confirmed by smears obtained from both mucosal surfaces (palate and dorsum of tongue) and from the fitting surface of the denture. Oral rinse or culture may be employed, but as denture wearers have a higher *Candida* carriage rate than non-denture wearers, interpretation of positive results needs to be judged in relation to clinical findings and the site from which the sample was obtained. Hematological investigations to assess any underlying systemic predisposing factors, e.g., iron, vitamin B_{12}, or folate deficiency or undiagnosed or poorly controlled diabetes mellitus, are important. In addition to antifungal treatment (see below), patients should be instructed to remove their dentures at night and, after cleaning them, to soak them in either 2% chlorhexidine gluconate or 1% sodium hypochlorite overnight. If the dentures are old, unstable, or unretentive, the patient should be encouraged to have new dentures made.

PLAQUELIKE/NODULAR CANDIDIASIS
Plaquelike/nodular candidiasis (also called chronic hyperplastic candidiasis or candidal leukoplakia) is characterized by irregular white plaques that cannot be removed by scraping (Fig. 3c). Lesions are generally bilateral and occur on the buccal mucosa near the commissures at the level of the occlusal plane. Local factors such as tobacco smoking, denture wearing, and occlusal friction imply a multifactorial etiology. Often biopsy is indicated to confirm the diagnosis because there may be worrying clinical signs (for example, induration, ulceration, etc.). The presence of *Candida* can be confirmed by microscopic examination of smears or by culture of swab or oral rinse samples. Hematological investigations are also important to assess any underlying systemic predisposing factors as described above. The frequency of epithelial dysplasia in plaquelike/nodular candidiasis is four or five times higher than that estimated for other oral leukoplakias, and 9 to 40% of lesions develop into oral cancer compared with 2 to 6% in leukoplakias in general. Frequently, treatment with antifungal agents alone (see below) does not result in complete resolution. Addressing the other contributory factors may help. Clinical review is necessary, and complete removal by surgical means (scalpel or laser) should be considered.

ANGULAR CHEILITIS
Angular cheilitis presents as erythema and crusting and cracking in the commissural regions of the lips (Fig. 3d). This *Candida*-associated lesion

frequently has a bacterial component. Associated factors include the deficiency states (iron, folate, or vitamin B_{12}), diabetes mellitus or HIV/AIDS, skin creasing due to age, poor dentures with reduced vertical dimension, and pooling of saliva in the affected areas. An intraoral *Candida* infection may also be present. Hematological investigations are appropriate, and the diagnosis may be confirmed by microscopic examination of lesional and intraoral smears or by culture of swabs or oral rinse. Treatment of both lesional tissue and the asymptomatic oral cavity is required.

MEDIAN RHOMBOID GLOSSITIS

Another *Candida*-associated lesion is median rhomboid glossitis, which often presents as a somewhat diamond-shaped lesion on the dorsum of the tongue near the junction of the anterior two-thirds and posterior one-third. An oral swab may confirm the mixed etiological microbiota. A biopsy is not necessary unless worrying clinical signs are present.

OTHER *CANDIDA* INFECTIONS

Other *Candida* infections occur rarely, usually in patients with underlying medical conditions (Table 4). These infections include cheilocandidiasis, mucocutaneous candidiasis, multifocal candidiasis, and *Candida* endocrinopathy syndrome.

TREATMENT

Treatment of people with oral *Candida* infections is usually topical (Table 5). Two useful polyenes, nystatin and amphotericin B, were discovered in the 1950s and are still of use today. Clinically, fungal polyene resistance is rare. Nystatin is highly toxic if it is administered parenterally and therefore is not suitable for systemic *Candida* infections. It is

TABLE 5 Treatment of candidiasis in the immunocompetent[a] host

Candida infection	Topical treatment	Other considerations
Pseudomembranous	10-mg amphotericin B lozenges sucked 4 times daily (qid), 10–28 days	If topical steroid-related, rinse mouth after inhaling and/or use of volumatic spacer
Erythematous	10-mg amphotericin B lozenges sucked qid, 10–28 days	If topical steroid-related, rinse mouth after inhaling and/or use of volumatic spacer
Plaquelike/nodular	10-mg amphotericin B lozenges sucked qid, 10–28 days, + miconazole oral gel[b] applied to lesions	Biopsy may be indicated if clinical appearance is "worrying"
Denture-associated *Candida* lesions	Miconazole oral gel[b] applied to fitting surface of denture + 10-mg amphotericin B lozenges sucked qid, 10–28 days	Remove denture(s) and soak overnight in 2% chlorhexidine gluconate or 1% hypochlorite
Angular cheilitis	Miconazole oral gel[b] applied to lesions + 10-mg amphotericin B lozenges sucked qid, 10–28 days	Remove denture(s) if present and soak overnight in 2% chlorhexidine gluconate or 1% hypochlorite
Median rhomboid glossitis	10-mg amphotericin B lozenges sucked qid, 10–28 days	Biopsy may be indicated if clinical appearance is "worrying"

[a]Systemic therapy with fluconazole or itraconazole is indicated for patients with immunosuppression.

[b]Miconazole oral gel potentiates the anticoagulant effect of warfarin with potentially fatal consequences and therefore must never be prescribed for patients taking warfarin.

not absorbed from the GI tract, and therefore it is used for topical application intraorally. Unfortunately, it has an unpleasant taste, so preparations for oral use contain flavoring agents. Nystatin comes in a number of forms, including a cream, an ointment, tablets, a suspension, a gel, a pessary, and a pastille.

Amphotericin B also is not absorbed very well from the GI tract and is generally used topically; it comes in similar formulations as nystatin. Amphotericin B can be given intravenously for the treatment of systemic candidiasis. Both antifungals are fungicidal and have been used successfully in the treatment of the forms of oral candidiasis described above. They can be used together, for example, nystatin ointment applied to the fitting surface of the denture and amphotericin B lozenges in the treatment of denture-associated chronic erythematous candidiasis, or nystatin ointment applied to the affected commissures and amphotericin B lozenges in the treatment of angular cheilitis. Not all forms of these agents are available in all countries. The use of antiseptic mouth rinses (e.g., chlorhexidine gluconate) for oral and denture hygiene should be considered, and for patients with xerostomia (dry mouth), sialagogues (e.g., pilocarpine) to stimulate salivary flow may be useful adjuncts.

More recently, imidazoles and triazoles have been used to treat oral candidiasis. They include miconazole, ketoconazole, clotrimazole, fluconazole, and itraconazole. Miconazole is not absorbed from the GI tract and is mainly used topically. It is reported to have a bacteriostatic effect in addition to being fungicidal and therefore is useful in the treatment of angular cheilitis. An important adverse reaction occurs if miconazole is absorbed topically in sufficient amounts in patients taking warfarin, an anticoagulant drug widely used to "thin the blood." Miconazole potentiates this effect, and the resultant internal hemorrhage is potentially fatal. Topical preparations of clotrimazole (oral troches) and itraconazole (solution) can also be used for oral candidiasis.

Ketoconazole was the first of the imidazoles developed that was systemically absorbed after oral administration. It is useful in the treatment of chronic mucocutaneous candidiasis and oral candidiasis in immunocompromised patients. It can have side effects such as nausea, cutaneous rash, pruritus, and hepatotoxicity. As alteration to liver function can occur, monitoring of liver enzymes is essential. The triazoles fluconazole and itraconazole, like the imidazoles, inhibit fungal biosynthesis of ergosterol, which is required for plasma membrane function. Fluconazole has been shown in a number of studies to be effective in treating HIV/AIDS-related oral candidiasis such as oropharyngeal candidiasis. More recently, however, fluconazole-resistant strains of *Candida* have emerged following the prophylactic use of fluconazole in HIV/AIDS patients.

Recently, a clinical trial has shown the echinocandin caspofungin to be as effective as amphotericin B for the treatment of patients with invasive candidiasis or candidemia, with significantly fewer adverse effects.

Aspergillosis

Oral aspergillosis is a rare infection consisting of three forms. It may be saprophytic, in which there is fungal growth without invasion into viable tissue. It may be allergic, that is, a hypersensitivity reaction to fungal hyphae develops, or it may be invasive in which case viable tissue is invaded by the fungus, resulting in severe necrosis. The saprophytic and allergic types have relatively low morbidity and mortality and affect the immunocompetent host. The invasive form occurs in immunocompromised individuals and has significant morbidity and mortality. Oral sites of involvement include soft palate, tongue, and gingiva. Lesions on the soft palate have generally been associated with upper respiratory tract involvement. The gingival lesions are seen in patients with hematological malignancy. Palatal lesions consist of oral ulceration surrounded by a margin of black tissue. The gingival lesions are painful, violaceous, and ultimately ulcerated with tissue necrosis.

Diagnosis can be made from cultures; however, this can take about a week. As the lesions are often clinically worrying in their appearance, biopsy is frequently performed and a pathology report is issued approximately a day later, i.e., before results of culture are known. Once the diagnosis is established, aggressive systemic antifungal treatment (e.g., intravenous amphotericin B) can be commenced.

Cryptococcosis

Cryptococcosis involves the oral cavity on rare occasions. The disease is caused by *C. neoformans,* and immunocompromised patients are at risk of disseminated disease. Oral lesion may present as ulceration or as a nodule. Sites of involvement include the tongue, palate, gingiva, and tooth socket following extraction. The differential diagnosis includes squamous cell carcinoma, tuberculosis, and traumatic ulcer. Diagnosis is confirmed by biopsy. Systemic treatment with amphotericin B, fluconazole, or itraconazole is indicated.

Histoplasmosis

Histoplasmosis is endemic in the United States in the Mississippi and Ohio River valleys, where 70 to 80% of adults have been infected (usually subclinically). Three forms of histoplasmosis are recognized: acute, chronic pulmonary, and progressive disseminated. Oral histoplasmosis may occur as either pulmonary or disseminated histoplasmosis or as a primary lesion in an otherwise healthy person. Oral histoplasmosis may be seen among patients with HIV/AIDS and may rarely be the initial manifestation of the disease. Oral lesions may present as single or multiple indurated ulcers or as nodular lesions. The palate, tongue, buccal mucosa, gingiva, and lips are the usual sites of involvement. Diagnosis can be established from histopathological examination of a biopsy specimen, culture, direct examination of smears, or complement fixation tests. Treatment with amphotericin B, ketoconazole, or itraconazole is effective.

Blastomycosis

Blastomycosis is a chronic fungal infection caused by *B. dermatitidis.* This condition mainly is found in North America and occasionally in Africa. Pulmonary involvement is common, and the patient may present with symptoms similar to those of tuberculosis, that is, low-grade fever, weight loss, cough, and purulent sputum. The most common extrapulmonary affected organ is the skin. Oral lesions may occur and are generally due to dissemination from pulmonary disease. Proliferative or ulcerated lesions may occur on the hard palate, gingiva, tongue, or lips. Bone involvement (maxilla or mandible) may occur. Males are more commonly affected than females. Diagnosis is based on culture, although organisms may be seen histologically on tissue obtained from a biopsy. Amphotericin B is the mainstay of treatment. Surgical removal and debridement may be required.

Paracoccidioidomycosis

Paracoccidioidomycosis (South American blastomycosis) is a chronic disease caused by *P. brasiliensis*. The disease is endemic in Brazil but also occurs in Argentina, Venezuela, Bolivia, Peru, Uruguay, Mexico, and Costa Rica. Adult males from rural farming areas are most commonly affected with lesions involving the mouth and pharynx. Oral lesions, which may be granular and present with ulceration, can result from either primary or secondary infection. Sites of involvement include the gingiva, palate, lips, and buccal mucosa. Gingival involvement may lead to tooth mobility. Palatal involvement may lead to perforation. Cervical lymphadenopathy can be the first sign of disease noted by the patient. Other forms of the disease include pulmonary, mucocutaneous-lymphangitic form, and disseminated disease. Often lesions are biopsied because of the worrying clinical appearance. Biopsy shows granulomas, multinucleated giant cells, and a mixed inflammatory cell infiltrate. Microabscesses and giant cells may contain fungal hyphae. Fungi can be more readily visualized on PAS-stained tissue sections. Smears can be taken and stained with either PAS or potassium hydroxide (KOH). Treatment is with either oral ketoconazole or intravenous amphotericin B.

Mucormycosis

Mucormycosis is rare but of significance, as it is frequently associated with a fatal outcome. It is an acute opportunistic infection usually involving debilitated individuals. The disease is caused by fungi of the family Mucoraceae, mainly *Rhizopus* and *Mucor* and rarely other species. Predisposing factors leading to debilitation include poorly controlled diabetes mellitus with ketoacidosis, hematological malignancies, burns, malnutrition, uremia, liver cirrhosis, HIV/AIDS, organ transplantation, oncological chemotherapy, and other causes of immunosuppression. The recognized forms of the disease are rhinocerebral, pulmonary, gastrointestinal, and disseminated. The rhinocerebral form is characterized by low-grade fever, general malaise, headache, sinus-associated pain, bloody nasal discharge, periorbital nasal or ocular swelling and edema, ptosis, and muscle paresis. Tissue necrosis may cause palatal ulceration and perforation. The differential diagnosis for rhinocerebral mucormycosis includes tertiary syphilis, tuberculosis, or malignant neoplasm (squamous cell carcinoma of the maxillary antrum or palatal mucosa). Biopsy and smears are appropriate laboratory tests, and computed tomography is useful in delineating the extent of the lesion. Treatment includes surgical debridement, systemic antifungal therapy, and management of predisposing factors.

KEY POINTS

Biology of fungi

Fungi are eukaryotic; they are structurally and metabolically distinct from bacteria. They are similar to mammalian cells but usually possess a cell wall.

Morphology. Fungi generally grow as yeast or hyphae. Those that can grow in both morphologies are termed dimorphic. *C. albicans* usually grows as yeast or hyphae but can grow as pseudohyphae and form chlamydospores.

Replication. Fungi can replicate sexually or asexually. Some fungi produce spores or conidia.

Pathogenesis of fungal infections

Acquisition of fungi from the environment. Fungi are prevalent in the environment, and several can colonize the human oral cavity. The fungi most commonly isolated from the oral cavity are *Candida* species.

Fungal virulence. Fungal factors associated with host damage include adherence, hydrolytic enzymes such as proteinases and phospholipases, evasion of the immune system, and melanin production.

Host defenses against fungal infection

Nonspecific defense mechanisms. The physical barrier or mucosae, salivary flow, salivary components, microbial competition, and phagocytes provide defenses against fungal colonization and invasion.

Specific defense mechanisms. Secretory IgA can prevent adhesion of fungi to oral surfaces. The cell-mediated immune response is important in preventing oral fungal infections.

Antifungal therapy

Growth and identification of fungi. Fungi can be identified by cellular and colony morphology, growth requirements, and specific DNA-based detection methods.

Principles of antifungal chemotherapy. Fungi present fewer specific drug targets than bacteria do. Currently, DNA synthesis is targeted by 5FC, plasma membrane integrity is targeted by polyenes, sterol biosynthesis is targeted by azoles, and glucan synthesis is targeted by candins. 5FC and polyenes are fungicidal and azoles are fungistatic. There is a clinical problem of azole resistance in oropharyngeal candidiasis.

Clinical conditions

Candidiasis. Oral candidiasis is the most common oral fungal infection. Presentations of oral candidiasis include pseudomembranous, erythematous, and plaquelike/nodular candidiases, angular cheilitis, and median rhomboid glossitis. Treatment involves amphotericin B lozenges and miconazole oral gel.

Aspergillosis. Oral aspergillosis may be saprophytic, allergic, or invasive and can affect the soft palate, tongue, and gingiva. Treatment is intravenous amphotericin B.

Cryptococcosis. Cryptococcosis rarely involves the oral cavity. Lesions present as ulceration or nodules on the tongue, palate, gingiva, or tooth socket. Systemic treatment with amphotericin B or itraconazole is indicated.

Histoplasmosis. Histoplasmosis is endemic in the United States and presents as acute, chronic pulmonary, or progressive disseminated disease. Treatment with amphotericin B, ketoconazole, or itraconazole is effective.

Blastomycosis. Blastomycosis mainly occurs in North America and occasionally in Africa. Proliferative or ulcerated oral lesions may occur on the hard palate, gingiva, tongue, or lips. Amphotericin B is the mainstay of treatment. Surgical debridement may be considered.

Paracoccidioidomycosis. Paracoccidioidomycosis is endemic in Central and South America. Oral lesions, which may be granular and present with ulceration, can result from either primary or secondary infection. Treatment is with either amphotericin B or an azole such as ketoconazole.

Mucormycosis. Mucormycosis is rare but of significance as it is frequently associated with a fatal outcome. The recognized forms of the disease are rhinocerebral, pulmonary, gastrointestinal, and disseminated. Treatment includes surgical debridement, systemic antifungal therapy, and management of predisposing factors.

FURTHER READING

Calderone, R. A. (ed.). 2002. Candida *and* Candidiasis. ASM Press, Washington, D.C.

Jacobs, P. H., and L. Hall. 1997. *Fungal Disease, Biology, Immunology, and Diagnosis.* Marcel Dekker Inc., New York, N.Y.

Kibbler, C. C., D. W. R. Mackenzie, and F. C. Odds (ed.). 1996. *Principles and Practice of Clinical Mycology.* John Wiley & Sons, Chichester, United Kingdom.

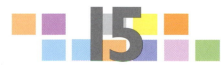

Endodontic Microbiology

Burton Rosan and Louis Rossman

INTRODUCTION

The dental pulp tissue is located within the dentin chamber and extends into the root canal. Dental pulp is undifferentiated connective tissue that is highly vascularized and rich in nerves and also contains immune cells. The blood vessels and nerves pass through one or more apical foramina at the apex of the tooth. Under normal conditions intact enamel and dentin protect the pulp, acting as a physical barrier to injury and microbial intrusion. Just as in other protected connective tissues, the enclosed, healthy, vital dental pulp is sterile. Thus, infections of the pulp are almost always secondary to other tooth infections, iatrogenic causes, or in some rare cases, traumatic occlusion. This contrasts markedly with the other major dental infections, caries and periodontal disease, that are directly associated with dental plaque. Because of this, the organisms that are the direct antecedent of the inflammatory process associated with pulp infections are endogenous oral bacteria (bacteria normally present in the oral cavity) that gain access to the pulpal connective tissues. This hospitable environment provides the nutrition that allows bacterial multiplication. More often than not, these bacteria lack, or cannot express, properties that can initiate invasion in their normal environment and therefore are usually considered of low virulence. Their "virulence" is usually only expressed when they can access connective tissues such as the dental pulp. For this reason they are called "opportunistic pathogens" and the infections they cause are called opportunistic infections. In this sense most pulpal and apical inflammatory diseases may be considered "endogenous opportunistic infections." This concept was understood by many of the pioneers in endodontics and dentistry who used a variety of techniques to achieve asepsis in treating root canals.

HISTORY

Although forms of root canal therapy were found in early Egyptian skulls, it was not until the 18th century that the preservation of teeth by treatment of the pulp was first attempted by Pierre Fauchard. This was accomplished by cauterizing the exposed pulp, following which the root canals were filled with lead. Despite these attempts, there was still a large segment of both the dental and medical profession that believed the "dead tooth" constituted a "focus of infection." This theory claimed that local infections such as pyorrhea and dental abscess were responsible for many chronic diseases. A renowned London physician, William Hunter, was a prominent advocate of this idea. In 1910, he lectured at the medical school of McGill University on the role of sepsis and antisepsis in medicine; he claimed that many chronic diseases were cured after extraction of infected teeth. Although the teeth he condemned never had root canal therapy, Hunter believed dead teeth, like other local infections, also represented a "focus of infection." The diseases that he claimed resulted from focal infections included arthritis, heart disease, and other diseases for which there was no satisfactory etiological explanation at the time.

This concept led to a stage in the history of dentistry in which the recommended treatment for gum and dental pulp diseases was tooth extraction, even for the simplest cases of gingivitis. This epidemic of mass extractions to cure many systemic diseases continued for more than half of the 20th century. The practitioners who advocated this treatment became known as "hundred per centers" because they would often extract all the teeth regardless of the extent of disease.

Fortunately, in the 1930s investigators began to question the anecdotal evidence that formed the basis of the theory of focal infection and thus initiated the modern phase of endodontic therapy. Additional factors that were essential to a rational approach to endodontics were the incorporation of radiology for diagnosis, measurement of canal length, and visual examination of hidden anatomy. Active research also provided evidence that the inflammatory lesions associated with teeth were manifestations of bacterial infections. On the basis of these studies, dentists began to apply the aseptic techniques used in surgery to reduce bacterial contamination of the operative field. In endodontics this meant isolating the tooth being treated with a rubber dam and swabbing the area to be treated with antiseptic agents. An additional precaution was the culturing of the infected root canals for bacteria in much the same way physicians took cultures to identify bacteria associated with infectious diseases. An obvious extension of this idea led to the sampling of the treated root canals to determine the effectiveness of the debridement. With these tools in place endodontic pioneers, like Louis Grossman, I. B. Bender, Edgar Coolidge, W. Clyde Davis, Jacob Freedland, George Hare, John Ingle, Harry B. Johnston, Henry Kahn, and George Stewart, were able to devise controlled experiments to show that root canals could be debrided to the point where sampling no longer detected viable bacteria. However, as techniques evolved, the availability of antibiotics, standardization of endodontic instruments, better chemotherapeutic agents as aids for debriding the root canals, cements for obturation (filling), and a much better understanding of the bacteria and their virulence properties have enabled endodontic therapy to become a safe and predictable treatment. Despite this progress, the concept of focal infection is still with us, albeit the approaches to studying it rely on modern epidemiological methods.

Although in the 1950s endodontists were practicing aseptic treatment, there were still many dentists who did not accept the idea of the infective nature of pulpal diseases despite the overwhelming clinical

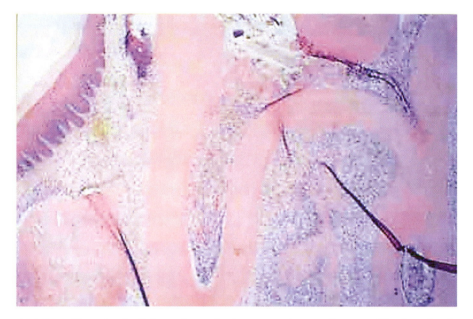

FIGURE 1 Dental pulp 7 days after pulpal exposure in germfree rats. The dental pulp remains viable even though food impaction is evident in the exposure site. Reprinted from S. Kakehashi, S. H. Stanley, and R. Fitzgerald, *Oral Surg. Oral Med. Oral Pathol.* **20:**342–349, 1965, with permission.

evidence supporting this concept. It was not until 1965 that the key experimental studies of Kakehashi et al. showed that pulpal exposure in germfree rats did not lead to inflammation (Fig. 1), whereas similar exposure in conventional animals invariably led to pulpal inflammation and pulp necrosis associated with endogenous oral bacteria (Fig. 2). In germfree animals, healing of the exposure occurred with the deposition of secondary dentin. Similar observations have been made in humans when pulp exposure to the contaminated oral environment rapidly resulted in inflammation of the pulp and/or periapical tissues. The success of antibiotics in reducing the severity of pulpal infections also points to a bacterial etiology. The final proof of the bacterial etiology led to a new chapter in endodontics in which clinical scientists have sought to improve the techniques for achieving asepsis in debridement of the root canal.

SOURCES OF INFECTION

Although the root canals represent distinct anatomic structures that present unique problems in treatment, superficially the treatment resembles that used for wounds that also become infected with bacteria that may be present in the local environment. Among the factors affecting the kinds of bacteria that are isolated from root canal infection are the route of infection, e.g., extension of caries, mechanical exposure, trauma, and association with periodontal disease. Invasion of the pulp as a result of direct extension of dental caries is probably one of the most common routes of infection, particularly in younger patients (Fig. 3). Results of studies that indicate the presence of cariogenic bacteria, e.g., streptococci and lactobacilli, in the dentinal tubules of advancing carious lesions suggest they

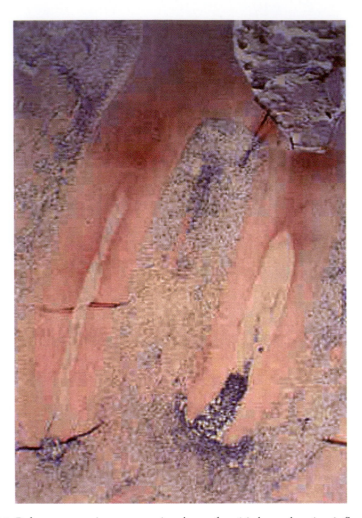

FIGURE 2 Pulp exposure in a conventional rat after 14 days, showing inflammation of pulp. Reprinted from S. Kakehashi, S. H. Stanley, and R. Fitzgerald, *Oral Surg. Oral Med. Oral Pathol.* **20**:342–349, 1965, with permission.

may be the first organisms present in the pulp after a carious exposure. Unfortunately, this idea is difficult to confirm scientifically because rarely, if ever, is there the opportunity to sample such "fresh" lesions. Study of samples that have been obtained immediately after a "mechanical exposure" of a root canal indicates that the majority of organisms are nonhemolytic streptococci. These probably consist of both α and γ streptococci, the most prevalent organisms in the oral cavity. However, unless precautions are taken to maintain aseptic conditions, e.g., use of a rubber dam, the open pulp is quickly exposed to the oral environment and infection with salivary bacteria follows rapidly. Another theory is that the initial invasion of tubules with lactic acid bacteria allows dissolution of some of the minerals of the dentin, leaving the organic matrix, composed of collagenlike material, open to attack by the anaerobic organisms whose metabolism is generally based on their proteolytic activities. Although this provides a reasonable teleological explanation for observations suggesting such bacterial succession, at present the evidence for such succession is limited. Other routes of infection, as well as environ-

FIGURE 3 Section through a tooth with dental caries (on left), showing penetration of bacteria into the dentinal tubules. Courtesy of Henry Trowbridge.

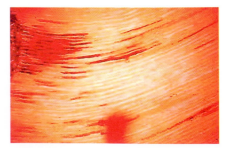

mental influences, can also alter the initial microbiota that may be present in the exposed pulp.

In addition to carious exposures, mechanical exposures probably constitute the other major cause of pulpal infection. Such exposure can be due to removal of thin layers of carious or noncarious dentin, the preparation of teeth for restorative dental procedures, and cracks or trauma. In the case of restorative procedures the inflammation that occurs is associated with the exposure of pulpal connective tissue to a contaminated environment. In addition to the direct contact with bacteria, the mechanical pressures exerted during tooth preparation may force bacteria present in the tubules into the pulp even without frank exposure. This could account for flare-ups well after the initial tooth preparation and the restorative procedures have been completed. Indeed, many kinds of occlusal trauma can lead to pulpal inflammation and the subsequent infection of the pulp by oral bacteria and other organisms leading to pulpal necrosis.

Some of these infections may occur through what has been called the "anachoretic" effect. It is well established that bacteremias can occur as a result of surgical and nonsurgical trauma in the oral cavity. Even chewing in patients with periodontal disease can force bacteria into tissues by simple mastication. These bacteria may circulate briefly in the bloodstream, and if there is an active site of inflammation, the bacteria may accumulate at this location. Although there is some experimental evidence to support this concept, clinically it is difficult to prove. However, there are other avenues that allow oral bacteria and particularly plaque bacteria to gain access to an inflamed pulp more directly.

In patients with periodontal disease, accessory canals on the lateral surfaces of the tooth may become exposed to the plaque bacteria. These organisms can multiply in the canals, resulting in inflammation and necrosis, and eventually the bacteria spread to infect the pulp chamber. Again, proving that this avenue is an important source of infection is problematic, but it remains a very real possibility. Certainly, infection of accessory canals often is a cause of apparent failure of root canal therapy. In addition, it is possible for bacterial plaque associated with periodontal disease to infect adjacent teeth through the apical foramen. It is also possible that bacteria can be forced into the apical foramina of neighboring teeth during surgical procedures. Although it would be expected that such differences in routes of infection might affect the kinds of organisms found, it is obviously very difficult to determine, because at the time of bacterial sampling of an infected canal there is invariably some contamination from oral bacteria.

BACTERIOLOGY OF ROOT CANAL INFECTIONS

Enumerable studies have been conducted in which attempts have been made to define the microbial composition of infected root canals. These are often divided by sampling site: chambers that still contain vital tissue, nonvital teeth, and apical areas. Although investigators have used a variety of techniques in attempts to ensure the integrity of the samples, it was and remains a daunting task. Thus, the data can be compromised by sampling errors as well as the failure of bacterial media to support the growth

TABLE I Bacteria cultivated most frequently in root canal infections

Genus or group	Frequency of isolation (%)
Bacteroides	70
Prevotella	60
Lactobacillus	51
Oral streptococci	41
Clostridium	36
Fusobacterium	33
Propionibacterium	29
Peptostreptococcus	25
Corynebacterium	25
Bifidobacterium	21
Eubacteria	20
Capnocytophaga	17
Actinomyces	16
Leuconostoc	13
Porphyromonas	10
Candida	10
Veillonella	9
Gamella	8
Staphylococcus	7
Aerococcus	5
Saccharomyces	3
Enterococcus	3

of all the organisms that are present in the various lesions. In the early days of bacterial sampling, most of the media employed did not support the growth of strict anaerobic bacteria; the organisms found were mainly those that could survive in the limited quantities of oxygen usually available in these media. Another source of sampling error involved the difficulty in obtaining a representative sample uncontaminated with salivary bacteria, despite efforts to isolate the sampled area from the oral cavity with a rubber dam and other aids. Perhaps a more basic problem was that the samples were incubated in a broth medium before streaking on solid medium to obtain individual isolates. This procedure leads to the selection for growth of the hardiest organisms rather than the spectrum of bacteria that may have been present originally. Thus, it is not surprising that the most frequently found species were the oral streptococci among the gram-positive bacteria, and the hardiest of the gram-negative bacteria that included species of *Neisseria, Bacteroides,* fusobacteria, and coliforms. Spirochetes were often observed in bacterial smears, but at the time these studies were conducted, these strictly anaerobic organisms could not be grown in the laboratory. More recent studies have utilized sampling and growth or genetic detection methods such as PCR, techniques that allow more sensitive detection and enumeration of the species originally present. Table 1 lists the kinds of bacteria that have been cultivated most frequently. Although a number of studies have been published that sought to find relationships between specific species and defined clinical conditions, no acceptable consensus has emerged that is equivalent to pathogenic groupings that have been defined for periodontal diseases (see chapter 12). Indeed, examination of Table 1 indicates the close relationship of endodontic microbiota to other ecological niches within the oral cavity and emphasizes the conclusion that endodontic infections are truly endogenous in nature.

These numbers represent the approximate percentage in which they are found in samples of root canals as collated from several different studies and they should not be taken as more than an approximation. They vary widely in the different studies and not all of the species are found in every instance. In addition, there are other organisms usually found less frequently that may in fact be more important in root canal infections. It is important to understand that just as in other studies of oral bacteria, many organisms that can be observed in microscopic examination of smears taken from the sample will not grow in the laboratory, and there is often a rather large sampling error, i.e., it generally requires the presence of a minimum number of bacteria to initiate growth. Indeed, results of recent studies, in which molecular detection systems were employed, have indicated a relatively high prevalence of spirochetes, particularly *Treponema denticola,* in infected root canals. The virulence properties of many of these organisms are presumably the same as those that are operative in other oral infections, and these factors will exert their effects in both the pulpal and the apical tissues of the tooth. Among these factors are endotoxins and other cell surface toxic components, along with spreading factors such as collagenase, hyaluronidase, and other enzymes that not only break down connective tissues but often are cytotoxic. In addition, the organisms and their products can induce immune reactions that intensify the inflammatory response. Both the kinds of virulence factors and their specific roles in the inflammatory process are described in detail elsewhere in this volume.

The inflammatory changes resulting from whatever cause are the same. As indicated above, endodontic infection is usually initiated in the pulp chamber from where it spreads to the root canals. The inflammation follows the same pathway with end stage of the inflammatory process characterized by pulp necrosis. The necrotic tissue in the canals remains infected and itself becomes the reservoir for the infectious agents. In the absence of treatment that consists principally of debridement, i.e., cleaning the canal with instruments and appropriate irrigating solutions, the bacteria and the accompanying inflammation spread to the apical area where it may develop into either acute or chronic inflammation. In the few studies that have been done, both organisms and virulence factors derived from them have been demonstrated in the apical area. Inflammation of the apex is often accompanied by excruciating pain linked to the confined area in which the accumulating inflammatory exudates and gases exert pressure on the sensitive nerve ending. Most often, the exudates are suppurative (purulent, i.e., containing pus) in nature, consisting of breakdown products of host cells, connective tissue elements, blood elements, and bacteria. Pain relief is obtained by relieving the pressure by providing drainage through the pulp chamber or through incision and drainage into the apical area. In some instances of long-standing chronic infection in the apex, a fistulous tract to the oral cavity that also relieves the pressure is created. One of the interesting microbiological aspects of this type of chronic apical inflammation is the presence of a facultative gram-positive coccus, *Enterococcus faecalis* (which is usually present only in low numbers in some ecological niches within the oral cavity). Although it is not clear why this organism is isolated so frequently in these suppurative infections, often in pure culture, it may be due to its very hardy nature. The organism grows well under a wide variety of harsh environmental conditions including high salt concentrations, both high and low pH, high temperatures (45°C), and the presence of certain heavy metals. It also grows well under both aerobic and anaerobic conditions. In addition, this species often contains numerous plasmids that carry a variety of antibiotic resistance genes, making the organism difficult to treat. Results of recent studies suggest that *E. faecalis* may survive in the dental tubules because of its ability to bind to collagen and thus may act as a nidus of infection even after the canal is sealed. This organism is often isolated from failed root canal treatments. In these cases, it is advisable to actually culture the lesion and determine antibiotic sensitivity during retreatment of the tooth. *E. faecalis* is also frequently found in patients with fatal endocarditis, and its appearance in suppurative exudates, particularly those associated with chronic apical infections, is a challenge for successful treatment.

Another organism that seems to be closely associated with root canal infection is *Porphyromonas endodontalis*. Originally described as a black-pigmented *Bacteroides* species, it is believed to have a pathogenic potential similar to that described for *Porphyromonas gingivalis*. Since its original isolation from root canals, the organism has been found in other ecological niches within the oral cavity, suggesting that its appearance in the root canal again reflects a selective mechanism that allows this opportunist to grow.

Although some investigators believe its presence is closely related to the type of inflammation observed in the infectious process, at present the evidence is merely anecdotal. Suffice it to say, the organism is often found in acute suppurative infections of the root apex. A more recent association of a new species of *Actinomyces (A. radicidentis)* with failed root canal treatment has been reported. All these observations lead to the inescapable conclusion that successful endodontic therapy is dependent on creating a "bacteria-free" environment in the root canal. This brings up two important questions that were alluded to earlier in this chapter, and still plague clinicians. First, how would we confirm the absence of bacteria, and second, if no bacteria can be detected, does this indicate the root canal is sterile?

TO CULTURE OR NOT TO CULTURE

The recognition of the importance of bacteria in the process led to the idea that culturing the canal before proceeding with its obturation could be used as a test for "sterility." This concept was espoused particularly by Louis Grossman of the University of Pennsylvania, one of the pioneers of endodontic therapy who some consider the "father" of modern endodontic practice. He also developed a polyantibiotic paste containing penicillin that was used widely before it became recognized that such applications could lead to allergic complications as well as selection of resistant strains, particularly when applied locally. Standard practice was to debride the canal with a solution of chlorine bleach and hydrogen peroxide as cleansing agents as well as a lubricant, apply the antibiotic paste, and when the patient returned for further treatment, flush the canal to remove as much antibiotic as possible. A paper point was inserted for a specified time to obtain adequate bacterial sample, and the point was transferred to a broth medium that usually contained a small amount of agar to render the medium "microaerophilic" and thus presumably encourage the growth of anaerobes. This standardization of therapy undoubtedly led to a much higher quality of endodontic practice. However, as endodontists became more proficient, the instruments available became more standardized, and our knowledge of oral microbiology much greater, questions were raised about both the basis for this approach and whether culturing the canals actually ensured success.

One of the first questions raised was whether the root canal could actually be "sterilized." Microbiologists correctly pointed out that "sterility, like pregnancy, was an absolute term"; something either is or is not sterile. Obtaining a negative culture does not ensure sterility but means only that no bacterial growth occurred. This could be due to a variety of reasons, including size of the inoculum, i.e., small numbers of bacteria in the sample often did not grow out in broth culture, and the carryover of the antibacterial agent that also could inhibit the growth of the organisms. More recently it has been shown that *E. faecalis* cells may be viable but do not grow when cultured. Perhaps the most important consideration was that the majority of organisms in the root canal were anaerobes that could not grow under the culture conditions used (see above). Thus, obtaining a negative culture was inconclusive. As these concepts became understood, many endodontists realized that in most cases they must have sealed bacteria within the canal. Since the success rate in modern endodontic therapy hovered around 90%, they concluded that the only purpose served by culturing was as a form of "debridement control" that did not guarantee success of root canal therapy. Indeed, several major investigations found that the success rate among cases that were cultured was the same as the rate among those not cultured, provided there was no evidence of active infection before obturation. This evidence consisted of the presence of a serous or suppurative exudate, pain, swelling, and/or fever. Thus, endodontic therapy has become more focused on achieving a thorough debridement of the root canal under aseptic conditions than on attempting to achieve "sterile" canals.

ONE-VISIT ENDODONTICS

In the treatment of vital teeth endodontists employed what was called "one-visit" endodontics. In those cases, since there was no active infection beyond the contamination associated with exposure of the pulp to the oral cavity, clinicians often extirpated the pulp, enlarged the canal, and sealed it in the same visit. Note that, except for location, this approach is identical to the treatment of wounds. In the case of fresh wounds, they are cleansed, the tissue tabs are removed, and if amenable to closure, the wounds are sutured (sealed) at the same time. One-visit endodontics, even in cases of necrotic pulps or chronic pulpitis, evolved as an extension of the one-visit concept for vital teeth.

The key issue in such approaches is thorough debridement of the root canal. If the patient is young, and the tooth has a minimal amount of restoration, access to the canal system and complete debridement can be accomplished and then the root canals may be obturated or sealed. However, there are many additional factors that determine whether the canals can be sealed in a single visit. These constraints include, for example, tooth anatomy, presence of calcifications in the canal, access to the tooth and its canals, patient management, and degree of discomfort.

MICROBIOLOGICAL CONSIDERATIONS FOR OBTURATION

No treatment is more dramatic than the pain relief that is achieved when a patient with a dental-alveolar abscess has the tooth opened for drainage. Through the 1970s, opening the tooth, prescribing antibiotics, and leaving it open for several days before continuing debridement was standard therapy. In such treatment, there was always a risk that superinfection with oral bacteria could occur. However, as it became clear that achieving sterility in the root canal was not a realistic goal, clinicians began to ask whether it would be advantageous to open the tooth, debride and enlarge the canal, prescribe systemic antibiotics, place an antibacterial dressing in the canal, and seal the canal with a temporary cement during the first visit. The major clinical concern was limiting the bacterial contamination that would occur if the canal were left open for drainage. Considering that saliva contains upward of 10^8 bacteria per milliliter and that chewing could act as a pump to force bacteria into the open canal, this was believed to be a potentially serious problem. If the patient experienced only minimal pain and no further suppuration or swelling, permanent obturation could be performed at the next visit. However, if pain is present, the clinician must judge whether it would be more efficacious to leave the tooth open for drainage or to seal a temporary antibacterial medication in the canal. When pain has subsided and there is no overt evidence of infection, temporary closure with an antibacterial agent can again be attempted. The faster the canal is completely debrided, the faster the infection will come under the clinician's control. Indeed, Longman et al. have stated, "The primary treatment of endodontic infections is to establish and maintain surgical drainage and to remove the cause of infection" (L. P. Longman, A. J. Preston, M. V. Martin, and N. H. F. Wilson, *J. Dent.* **28**:539–548, 2000). Certainly, in the case of intractable pain, maintaining drainage in combination with antibiotics is the correct treatment. There have been reports indicating that the failure to provide adequate local drainage in suppurative endodontic infections has resulted in brain abscesses with fatal outcomes. It should be kept in mind that in the treatment of abscesses in other areas of the body, including the gastrointestinal tract, the antibiotic is considered as an adjunct to the surgical drainage that is deemed essential for successful treatment. The problem with many studies that have attempted to evaluate objectively whether healing in root canal therapy is retarded or aided by allowing drainage to occur is that there really are no good objective criteria by which to evaluate healing. Certainly persistent pain is an indication for continuing to obtain drainage, but true endodontic success can only be measured after a sufficient time to allow apical healing. In some patients this can be measured in months; others may take much longer. Thus, determination of when and how much drainage is necessary for a specific case depends almost totally on clinical acumen developed in practice and truly reflects part of the art of the practice of dentistry.

ANTIBACTERIAL AGENTS USED IN ENDODONTICS

As indicated above, Grossman was among the first to use a combination of hydrogen peroxide and sodium hypochlorite (chlorine bleach) to irrigate the canal during debridement. These solutions were washed out with water. Following the debridement, Grossman placed a polyantibiotic paste containing penicillin in root canals. Although this mixture was efficacious, with increasing understanding of the properties of antibiotics and the hazards when antibiotics are used for local applications, clinicians sought a more general type of antibacterial agent. The phenolic disinfectants were also used as aids in debriding the root canals. Indeed, dentists had been using similar agents long before the advent of antibiotics. Camphorated derivatives of these compounds were believed to be less toxic. Nonetheless, these preparations were sufficiently toxic for host tissues to outweigh their usefulness as antibacterial agents in root canal therapy and thus most clinicians have discarded them today. The same is true for the formaldehyde preparations that have been used for "sterilizing" root canals, although there is a group of practitioners who still advocate the idea of "pulp mummification" (Sargenti method) using formaldehyde, or in essence "pickling" the residual pulp or necrotic tissue, much as is done with preserving tissues for histological study. For a variety of reasons beyond the scope of this text, this method is not approved for use by any dental school in the United States.

Calcium hydroxide has become the drug of choice as antibacterial agent for temporary seals. It is usually prepared as a water paste because the compound is insoluble and therefore the concentration of hydroxyl ions is low, but nevertheless the solution is highly alkaline without being caustic. Over time the alkalinity of the calcium hydroxide is toxic to most bacteria, even *E. faecalis*. The compound appears to be well tolerated by host tissues and has been used for years in pulp capping, in which it appears to stimulate the formation of secondary dentin over an exposed pulp. Calcium hydroxide also appears to inactivate bacterial endotoxins, although the mechanism has not been elucidated. Results of animal studies have shown that endotoxins are found within infected canals and cause inflammatory reactions in the surrounding tissues.

FOCAL INFECTION TODAY

In recent years there has been a resurgence of the idea of focal infection, although it has taken on new perspectives. Chapter 16 describes in detail the various mechanisms and diseases and the epidemiological evidence that associates these diseases with "focal infection." Results of epidemiological studies suggest that patients with periodontal disease show a higher frequency of coronary artery disease. Bacterial culture of atheromatous plaques indicated the presence of oral bacteria, suggesting that bacteremias created from oral foci could deposit bacteria directly on coronary vessels or in plaque already present. Subsequently, it was shown that certain oral microbes can adhere to and invade endothelial cells. Results of additional studies suggest that periodontal disease could also be related to preterm labor and low birth weight of babies. Results of recent epidemiological studies have also suggested that endodontic foci may be the source of similar depositions of oral bacteria. Despite this epidemiological evidence, however, there are still many investigators and cardiologists who are skeptical that the currently available data are sufficiently robust to implicate oral infections as important mechanisms of coronary artery disease or preterm labor and low-birth-weight babies. If a true association is eventually demonstrated, both the medical and dental professions will have to pay more attention to dental health as a source of serious cardiovascular disease.

SUMMARY

It is clear that bacterial infection is the major cause of endodontic pathology. It is equally clear that just as in the other major infections of the oral cavity, i.e., dental caries and periodontal disease, the bacterial microbiota involved is complex. Indeed, the spectrum of bacterial species associated with root canal and apical infections is similar to those associated with the latter diseases. The question remains whether there are specific pathogens or even specific virulence factors that make the root canal or apical area more likely to experience severe symptoms. As indicated, numerous studies have been conducted in an attempt to resolve these issues, but as yet the evidence is still rather soft. However, *E. faecalis* does stand out in terms of the number of studies and the frequency in which it is found in both pure and mixed cultures of chronic and acute dental alveolar abscesses. As indicated above, this may not be because it possesses potent virulence factors but because of its resistance to environmental stress and antibiotics. Thus, it is evident that just as successful treatment of wound infection requires careful debridement before closure, so too success in endodontics requires meticulous attention to cleaning and preparation of the canals before sealing.

KEY POINTS

Root canal infections are usually caused by contamination of the endodontic tissues by oral bacteria (endogenous infections).

Although these bacteria are usually of low virulence, i.e., noninvasive, occasionally more virulent organisms such as *E. faecalis* infect the canal. This organism is particularly difficult to eliminate because it is resistant to many antibiotics and can survive at high pH and salt concentrations.

Occasionally, specific organisms have been identified with root canal infections, e.g., *A. radicidentis* and *P. endodontalis*.

Root canals cannot be "sterilized," since the complete absence of viable organisms is impossible to obtain in this environment. Thus, though useful, particularly for the neophyte, a negative culture does not guarantee success of treatment.

Treatment of endodontic infections is directed at debriding the canal thoroughly before sealing it. This treatment is analogous to the treatment of wound infections, i.e., debridement followed by closure.

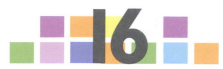

16

Systemic Disease and the Oral Microbiota

Susan Camp, Yu Lei, Massimo Costalonga, Yongshu Zhang, Alexandre Zaia, Reka Vajna, Karen F. Ross, and Mark C. Herzberg

INTRODUCTION

The oral microbiota comprises species that span the continuum from commensal to pathogenic. The pathogens are best known for their ability to cause infections that are normally limited to the oral cavity, including dental caries and periodontitis. However, when these organisms or their components enter the circulation or connective tissues or encounter the mucosal immune system, they may be linked to the occurrence of systemic disease. A strong causal association has been suggested for oral bacteria in the systemic diseases infective endocarditis and disseminated intravascular coagulation (DIC). Both are life-threatening diseases. Oral microorganisms have also been associated with pathogenic mechanisms in nephritis, rheumatoid arthritis, and Behçet's disease. In some epidemiological studies, oral infections, such as periodontal diseases, have been associated with the occurrence of diverse diseases such as atherosclerosis and preterm low-birth-weight infants. Principles of entry from the oral cavity into the systemic compartment, systemic dissemination of microbes, and subsequent host responses that have been learned from molecular, animal, and human studies of infective endocarditis may be applicable to other systemic infections. This chapter explores the underlying biological plausibility that oral microbes may contribute more generally to systemic disease.

ROUTES FROM ORAL TO SYSTEMIC COMPARTMENTS

Breaches in the Oral Mucosa

Oral microbes reside in saliva and dental plaque, and on and within the mucous membranes and epithelium of the gingival crevice. Oral microorganisms enter systemic compartments when dental procedures or injuries, or infections of the oral soft tissues, create a breach. For example, in healthy individuals, certain microbes from dental plaque may promote ulcerative lesions in the gingival crevicular epithelium. Through these ulcerative lesions, personal oral hygiene procedures can inoculate dental plaque bacteria into the circulation, resulting in bacteremias. Similarly, ulcerative lesions form on the mucous membranes (mucositis) in immunocompromised individuals. Through these breaches in mucosal integrity, oral commensals enter the blood, resulting in polymicrobial bacteremias, fungemia, and viremia.

Transport and Translocation of Microbes

Oral microbes can also enter the systemic compartment when processed and transported by the mucosal immune system. Prominent in the oral cavity and the intestines, the mucosal immune system provides surveillance against ingested environmental pathogens. Continuously swallowed at 10^5 cells per milliliter of saliva per minute, oral microbes can interface with the systemic compartment in the intestines, or "gut." In the gut, particulate and soluble antigens are processed in the Peyer's patches, which can result in stimulation or suppression of a systemic antigen-specific immune response. Proximal to the Peyer's patches, the M cells can translocate whole bacteria from the intestinal lumen to specialized phagocytic cells on the systemic side. These bacteria can then be processed, regulating an antigen-specific systemic immune response. The mucosal immune system therefore facilitates entry of whole or processed microbes into the systemic compartment as part of a mechanism to foster systemic defense.

THE POTENTIAL OF COMMENSALS TO BEHAVE AS PATHOGENS

Several hundred species of bacteria reside in the oral cavity. Most are benign, causing no known disease in the mouth and surrounding tissues and coexisting peacefully with the host as commensals. When these bacteria enter the blood and other systemic compartments, the constitutively expressed genes may be sufficient to engender pathogenicity, for example, with an organism like *Streptococcus sanguinis* (formerly *S. sanguis*). In 1948, the eminent microbiologist Theodor Rosebury, working at Columbia University, identified oral streptoccci as "endogenous pathogens," able to cause disease in a nonnative environment. Whether oral bacteria rely solely on constitutively expressed genes to cause disease in nonnative compartments is less clear.

Microbial virulence can change as new environmental stressors influence the pattern of expressed genes. Indeed, upon transition to a new environment, survival may require the regulated expression of genes. In some cases, expression of environmentally regulated genes may increase pathogenic potential or cause a harmless commensal to behave as a pathogen. To ensure survival in a foreign environment, benign commensal bacteria may be genetically programmed to become virulent.

Conventional wisdom holds that most bacteremias, viremias, and fungemias originating from oral foci are cleared uneventfully by the reticuloendothelial system, suggesting that their virulence in systemic compartments is insufficient to overcome the antimicrobial defenses of a healthy host. To survive in a nonoral environment, the oral bacteria typically locate in a hospitable niche in an abnormal or injured anatomic site, or an immunocompromised host. Consequently, oral microorganisms often cause systemic opportunistic infections by colonizing abnormal anatomic sites, such as damaged heart valves, or by avoiding immune recognition and clearance in immunodeficient individuals. Hence the association of oral microbiota with systemic diseases would often require the coincidence of transient bacteremias and underlying anatomical abnormalities and immunodeficiency. Alternatively, oral microbial infections of healthy cells and tissues in the systemic compartment could cause subclinical pathology or superimpose secondarily on other subclinical disease. Oral bacteria, such as *S. sanguinis*, *Streptococcus oralis*, *Streptococcus mutans*, and *Streptococcus salivarius*, have been isolated from foreign anatomic locations in systemic infections. Given these several scenarios, the precise mechanisms by which oral bacteria become virulent and capable of causing disease upon infection of other organs and tissues remain unclear.

Microbial Chameleons: Changing Gene Expression in Response to Environmental Signals

To adapt to changing ecological niches, bacteria have evolved the capacity to change profiles of expressed genes. Environmentally regulated genes are modulated by intracellular signaling pathways "activated" when bacteria "sense" environmental signals using biochemically specific receptors. Altered expression of some genes may increase virulence and pathogenicity of bacteria.

Gene expression in oral bacteria is regulated by many factors including changes in pH, oxygen level, ion concentrations, carbohydrate source, osmolarity, temperature, and access to protein substrates (Fig. 1). When oral bacteria gain access to the blood or other tissues, the new environment is dramatically different from the oral cavity. For example, most sites in the mouth are slightly acidic with a pH near 6. In dental plaque, the pH can dip below 5.0. However, in blood and other tissue fluids, pH is near neutral, about 7.4. At pH 6.5 to 7.0, oral streptococci release a histone-like protein (HlpA) into the medium. Release is not observed at or below pH 6.0. HlpA can complex with soluble lipoteichoic acid. When recognized by specific antibodies, the resulting immune complex may promote inflammation and increase the pathogenicity of the bacteria.

Other genes regulated by changes in environmental pH may also change oral bacterial virulence. When pH increases from 6.2 to 7.3, *Streptococcus gordonii* upregulates expression of *msrA*, which encodes the enzyme methionine sulfoxide reductase. Methionine sulfoxide reductase protects organisms against oxidative damage and has potential roles in bacterial multiplication, stress resistance, and survival. As the oral streptococci accommodate to a more alkaline environment and respond to host proteins, the spectrum of expressed proteases also changes. Upon pH elevation from 5.5 to 7.5, the oral streptococci increase expression of thrombin-like activity. Since thrombin promotes polymerization of fibrinogen into fibrin and triggers platelet aggregation, oral streptococci exposed to an alkaline shift in pH may become increasingly thrombogenic. Thrombogenicity of oral streptococci may facilitate infection and lesion formation on damaged heart valves during infective endocarditis.

Still other environmental factors change bacterial gene expression. For example, extracellular matrix proteins become available to oral streptococci that have infected damaged heart valves. When exposed to the extracellular matrix proteins laminin and collagen, oral streptococci express new or modified proteins. A laminin-binding protein from *S. gordonii* is up-regulated in the presence of laminin, increasing bacterial adhesion to the injured valve

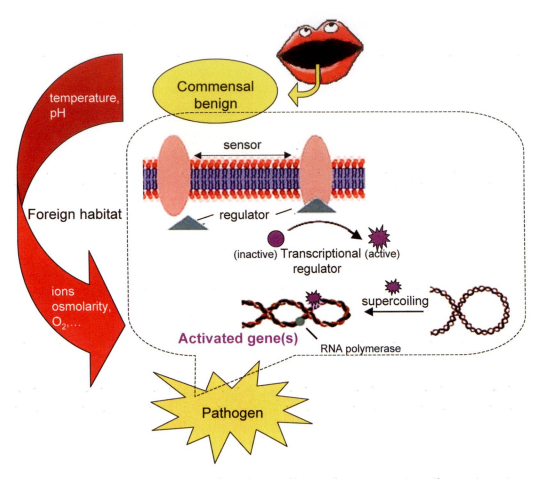

FIGURE I Environmental regulation of bacterial gene expression. Changes in environmental stressors such as temperature, pH, ion concentration, osmolarity, oxygen tension, and metabolic substrate can regulate bacterial gene expression.

surface. Consistent with a regulated virulence factor, the streptococcal laminin-binding protein is a major serum antigen in patients with infective endocarditis, in contrast to patients with noninfected valvulopathies. On its cell wall, *S. sanguinis* expresses a platelet aggregation-associated protein (PAAP), which enables the bacteria to induce platelet aggregation. When isolated from *S. sanguinis* cells, PAAP cannot induce platelet aggregation. In contrast, isolated, cell-free PAAP from cells grown with type I collagen can induce platelet aggregation, and hence the *S. sanguinis* cells may be more thrombogenic. Since platelet aggregation is pivotal to the development of valvular vegetations in infective endocarditis, altered expression of PAAP may reflect environmentally regulated pathogenicity.

How can we learn if specific genes are expressed in selective environments? As discussed in chapter 8, several approaches have been developed to identify genes expressed in vivo but not in vitro. In vivo expression technology uses a mutational library of a randomly inserted promoterless reporter gene to identify genes induced by an upstream promoter in a specific environment. Signature-tagged mutagenesis uses comparative hybridization to isolate mutants unable to survive in specified environmental conditions. An in vivo expression technology mutational library of *S. gordonii* has been used in an animal model of infective endocarditis. In experimental endocarditis, genes found to be induced by *S. gordonii* infecting heart valves include *msrA*. Up-regulation of *msrA* during infective endocarditis is consistent with a shift in environmental pH from acidic to neutral.

Whether oral bacteria alter expression of a unique set of genes in response to changes in pH, or whether other environmental stressors induce a similar set of genes, remains unclear. Certainly the expression of some virulence genes appears to be globally regulated. For example, a common stimulus-response coupling mechanism in bacteria is a two-component system. Environmental stress signals are "sensed" by a sensor histidine kinase and transduced into the cell by a cognate response regulator protein (Fig. 2). Most sensor histidine kinases are membrane proteins with an N-terminal transmembrane region and an independent C-terminal autokinase domain. However, most response regulators are cytosolic proteins containing an N-terminal receiver domain and a C-terminal effector domain with transcription factor activity. The periplasmic domain of a sensor histidine kinase can bind directly with extracellular signals. Binding of a specific extracellular stress signal results in autophosphorylation of a conserved histidine residue on the kinase. Next, the autokinase domain of the sensor transfers a phosphate moiety to an aspartate residue on the receiver domain of the cognate regulator. The regulator may control this phosphoryl transfer reaction. Phosphorylation activates the effector domain of the regulator. Activation of the regulator can then turn on or turn off specifically targeted genes and

FIGURE 2 The typical two-component system. A transmembrane protein sensor binds to an extracellular signal via its N-terminal region, resulting in autophosphorylation of a histidine in the C-terminal kinase. The N terminus of the specific cytosolic response regulator is the target of phosphoryl transfer. This activates the regulator's C-terminal domain, and the specific target gene is activated or deactivated.

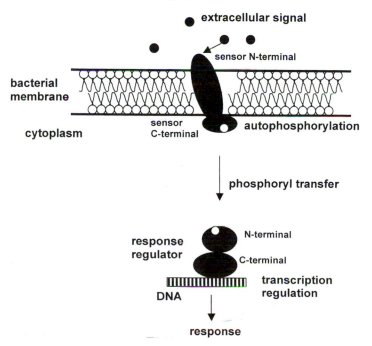

trigger the corresponding response pathway. Many sensor kinases also have phosphatase activity and can dephosphorylate regulators, particularly in absence of the signal. In this way, a sensor and its mated regulator can coordinate their behaviors during signal transduction.

Another response to environmental signals involves changes in DNA topology, which makes the promoter region of target genes accessible to transcriptional regulators. As a result, environmental stresses can activate previously inactive virulence genes. *Escherichia coli* regulates pilus expression by a flip-flopping on-off genetic switch. The promoter for the pilus gene is a spontaneously invertible segment of the chromosome. Under colonizing conditions, the promoter segment flips to produce piliated organisms, which can stick to the mannose molecules on the surface of epithelial cells, increasing virulence.

Clearly, altered expression of genes modifies the behaviors of bacteria to fit various environmental conditions. Differential gene expression can be anticipated to be widespread among the oral bacteria. For example, the anaerobic periodontal pathogen *Porphyromonas gingivalis* regulates expression of its major fimbrial adhesin in response to temperature. Moreover, the organism regulates expression (both up and down) of almost 500 proteins when exposed to host epithelial cells. As we learn to model environmentally specific stressors and identify specific and globally regulated genes, we may be able to explain better how oral microbes behave as endogenous pathogens.

HOST DEFENSES

Microorganisms have evolved many mechanisms to adapt to changing environmental conditions, but the host is not defenseless. Since the antigenic load within the oral cavity is large, the mucous membranes have evolved to distinguish between pathogenic and commensal microorganisms, and food molecules. The squamous epithelial cells and resident intraepithelial and lamina propria immune cells form a sophisticated system of pathogen recognition, barrier protection, and immune response.

When microorganisms enter the mouth, they encounter a number of nonspecific defense mechanisms that help prevent them from binding to and penetrating the oral mucosa (see chapter 10). Saliva has a flushing effect, physically removing microbes to the gut by swallowing. Saliva contains a supply of nonimmune and immune factors, including mucin glycoproteins and salivary agglutinin, which bind and clear bacteria more efficiently by swallowing. A mucinous salivary film coats the oral soft and hard tissue surfaces. Constituents of the film may form a protective coating, including blockade of epithelial cell receptors for bacterial adhesion and invasion.

Saliva contains antimicrobial peptides such as histatins, lysozyme, and lactoferrin. Other antimicrobial peptides are released into the saliva by epithelial cells and neutrophils. The epithelial- and neutrophil-derived antimicrobial peptides are present in higher concentrations on the mucosal surfaces, where they may be most active. Examples of these innate immune molecules include the defensins, which protect against harmful colonization by a wide variety of microorganisms. In the oral cavity, keratinocytes also express an antimicrobial protein, calprotectin, which appears to protect oropharyngeal mucosa from colonization by highly invasive pathogens such as *Candida albicans, Listeria monocytogenes,* and *P. gingivalis.*

The mucosal epithelium also protects the underlying connective tissues against microbial entry by forming a tight and strong physical barrier. The keratins cornify as cells mature, making an abrasion-resistant epithelium. As the superficial cells bind microbes, the keratin-rich mucosal surface cells are shed by desquamation and replaced by cells from underlying layers. The extensive innate antimicrobial mechanism notwithstanding, superficial mucosal keratinocytes contain oral bacteria that have invaded. By shedding the mature superficial cells, the mucosa limits colonization and invasion by pathogenic microorganisms. Furthermore, mucosal epithelial cells restrict access of microbes from the oral cavity to the connective tissues by forming intercellular attachments. Keratinocytes attach to one another with specialized intercellular junctions, which prevent passage of water, solutes, and surface microbes between the oral cavity and interior tissue compartments. Healthy mucosal epithelium tends to protect against intercellular passage and transcytosis of microbes. Invasive pathogens cannot penetrate deeper into the tissue.

If the infectious agent manages to penetrate the mucosal surface and invade the epithelium, the damaged cells secrete interleukin-1 (IL-1), IL-6, IL-8, and macrophage chemoattractant protein (MCP-1). These cytokines recruit phagocytic cells to the site of bacterial invasion. Blood monocytes, neutrophils, tissue macrophages, dendritic cells, and Langerhans cells internalize (phagocytose), kill, and digest whole microorganisms, protecting the underlying tissues by creating a phagocytic barrier against further microbial invasion. These phagocytes of the innate immune system react to a wide variety of pathogens without requiring prior sensitization.

How do mucosal keratinocytes recognize infectious agents? Microbes express certain highly conserved molecular structures that are distinct from self (the host). The innate immune system recognizes these pathogen-associated molecular patterns (PAMPs). For example, the general structure of lipopolysaccharide (LPS) is common to all gram-negative bacteria. Recognition of LPS by a host cell receptor would allow any gram-negative bacteria to be detected. In addition to LPS, common PAMPs include peptidoglycan, lipoteichoic acid, mannans, bacterial DNA, double-stranded RNA, and glucans. These patterns are recognized by host cell pattern recognition receptors expressed by the phagocytic cells and other cells of the innate immune system. Pattern recognition receptors include CD14, mannose receptor, DEC205, and molecules of the Toll-like receptor (TLR) family. Binding of these receptors with a PAMP directly induces the expression of inflammatory cytokines, especially IL-1, IL-6, and tumor necrosis factor alpha (TNF-α), to alert the host to the presence of infection. These soluble signals then recruit and activate antigen-specific lymphocytes and initiate an adaptive immune response.

Gingival keratinocytes express proinflammatory cytokines in response to LPS and other PAMPs by signaling through TLRs. The TLRs are up-regulated by interferon-γ, another cytokine, increasing the response to PAMPs. Unlike leukocytes and dermal keratinocytes, gingival keratinocytes do not appear to express CD14, nor does saliva appear to contain sufficient LPS-binding protein to serve as a required cofactor for CD14-mediated

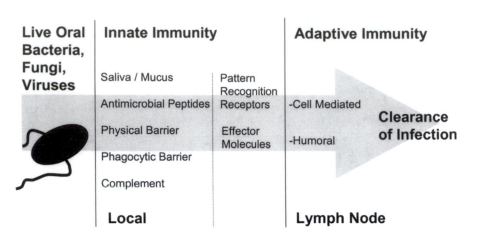

FIGURE 3 Levels of protection against systemic infection by oral microbes. A local innate immune response helps contain the infection and delivers the antigen to local lymph nodes, leading to initiation of adaptive immunity and clearance of infection.

signaling and cytokine expression. Hence gingival keratinocytes probably respond to microorganisms through TLRs and not CD14.

Together the innate and adaptive immune systems interact and cooperate to produce an effective response against foreign invaders. Host defenses are summarized in Fig. 3.

SYSTEMIC DISEASES ASSOCIATED WITH ORAL MICROBES

Infective Endocarditis

Perhaps the best-known example of a systemic infection that can be caused by oral bacteria is infective endocarditis. This is a disease of injured or abnormal heart valves, which are typically asymptomatic until infection, often by oral streptococci. Infections of the oral tissues such as periodontitis and periapical abscesses allow entry and dissemination of a mixture of oral pathogens and commensal bacteria by way of the circulating blood. These polymicrobial bacteremias may occur spontaneously during innocent activities such as routine oral hygiene, or can result from invasive dental procedures. Once in the blood, even organisms that are harmless in the oral cavity can behave as pathogens and infect susceptible heart valves.

The valves and endocardial tissues at risk of infection are abnormal, generally because of earlier disease, injury, or developmental abnormality. Conditions creating risk of infective endocarditis include rheumatic fever with heart valve damage, prior heart valve surgery, mitral valve insufficiency with regurgitation, or use of intravenous narcotics or diet drugs such as "fen-phen." As a consequence of these conditions, the valvular endothelium can slough. On the denuded valve, underlying connective tissues are exposed and circulating platelets are activated to repair the wound (Fig. 4). Platelets adhere and spread on the exposed connective tissues.

The adherent platelets and exposed connective tissues bind bacteria, usually commensal oral streptococci, during polymicrobial bacteremias. In this new environment certain streptococci induce platelets to bind fibrinogen, aggregate, and form a thrombus or platelet clot (Fig. 4). These

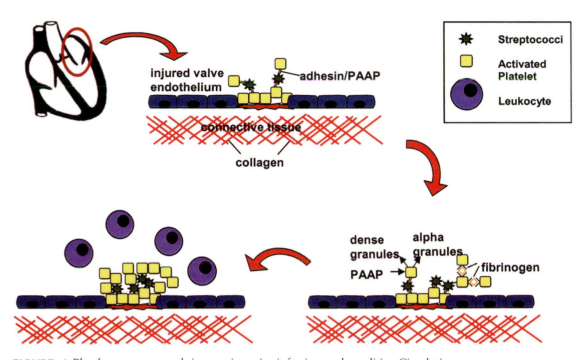

FIGURE 4 Platelet streptococcal interactions in infective endocarditis. Circulating platelets adhere to collagen exposed on damaged heart valves. During polymicrobial bacteremia, oral streptococci bind to the activated adherent platelets through expressed adhesins and PAAP. PAAP activates and induces additional platelets to aggregate on the heart valve. Aggregation requires the cross-linking of platelets to one another by fibrinogen molecules. The fibrinogen molecules are polymerized into fibrin by thrombin, forming an insoluble thrombus or platelet clot. Released platelet granules contain innate antimicrobials, including platelet microbicidal protein, which may limit the valvular infection by sensitive bacteria. Leukocytes accumulate on the exterior of the septic thrombus as an inflammatory response is initiated.

streptococci express PAAP. Near the forming septic valvular thrombus, damaged endothelial cells and activated mononuclear cells express tissue factor in response to LPS from gram-negative bacteria, which are also present in the blood during polymicrobial bacteremias. Tissue factor activates the coagulation cascade, a major pathway promoting the polymerization of clot-forming fibrin. The mass of microorganisms, platelets, and fibrin on diseased or injured heart valves or other endocardial surfaces constitutes a vegetation, which is characteristic of infective endocarditis. Protected from the immune system within the vegetation, the infections expand as the bacterial colonies grow. In this nonnative changing environment, the streptococci shift from commensal into pathogenic microorganisms by environmental regulation of gene expression.

The vegetation itself is significant to the outcome of infective endocarditis. Shielded within a thrombus-like mass of platelets and fibrin on the heart valve, the colonizing bacteria resist the action of the adaptive immune system and antibiotic therapy. Some infections may resolve if the infecting bacteria are sensitive to platelet microbicidal protein, an innate antibacterial defense protein released by activated platelets. If the colonizing bacteria are resistant to platelet microbicidal protein, the infection can prove intractable. Without treatment, infective endocarditis can lead to valvular insufficiency. With septic embolization, infection and infarction of other organs can result in loss of function, and mortality can approach 100%. Consequently, health care professionals are advised by the American Heart Association and other agencies internationally to reduce the risk of infective endocarditis among dental patients at risk by prescribing specific antibiotic prophylaxis regimens before performing procedures that induce bacteremia.

Disseminated Intravascular Coagulation

In immunocompromised individuals, alpha-hemolytic oral streptococci cause DIC. DIC associated with alpha-hemolytic streptococci is a major cause of mortality in pharmacologically immunosuppressed individuals awaiting organ transplantation. As with infective endocarditis, oral streptococci must gain access into the systemic compartment to cause DIC. In DIC in the immunocompromised, the most common portal of entry is the painful, erosive lesions of the oral and oropharyngeal mucous membranes known as mucositis. After translocating through the mucous membranes, the oral microbes induce disseminated activation of the coagulation cascade. Fibrin becomes deposited in capillary beds and in small blood vessels, occluding the flow of blood to the major organs and tissues. If occlusion is prolonged, tissue and organ ischemia and infarction can result. With alpha-streptococci, DIC is usually not accompanied by febrile illness, and the clinical outcome is often fatal. DIC and infective endocarditis illustrate the potential of otherwise benign oral, commensal streptococci to cause life-threatening disease in susceptible individuals.

OTHER POSSIBLE ASSOCIATIONS BETWEEN ORAL MICROBES AND SYSTEMIC DISEASE

Heat Shock Proteins

Molecular mimicry is among the most intriguing mechanisms whereby commensal bacteria may contribute to systemic disease. Bacteria, fungi, and mammalian hosts express the family of heat shock proteins (HSPs). These proteins are highly conserved, showing nearly identical primary amino acid sequences across species. In humans, some heat shock proteins are cryptic, hidden from the view of the adaptive immune system. For example, HSP60 resides in mitochondria and is normally shielded from host immune surveillance. Consequently, the mammalian immune system considers HSP60 to be foreign. Upon exposure to HSP60, an immune response is initiated. Microbes that express HSP60 homologues, therefore, may trigger an autoimmune response upon infection.

HSPs are found in microorganisms and host cells during normal growth. Cellular expression increases in response to heat shock and other stressors. HSP60, HSP70, and HSP90 are the most significant HSP families. During heat shock and other stresses, newly synthesized proteins tend to unfold, complex, and become insoluble. After protein synthesis and translocation of proteins into intracellular compartments, HSPs bind or chaperone new unfolded or partially folded proteins. Chaperoned, newly synthesized proteins retain their native conformation and are protected against complexing into unwanted, insoluble globular aggregates.

Molecular chaperones, therefore, form a wax paper-like protein layer to ensure that proteins destined for export will be able to assume a fully functional shape.

The structural similarity between HSPs of prokaryotic and eukaryotic origins is remarkable. Indeed, the host adaptive immune system may not distinguish between host and foreign HSP antigens. Human HSP60 expressed during normal growth is highly homologous to bacterial HSPs such as *Mycobacterium* HSP65, *S. sanguinis* HSP65, and *Helicobacter pylori* HSP60. Antibodies elicited by a bacterial HSP will generally cross-react with the others and with the human orthologue. During bacteremia, HSP concentrations increase in the blood. The presence of small amounts of bacterial HSPs induces low titers of anti-HSP antibodies. Anti-HSP antibodies apparently produced against gram-negative bacteria can be detected in serum and gingival crevicular fluid of dental patients. Antibodies to bacterial HSPs cross-react and block human HSP60 when accessible.

Oral bacterial HSP antigens eliciting antibodies that react with self- or foreign HSPs will form immune complexes. Immune complexes will then activate the complement cascade. Anti-HSP antibodies in the blood and gingival crevicular fluid are associated with inflammation in the periodontal tissues. By reacting with cross-reactive self-antigens, therefore, immune complexes can form and deposit in different tissues of the body and contribute to systemic inflammation. The accumulation of immune complexes and activation of the complement system suggest a role for HSPs in some systemic diseases, including Behçet's disease, which is a syndrome of immune-mediated ulcers and eruptions of the mucous membranes of the eye, genitals, and oral cavity of young adult males.

In summary, HSP-specific antibodies produced in response to a localized increase in oral bacterial HSPs may gain access to the circulation. Antibodies against oral microbial HSPs can cross-react with self-HSP antigens. Immune complexes form, activating the complement system. If deposited in the arterial wall (atherogenesis), joints (arthritis), or the mucous membranes (Behçet's disease), HSP mimicry can contribute to systemic disease.

Autorecognition Induced by Oral Microorganisms

In the epithelium of inductive sites such as the tonsils or the junctional epithelium, oral microorganisms interact with immune cells to activate antigen-specific T cells. Microbes can express antigens that mimic endogenous or "self" structural proteins. When presented to the mucosal or systemic immune system, these molecular mimics stimulate the naturally anergic T cells specific for the self-proteins and induce T-cell activation. These activated T cells recirculate, not only between the blood and the lymphoid organs, but also through peripheral tissues. In the peripheral tissues, activated T cells can encounter these same self-antigens and initiate autoimmune recognition.

S. sanguinis, for instance, can enter the blood periodically through breaches in the dentogingival junction or the oral mucosa. Some *S. sanguinis* strains express a collagen-like epitope within the PAAP. The PAAP epitope is partially homologous to the arthritogenic epitope of type II collagen. In rodents, primates, and patients with rheumatoid arthritis, type

II collagen is a candidate antigen in autorecognition. *S. sanguinis* does not appear to activate naïve type II collagen-specific T cells but can stimulate primed type II collagen-specific T cells in vitro. In a murine arthritis model, *S. sanguinis* infection exacerbates arthritis in type II collagen-primed mice. PAAP+ *S. sanguinis*, therefore, can activate memory T cells specific for type II collagen in vitro. In susceptible mice, PAAP+ *S. sanguinis* exacerbates type II collagen-induced autoimmune arthritis.

On the other hand, mucosal exposure of PAAP+ *S. sanguinis* to arthritis-susceptible neonatal mice (strain DBA/1J) inhibited the development of autoimmune arthritis in the adult. These results suggest that commensal bacteria can induce oral tolerance early in life and that the same bacteria can trigger autorecognition when memory autoreactive T-cell clones are already present. To extrapolate from these conclusions to rheumatoid arthritis-susceptible individuals, early colonization of newborns and infants by PAAP+ *S. sanguinis* strains may be protective. Colonization or infection later in development could exacerbate arthritic episodes.

The oral microbial environment can also interfere with the adaptive immune response by activating a large number of T cells independently of their specificities. Some streptococcal molecules have superantigen-like function. The result is a polyclonal activation of CD4+ T cells. Superantigens subvert the ordered T-cell response by nonspecifically activating T cells. The lymph nodes clog with the high density of proliferating T cells, which lack the specificities needed to direct B cells toward an efficient antibody response. The large ulcerative lesions seen in the oral mucosa of patients with Behçet's disease appear to result from local polyclonal activation of T cells by oral streptococcal superantigen-like molecules. Some nonspecifically activated T cells activate specific B cells. When superantigens activate T cells that are specific for local self-antigens or HSPs, the activated T-helper cells can direct the production of autoantibodies and cytotoxic T cells. If directed against HSPs, autoantibodies and cytotoxic T cells may destroy HSP-expressing epithelial cells. The presence of bacterial superantigens may augment the self-directed immune response to destroy the epithelial layer, creating the painful ulcer seen in the oral cavity of patients with Behçet's disease.

Inflammation—a Link between Local Dental Disease and Systemic Pathology?

Oral infections have come under scrutiny as possible risk factors for systemic conditions such as cardiovascular disease, cerebrovascular events, and preterm low-birth-weight infants. Several epidemiological studies show that there is an association between dental health and cardiovascular disease. Those with the worst dental health were most likely to have cardiovascular disease. This association is apparent in both retrospective and case-control studies and is specific for periodontal disease, not dental caries.

Periodontal disease is characterized by repeated episodes of inflammation. The predominant bacteria associated with periodontal disease (*P. gingivalis*, *Tannerella forsythensis*, *Actinobacillus actinomycetemcomitans*, and *Treponema denticola*) have LPS in their cell walls. Bacterial toxins including LPS diffuse into ulcerated gingival tissue in the gingival sulcus. Monocytes are among the early immune cells that react to this local presence of bacteria. LPS is an especially potent activator of monocytes/macrophages, which respond by secreting soluble mediators of inflammation, TNF-α and IL-1β. When activated, monocytes also release prostaglandin E_2 (PGE_2), an arachidonic acid metabolite, which promotes vasodilation of the local microvasculature, adding to the inflammation. Locally, IL-1β and TNF-α increase cellular adhesion molecule expression by endothelial cells, which facilitates binding of neutrophils to the vessel wall before extravasation into the affected tissues. When local concentrations of IL-1β and TNF-α are high, these soluble mediators can enter the circulatory system. IL-1β and TNF-α induce the liver to produce acute reactants, including C-reactive protein (CRP) (Fig. 5).

CRP binds specifically to C-polysaccharide, a membrane component of bacteria and fungi, and acts as an opsonin, promoting phagocytosis by macrophages. CRP also binds to damaged cells and complexed CRP can activate complement. When stimulated by CRP, macrophages produce tissue factor, an initiator of coagulation. Elevated serum CRP is a normal occurrence during the body's response to infection and inflammation. Levels return to normal as the infection is cleared, so serum CRP can be used as a marker of infection or inflammation. In healthy subjects at risk for cardiovascular disease, those with high serum CRP levels were more likely to develop cardiovascular disease. Interestingly, it has been reported that periodontal patients have higher serum CRP levels than periodontally healthy patients.

There is increasing evidence that inflammatory events contribute to atherogenesis and cardiovascular disease. Monocytes which have infiltrated the blood vessel intima and taken up lipids (cholesterol) play a critical role in the formation of atherosclerotic plaques. In the presence of IL-1β and TNF-α, these monocytes may be induced to ingest more lipid and to continue to secrete inflammatory cytokines. IL-1β can also promote smooth muscle cell proliferation, which may be responsible for thickening of the vessel wall associated with the atherosclerotic lesion.

Periodontal microorganisms may contribute to the proinflammatory infectious load created by other chronic infectious organisms such as *Chlamydia pneumoniae* and cytomegalovirus, which are often associated with atherosclerotic plaques. These organisms are endemic in otherwise healthy populations, potentially adding to systemic pathogen burden. Among the endemic periodontal microbiota, *P. gingivalis* has been detected in specimens of human atherosclerotic plaques. Known to invade and induce expression of proinflammatory cytokines by endothelial cells in culture, *P. gingivalis* may also challenge the health and integrity of the endothelial lining of blood vessels by modulating the expression of cellular adhesion proteins. If it gains entry to the subendothelial myointima, *P. gingivalis* may also induce formation of lipid-filled foam cells from macrophages. The formation of foam cells in vitro simulates a key step in atherogenesis. Finally, like *S. sanguinis* and certain other microorganisms that have been localized to atherosclerotic plaques from humans, *P. gingivalis* induces human platelets to aggregate in vitro. Hence, *P. gingivalis* and other microbes that chronically enter the blood circulation during mucosal infections may express similar pathogenic characteristics. To determine how, and to what extent, each infection and associated microorganisms contribute to cardiovascular disease outcomes is a difficult challenge for scientists to solve.

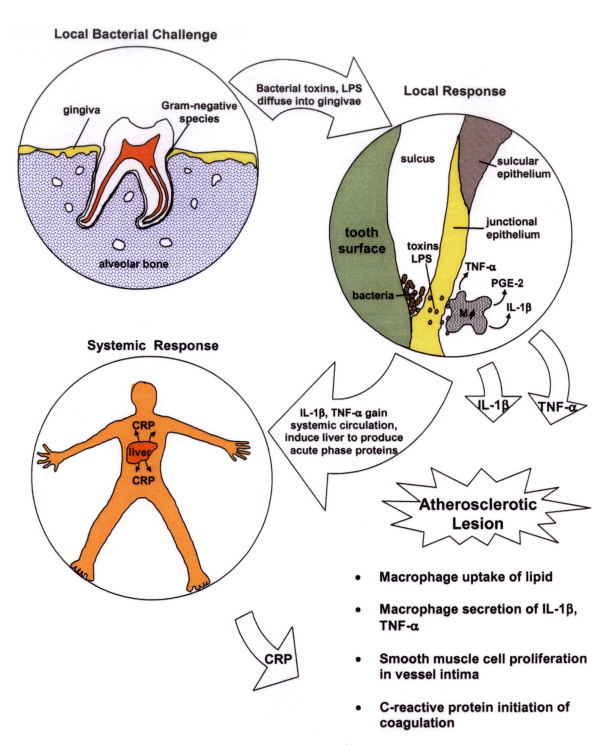

Local Bacterial Challenge

gingiva

Gram-negative species

alveolar bone

Bacterial toxins, LPS diffuse into gingivae

Local Response

sulcus

sulcular epithelium

junctional epithelium

tooth surface

toxins LPS

bacteria

TNF-α

PGE-2

IL-1β

IL-1β   TNF-α

Systemic Response

CRP

liver

CRP

IL-1β, TNF-α gain systemic circulation, induce liver to produce acute phase proteins

Atherosclerotic Lesion

CRP

- **Macrophage uptake of lipid**

- **Macrophage secretion of IL-1β, TNF-α**

- **Smooth muscle cell proliferation in vessel intima**

- **C-reactive protein initiation of coagulation**

FIGURE 5 How oral microbes produce local inflammation to influence systemic pathology. In the gingival sulcus, bacteria and their PAMPs such as LPS affect underlying tissues, causing local inflammation. High levels of the inflammatory mediators TNF-α and IL-1β may enter the circulation and induce the liver to produce acute-phase reactants, such as CRP. IL-1β and TNF-α may also act on monocytes in existing atherosclerotic plaques, causing exacerbation of existing disease.

When present simultaneously or intermittently in the blood over time, however, the systemic pathogen burden represents the aggregate risk of atherosclerosis and thrombosis formed by the redundant pathogenicity of microorganisms such as *C. pneumoniae* and cytomegalovirus, and *S. sanguinis* and *P. gingivalis*.

Some studies have also shown associations between periodontal disease and preterm low-birth-weight babies. Soluble inflammatory mediators, such as PGE_2, could be the molecular link from a local infection (periodontitis) to a distal event, parturition. Uterine levels of PGE_2 normally rise as gestation nears completion. If some threshold PGE_2 level triggers the onset of labor, it is possible that the combined PGE_2 from a distant infection and uterine tissue may induce premature labor and delivery of a low-birth-weight baby.

Thus, the microbes associated with periodontal disease may induce local monocytes to express inflammatory mediators. These mediators enter the systemic circulation and may exacerbate existing pathology at distant sites, such as atherosclerotic plaques, or trigger abnormal vascular function in specific tissues. For example, PGE_2 generated at the site of periodontal infection could enter the systemic circulation to increase uterine levels to trigger premature labor. The associations between periodontal disease and both cardiovascular disease and preterm low-birth-weight infants are subjects of current investigations.

KEY POINTS

Commensal oral bacteria can become pathogenic when they gain access to environments other than the oral cavity. A breach in the integrity of the soft tissues of the oral cavity can be caused by dental procedures, injuries, or infections. The new environmental conditions that are found systemically induce changes in bacterial gene expression, which may increase virulence.

Oral streptococci that are benign in the oral cavity are often causative in infective endocarditis. In the systemic compartment the streptococci locate on damaged or developmentally abnormal heart valves. The valvular endothelium can then slough, leaving the underlying connective tissues exposed. Circulating platelets are activated to repair the wound, and the platelets adhere and spread on the exposed connective tissues. The streptococci then induce the platelets to bind fibrinogen, aggregate, and form a thrombus or platelet clot. The mass of microorganisms, platelets, and fibrin on diseased or injured heart valves or other endocardial surfaces constitutes a vegetation, which is characteristic of infective endocarditis.

Cross-reactivity of antibodies to bacterial HSPs with self-HSPs may contribute to systemic diseases such as arthritis and Behçet's disease.

Bacterial mimicry of self-peptides such as a collagen fragment by PAAP epitope of *S. sanguinis* may lead to autorecognition and autoimmune arthritis.

Local intravascular inflammation caused by oral bacteria may be implicated in premature labor and the progression of systemic diseases such as atherosclerosis. Periodontal bacteria such as *P. gingivalis* may contribute more directly to atherosclerosis by invading artery endothelial cells and inducing inflammation. *P. gingivalis* can also induce formation of lipid-filled foam cells from macrophages, a key step in atherosclerosis.

FURTHER READING

Herzberg, M. C. 2000. Persistence of infective endocarditis, p. 357–374. *In* J. P. Nataro, M. J. Blaser, and S. Cunningham-Rundles (ed.), *Persistent Bacterial Infections*. ASM Press, Washington, D.C.

SECTION III CONTROL OF ORAL INFECTIONS

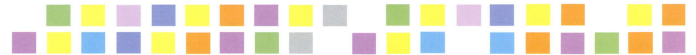

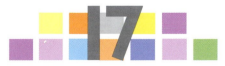

17

Antibiotics and the Treatment of Infectious Diseases

DONALD J. LEBLANC, THOMAS R. FLYNN, CONSTANTINE SIMOS, AND MARILYN S. LANTZ

ANTIBIOTICS: A CLASS OF THERAPEUTIC AGENT

Chemotherapeutic agents are chemical compounds used to treat diseases. A subgroup of these compounds are the antimicrobial agents, which are used in the treatment of infectious diseases. The focus of this chapter is antibiotics, which are either toxic or growth-inhibitory for bacteria. Antibiotics represent a separate class of antimicrobial agent, distinguished from antifungals, which are used to treat yeast and fungal infections, and antivirals, which aid in the treatment of viral infections. The distinction between antibiotics and antivirals is particularly important, because antibiotics are never effective against viral infections, whereas some antibiotics may also be effective in the treatment of certain fungal, and occasionally, parasitic infections.

Initially, all known antibiotics were natural products of microbial metabolism (fungal, actinomycete, or bacterial) that possessed killing or inhibitory activity against bacteria, e.g., penicillins; tetracyclines; aminoglycosides, such as streptomycin; macrolides, such as erythromycin; and glycopeptides, such as vancomycin. Most classes of antibiotics in clinical use today are still either natural products or semisynthetic derivatives of these products. In fact, there are only three classes of totally synthetic antibiotics used clinically: the quinolones (e.g., ciprofloxacin), which were first introduced in the 1960s; the oxazolidinones, the first representative of which, linezolid, was approved for clinical use in the United States only in 2000; and the sulfa drugs, predating even penicillin, which were introduced into clinical practice in the 1930s. The sulfa drugs have been used to treat parasitic and bacterial infections. A few other antimicrobial agents, such as the prodrug metronidazole, may also be used to treat infections caused not only by bacteria but by eukaryotic parasites as well.

There are several ways by which antibiotics may be classified, the three most common being (i) type of antimicrobial activity, i.e., microbicidal or microbiostatic; (ii) their antimicrobial spectrum, usually either narrow or broad; and (iii) their mechanism of action, i.e., the cellular target of inhibition. The first classification can be misleading because a particular antibiotic may be bactericidal (lethal) for some bacterial species or strains but have only bacteriostatic (inhibiting growth without killing) activity against others. In addition, an antibiotic may be bactericidal for a particular species at one concentration, but bacteriostatic for the same species at lower concentrations. The spectrum of an antibiotic may be very narrow, i.e., effective against only one or a few species of bacteria, or relatively narrow, in that it may act against only gram-positive or only gram-negative bacteria. A broad-spectrum antibiotic is one that is effective against a variety of gram-positive and gram-negative bacterial species. One of the most useful methods of antibiotic classification is based on the bacterial target(s) of inhibition, i.e., a step in cell wall biosynthesis, a component of the protein synthetic machinery, nucleic acid synthesis, cell membrane function, or a step in intermediary metabolism, e.g., the so-called antimetabolites. The more common antibiotic targets, and examples of the types of antibiotics that inhibit them, are listed in Table 1. The mechanisms by which antibiotics inhibit these targets are the topic of the next several sections of this chapter.

Inhibitors of Cell Wall Synthesis

The pathway of bacterial peptidoglycan (PG) (cell wall) synthesis, key enzymes that catalyze the various steps in its synthesis, and antibiotics known to inhibit one or more of these steps are illustrated in Fig. 1. Most of the enzymes involved in (PG) synthesis are unique to this pathway and are thus ideal antibiotic targets, since mammalian cells do not have cell walls. Many cell wall inhibitory agents are thus specific for bacteria and, ideally, nontoxic to the human patient. Inhibitors of cell wall synthesis function only against growing bacterial cells that are actively incorporating precursors into the PG layer.

The backbone of PG (also referred to as murein) consists of two sugar moieties, *N*-acetylglucosamine (Glc-NAc) and *N*-acetyl muramic

TABLE 1 Common targets of antibiotics[a]

Target	Antibiotic(s)
Protein synthesis	
30S ribosomal subunit	Aminoglycosides, tetracyclines
50S ribosomal subunit	Macrolides, chloramphenicol, oxazolidinones
tRNA^{Ile}	Mupirocin
Elongation factor G	Fusidic acid
Nucleic acid synthesis	
DNA gyrase and topoisomerase IV	Nalidixic acid, fluoroquinolones, novobiocin
RNA polymerase β subunit	Rifampin
DNA	Metronidazole (prodrug)
Cell wall (peptidoglycan) synthesis	
Transpeptidases	β-lactams (penicillins, cephalosporins, etc.)
D-Ala–D-Ala	Glycopeptides (vancomycin, teicoplanin)
Antimetabolites	
Dihydrofolate reductase	Trimethoprim
Dihydropteroate synthetase	Sulfonamides
Mycolic acid synthesis	Isoniazid
Membranes	Polymyxins

[a]Adapted and updated from D. T. Moir, K. J. Shaw, R. S. Hare, and G. F. Vovis, *Antimicrob. Agents Chemother.* **45**:439–446, 1999.

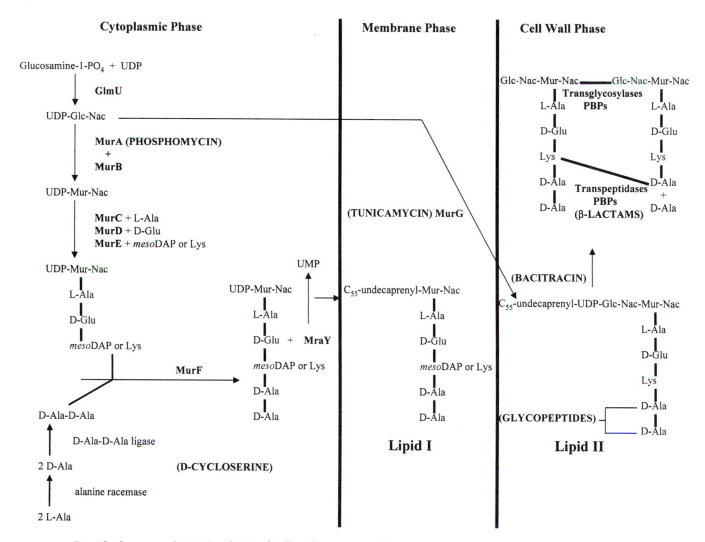

Cytoplasmic Phase   **Membrane Phase**   **Cell Wall Phase**

FIGURE 1 Peptidoglycan synthesis. Synthesis of cell wall precursor, UDP-Mur-Nac-pentapeptide, occurs in the bacterial cytoplasm. Precursor molecules are transported to the cytoplasmic membrane by the attachment of C_{55}-undecaprenyl in the formation of lipid I. Subsequently, lipid I is transported to the exterior side (periplasmic space in gram-negative bacteria) of the cytoplasmic membrane, and the disaccharide (UDP-Glc-Nac-Mur-Nac)-pentapeptide, designated lipid II, is formed. Subsequently, the C_{55}-undecaprenyl moiety is released for subsequent cycles, and the cell wall continues to grow on the exterior of the cytoplasmic membrane due to the transglycosylase and transpeptidase activities of penicillin-binding proteins (PBPs). Enzymes catalyzing the peptidoglycan synthetic steps are in bold letters, and antibiotics that target the various steps in peptidoglycan synthesis are indicated in bold capital letters surrounded by parentheses. See the text for further details on peptidoglycan synthesis and antibiotics that inhibit it. Adapted from I. Chopra, L. Hesse, and A. J. O'Neill, *J. Appl. Microbiol.* **92**(Suppl.):4S–15S, 2002.

acid (Mur-NAc). These precursors are synthesized in the bacterial cytoplasm, as are the amino acids that make up a pentapeptide molecule that is attached to Mur-NAc. The first reaction that occurs in the cytoplasm is catalyzed by a bifunctional enzyme, GlmU, which acetylates glucosamine-1-phosphate and subsequently adds UDP to it to form UDP-Glc-NAc. Subsequent steps are catalyzed by a series of enzymes referred to as MurA-F. Mur-NAc is synthesized from UDP-Glc-NAc via the activities of two enzymes, MurA and MurB, resulting in the uridylated product, UDP-Mur-NAc. MurA is inactivated by fosfomycin, an antibiotic recommended for the treatment of urinary tract infections. The next series of cytoplasmic steps involves the synthesis of UDP-muramyl tripeptide by the sequential addition to UDP-Mur-NAc of L-Ala, D-Glu, and *meso*-diaminopimelic acid (*meso*-DAP), catalyzed by MurC, MurD, and MurE, respectively. DAP is replaced by lysine in a number of gram-positive bacterial species. Subsequently, a pentapeptide is formed by the addition to the UDP-muramyl tripeptide of the dipeptide D-Ala–D-Ala, catalyzed by MurF. Two enzymes are involved in the formation of D-Ala–D-Ala. First, an alanine racemase converts the naturally occurring L-Ala to D-Ala, and the dipeptide is synthesized by D-alanyl–D-alanine ligase. The racemase and ligase are both inhibited by D-cycloserine, but toxicity issues have precluded the clinical use of this agent except as a second-line antibiotic in the treatment of tuberculosis.

The next steps in PG synthesis consist of the formation of two cytoplasmic membrane-bound lipid intermediates, lipid I and lipid II. The formation of lipid I involves MraY, an enzyme that catalyzes the removal of UDP from the muramyl pentapeptide and its replacement by the membrane component, C_{55}-undecaprenyl-phosphate. MurG catalyzes the addition of GlcNAc to lipid I, using UDP-GlcNAc as a cosubstrate, yielding the lipid-disaccharide-pentapeptide, lipid II, and resulting in the translocation of the disaccharide-pentapeptide from the inside of the cytoplasmic membrane to the outside, but still anchored to it by C_{55}-undecaprenyl-phosphate. In gram-negative bacteria, which have an outer membrane, lipid II is located in the periplasmic space. The antibiotic tunicamycin is an inhibitor of MurG, but it is too toxic for clinical use, due to its inhibition of a step in eukaryote glycoprotein synthesis.

Once exposed to the outer surface of the cytoplasmic membrane, the disaccharide pentapeptide subunits of the growing PG become substrates for two types of enzymatic activities, transglycosylases and transpeptidases, which form covalent linkages between adjacent disaccharides (GlcNAc–Mur-NAc) and pentapeptides, respectively, ultimately producing the mature, rigid PG layer. The transpeptidases form peptide bonds between the third amino acid in one pentapeptide (usually *meso*-DAP or lysine) and the fourth amino acid (D-Ala) in an adjacent pentapeptide, accompanied by the release of the second D-Ala. The joining of two disaccharide subunits, via transglycosylase activity, is accompanied by the hydrolysis of the pyrophosphate linkage, which results in release of the C_{55}-lipid phosphate for subsequent transport of disaccharide-pentapeptide subunits to the cytoplasmic membrane. Several antibiotics interfere with release of the C_{55}-lipid phosphate from lipid II, preventing further rounds of lipid I and lipid II synthesis and, thus, PG maturation. Only one such antibiotic, bacitracin, which prevents the recycling of the C_{55}-lipid phosphate moiety of lipid II, is of clinical significance. However, because of toxicity, it is used topically only.

The transglycosylase and transpeptidase activities associated with PG synthesis reside in a group of cytoplasmic membrane-associated proteins collectively referred to as penicillin-binding proteins, or PBPs. Bacteria synthesize a variety of PBPs and may contain as many as eight or more.

The lower-molecular-weight PBPs tend to possess transpeptidase activity only, whereas those with higher molecular weights may be bifunctional, expressing both transpeptidase and transglycosylase activities. The best-known class of antibiotics, i.e., the β-lactams, bind to the PBPs and block their transpeptidase activity. The β-lactams include the penicillins (hence the name penicillin-binding proteins), the cephalosporins, the carbapenems, and the monobactams, and as the name implies, all contain the four-membered β-lactam ring, illustrated in Fig. 2.

Normally, the cross-linking transpeptidases form one DAP-D-Ala or Lys-D-Ala peptide bond and cleave one D-Ala–D-Ala peptide bond, releasing a free D-Ala. However, β-lactam antibiotic structures resemble the D-Ala–D-Ala terminus of the pentapeptide, and thus bind to the PBP instead of the normal substrate. An acyl enzyme intermediate, in which the β-lactam ring is opened, is formed. Thus the enzyme is not free to add further cross-links to the maturing PG, and the cell eventually lyses, due in part to the concomitant release by several bacterial species of autolysins that destroy existing mature PG.

The first β-lactams to be used clinically were the natural penicillins penicillin G (which is acid labile) and penicillin V (which is acid stable), which had activity against the staphylococci, streptococci, enterococci, some gram-negative cocci, and spirochetes. The aminopenicillins amoxicillin and ampicillin were effective against the same bacterial species as the natural penicillins but also had activity against many gram-negative bacterial species, and thus they were effective in the treatment of urinary tract infections. As *Staphylococcus aureus* became resistant to the penicillins, due to the production of β-lactamase activity (see sections on antibiotic resistance below), the antistaphylococcal or β-lactamase-resistant penicillins, e.g., methicillin, were developed. The last of the penicillins to be introduced were the so-called broad-spectrum penicillins, also referred to as the antipseudomonal penicillins. These included pipericillin, mezlocillin, and

FIGURE 2 β-lactam antibiotics. Core structures of the four major classes of β-lactams: penicillins, cephalosporins, carbapenems, and monobactams. Cleavage of the β-lactam ring by β-lactamases is illustrated in the center of the figure.

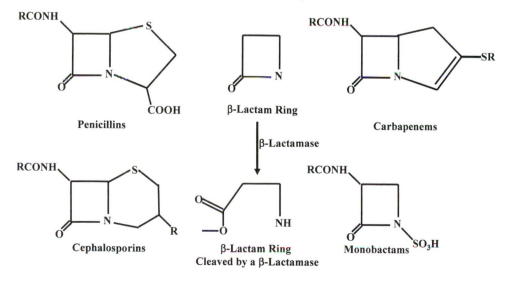

ticarcillin, which exhibited activity against a broad spectrum of gram-negative bacilli, including *Pseudomonas* species, a number of anaerobic species, and enterococci.

Next among the β-lactam antibiotics were the cephalosporins, which are derivatives of cephalosporin C, produced by the fungal genus *Cephalosporium*. The cephalosporins, four generations of which have been introduced into clinical practice, are active against most organisms that are susceptible to penicillins, and in general, are useful alternatives for patients who are allergic to penicillin. Approximately 8% of individuals who are treated with a penicillin become allergic to all penicillins. Like the penicillins, the cephalosporins are relatively nontoxic, and fewer individuals become hypersensitive. The first-generation cephalosporins, e.g., cephazolin, cephalothin, and cephalexin, are active against staphylococci and streptococci, but not enterococci or most gram-negative pathogens. Most importantly, when first introduced, they were effective against β-lactamase-producing bacterial strains and became widely used prophylactically before surgery. As with the penicillins, resistance to the cephalosporins began to emerge, due to a large extent to β-lactamases, referred to as cephalosporinases.

The second-generation cephalosporins, such as cefamandole, cefuroxime, cefaclor, cephamycins, and cefoxitin, were unaffected by cephalosporinases produced by gram-negative rods and had some activity against anaerobic species but were much less effective against gram-positive bacteria than the first-generation cephalosporin molecules. Like the first-generation cephalosporins, they have been used prophylactically before surgery and found a use in the treatment of mixed aerobic/anaerobic infections.

Third-generation cephalosporins, e.g., cefotaxime, ceftazidime, ceftriaxone, ceftizoxime, and cefoperazone, exhibited a broader activity against gram-negative rods, especially members of the family *Enterobacteriaceae* and *Pseudomonas* species, but had reduced activity against gram-negative cocci and very little gram-positive antibacterial activity. They were also useful for treatment of sexually transmitted diseases such as gonorrhea (which is caused by *Neisseria gonorrhoeae*) and syphilis (caused by *Treponema pallidum*), as well as Lyme disease (caused by *Borrelia burgdorferi*), and they were the only cephalosporins that could cross the blood-brain barrier.

The only fourth-generation cephalosporin approved for use in the United States, cefepime, is resistant to inactivation by a large array of β-lactamases produced by gram-negative bacteria and can readily pass through outer membrane porins.

Two newer classes of β-lactam antibiotics include the monobactams and carbapenems. The monobactam aztreonam has activity against a broad spectrum of gram-negative bacteria, including *Pseudomonas* species, but virtually no activity against gram-positive bacteria. It is also useful for treatment of patients allergic to β-lactams, since it is the least likely of the β-lactam antibiotics to trigger a hypersensitivity response. The carbapenems imipenem and meropenem exhibit the broadest spectrum of activity of all the β-lactams, including gram-positive and gram-negative bacteria.

Another group of β-lactams are the so-called β-lactamase inhibitors, e.g., clavulanic acid, sulbactam, and tazobactam. These compounds are not antibiotics as such, but they bind to β-lactamases almost permanently (they are very slowly released by the β-lactamases), preventing the binding of the β-lactamases to true β-lactam antibiotics such as penicillins, if present in the same environment. Combinations of β-lactamase inhibitors and β-lactamase-susceptible β-lactams currently are used therapeutically. The first of these combinations was Augmentin (amoxicillin plus clavulanic acid), and subsequently, Unasyn (ampicillin plus sulbactam), Timentin (ticarcillin plus clavulanic acid), and Zosyn (piperacillin plus tazobactam) were introduced.

The glycopeptide antibiotics vancomycin and teicoplanin are naturally occurring secondary metabolites of the bacteria *Amycolatopsis orientalis* and *Actinoplanes teichomyceticus*, respectively. These antibiotics bind to the D-Ala–D-Ala terminus of the UDP-muramylpentapeptide after transfer out of the cytoplasm while they are still lipid-linked. When bound to the murein, the glycopeptides block the binding of PBPs, inhibiting transpeptidation and transglycosylation reactions. Vancomycin is the only glycopeptide antibiotic licensed for use in the United States, whereas teicoplanin is used extensively in Europe. The glycopeptides are active only against gram-positive bacteria, being unable to penetrate the outer membranes of gram-negative cells. They are administered intravenously for the treatment of infections caused by gram-positive cocci, such as species of *Enterococcus* and *Staphylococcus*, that are resistant to all other clinically useful antibiotics.

Inhibitors of Translation

The protein biosynthetic process, i.e., translation, and some inhibitors of the process are depicted in Fig. 3. The platform on which proteins are synthesized, i.e., on which mRNA cistrons are translated into polypeptides, is the ribosome. Bacterial 70S ribosomes are composed of two large complexes designated the 30S and 50S ribosomal subunits, each of which contains RNA and proteins. The 30S subunit consists of 16S rRNA and approximately 20 proteins, whereas the 50S subunit consists of 5S and 23S rRNA plus approximately 30 proteins.

Translation begins with the formation of an initiation complex consisting of mRNA, a 30S ribosomal subunit, and a charged fMet-tRNA^{fMet}, and the binding and release of three initiation factors, IF1, IF2, and IF3. Formation of an initiation complex involves the binding of a 30S ribosomal subunit to the ribosomal binding site on mRNA, approximately 5 bases upstream of the start codon (usually AUG) of a gene (cistron). Premature binding of the 50S ribosomal subunit to the 30S subunit is prevented by the presence of IF1 and IF3. A charged fMet-tRNA^{fMet}, following activation by IF2 and GTP, then binds to the start codon on the mRNA via base pairing to the anticodon on the tRNA. In a step involving the hydrolysis of GTP, the three initiation factors dissociate from the 30S initiation complex, which now binds to a 50S ribosomal subunit, producing a 70S initiation complex in which the charged tRNA^{fMet} is situated at the P (peptide) site, which is flanked on one side by the empty A (amino acid acceptor) site for binding of the next aminoacyl-charged tRNA encoded by the mRNA, and

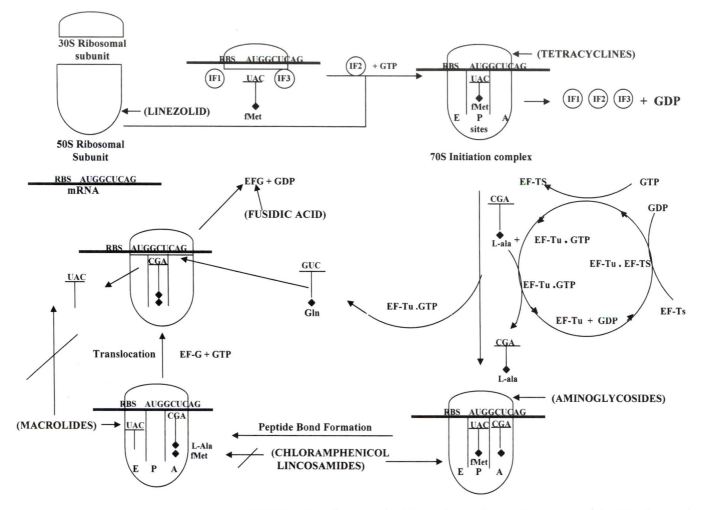

FIGURE 3 Translation and inhibition by antibiotics. Formation of the 70S ribosomal initiation complex, containing an mRNA molecule and fMet-tRNA, is followed by subsequent steps in the cycle by which each additional amino acid is added to the growing polypeptide chain via the formation of a peptide bond with its predecessor. Specific antibiotics, or antibiotic classes, inhibiting individual steps in translation are shown in bold capital letters surrounded by parentheses. See the text for further details. Adapted from I. Chopra, L. Hesse, and A. J. O'Neill, *J. Appl. Microbiol.* 92(Suppl.):4S–15S, 2002, and from J. W. Lengeler, G. Drews, and H. G. Schlegel, *Biology of the Prokaryotes* (Blackwell Science/Thieme, Stuttgart, Germany, 1999).

on the other side by the empty E (peptide exit) site. The oxazolidinone linezolid inhibits bacterial protein synthesis at the initiation stage by binding to the 50S ribosomal subunit, and is thought to inhibit the formation of the 70S initiation complex. Linezolid is used to treat infections caused by multidrug-resistant gram-positive pathogens such as methicillin-resistant *S. aureus* (MRSA), vancomycin-resistant enterococci (VRE), and penicillin-resistant *Streptococcus pneumoniae*. Translation continues via a series of elongation cycles, each of which results in the addition of a single amino acid to the growing polypeptide chain. Each cycle begins with the binding of an EF-Tu · GTP-activated and charged tRNA to the A site, the specific aminoacyl-tRNA bound being determined by the codon at that site. Tetracyclines bind to the 30S ribosomal subunit and interfere with the binding of aminoacylated tRNA molecules to the ribosomal A site. They pass through porins on the outer membranes of gram-negative bacteria and through cytoplasmic membranes of all bacteria by energy-dependent, carrier-mediated processes. Their selective action against bacteria is based on greater uptake by bacteria than by human cells. Tetracycline use is contraindicated in pregnant women and children under the age of 8 years because it interferes with bone development and it stains teeth brown in fetuses and children. These antibiotics are usually administered orally, with doxycycline and minocycline being more completely absorbed than tetracycline, oxytetracycline, or chlortetracycline. Mupirocin is a topical antibiotic used to treat skin infections, e.g., impetigo caused by staphylococci and streptococci. Mupirocin inhibits tRNA^{Ile} synthase, thus halting protein synthesis at an elongation cycle that calls for the incorporation of isoleucine into the growing peptide chain.

Activation of the tRNA molecules requires the hydrolysis of GTP to GDP + P$_i$, resulting in the formation of an EF-Tu · GDP complex. Ribosomal protein S12 is responsible for ensuring that the correct aminoacyl-tRNA has been bound to the A site. Streptomycin, an aminoglycoside, interferes with this process and contributes to translational misreading. All aminoglycosides (amikacin, gentamicin, kanamycin, neomycin, tobramycin) bind to the 30S subunit of the 70S ribosome, causing distortion of the A site and ultimate irreversible inhibition of protein synthesis. These antibiotics, which (except for semisynthetic derivatives such as amikacin) are produced by various species of actinomycetes found in the soil, pass through the outer membranes of gram-negative bacteria due to disruption of membrane cross-bridges. They are actively transported through bacterial cytoplasmic membranes by mechanisms dependent on electron transport. Aminoglycosides are inactive against anaerobes, and are used primarily to treat infections caused by gram-negative bacteria. They are occasionally used to treat gram-positive bacterial infections, in conjunction with a cell wall inhibitor such as a β-lactam or glycopeptide (see discussion of antibiotic synergy under "Antibiotic Combinations" below). All of the aminoglycosides are potentially nephrotoxic and ototoxic, and have relatively narrow therapeutic indexes, i.e., antibacterial concentration to toxic concentration ratios.

Before each successive elongation cycle, with the addition of the next amino acid encoded by the mRNA, EF-Tu · GTP is regenerated from the EF-Tu · GDP complex by EF-TS and GTP. The next step in an elongation cycle involves the formation of a peptide bond between the α-amino group of the amino acid just added to the A site and the activated carboxyl group of either fMet or the last amino acid that was added to a growing peptide chain. Formation of each peptide bond is catalyzed by peptidyl transferase activity of the 50S ribosomal subunit. Chloramphenicol and the lincosamides bind to the 50S ribosomal subunit and inhibit peptidyl transferase activity. Chloramphenicol, a very-broad-spectrum antibiotic, penetrates the cytoplasmic membrane via an energy-dependent influx mechanism. However, it is used in developed countries with extreme caution, and only if deemed absolutely necessary, because it has been associated with rare but fatal cases of aplastic anemia. In underdeveloped countries, chloramphenicol is usually the least expensive and most widely available of antibiotics. Clinically, clindamycin is the most commonly used member of the lincosamides. It exhibits good activity against gram-positive and gram-negative anaerobes and is particularly effective against *Bacteroides* spp. It is also effective against gram-positive aerobes and is often used in the treatment of osteomyelitis because of its tendency to concentrate in bone.

Peptide bond formation is followed by the translocation of the ribosomal complex to the next codon on the mRNA molecule, which is mediated by elongation factor EF-G with the necessary energy supplied by the hydrolysis of GTP. Translocation of the ribosomal complex results in the movement of the growing peptide chain to the P site, the release of the uncharged prior tRNA molecule as well as EF-G through the E site, and a now-empty A site for initiation of the next elongation cycle that will result in the addition of the next amino acid to the growing peptide chain. Macrolides bind to 23S rRNA in the 50S ribosomal subunit and block peptide translocation and release of tRNA after peptide bond formation. They also inhibit the formation of the 50S ribosomal subunit. Erythromycin is the best known and still the most widely used of the macrolides. It has activity against gram-positive cocci and is an important alternative to penicillin for allergic patients for the treatment of streptococcal infections. It also is used to treat infections of the upper and lower respiratory tract, skin, and soft tissues, as well as urinary tract infections, sexually transmitted diseases such as syphilis and gonorrhea, and intestinal parasitic infections. The macrolides are relatively nontoxic but cause nausea and vomiting after oral administration in some patients. Such gastrointestinal disturbances tend to be less common with the newer macrolides, clarithromycin and azithromycin. Fusidic acid binds to EF-G, forming a stable complex with EF-G, GDP, and the ribosome. EF-G is not released for subsequent rounds of translocation and GTP hydrolysis. Fusidic acid is active against gram-positive but not gram-negative bacteria. One of the few indications for fusidic acid is infection with penicillin-resistant *Staphylococcus*, especially osteomyelitis, since fusidic acid is concentrated in bone. However, a second antistaphylococcal agent is also required to prevent the development of resistance. Recently, fusidic acid, formulated as a cream, has shown promise for the treatment of impetigo in children 12 years old or younger.

The elongation cycles continue until a translocation step results in movement of the ribosomal complex to a stop codon on the mRNA, at which point release factor RF3, plus either RF1 or RF2, depending on the stop codon, binds at the empty A site, forming a termination complex. The 50S-mediated peptidyl transferase activity then releases the polypeptide chain, which causes dissociation of the mRNA, release factors, and the 70S ribosome. Initiation factors IF1 and IF3, at the expense of GTP hydrolysis, cause the dissociation of the 70S ribosome into its 50S and 30S subunits.

Inhibitors of Transcription and Replication

The rifamycins bind to the β-subunit of DNA-dependent RNA polymerase and are the only antibiotics that block transcription, specifically the initiation of mRNA synthesis. Rifamycins are natural products of bacterial (*Streptomyces mediterranei*) fermentation, but only semisynthetic derivatives, such as rifampin, rifapentine, and rifamide, are used clinically. They exhibit a broad spectrum of activity, which includes gram-positive bacteria, some gram-negative species (primarily cocci), some anaerobes, and chlamydiae. The rifamycins are seldom used as single antimicrobial agents, due to high frequencies of bacterial mutation resulting in resistance to these drugs. The most important use of rifampin is in the treatment of tuberculosis, but always in combination with at least two other drugs. Rifampin may often color urine, feces, saliva, sputum, sweat, and tears orange-red and can permanently stain contact lenses. Long-term treatment may cause a flulike syndrome, and some patients develop hepatotoxicity and thrombocytopenia.

All inhibitors of bacterial DNA replication interfere with the activities of one or both of the type II topoisomerases, either DNA gyrase only or DNA gyrase and topoisomerase IV. DNA gyrase, a heterotetramer composed of two GyrA and two GyrB subunits, is the only bacterial enzyme able to introduce negative superhelical turns into DNA, and is required for both the initiation and continuation of DNA replication. At the termination of replication, topoisomerase IV catalyzes the separation (decatenation) of the two daughter DNA molecules in order to permit their segregation to daughter cells during cell division. Topoisomerase IV, like DNA gyrase, is also a heterotetramer, consisting of two ParC and two ParE subunits. GyrB and ParE each have ATPase activity, providing energy for the activities of gyrase and topoisomerase IV, respectively.

The coumerins, such as novobiocin and coumermycin, are fermentation products of *Streptomyces* species and were the first topoisomerase inhibitors to be studied. They compete with ATP for binding to GyrB and are active against gram-positive but not gram-negative bacteria. Because of numerous toxic side effects and high frequencies of mutation to resistance, the coumerins are not clinically useful. The quinolones, on the other hand, have become major players in the arsenal of antimicrobial agents.

Quinolones bind to DNA-gyrase and DNA-topoisomerase IV complexes, stabilizing DNA strand breaks created by these enzymes such that religation cannot occur, resulting in the accumulation of replication intermediates and the eventual death of the cell. Although the quinolones have activity on both enzymes, the major target in gram-negative bacteria is GyrA, whereas in gram-positive bacteria it tends to be ParC. The first of this family of synthetic agents, nalidixic acid, introduced in 1962, is active only against the *Enterobacteriaceae* and is used only for the treatment of urinary tract infections. Bacteria also have high frequencies of mutation to resistance to nalidixic acid.

The addition of a fluoride atom to quinolones produced increased potency and an expanded spectrum, resulting in the introduction of a whole new family of fluoroquinolones into clinical practice, such as norfloxacin (1986), ciprofloxacin (1987), levofloxacin (1996), and gatifloxacin and moxifloxacin (1999). Not only do the fluoroquinolones have greater activity against the *Enterobacteriaceae*, but they are also active against other gram-negative and gram-positive bacteria. Some of the fluoroquinolones also have activity against *Pseudomonas aeruginosa* and *Mycoplasma*, *Chlamydia*, and *Mycobacterium* species. Approximately 5% of patients experience gastrointestinal problems, but serious side effects are very uncommon with the fluoroquinolones. However, possible inhibition of cartilage development has precluded their licensing for use in children.

Miscellaneous Antibiotics

The first clinically effective antibacterial agent was the sulfa drug sulphanilamide, introduced in 1935 as Prontosil. These sulfonamides are similar in structure to *para*-aminobenzoic acid, a precursor of folic acid (Fig. 4), and function as competitive inhibitors of dihydropteroate synthetase, which catalyzes the synthesis of dihydropteroic acid from *para*-aminobenzoic and pteridine. The sulfa drug most commonly prescribed today is sulfamethoxazole, which, although generally used in combination with trimethoprim (see below), is active against many gram-positive and gram-negative bacteria, as well as chlamydiae, *Plasmodium falciparum*, *Pneumocystis carinii*, and *Toxoplasma gondii*. Trimethoprim is a pyrimidine-like structure resembling the aminohydroxypyrimidine moiety of folic acid; it functions as a competitive inhibitor of dihydrofolate reductase. It may still be used as a single antimicrobial agent in the treatment of urinary tract infections and traveler's diarrhea, but its primary application is in combination with sulfamethoxazole.

Metronidazole (Flagyl), a member of the nitroimidazole class of antimicrobials, is an antibacterial and antiparasitic agent that is used to

FIGURE 4 The folate biosynthetic pathway. Enzymatic steps involved in the bacterial synthesis of tetrahydrafolic acid (THF) are illustrated, as are two antibiotics, sulfamethoxazole and trimethoprim, that inhibit two key enzymes involved in THF synthesis, dihydropteroate synthetase (DHPS) and dihydrofolate reductase (DHFR), respectively. Reprinted with permission of Wiley-Liss, Inc., subsidiary of John Wiley & Sons, Inc., from A. Bermingham and J. P. Derrick, *Bioessays* **24:**637–648, 2002. © 2002 John Wiley & Sons, Inc.

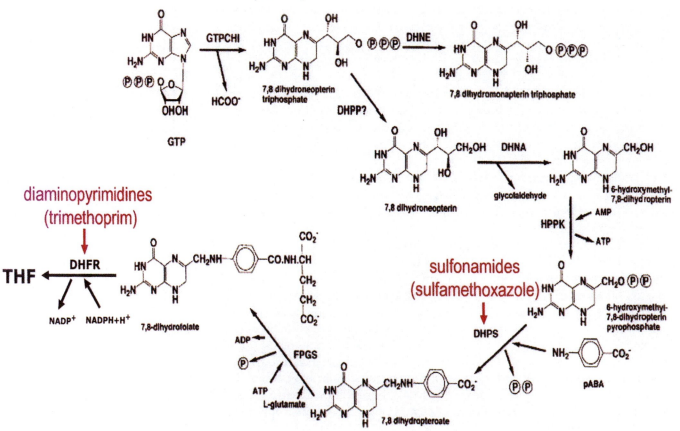

treat infections caused by anaerobes and some microaerophiles. It is effective against *Bacteroides* species, *Helicobacter pylori,* and such parasites as *Trichomonas vaginalis, Giardia lamblia,* and *Entamoeba coli.* Metronidazole itself is a prodrug and has no antibacterial activity, but under anaerobic conditions the nitro group is reduced to produce radicals that cause DNA damage. Nitro group reduction requires enzymes that function at very low redox potential, as are present only in anaerobes and some microaerophiles.

Polypeptide antibiotics such as polymyxins and gramicidins appear to interact with phospholipids in cytoplasmic membranes, resulting in disruption of the membrane and leakage of cellular contents. They are used topically for treatment of severe infections caused by certain gram-negative bacteria, systemic use being precluded by their toxicity.

Treatment of Tuberculosis

Due largely to the long generation time of *Mycobacterium tuberculosis,* the location of the organism in infected individuals, and the long latencies associated with tuberculosis, treatment of patients with single antibiotics results in the emergence of strains resistant to those antibiotics. Therefore, treatment must be initiated with multiple antimicrobial agents. Such treatment may involve three or more of such first-line drugs as isoniazid, rifampin, pyrazinamide, ethambutol, and streptomycin or of such second-line antibiotics as *p*-aminosalicylic acid, ethionamide, D-cycloserine, fluoroquinolones, the aminoglycosides, kanamycin, and amikacin, as well as other lesser-known drugs. The first-line agents have higher efficacies and lower toxicities than the second-line agents. Isoniazid and ethionamide are prodrugs that once activated via oxidation inhibit an enzyme involved in mycolic acid synthesis. Pyrazinamide is also a prodrug that must be activated, in this case by enzymes unique to *M. tuberculosis,* prior to inhibition of its target, which is unknown. The targets of ethambutol appear to be several arabinosyltransferases involved in the synthesis of arabinans, which are unique to the cell walls of mycobacteria. *p*-Aminosalicylic acid is an inhibitor of folic acid synthesis.

Antibiotic Combinations

Occasionally, the combined activity of two antibiotics is greater than the activity expected from the effect of each individual antibiotic, a phenomenon referred to as synergism. The classic example of synergism is the simultaneous use of a β-lactam antibiotic, such as penicillin, and an aminoglycoside, such as streptomycin. The synergistic effect is thought to derive from an enhancement of cell permeability to the aminoglycoside due to the inhibition of cell wall synthesis by the β-lactam. The combined use of trimethoprim and sulfamethoxazole, also known as co-trimoxazole, is also thought to be synergistic. Combination treatment need not involve antibiotic synergism. For example, such combinations may be used to prevent or delay the emergence of resistant microorganisms, as in the combined use of isoniazid, rifampin, and ethambutol for the treatment of tuberculosis; to overcome polymicrobial infections, such as intra-abdominal abscesses in which the different bacteria involved may be susceptible to different antibiotics; or to treat particularly serious infections at a stage before the identification of the infectious agent(s).

There are some instances in which the combined effect of two antibiotics is less than that of either antibiotic alone. Such antagonism is typically associated with the combined use of a bacteriostatic, e.g., chloramphenicol, and a bactericidal antibiotic, e.g., streptomycin. Macrolides, lincosamides, and chloramphenicol are antagonistic because of their overlapping binding sites on the ribosome.

Measurements of Antibiotic Potency

The strength or potency of any antibiotic against bacteria varies from species to species, and even from strain to strain within the same species. The degree of potency of an antibiotic is measured in terms of the minimal concentration of that agent required to completely inhibit the growth of a bacterial strain in question, and is designated the minimal inhibitory concentration (MIC), usually in micrograms per milliliter. MICs can be measured precisely by setting up a series of antibiotic solutions, usually in twofold increments, made up in a growth medium determined by the particular species being examined; adding to these solutions a predetermined number of bacterial cells, e.g., 10^5, per solution; and then incubating the inoculated solutions at a temperature, and for a period, generally 24 to 48 h, also determined by the species under study. If, in a particular test, the bacteria were able to grow in solutions containing 1, 2, and 4 µg of the antibiotic per ml but did not grow in solutions containing 8, 16, 32, 64, or 128 µg/ ml, then the MIC of that antibiotic for that particular bacterial isolate would be reported as 8 µg/ml (Fig. 5). The MIC provides an indication of the concentration of antibiotic required to prevent the growth of the test organism but does not indicate the concentration of the antibiotic required to kill the strain, i.e., the minimal bactericidal concentration (MBC), or whether the antibiotic is able to kill bacteria at any concentration. If the experiment illustrated in Fig. 5 is carried one step further, the MBC can be determined. In this case, aliquots of the cultures from which the MIC was read are subcultured on petri dishes containing agar-based media devoid of any antibiotic. The plates are then incubated for 24 to 48 h and examined for the presence of bacterial colonies. In this case, the lowest concentration of antibiotic in the original solution that did not produce any colonies on the antibiotic-free plates, 16 µg/ml, would be designated the MBC. Methods of MIC determination have been standardized and updated over time for all clinically available antibiotics and all relevant bacterial species. These standards are published by the Clinical Laboratory Standards Institute so that results obtained in different laboratories can be compared.

Often, it is only necessary to know whether the organism(s) likely causing a particular infection is susceptible or resistant to one or more of the antibiotics normally used to treat such infections. In such cases, particularly in the hospital setting, a quantitative disk diffusion test is employed. A disk impregnated with a standard amount of antibiotic is placed on a petri dish containing an agar-based medium (usually Mueller-Hinton agar) that has been inoculated with a standard concentration of the bacterial isolate to be tested. The plate is incubated for a specified time and then examined for zones of inhibition of bacterial growth around the disk. If the strain is resistant to the antibiotic on the disk, it will have grown up to or very close to the edge of the disk. If it is susceptible to the antibiotic, there will be a clear zone around the disk within which growth of the

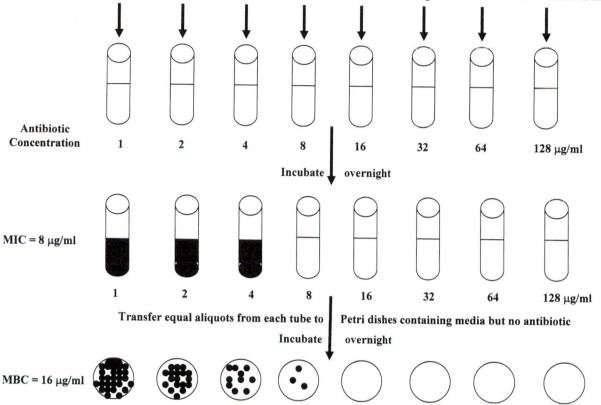

Inoculate each tube of media containing the indicated concentration of antibiotic being tested with the same amount of bacterial culture

FIGURE 5 Determination of the MIC and MBC of an antibiotic. A series of sterile test tubes (or wells in a microtiter plate) are set up, each containing a broth medium that will permit the growth of the bacterial pathogen of interest, as well as twofold dilutions of the antibiotic of which the MIC is to be determined. Each tube is inoculated with a specific number of bacteria, e.g., 10^5, in an overnight culture. All tubes are incubated overnight or longer, depending on the bacterial species. Each tube is then examined for growth (increased turbidity, e.g., optical density at a specific wavelength in a spectrophotometer). The concentration of antibiotic that completely inhibits the growth of the bacterium, in the instance illustrated, 8 µg/ml, is recorded as the MIC. To determine what concentration of the antibiotic is necessary to kill the bacterium if the antibiotic is bactericidal, an aliquot, e.g., 0.1 ml, of each culture used to determine the MIC is spotted on a petri dish containing an agar-based medium, but lacking antibiotic, and spread over the entire surface of the medium. All petri dishes are incubated overnight or longer, and then examined for the presence of bacterial colonies. That plate on which no colonies can be detected is used to determine the MBC of the antibiotic under study. In the case illustrated, the first plate in the series that contained no colonies had been inoculated with medium from the tube containing 16 µg of antibiotic per ml, which is thus designated as the MBC.

strain has been inhibited. Based on previously determined results published in tables, the diameter of the zone is interpreted as an indication of a susceptible, intermediate, or resistant bacterial strain.

USE OF ANTIBIOTICS IN THE PRACTICE OF DENTISTRY

Antibiotics are used in several ways in the treatment and management of oral and orofacial infections in the practice of dentistry. Acute and chronic infections that are associated with and arise from the teeth (odontogenic infections) can be localized to the alveolar bone adjacent to the apex of the root of a tooth (periapical infections), can spread beyond this area deeper into the alveolar bone and/or basal bone of the mandible or maxilla, can exit the bone and spread into adjacent areas such as the parapharyngeal spaces, or can exit the bone and spread to adjacent soft tissues, resulting in dental abscesses or cellulitis. Occasionally, infections in the maxilla and mandible progress to osteomyelitis. Antibiotics are used systemically to treat odontogenic infections in much the same way that antibiotics are used to treat exogenous infections at other body sites, with the goal of permanently eliminating the causative organism from the infected site. The use of antibiotics in the treatment of odontogenic infections is considered in more detail below.

Antibiotics may also be used in the treatment of periodontitis (see chapter 12). These infections occur in the periodontal tissues, which include the epithelium, connective tissues, and alveolar bone that surround the roots of the teeth and constitute the attachment apparatus that anchors teeth to the alveolar bone. Periodontitis results in the progressive loss of the periodontal attachment apparatus from around the roots of the teeth and may ultimately progress to tooth loss. For reasons discussed below, antibiotics are not usually used in the treatment of chronic adult periodontitis, the most common form of periodontitis. However, there are situations in which the use of antibiotics is helpful in the treatment of periodontitis. In these situations, antibiotics are used as adjuncts to conventional mechanical therapy (scaling and root planing, with or without surgical access) and excellent home care. With a few possible exceptions, periodontal infections are considered to be opportunistic infections; hence the goal of therapy is to disrupt the pathogenic subgingival plaque biofilm to foster the reestablishment of a commensal subgingival biofilm associated with health (see chapter 12 for more detail). Because most of the bacterial species associated with progression of periodontitis are members of the indigenous microbiota, suppression of these species rather than elimination of them from subgingival sites may be the goal of treatment. When antibiotics are used as adjuncts to conventional therapy, dentists must decide whether to administer antibiotics to these patients systemically or locally to specific periodontal pockets. This topic is considered in more detail below.

Finally, antibiotics are sometimes used in the practice of dentistry to prevent oral bacteria introduced into the bloodstream during dental procedures from disseminating to extraoral body sites and colonizing there. Certain patients require antibiotic prophylaxis (administration of antibiotics systemically) before receiving any type of invasive dental care, that is, dental care that could cause bleeding and/or introduce oral bacteria into the bloodstream. Antibiotic prophylaxis is used to prevent infections and is also considered in more detail below.

Use of Antibiotics in the Treatment of Odontogenic Infections

PERIAPICAL INFECTIONS

Odontogenic infections may begin when bacteria in carious lesions gain access to the dental pulp or when oral bacteria gain entry into the pulpal tissues by some other means. Pulpal infection is accompanied by inflammation and may result in pulp necrosis (see chapter 15 for more details).

Acute and chronic periapical infections result from the spread of an infection from the root canals of a tooth into the periapical region of the alveolar bone. The first line of treatment for periapical infections is through debridement, endodontic therapy, or extraction of the tooth. Generally, antibiotics are not used in the treatment of periapical infections. However, in cases where endodontic infections have spread beyond the alveolar bone (see below) penicillin VK is the empiric antibiotic of choice for treatment, and clindamycin is the antibiotic of choice for patients allergic to penicillin.

ODONTOGENIC INFECTIONS THAT HAVE SPREAD BEYOND THE TEETH AND ALVEOLAR BONE

In spite of the fact that caries is caused by gram-positive aerobic and facultative organisms (oral streptococci and *Actinomyces* species), odontogenic infections that spread beyond the teeth and alveolar processes are polymicrobial (mixed) infections that are caused by aerobic, facultative, and anaerobic microorganisms. Approximately 56% of specimens obtained from odontogenic abscesses have been shown to contain both facultative and anaerobic bacteria. The concept of the progression from facultative streptococci to anaerobic gram-negative rods in orofacial infections has been supported by the finding of a predominance of streptococci in early infections (in the first 3 days of symptoms) and a predominance of anaerobes in late infections. Table 2 charts the characteristics of the three different stages of infection. During the inoculation stage, which may last up to 3 days, aerobic bacteria predominate and the clinical picture may not be very much affected. The infection becomes more established in the cellulitis stage and the involved pathogens are likely to be both aerobic and anaerobic. It is during this period of 3 to 7 days that the patient starts to develop erythema and edema, which may be diffuse and very tender. If the infection continues to go untreated, anaerobes predominate and eventually abscess formation occurs. In the abscess stage, the patient's edema is more localized and perhaps fluctuant or indicative of pus formation within the abscess cavity. At this late stage the microorganisms have caused a significant amount of tissue destruction, and it is unlikely that antibiotics alone can

TABLE 2 Stages of odontogenic infections[a]

Parameter	Inoculation	Cellulitis	Abscess
Time	0–3 days	3–7 days	>5 days
Pain	Mild to moderate	Severe and generalized	Moderate to severe and localized
Size	Small	Large	Small
Location	Diffuse	Diffuse	Circumscribed
Palpation	Soft, doughy, mildly tender	Hard, exquisitely tender	Fluctuant, tender
Appearance	Normal coloration	Reddened	Peripherally reddened
Skin quality	Normal	Thickened	Centrally undermined and shiny
Surface temperature	Slightly heated	Hot	Moderately heated
Loss of function	Minimal or none	Severe	Moderately severe
Tissue fluid	Edema	Serosanguineous, flecks of pus	Pus
Level of malaise	Mild	Severe	Moderate to severe
Degree of seriousness	Mild	Severe	Moderate to severe
Predominant bacteria	Aerobic, facultative	Mixed	Anaerobic

[a]Adapted from L. J. Peterson, p. 417, *in* L. J. Peterson (ed.), *Contemporary Oral and Maxillofacial Surgery*, 2nd ed. (Mosby Co., St. Louis, Mo., 1993).

sufficiently penetrate the involved areas. Thus, surgical intervention may be required to resolve the infection.

Selection of Antibiotics for the Treatment of Odontogenic Infections

β-LACTAM ANTIBIOTICS

The narrow-spectrum, penicillinase-sensitive agents such as penicillin G and penicillin V and the broad-spectrum aminopenicillins, e.g., ampicillin and amoxicillin, are of primary interest to the dental practitioner. Penicillin V is orally administered and active against streptococci and most oral anaerobes. Absorbed from the small bowel, peak serum levels are reached within 60 min and maintained for about 4 h. For most dental indications, 500 mg of penicillin V is administered orally every 6 h. Penicillin is primarily excreted by the kidneys, and in patients with severe renal dysfunction, daily dosages must be adjusted.

The aminopenicillins owe their extended spectrum to an increased ability to penetrate the outer membrane of gram-negative bacteria. This increased activity against organisms such as *Haemophilus influenzae* is occasionally useful, whereas the spectrum against gram-negative enteric rods such as *Escherichia coli* and *Salmonella, Shigella,* and *Proteus* species is rarely needed in odontogenic infections. Amoxicillin is indicated for subacute bacterial endocarditis prophylaxis because of its predictable and reliable absorption after oral administration rather than its increased spectrum. Cross-allergenicity between natural and semisynthetic penicillins can be expected, so all penicillins should be avoided in patients with a history of allergy.

Cephalosporins are rapidly and thoroughly absorbed after oral administration. Similar to penicillins, they are excreted in the urine and dosing adjustments need to be made for patients with renal failure. Allergic reactions to cephalosporins have an overall incidence of 1 to 3% of the patients who receive the drugs. There is cross-allergenicity between penicillins and cephalosporins, and patients who are allergic to penicillin are four times more likely to have an allergic reaction to a cephalosporin. Accordingly, cephalosporins should not routinely be prescribed for patients with penicillin allergy.

CLINDAMYCIN

Clindamycin is rapidly absorbed from the gut, and it is not affected by the presence of food in the stomach. It is widely distributed and reaches high levels in most tissues, including bone. However, it does not effectively cross the blood-brain barrier, making it ineffective for the treatment of meningitis, brain abscess, or cranial extension of odontogenic infections. The half-life of clindamycin is about 2.5 h and it is metabolized by the liver and excreted into the urine and bile. Clindamycin and its metabolites are involved in the enterohepatic circulation and can remain present for several weeks after the cessation of drug administration.

Clindamycin's main spectrum of activity is against anaerobes, including most strains of *Bacteroides, Porphyromonas, Prevotella, Fusobacterium,* and *Peptostreptococcus,* but *Eikenella corrodens* is uniformly resistant. Clindamycin is indicated in the treatment of patients with serious odontogenic infections or patients who present several days after the onset of symptoms. It is also used as a first-line agent in patients who are allergic to penicillins and as a key alternative for prophylaxis in such patients. Diarrhea is a common side effect of clindamycin as well as many other oral antimicrobial agents. *Clostridium difficile* colitis is a severe complication that has been most associated with the administration of clindamycin, although many antibiotics can precipitate this condition. Previously known as pseudomembranous colitis, it is now more appropriately referred to as antibiotic-associated colitis. This complication is described in greater detail later in the chapter. Less common complications include rash, drug- associated fever, and anaphylaxis, with the overall rate thought to be less than 1%.

MACROLIDES

Erythromycin and clarithromycin are the macrolide antibiotics with dental indications, having activity against streptococci, staphylococci, and some oral anaerobes. Erythromycin base is unstable in gastric acid and must be formed into an ester or ester salt for oral administration. The normal serum half-life is 1.4 h and blood serum levels are maintained for approximately 6 h. It is primarily excreted in the bile and only 2 to 5% is excreted in the urine. Adverse effects of erythromycin include nausea, vomiting, abdominal cramps, diarrhea, and skin rash, and it must be prescribed with caution in patients taking other medications because of potential drug-drug interactions. The hepatic cytochrome P-450 enzyme system can be inhibited by erythromycin, causing increased blood levels of medications that are metabolized by this pathway.

Clarithromycin differs from erythromycin in that it is stable in acid and very well absorbed from the gut, even in the presence of food. Clarithromycin is also extensively metabolized in the liver, but it is excreted in the urine and dose adjustments are suggested in patients with decreased renal function. Clarithromycin has fewer gastrointestinal side effects than erythromycin; however, the potential drug-drug interactions are still present. Along with azithromycin, clarithromycin is indicated as an option for patients allergic to penicillin who need prophylaxis for subacute bacterial endocarditis.

FLUOROQUINOLONES

Ciprofloxacin is indicated for some dental applications. It is absorbed readily from the gastrointestinal tract and has excellent tissue penetration. Dosage adjustments must be made for patients with impaired renal function, as some renal excretion occurs. Fluoroquinolones have been found to cause chondrocyte toxicity in animal studies and therefore should not be prescribed for dental indications to women who are pregnant or nursing, or to children.

METRONIDAZOLE

Originally indicated as an antiprotozoan agent, metronidazole was later shown to be effective against anaerobic bacteria. It is often indicated for moderate to severe odontogenic infections, frequently in combination with penicillin. Metronidazole has a relatively low side effect profile, its main adverse effect being a disulfiram-type reaction and interaction with warfarin (Coumadin). These are discussed in further detail below.

TETRACYCLINES

Tetracycline, doxycycline, and minocycline are the best-known members of this family of antibiotics. Although the tetracyclines have widespread medical indications, including atypical pneumonias, genital infections, Lyme disease, and others, they do not have specific indications for treatment of odontogenic infections.

EMPIRIC ANTIBIOTICS OF CHOICE FOR THE TREATMENT OF ODONTOGENIC INFECTIONS

Recommendations for empiric antibiotic therapy of odontogenic infections are listed in Table 3. A distinction can be made between the antibiotic therapy of early odontogenic infections that have spread beyond alveolar bone, i.e., within the first 3 days of symptoms in adjacent soft tissues, and soft tissue infections of longer duration. Such early infections have been associated with the oral streptococci, especially the *Streptococcus milleri* group. These microorganisms may be responsible for initial tissue invasion because of their elaboration of hyaluronidases. These enzymes break down the ground substance of connective tissue, thereby allowing the bacteria to penetrate into the tissues beyond the alveolar process. Fortunately, these organisms are still highly susceptible to penicillin, which should be effective for treatment of these odontogenic infections early in their course, before the appearance of the anaerobic gram-negative rods, such as *Fusobacterium nucleatum*, in which penicillin resistance has been on the rise. The reported rate of penicillin-resistant odontogenic infections among outpatients is low, in the 6 to 12% range. For this reason, penicillin V should be the empiric antibiotic of choice for treatment of outpatient odontogenic infections early in their clinical course. Three or more days after the onset of symptoms anaerobic gram-negative rods, such as *Prevotella* and *Porphyromonas* species, begin to appear in odontogenic infections. Roughly 25% of the strains of these two genera are penicillin resistant, although higher resistance rates have

TABLE 3 Empiric antibiotics of choice for odontogenic infections[a]

Type of infection	Antibiotic of choice
Mild or early infections	Penicillin
	Clindamycin, cephalexin (or other first-generation cephalosporin)
In case of penicillin allergy	Clindamycin, cephalexin (if penicillin allergy not the anaphylactoid type, use caution)
Severe or chronic infections	Clindamycin
	Ampicillin plus metronidazole
	Ampicillin plus sulbactam
In case of penicillin allergy	Clindamycin
	Cephalosporin (if penicillin allergy not the anaphylactoid type, use caution)
	Metronidazole alone (if neither clindamycin nor cephalosporins can be tolerated)
	Ciprofloxacin (especially for staphylococcal osteomyelitis or *E. corrodens*)

[a]Empiric antibiotic therapy is used before culture and sensitivity reports are available. Cultures should be taken in cases of severe infections that threaten vital structures.

been reported in some studies. Therefore, penicillin-resistant organisms are likely to be present in significant numbers in odontogenic infections that are mature (3 or more days after the onset of symptoms) or severe, requiring hospitalization. Under these conditions, clindamycin should be considered the empiric antibiotic of choice.

Erythromycin and the other macrolide antibiotics have been eliminated as antibiotics of choice for the treatment of soft tissue odontogenic infections in patients allergic to penicillin. *Prevotella* and *Porphyromonas* species are now largely resistant to the macrolides, including the newer ones such as clarithromycin and azithromycin. In fact, many oral streptococci have become resistant to this class of antibiotics. The fact that azithromycin is actively concentrated in phagocytes may make it more effective against the microbiota of odontogenic infections than would be suggested by in vitro susceptibility testing methods. Therefore, clinical studies are required, which may indicate that the newer macrolide antibiotics are indeed effective against odontogenic infections.

The oral cephalosporins remain effective against the oral streptococci, but as some *Prevotella* and *Porphyromonas* strains have acquired cephalosporinases, the advantages of these antibiotics in the treatment of odontogenic infections have decreased. The issue of cross-allergy between the penicillins and the cephalosporins must always be considered, although it appears that cross-allergy is generally limited to those individuals who have had an anaphylactic or anaphylactoid reaction (urticaria, bronchospasm, angioedema, or hypotension) in response to the penicillins. It may be appropriate to use oral cephalosporins for treatment of a patient with an odontogenic infection who is intolerant of clindamycin and has experienced either gastrointestinal intolerance or a nonanaphylactoid reaction to the penicillins.

Metronidazole remains an excellent antimicrobial agent for obligate anaerobes, with few resistance problems to date. Ornidazole, also a member of the nitroimidazole class that is available in the United Kingdom, has been used alone with good success to treat odontogenic infections. In the United States, however, metronidazole is generally used in combination with penicillin or another antibiotic that is effective against the oral streptococci.

The fluoroquinolones have seen some use in dentistry, although the spectrum of this class of antibiotics does not generally include the oral facultative and anaerobic flora. The major uses of these antibiotics in oral and maxillofacial infections would be for *E. corrodens* in a patient allergic to penicillin and perhaps in staphylococcal osteomyelitis. *E. corrodens* is uniformly resistant to clindamycin and is an occasional pathogen that may survive initial surgical and antibiotic therapy. Amoxicillin or ampicillin, with or without a β-lactamase inhibitor, is the antibiotic of choice for this organism, except in penicillin allergy. The use of a fluoroquinolone such as ciprofloxacin may allow a patient with staphylococcal osteomyelitis of the mandible, for example, to receive oral outpatient antibiotic therapy if cultures have shown that the staphylococci are susceptible to this antibiotic. This is because of the excellent oral absorption and bone penetration of ciprofloxacin. Ciprofloxacin is also used in the treatment of some forms of periodontitis (discussed below).

PERICORONITIS

Like most oral infections, pericoronitis is typically a polymicrobial infection. The periodontal pathogens, *Prevotella* and *Porphyromonas* species and oral spirochetes, such as *Treponema denticola,* are frequently the causative organisms. Recently, the *S. milleri* group has also been found to have a significant role in acute pericoronitis. These organisms usually are susceptible to penicillin or penicillin in combination with metronidazole.

Lower third molars lie in proximity to the pterygomandibular space, a portion of the masticator space. When these pericoronal infections spread to involve this space, trismus results, obscuring the infection to clinical examination. Therefore, the presence of trismus with a history of pain in the third molar region is an ominous sign of infection involving the masticator space, which, although not manifested by external facial swelling, may begin to involve the deeper parapharyngeal spaces. These infections may become life-threatening. The lower third molar is the most frequent offending tooth in severe odontogenic infections requiring hospitalization, and these infections occur most frequently in adolescents and young adults. Immediate removal of the involved tooth hastens resolution of the infection and should be done whenever possible. However, trismus or a suspected difficult extraction may require reliance on antibiotics until the infection is resolved and the tooth can be removed. In mild cases of pericoronitis (those without trismus, purulence, edema, or systemic manifestations), antibiotic therapy is rarely necessary, and extraction is the treatment of choice. In moderate and severe cases of pericoronitis, penicillin with or without metronidazole and clindamycin are good choices for empiric therapy and extraction is performed as soon as possible.

Use of Antibiotics in the Treatment of Periodontitis

Periodontal infections are considered to be endogenous or opportunistic infections because most putative periodontal pathogens are members of the indigenous microbiota. Generally, periodontitis lesions contain a mixture of these putative pathogens rather than a single pathogenic species (for a review, see chapter 12). Most patients with periodontitis respond well to conventional mechanical therapy (scaling and root planing, with or without surgical access) coupled with meticulous home care to control their disease and prevent future inflammation and loss of periodontal attachment. As a result, it is generally not necessary to use antibiotics to control loss of periodontal attachment in most patients, and they would derive little or no additional benefit if antibiotic therapy were added to conventional mechanical therapy. However, patients who continue to lose periodontal attachment despite diligent mechanical therapy and meticulous home care (patients with refractory periodontitis), patients with impaired host resistance, patients with localized juvenile periodontitis or other forms of early-onset periodontitis, patients with systemic diseases that predispose to periodontitis, and patients with certain acute or severe periodontal infections (periodontal abscess, acute necrotizing ulcerative gingivitis, or periodontitis) may derive additional benefit from antibiotic therapy.

The fact that subgingival dental plaque is a biofilm is important to take into account when considering therapies to control the bacteria that cause periodontitis. Early studies that did not take this form of growth into account suggested that most antibiotics can achieve therapeutic concentrations in periodontal pockets after oral administration. In these studies, bacteria were grown planktonically and exposed to antibiotics. More recent in vitro studies suggest that the biofilm mode of growth confers certain survival advantages to plaque bacteria, particularly significantly increased resistance to antibiotics. Therefore it is likely that earlier studies significantly overestimated the effect of the antibiotics on the subgingival microbiota. It has been suggested that conventional mechanical therapy is effective for most patients because it physically disrupts the pathogenic subgingival plaque biofilm and allows recolonization of periodontal pockets with a commensal microbiota. When considering treatment options for patients who do not respond well to mechanical therapy, dentists must consider all possible factors that contribute to this treatment outcome and should be sure that debridement has been meticulous and that the patient's home care has been excellent before considering the adjunctive use of antibiotics. When the dentist determines that a patient is not responding well to mechanical therapy and excellent home care, or when a patient presents with an aggressive form of periodontitis or early-onset periodontitis, or other systemic factors as described above, adjunctive antibiotic therapy should be considered.

Selection of an appropriate antibiotic should depend on the diagnosis, the patient's history of antibiotic use, the identity of the putative periodontal pathogens found, and in some cases, the sensitivity of these organisms to antibiotics. All of the following antibiotics have been used systemically as adjuncts to mechanical periodontal therapy: tetracyclines, penicillins (including amoxicillin and amoxicillin with clavulanic acid [Augmentin]), clindamycin, azithromycin, metronidazole, metronidazole with amoxicillin, metronidazole with Augmentin, and metronidazole with ciprofloxacin. It is clear from a large number of studies that no single antibiotic produces a reliable and beneficial response for every patient. Each antibiotic has its advantages and disadvantages. Tetracyclines have a broad spectrum, but resistance to them is relatively common among members of the subgingival microbiota. Penicillins, even combined with clavulanic acid, are not particularly good antibiotics for adjunctive use because many members of the subgingival microbiota are β-lactamase producers. Clindamycin is active against most gram-positive bacteria and is very active against most of the gram-negative anaerobic putative periodontal pathogens. However, both *E. corrodens* and *Actinobacillus actinomycetemcomitans* are resistant to clindamycin, so it should only be used after it is established that these microorganisms are not part of the disease-associated microbiota of the patient. Metronidazole is specifically active against obligate anaerobes and is helpful as an adjunctive treatment for patients who do not harbor *A. actinomycetemcomitans* as part of the disease-associated microbiota. Metronidazole together with amoxicillin appears to be effective against *A. actinomycetemcomitans* and is an appropriate treatment for aggressive periodontitis associated with this microorganism.

Both tetracyclines and metronidazole have been incorporated into subgingival delivery systems and used locally to treat individual periodontal sites that do not respond to mechanical therapy. They are particularly helpful when a patient's response to mechanical therapy is generally good but some sites continue to be inflamed. Local delivery of these antibiotics can be advantageous because much higher concentrations of antibiotic can be administered directly to the inflamed site than can be achieved with systemic antibiotics, there is almost no systemic load so adverse reactions can be avoided, selection for multiply resistant strains is largely avoided, and concerns about patient compliance are eliminated. On balance, systemic administration of antibiotics may allow suppression or elimination of a periodontal pathogen from the entire mouth, reducing the risk for future recolonization. Moreover, systemic antibiotic therapy is easy to administer and is much lower in cost.

A growing body of evidence suggests that patients with chronic periodontal infections are at higher risk for developing certain chronic systemic diseases, including diabetes and heart disease. There is also evidence suggesting that women with chronic periodontitis are at higher risk for preterm labor than periodontally healthy women. If these oral-systemic disease connections are confirmed, then control of inflammatory periodontitis will become a major health need for all people.

Use of Antibiotics for the Prevention of Infection (Antibiotic Prophylaxis)

Antibiotics are administered prophylactically to select patients prior to dental treatment to prevent bacterial endocarditis or infection of an orthopedic prosthesis. There are other indications for the use of prophylactic antibiotics, such as vascular prostheses and a suppressed immune system, which are not as common and need to be reviewed with a patient's physician prior to dental treatment. Knowledge of the indications and medications to be administered to prevent bacterial endocarditis is compulsory for all dental practitioners. Table 4 lists the indications for antibiotic prophylaxis and the conditions for which prophylaxis is not indicated. Infective endocarditis is most frequently associated with streptococci and staphylococci. The general recommendations for antibiotic prophylaxis in most patients are outlined in Table 5. In addition to these guidelines, the patient's history of drug allergies, current medications, and overall physical status must be taken into consideration when selecting an antibiotic.

Additional Considerations for the Use of Antibiotics in Dental Practice: Drug Interactions

An enumeration of all possible antibiotic and drug interactions known is not within the scope of this chapter. The following discussion highlights some key antibiotic and drug interactions and the practitioner is cautioned to be aware of product information when prescribing medications. A mechanism that explains a multitude of drug interactions has recently been more fully elucidated. The cytochrome P-450 system is a large set of isoenzymes located in the liver and gut wall. One isoenzyme, CYP3A4, accounts for 60% of the cytochromes in the liver and 70% of them in the intestinal wall. CYP1A2 is another important cytochrome that metabolizes the theophylline drugs. When these enzymes are inhibited by certain drugs, including macrolides and the antifungals ketaconazole, fluconazole, and itraconazole, the metabolism of other drugs using the same cytochrome is inhibited. Therefore, the bioavailability of the second drug increases, augmenting the desired effects and the unintended side effects of

TABLE 4 Cardiac conditions associated with endocarditis[a]

Part I. Endocarditis prophylaxis recommended

High-risk category
- Prosthetic cardiac valves (bioprosthetic and homograft valves)
- Previous bacterial endocarditis
- Complex cyanotic congenital heart disease (e.g., single ventricle states, transposition of the great arteries, tetralogy of Fallot)
- Surgically constructed systemic pulmonary shunts or conduits

Moderate-risk category
- Most other congenital cardiac malformations
- Acquired valvular dysfunction (e.g., rheumatic heart disease)
- Hypertrophic cardiomyopathy
- Mitral valve prolapse with valvular regurgitation and/or thickened leaflets

Part II. Endocarditis prophylaxis not recommended

Negligible-risk category
- Isolated secundum atrial septal defect
- Surgical repair of atrial septal defect, ventricular septal defect, or patent ductus arteriosus (without residua beyond 6 months)
- Previous coronary artery bypass graft surgery
- Mitral valve prolapse without valvular regurgitation
- Physiologic, functional, or innocent heart murmurs
- Previous Kawasaki disease without valvular dysfunction
- Previous rheumatic fever without valvular dysfunction
- Cardiac pacemakers (intravascular and epicardial) and implanted defibrillators

[a]Reprinted with permission from A. S. Dajani, K. A. Taubert, W. Wilson, A. F. Bolger, P. Ferrieri, M. H. Gewitz, S. T. Shulman, S. Nouri, J. W. Newburger, C. Hutto, T. J. Pallasch, T. W. Gage, M. E. Levison, G. Peter, and G. Zuccaro, Jr., *Clin. Infect. Dis.* **25**:1448–1458, 1997.

TABLE 5 Prophylactic regimens for dental, oral, respiratory tract, or esophageal procedures[a]

Situation	Agent	Regimen[b]
Standard general prophylaxis	Amoxicillin	Adults: 2.0 g Children: 50 mg/kg orally 1 h before procedure
Unable to take oral medications	Ampicillin	Adults: 2.0 g intramuscularly (IM) or intravenously (IV) Children: 50 mg/kg IM or IV within 30 min of procedure
Allergic to penicillin	Clindamycin	Adults: 600 mg Children: 20 mg/kg orally 1 h before procedure
	or	
	Cephalexin or cefadoxil[c]	Adults: 2.0 g Children: 50 mg/kg orally 1 h before procedure
	or	
	Azithromycin or clarithromycin	Adults: 500 mg Children: 15 mg/kg orally 1 hr before procedure
Allergic to penicillin and unable to take oral medications	Clindamycin	Adults: 600 mg Children: 20 mg/kg IV within 30 min of procedure
	or	
	Cefazolin	Adults: 1.0 g Children: 25 mg/kg IM or IV within 30 min of procedure

[a]Reprinted with permission from A. S. Dajani, K. A. Taubert, W. Wilson, A. F. Bolger, P. Ferrieri, M. H. Gewitz, S. T. Shulman, S. Nouri, J. W. Newburger, C. Hutto, T. J. Pallasch, T. W. Gage, M. E. Levison, G. Peter, and G. Zuccaro, Jr., *Clin. Infect. Dis.* **25**:1448–1458, 1997.

[b]Total children's dose should not exceed adult dose.

[c]Cephalosporins should not be used in individuals with immediate-type hypersensitivity reaction (urticaria, angioedema, or anaphylaxis) to penicillins.

the second drug. The most important of these interactions include erythromycin and itraconazole with theophyllines (seizures); alfentanil (increased respiratory depression); erythromycin, itraconazole, and ketaconazole with astemizole or terfenadine (cardiac dysrhythmias and death); cisapride (Propulsid) and disopyramide (cardiac dysrhythmias and death); carbamazepine (vertigo, drowsiness, confusion); and triazolam or oral midazolam (increased sedation).

Another important antibiotic drug interaction is with the oral contraceptives. To minimize the side effects of estrogen in contraceptives, such as thrombophlebitis, pulmonary embolism, and induction of breast cancers, the amount of estrogen in modern contraceptives has been reduced to a point such that the serum level of the estrogen component is supported by enterohepatic recirculation. Essentially, when estrogen passes through the liver, it is conjugated with glucuronide and excreted through the bile into the gut. The gut flora, in turn, is able to detach the glucuronide from the estrogen molecule, thus allowing it to be reabsorbed by the gut. When an antibiotic eliminates enough of the gut flora, the enterohepatic recirculation of estrogen is inhibited, and therefore the serum level of estrogen falls. This may account for breakthrough menstrual bleeding and unwanted pregnancies. Rifampin is the only drug clinically proven to have this effect. The evidence supporting such a role for other antibiotics is less clear, but the penicillins, cephalosporins, metronidazole, macrolides, and tetracyclines have been implicated to some degree. Therefore, it is wise to advise patients taking oral contraceptives to use a backup birth control method for at least the remainder of the current menstrual cycle.

Some antibiotics can interact with anticoagulants. The macrolides and metronidazole decrease the metabolism of warfarin; this can raise blood levels and enhance bleeding. Other broad-spectrum antibiotics, including the tetracyclines and occasionally clindamycin, may reduce the population of gastrointestinal bacteria that synthesize vitamin K, an antagonist of warfarin. In this situation, the anticoagulant effect of warfarin may increase.

Both metronidazole and the tetracyclines interfere with the renal excretion of lithium. Therefore, patients taking lithium may experience lithium toxicity, symptoms of which include confusion and ataxia, as well as kidney damage, when taking these antibiotics. Metronidazole also has a well-known disulfiram (Antabuse) effect when combined with alcohol. Patients prescribed metronidazole should be cautioned not to consume alcohol. Patients who use alcohol while taking metronidazole may experience flushing, headache, palpitations, and nausea, due to an accumulation of acetaldehyde, a metabolic by-product of alcohol.

The fluoroquinolones have been found to irreversibly damage newly forming cartilage in animals, and thus are contraindicated in children. The fluoroquinolones also interfere with theophylline metabolism via the cytochrome P-450 system, possibly causing seizures.

Antibiotic-associated colitis is caused by an exotoxin produced by C. *difficile*, an obligate gram-positive enteric anaerobe. Patients at risk for this complication are generally debilitated. Their profile includes multiple prior therapies with antibiotics, inflammatory bowel disease, abdominal surgery, and hospitalization. The only risk factor commonly found in dental outpatients is feminine gender. Symptoms include abdominal cramping and five or more episodes of diarrhea per day, or mucoid or bloody diarrhea, and a positive stool assay for *C. difficile* exotoxin is diagnostic. The treatment of choice is withdrawal of the antibiotic. In cases that do not resolve after discontinuation of the original antibiotic, oral metronidazole is indicated as a first-line agent. Any patient suspected of having this complication must be immediately referred to a physician for prompt diagnosis and treatment.

ANTIBIOTIC RESISTANCE

Resistance to Antibiotics Follows Their Introduction into Clinical Practice

By 1939, Howard Florey, Ernst Chain, and Norman Heatley, working in England, had devised methods for the production of large quantities of penicillin, a feat that had eluded Alexander Fleming after his discovery of the antibiotic in 1928. Subsequently, Florey and Chain were invited to the United States to help in a joint effort by Great Britain, Canada, and the United States to mass produce penicillin. By 1941, sufficient quantities were available to treat Allied troops injured in battle, which, for the first time, lowered significantly the numbers of military casualties due to wound infections. Penicillin was used to treat infections exclusively by the military until 1942, when it was shipped to Massachusetts General Hospital for the treatment of more than 200 badly burned survivors of a major fire in Boston, most of whom were saved from fatal infections. Shortly thereafter, penicillin became readily available to the general public, and until the mid-1950s, without prescription. Individuals began to use the antibiotic for numerous ailments, both appropriate and inappropriate, and often at inappropriate doses.

Strains of *S. aureus* resistant to high levels of penicillin were isolated from patients as early as 1942, and by 1946, in one particular hospital, approximately 14% of *S. aureus* isolated from patients were resistant. Today, greater than 90% of *S. aureus* isolates from hospitals and the community are resistant to penicillin. Similar stories have played out over and over again, such that the introduction of every new antibiotic, or class of antibiotic, into clinical practice has been followed by the emergence of bacterial pathogens exhibiting resistance to clinically relevant levels of that antibiotic, often within 1 to 3 years of its introduction (Table 6).

R Factors and Other Antibiotic Resistance Plasmids

Beginning in the mid-1930s, sulfonamides were the only drugs available for the treatment of dysentery. However, by 1950, virtually 100% of *Shigella* strains isolated from such patients in Japan were resistant to these drugs. Fortunately, also by 1950, the antibiotics streptomycin, tetracycline, and chloramphenicol had become available for the treatment of these *Shigella* infections. Due in large measure to their experience with the sulfonamides, the Japanese began to monitor *Shigella* isolates for their susceptibility to these three antibiotics, as well as sulfonamides. Strains resistant to the antibiotics began to emerge at very low frequencies, with five isolates resistant to streptomycin and only two resistant to tetracycline out of nearly 5,000 examined in 1953, and resistant strains continued to appear at low frequencies through 1956 (Table 7).

TABLE 6 Introduction of antibiotics into clinical practice followed by emergence of resistance in key bacterial species

Antibiotic	Yr introduced	Emergence of resistance in:	Resistance first reported in:
Sulfonamides	1935	*Shigella dysenteriae*	1940s
Penicillin	1941	*Staphylococcus aureus*	1942
		Streptococcus pneumoniae	1970
Streptomycin	1943	*Enterobacteriaceae*	1940s
Tetracycline	1948	Numerous genera and species	1950s
Erythromycin	1952	*Streptococcus* species	1960s
Vancomycin	1956	*Enterococcus faecalis*	1988
		Staphylococcus aureus	2002
Trimethoprim	1956	*Salmonella enterica* serovar Typhimurium	1959
Methicillin	1960	*Staphylococcus aureus*	1961
Ampicillin	1963	*Escherichia coli*	1963
		Haemophilus influenzae	1974
		Neisseria gonorrhoeae	1976
Gentamicin	1964	*Enterococcus faecalis*	1983
Fluoroquinolones	1984	*Enterobacteriaceae*	1990s
Linezolid	2000	*Enterococcus* species	2001

Beginning in 1957, not only did the number of isolates resistant to one of the three antibiotics increase, but strains resistant to two and even all three of these antibiotics emerged, and frequencies of isolation of such multiply resistant strains also increased over the next 3 years. These isolates were also resistant to sulfonamides. Assuming that resistance to each of these antimicrobial agents was encoded by a different gene, and that the frequency of mutation to resistance for each gene could be as high as one per 10^6 bacteria per generation, Japanese investigators calculated that the highest frequency at which a relevant mutation could have occurred in each of the four genes in the same bacterial cell was one in 10^{24} bacteria. Clearly, such multiple antimicrobial resistance could not be explained on the basis of mutation. These investigators had also observed that multiply resistant and totally susceptible *Shigella* strains could be isolated from the same patient, and that both *Shigella* and *Escherichia coli* strains exhibiting the same multiple resistance phenotype could also

TABLE 7 Emergence of antibiotic-resistant *Shigella* species in Japan[a]

Year	No. of isolates tested	No. of isolates resistant to:						
		Sm[b]	Tc[b]	Cm[b]	Sm, Cm	Sm, Tc	Cm, Tc	Sm, Cm, Tc
1953	4,900	5	2	0	0	0	0	0
1954	4,876	11	0	0	0	0	0	0
1955	5,327	4	0	0	0	0	0	0
1956	4,399	8	4	0	0	0	0	0
1957	4,873	13	46	0	2	2	0	37
1958	6,563	18	20	0	7	0	0	193
1959	4,071	16	32	0	71	0	0	74
1960	3,396	29	36	0	61	9	7	308

[a]Adapted from S. Falkow, *Infectious Multiple Drug Resistance* (Pion Limited, London, United Kingdom, 1975).
[b]Sm, streptomycin; Tc, tetracycline; Cm, chloramphenicol.

be obtained from the same patient. They postulated that the resistance genes might be transferred together between these two species in the intestinal tracts of patients, and demonstrated such transfer in the laboratory by mixed incubation of susceptible *Escherichia coli* and multiresistant *Shigella* strains, and vice versa. They also demonstrated a requirement for cell-to-cell contact between donor and recipient strains, as had been demonstrated for the F factor. The investigators proposed a new term, "R factor," for a genetic element able to transfer antibiotic resistance from one bacterial cell to another by conjugation. Subsequently, it was shown that R factors were conjugative plasmids that encoded one or more antibiotic resistance genes. Throughout the 1960s and into the early 1970s, it appeared that resistance to antibiotics among clinical isolates of the *Enterobacteriaceae* was almost exclusively plasmid-mediated, either by large conjugative plasmids (R factors) or smaller nontransmissible plasmids that were often mobilizable by conjugative plasmids present in the same cells.

Penicillin resistance in *S. aureus* was shown to be mediated by a large, nonconjugative plasmid, and the gene responsible for penicillin resistance of *S. aureus* codes for the production of an enzyme, penicillinase (later designated β-lactamase), that inactivates penicillin by cleavage of its β-lactam ring. The macrolide erythromycin became available in 1952 for treatment of infections caused by gram-positive bacteria, and by the 1960s strains of *S. aureus* and *Streptococcus pyogenes* resistant to this antibiotic were being isolated from patients. Resistance to trimethoprim, a totally synthetic antibiotic, was first observed in England among isolates of *Salmonella enterica* serovar Typhimurium in 1959, just 3 years after its introduction (Table 6). These resistance traits were also shown to be plasmid-mediated, at least among the early isolates.

Acquired Antibiotic Resistance

Pathogenic bacterial species that were becoming resistant to antibiotics were said to have acquired these resistance traits, since initially, these species had been shown to be intrinsically susceptible to those antibiotics, and their resistance traits were due to specific genes carried on plasmids, as opposed to mutations in chromosomal genes. These plasmid genes coded for proteins that rendered the host bacterium resistant by one of four basic mechanisms, i.e., by enzymatic detoxification of the antibiotic; by alteration of the antibiotic target site; by altered uptake or retention of the antibiotic; or via a bypass of the antibiotic target. Examples of enzymatic detoxification include the hydrolysis of the β-lactam ring of penicillins and other β-lactam antibiotics by β-lactamases, the acetylation of chloramphenicol by a chloramphenicol-specific acetyltransferase, and the phosphorylation, adenylylation, or acetylation of different residues of an aminoglycoside.

The earliest example of alteration of an antibiotic target site was the methylation of an adenine residue of 23S rRNA encoded by an *erm* gene that results in resistance to macrolides, such as erythromycin; lincosamides, such as lincomycin or clindamycin; and streptogramin B type antibiotics, such as virginiamycin, the so-called MLS resistance phenotype. The classic example of altered uptake or retention of an antibiotic is active efflux from the cell of tetracycline, encoded by some *tet* genes, e.g., *tet*A and *tet*B, common to many gram-negative bacteria, or the gram-positive bacterial determinant, *tet*K. The sulfonamides and trimethoprim inhibit specific enzymes in the folate pathway, and acquired resistance to these antimicrobials involved bypassing these sensitive steps via plasmid-mediated production of sulfonamide-resistant dihydropteroate synthase or trimethoprim-resistant dihydrofolate reductase.

Transposons and Other Mobile Genetic Elements Carry Antibiotic Resistance Genes

The amino penicillin, ampicillin, with a broader gram-negative bacterial spectrum than penicillin G, was introduced into clinical practice in 1963, and in the same year *Escherichia coli* strains resistant to this antibiotic began to emerge. Antibiotic resistance transposons, i.e., individual resistance genes flanked by insertion sequences (see chapter 7), were being discovered and analyzed by several laboratories in the early 1970s. One such transposon, designated Tn3, encodes TEM β-lactamase activity that destroys penicillin and ampicillin. Initially, Tn3 was shown to be present on a variety of plasmids isolated, not only from *Escherichia coli* but also from several different species of *Enterobacteriaceae*. Ampicillin was also effective for the treatment of infections caused by *H. influenzae* and was safe to use on children. However, in 1974, three infants died from bacterial meningitis following treatment with ampicillin. All had been infected by ampicillin-resistant strains of *H. influenzae*. Subsequently, it was shown that the strains harbored plasmids that carried approximately one-third of Tn3, but that the rest of each plasmid was unrelated to any known plasmid from the *Enterobacteriaceae*.

One scenario to explain how this may have occurred is as follows. A plasmid carrying Tn3 had been transferred from a bacterial species, e.g., *E. coli*, to a strain of *H. influenzae*, but the introduced plasmid could not replicate in the new host. However, the incoming plasmid survived long enough for the transposon to relocate on an indigenous *H. influenzae* plasmid, creating a new R-plasmid and broadening the spectrum of species now resistant to penicillins.

Two years after the emergence of ampicillin resistance in *H. influenzae*, strains of ampicillin-resistant *N. gonorrhoeae* began to appear. In this case, resistant isolates were shown to harbor a small, β-lactamase-encoding plasmid with greater than 90% homology to a plasmid isolated from a strain of *Haemophilus parainfluenzae*, each containing approximately 40% of Tn3. Subsequently, it was shown that small β-lactamase-encoding plasmids could be mobilized from strain to strain by a conjugative plasmid indigenous to *N. gonorrhoeae*. Thus, although the first resistant strains of *N. gonorrhoeae* may have received this trait from an unrelated bacterial species, possibly via conjugation or transformation, penicillin resistance was now being spread among *N. gonorrhoeae* strains via conjugative mobilization.

From the early 1970s through the mid-1980s, transposons encoding a variety of antibiotic resistance traits were discovered and studied in gram-positive and gram-negative bacterial species. It was also observed that transposons often had a tendency to insert in a plasmid adjacent to other transposons, such that resistance regions of R-plasmids evolved by the successive addition of individual transposons, often forming new transposons encoding multiple resistance traits, as illustrated in Fig. 6.

Throughout the 1970s, and into the 1980s, it became a popular belief that all acquired antibiotic resistance was plasmid-mediated and that the dissemination of resistance plasmids among bacterial strains was by the transfer of a conjugative plasmid, or via the mobilization by such a plasmid of a nonconjugative plasmid, and maybe occasionally via plasmid transformation. Furthermore, multiple resistance plasmids, whether conjugative or not, evolved by the acquisition of transposons. There was, however, a growing body of anecdotal "data" to suggest the existence of bacterial strains that expressed acquired resistance phenotypes, but from which no plasmid DNA could be isolated. In some instances, these traits could be transferred from one strain to another by a process that required cell-to-cell contact, but with no evidence for the presence of plasmid DNA in either donor or transconjugant strains. In 1982, an explanation for such results was forthcoming with the first published description of a conjugative transposon, Tn916. This transposon, 18 kb in size, carried not only a *tet*M determinant of tetracycline resistance, but it also encoded all the information required for its excision from the host chromosome, circularization, conjugative transfer, and reinsertion into the chromosome of its new host, all in the absence of plasmid DNA. Conjugative transposons of various sizes, and encoding multiple resistance traits, have since been described, and such transposons are known to be capable of

FIGURE 6 Evolution of a multiple antibiotic resistance plasmid by acquisition of transposons. The plasmid illustrated encodes resistance to six different antibiotics: chloramphenicol (Cm), streptomycin (Sm), sulfonamides (Su), ampicillin (Ap), kanamycin (Km), and neomycin (Nm). The acquisition of the genes encoding these traits apparently occurred via the insertion of three different transposons, TnA, a well-studied β-lactamase-encoding transposon; a second transposon, Tn4, encoding resistance to Sm and Su; and yet a third transposon, TnX, encoding resistance to Cm, Km, and Nm, that inserted on either side of the two other transposons, or into which TnA and Tn4 inserted.

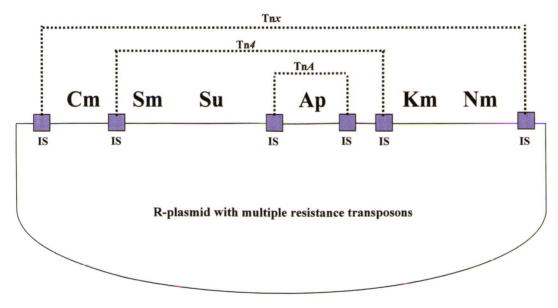

inserting into any type of bacterial replicon, chromosome, phage, or plasmid. Unlike previously described tetracycline resistance determinants, *tet*M did not encode resistance by an efflux mechanism, but rather the product of *tet*M was shown to protect the ribosome from the inhibitory activity of not only tetracycline, but also of the newer tetracycline, minocycline, resistance to which is not provided by the efflux-encoding genes. In addition, whereas each tetracycline efflux-mediating gene was found exclusively in gram-positive or gram-negative species, ribosomal protection determinants, *tet*M, and later several others were detected and shown to express in gram-positive and gram-negative bacteria, as well as the cell wall-free *Mycoplasma* species.

Vancomycin has been available for the treatment of serious nosocomial infections caused by gram-positive bacteria since 1956, and no resistance was encountered until 1988, when isolates of VRE began to appear in France, soon to be followed in the United States. The mechanism of resistance involved alteration of the target of vancomycin, the D-Ala–D-Ala portion of UDP-muramylpentapeptide. The terminal D-Ala residue in resistant isolates is replaced by D-lactate. While vancomycin binds to D-Ala–D-Ala, it cannot bind to D-Ala–D-Lac. In 1989, resistance to vancomycin was shown to be mediated by a conjugative plasmid isolated from a strain of *Enterococcus faecalis*, and in 1993, the genes responsible for resistance were located on a transposon, Tn*1546* (illustrated in Fig. 7), carried on a conjugative plasmid. The genes encoding enzymes directly involved in vancomycin resistance are *vanH, vanA, vanX,* and *vanY*. A dehydrogenase, which converts pyruvate to D-lactate, is encoded by *vanH*. A ligase, encoded by *vanA*, joins D-Lac to a D-Ala residue to form D-Ala–D-Lac, which is added to UDP-muramyl tripeptide in place of D-Ala–D-Ala. The *vanX* gene encodes a carboxypeptidase, which breaks any D-Ala–D-Ala dipeptides that have been formed, and *vanY* encodes a carboxypeptidase to hydrolyze any pentapeptides that contain D-Ala–D-Ala. The function of *vanZ* remains unknown. The *vanS* and *vanR* genes encode proteins of a two-component regulatory system through which expression of the *van* genes is induced in the presence of

FIGURE 7 Organization of genes on VanA transposon Tn*1546*. Depicted are the genes encoded by the transposon. ORF1 and ORF2, which are not part of the *vanA* operon, encode enzymes involved in the transposition process. *vanR* and *vanS* encode the two-component regulatory system by which the expression of the operon genes are induced in the presence of vancomycin. *vanH, vanA, vanX, vanY,* and *vanZ* encode enzymes involved in the replacement of D-Ala–D-Ala with D-Ala–D-Lac in the cell wall precursor pentapeptide, as described in greater detail in the text. Adapted from M. Arthur, F. Depardieu, G. Gerbaud, M. Galimand, R. Leclercq, and P. Courvalin, *J. Bacteriol.* **179:**97–106, 1997.

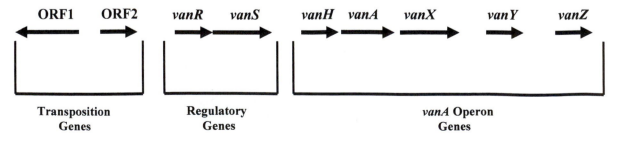

vancomycin. ORF1 and ORF2 are genes that encode proteins involved in transposition. Transposons encoding similar vancomycin resistance operons, mediating the so-called VanB, VanD, and VanG phenotypes, have also been described. More recently, in 1995, a >25-kb conjugative transposon, Tn*5482*, encoding a VanB phenotype, was identified in a strain of *Enterococcus faecium*.

Vancomycin has been the drug of choice for the treatment of MRSA (see below) since the 1960s. A strain of *S. aureus* resistant to intermediate concentrations of vancomycin (4 to 8 μg/ml), termed VISA, was isolated from a patient in Japan in 1996, and similar strains appeared throughout the world shortly thereafter. The VISA strains were shown to produce three to five times as much PBP2 or PBP2′ as wild-type *S. aureus* and to accumulate intracellularly three to eight times as much murein monomer precursors as wild-type strains. Microscopically, the cell walls of these strains were much thicker than normal. Infections caused by VISA strains were still treatable by higher concentrations of vancomycin. The real fear, for some time, was that *S. aureus* might obtain a vancomycin resistance operon from a resistant enterococcal strain, and in fact, transfer of a plasmid carrying a *vanA* transposon from a strain of *E. faecalis* to *S. aureus* was demonstrated in the laboratory in 1992. However, it was not until 2002 that the first clinical isolate of *S. aureus* harboring a conjugative plasmid that encoded the VanA phenotype was obtained in Michigan. The plasmid in that isolate had clearly come from an *Enterococcus*. A similar strain of *S. aureus*, with a 120-kb VanA-encoding plasmid, was isolated from a patient in Pennsylvania later in the same year, and in 2004, another isolate was obtained from a patient in New York. The MIC of vancomycin against these resistant *S. aureus* strains is ≥32 μg/ml.

The gene responsible for β-lactamase production by *S. aureus* isolates obtained from patients in the 1940s was designated *blaZ*. The gene is part of a transposable element found on a large plasmid that often encodes resistance to other antibiotics, such as gentamicin and erythromycin, and is present in an overwhelming majority of *S. aureus* strains isolated from patients in hospitals and in the community. Methicillin, the first of the semisynthetic penicillins, and resistant to the activity of the β-lactamase encoded by *blaZ*, was introduced into clinical practice in 1961. As was true with penicillin-resistant *S. aureus*, MRSA began to appear almost immediately, first in the hospital setting, followed much later (2000) in the community. Methicillin resistance is encoded by the *mecA* gene, which is part of a chromosome-borne mobile genetic element found only in MRSA. Although methicillin resistance is common in hospitals and in the community, only a few clones of *S. aureus* carry it, transfer of *mecA* being relatively rare. The *mecA* gene encodes a penicillin-binding protein, PBP2a (also called PBP2′), that has a very low affinity for all β-lactam antibiotics. PBP2a is not found in methicillin-susceptible *S. aureus*. Methicillin resistance equals resistance to all β-lactam antibiotics, including cephalosporins.

A new type of genetic element, the integron, was identified in the late 1980s. There are two types of integrons, the so-called super integrons, which can encode more than 100 genes, and the resistance integrons, which can carry up to 10 different genes encoding resistance to antibiotics or disinfectants. All integrons are composed of three essential elements, illustrated in Fig. 8. The first of these elements is a gene *(int)* encoding an integrase, which mediates the insertion, by a *recA*-independent mechanism, of circularized segments of DNA-designated gene cassettes at the second essential integron element, the attachment site *(att)*. Gene cassettes are open reading frames without promoters. However, they are inserted within an integron downstream of the third essential element of the integron, a strong promoter, designated P_C, which controls the expression of all the open reading frames in a given integron. Integrons may be located on plasmids or in the host chromosome, and some are located within transposons. Initially, integrons were identified only in gram-negative bacterial species, but more recently they have been detected in such gram-positive bacterial genera as *Corynebacterium*, *Mycobacterium*, and *Enterococcus*. It has been discovered that the R-factor-mediated resistance to sulfonamides, tetracycline, streptomycin, and chloramphenicol in one of the multiply resistant *Shigella dysenteriae* strains isolated in Japan in the 1950s was encoded by an integron.

The Role of Mutations in Antibiotic Resistance

Resistance to fluoroquinolones in most bacterial species can be traced to mutations that result in amino acid changes in either DNA gyrase or topoisomerase IV. Such mutations are usually identified in the *gyrA* gene of DNA gyrase, or the *parC* gene of topoisomerase IV, although occasionally mutations contributing to resistance have been identified in the *gyrB* or *parE* genes. Low-level resistance can, for the most part, be traced to one or more mutations in the genes encoding the primary target of the fluoroquinolones to which resistance is exhibited, usually gyrase in gram-negative bacteria and topoisomerase IV in gram-positive bacteria. Mutations resulting in fluoroquinolone resistance are located in a specific region of the gene referred to as the quinolone resistance-determining

FIGURE 8 Building of an integron. The top box depicts a simple integron composed of an integrase gene, *int*; a strong constitutively expressed promoter, P_C; an attachment site for insertion of resistance gene cassettes just downstream of the promoter; and one resistance gene, *RA*. The two bottom boxes depict the addition of new cassettes to the integron, catalyzed by the integrase, Int. Expression of the three resistance cassettes depicted in the bottom box is controlled by the single promoter. Adapted from D. Mazel, *ASM News* 70:520–525, 2004.

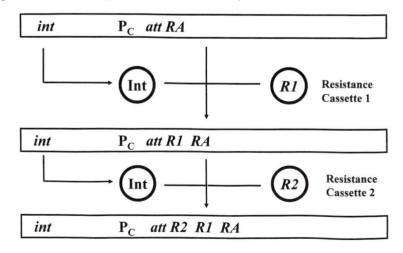

region (QRDR). Mutations in the primary target of a fluoroquinolone lower the sensitivity of that target to the antibiotic such that subsequent mutations, resulting in higher levels of resistance, may be in either *gyrA* and/or *parC* or, to a lesser extent, in *gyrB* or *parE*.

Penicillin-resistant strains of *S. pneumoniae* were isolated for the first time in the late 1970s in South Africa and in the United States. Coincident with the isolation of penicillin-resistant *S. pneumoniae* in South Africa, resistant viridans group streptococci, such as *Streptococcus mitis* and *Streptococcus sanguinis* (formerly *S. sanguis*), were being isolated from the nasopharynxes of the same children. Resistance to penicillin in *S. pneumoniae* and in the viridans group of streptococci has been traced to the presence of multiple mutations in the region of the genes associated with the binding affinity for penicillin of the larger PBPs, such that their affinities for these antibiotics are lowered considerably. Once such strains emerged, their resistance could easily have been disseminated among several members of the viridans group of streptococci, or strains of *S. pneumoniae*, due to the ability of these species to achieve a state of natural competence for transformation. That the exchange of PBP-encoding genes has actually occurred in nature was clearly demonstrated in two types of studies. First, the genes encoding PBP2b from several penicillin-resistant isolates of *S. pneumoniae* were shown to have a mosaic structure with large blocks of DNA sequence clearly derived from *S. mitis*. These mosaic genes likely arose via localized recombinational events between an incoming gene and its resident chromosomal homolog in the transformed recipient strain. In another study, PBP2b-encoding genes from penicillin-resistant isolates of *Streptococcus oralis* were shown to be greater than 99% identical in sequence to the homolog from a penicillin-resistant strain of *S. pneumoniae*. Thus, although it very likely required several years for a few strains of viridans group streptococci and/or *S. pneumoniae* to accumulate a sufficient number of mutations in a PBP-encoding gene to render the bacterium resistant, such resistance has been and continues to be broadly disseminated among these streptococcal species via transformation.

That a scenario similar to that occurring among penicillin-resistant naturally transformable streptococci might also apply to resistance to the fluoroquinolones among these bacterial species has been demonstrated in the laboratory. It has been possible to transfer to *S. pneumoniae* resistance to fluoroquinolones with DNA obtained from resistant strains of *S. oralis*, *S. mitis*, *S. sanguinis*, and *Streptococcus constellatus* containing mutations in *parC*. Similarly, DNA from a *S. pneumoniae* transformant could be used to transform *S. mitis* to resistance. Even more significantly, high-level fluoroquinolone resistance was transferred to *S. pneumoniae* with DNA obtained from a strain of *S. mitis* that had mutations in both *gyrA* and *parC*. Since these two genes are separated by a considerable distance on the chromosome, such a transformation required two independent events in a single transformation, and occurred at a very low frequency, but it did occur, and likely could occur in nature.

Linezolid, an oxazolidinone, was approved by the FDA for the treatment of infections caused by gram-positive bacteria in 2000. As mentioned above, linezolid represented the first new class of antibiotics to be introduced into clinical practice in more than 30 years. Although its bacterial target, the 50S ribosomal subunit, was not new, its mechanism of action, inhibition of formation of the translational initiation complex, was. In addition, all enterococcal and staphylococcal strains in a panel of clinical isolates tested were susceptible to this antibiotic, and frequencies of spontaneous mutation to resistance were extremely low, less than one in $>10^{10}$ bacteria for all relevant species tested. All of the above data suggested that the emergence of resistance to linezolid in the clinical setting would be rare. However, during clinical trials, prior to its approval by the FDA, linezolid-resistant enterococci were isolated from 2 of 169 patients with VRE infections who had been treated with the antibiotic in a compassionate use program. SENTRY, a worldwide (North and South America, Europe, Asia, Australia, and South Africa) antimicrobial surveillance program that monitors the susceptibility of major bacterial pathogens to relevant antibiotics, reported that of 9,833 gram-positive clinical isolates obtained from January 2001 to June 2002, 8 were resistant to linezolid. Only three of the eight patients from whom the resistant isolates had been obtained had received linezolid. The appearance of linezolid-resistant enterococci was reported for the first time in several countries from 2002 to 2004. Among all isolates studied, resistance was attributed to a mutation in residue 257 in domain V of 23S rRNA that results in a change from guanine to uridine, or to thymidine, in the DNA. Most bacterial species have multiple 23S rRNA genes, and results of one study have demonstrated a correlation between the level of resistance to linezolid and the percentage of 23S rRNA genes that contain the G257T mutation.

Resistance to metronidazole among anaerobic and microaerophilic bacteria can usually be attributed to mutations that result in the alteration or loss of the reductase or hydrogenase, or a cofactor such as flavodoxin, involved in the conversion of the prodrug to an active antibacterial compound within the cell. However, in some resistant isolates of *Bacteroides* species, resistance is due to the activity of the product of one of at least four known genes designated *ninA, ninB,* etc. The actual mechanism of resistance is not known. However many *nin* genes have been shown to be carried on plasmids, some of which are transmissible.

Efflux Pumps: Association with Acquired and Intrinsic Resistance and Mutation to Resistance

One mechanism of resistance to some antibiotics, as already mentioned with regard to tetracycline, involves the acquisition of genes encoding proteins able to pump the antibiotic out of the cell. In addition, virtually all bacterial species encode on their chromosomes one to several transport systems that are or can become involved in efflux from the cell of single to multiple antibiotics, thus contributing to their antibiotic resistance phenotypes. To date, five families of bacterial efflux transporters, or pumps, have been described, and their arrangements on the surfaces of bacterial cells are illustrated in Fig. 9.

The ATP-binding cassette superfamily of efflux pump proteins, i.e., the chromosomally encoded ABC transporters, for which the energy for transport is derived from ATP, is primarily involved in the transfer in and/or out of the bacterial cell of sugars, polysaccharides, amino acids, proteins, ions, and iron complexes. Several ABC transporters, mostly putative, but several previously characterized, have been identified in

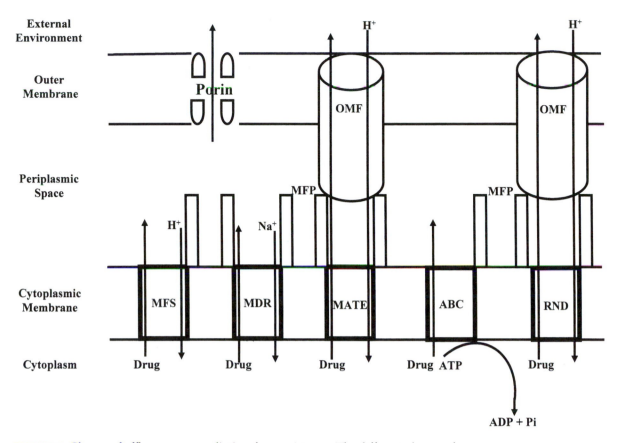

FIGURE 9 Classes of efflux pumps mediating drug resistance. The different classes of efflux pumps are explained in detail in the text. Gram-positive bacteria require only the cytoplasmic membrane component for transport to the environment, whereas gram-negative bacteria also employ periplasmic membrane fusion proteins (MFP) and outer membrane factor (OMF), also referred to as outer membrane protein, or a porin. Adapted from X.-Z. Li and H. Nikaido, *Drugs* **64:**159–204, 2004, and from K. Poole, *Curr. Pharm. Biotechnol.* **3:**77–98, 2002.

every bacterial species whose genome has been sequenced. However, the MacAB system of *E. coli* is the only one that has actually been shown to mediate the efflux of antibiotics in a gram-negative bacterium. This *macAB*-encoded system, composed of the periplasmic membrane fusion protein (MFP), MacA, and an integral cytoplasmic membrane protein, MacB, transports macrolides into the periplasmic space where they are then transferred out of the cell through the multifunctional outer membrane channel, TolC.

The major facilitator superfamily (MFS) of transporters includes many intrinsically encoded symporters and antiporters of sugars, anions, and various metabolites, which generally function as single-component protein pumps. The transport energy for the MFS pumps is derived from the cell's electrochemical gradient, i.e., proton motive force (PMF). Examples of single-component MF transporters are the fluoroquinolone efflux pumps, NorA of *S. aureus* and PmrA of *S. pneumoniae*. Also included in this family are the macrolide efflux pumps, MefA (first identified in *S. pyogenes*) and MefE (found first in *S. pneumoniae*), which mediate resistance to macrolides, but not to lincosamides or streptogramins. The *mefA* and *mefE* genes are both encoded by conjugative transposons, and in some strains of *S. pyogenes*, the *mefA*-encoding transposon is located within the genome of a lysogenic bacteriophage. Thus, dissemination of these macrolide resistance elements can occur via conjugation, transformation, or transduction (at least among strains of *S. pyogenes*). The EmrAB-TolC pump of *Escherichia coli* consists of the MFP EmrB and the MFP EmrA, which act in conjunction with TolC to transport nalidixic acid and hydrophobic toxic compounds out of the cell. The plasmid- or transposon-mediated tetracycline resistance efflux pumps, such as TetL and TetK of gram-positive bacteria, and TetA (initially described in Tn*10*) and TetB of gram-negative bacteria, are also members of the MF family of transporters.

The multidrug and toxic compound extrusion (MATE) family comprises a group of electrochemical gradient-dependent transport proteins, similar to the MF proteins. However, the energy source for transport in these cases is usually a Na^+ gradient rather than the H^+ gradient. Examples are the chromosomally encoded NorM and YdhE pumps of *Vibrio parahaemolyticus* and *Escherichia coli*, respectively, that mediate resistance to aminoglycosides and fluoroquinolones, as well as cationic dyes.

A fourth family of efflux pumps, the small multidrug resistance transporters, like the MF transporters, are driven by the PMF. However, these pumps transport only antiseptics and disinfectants, and include the Smr protein of *S. aureus* and the EmrE protein of *E. coli*.

The resistance-nodulation-cell division (RND) family of efflux pumps, which are usually chromosomally encoded, play a major role in the intrinsic resistance to antibiotics of several gram-negative bacterial species, such as *P. aeruginosa*, *Acinetobacter baumannii*, *H. influenzae*, many species of *Enterobacteriaceae*, and the anaerobic periodontal pathogen *Porphyromonas gingivalis* (Table 8). The RND pumps are usually complexes of proteins consisting of a PMF-driven cytoplasmic membrane transporter, a periplasmic MFP, and an outer membrane channel, and mediate the efflux of multiple classes of antibiotics. The constitutively expressed MexAB-OprM pump of *P. aeruginosa* renders this bacterium resistant to members of such antibiotic classes as the β-lactams, aminoglycosides, macrolides, sulfonamides, and tetracyclines; to chloramphenicol, novobiocin, and trimethoprim; to toxic dyes such as acridine orange, ethidium bromide, and crystal violet; to several organic solvents; and to the biocide triclosan found in many household products such as antibacterial soaps and toothpastes. At least five other chromosomally encoded RND efflux systems have been identified in *P. aeruginosa*, making this opportunistic pathogen one of the most highly antibiotic resistant of all bacteria.

Oral Microbial Resistance

Much of the early work on antibiotic resistance in members of the oral microbiota concentrated on the oral streptococci. One of the earliest reports of antibiotic resistance in oral bacteria described, in 1974, isolates of *Streptococcus mutans* from endocarditis patients that were resistant to penicillin (one isolate; MIC, ~1.3 μg/ml), vancomycin (five isolates; MIC, 5 μg/ml), chloramphenicol (nine isolates; MIC, 4 to 8 μg/ml), and tetracycline (three isolates; MIC, 16 μg/ml). Another report in 1980 described the effects of tetracycline therapy of periodontal patients on the resistance of the viridans group streptococci to this antibiotic. The results of this study

TABLE 8 RND family multidrug efflux pumps in representative gram-negative species[a]

| Bacterial species | Efflux system component | | | Substrates[b] |
	MFP	RND	OMP	
Acinetobacter baumannii	AdeA	AdeB	AdeC	AG, Ct, Tc, Em, Cm, Tp, FQ
	AdeI	AdeJ	AdeK	BL, Tc, Cm, SG, Rf
Enterobacter aerogenes	AcrA	AcrA	TolC	Ac, Cm, FQ, Mc, Nv, SDS, Tc
Escherichia coli	AcrA	AcrB	TolC	Ac, BL, BS, Cm, Cv, Eb, FA, ML, Nv, OS, Rf
	SDS AcrA	AcrD	TolC	AG, Dc, Fu, Nv
	AcrE	AcrF	TolC	Similar to AcrA- AcrB-TolC
	MdtA	MdtBC	TolC	Dc, Nv
	YhiU	YhiV	TolC	Dc
Haemophilus influenzae	AcrA	AcrB	TolC	Ac, Cv, Eb, Em, Nv, Rf, SDS
Porphyromonas gingivalis	XepA	XepB	XepC	Ac, Eb, Pu, Rf, SDS
Pseudomonas aeruginosa	MexA	MexB	OprM	Ac, AG, BL, Cm, Cv, Eb, ML, Nv, OS, SDS, Sf, Tc, Tp, Tr
	MexC	MexD	OprJ	Cm, CP, FQ, Tc, Tr
	MexE	MexF	OprN,	Cm, FQ
	MexX	MexY	OprM	AG, ML, Tc
	MexH	MexI	OpmD	Vanadium
	MexJ	MexK	OprM	Em, Tc, Tr
Serratia marcescens	?	MexF-like	?	FQ
Salmonella enterica serovar Typhimurium	AcrA	AcrB	TolC	BL, FQ

[a]Adapted and updated from X.-Z. Li and H. Nikaido, *Drugs* **64:**159–204, 2004.

[b]Ac, acriflavin; AG, aminoglycosides; BL, β-lactams; BS, bile salts; Cm, chloramphenicol; CP, cephalosporins; Ct, cefotaxime; Cv, crystal violet; Dc, doxycychloate; Eb, ethidium bromide; Em, erythromycin; FA, fatty acids; FQ, fluoroquinolones; Fu, fusidic acid; Mc, mitomycin; ML, macrolides; Nv, novobiocin; OS, organic solvents; Pu, puromycin; Rf, rifampin; SF, sulfonamides; SDS, sodium dodecyl sulfate; Tc, tetracycline; Tp, trimethoprim; Tr, triclosan.

showed that the proportion of resistant streptococci isolated from the gingiva of patients usually increased dramatically during treatment, but in most patients decreased to pretreatment levels within a few months following the cessation of treatment. This report was one of the first to demonstrate the low proportion of viridans group streptococci that harbored plasmids (<14%), and in no instance was the resistance to tetracycline shown to be plasmid-mediated. In 1992, the results of a study in France indicated that approximately 5% of viridans group streptococci expressed high-level resistance (MICs, >2,000 μg/ml) to aminoglycosides. Some of the isolates obtained in the latter study were able to transfer their resistance to the aminoglycosides kanamycin and streptomycin, as well as their MLS and tetracycline resistance phenotypes, en bloc to susceptible streptococcal species via mating on solid surfaces. Finally, in 1984, an *S. sanguinis* II isolate from a patient with bacteremia was shown to have a vancomycin MIC of >128 μg/ml. Unfortunately, the mechanisms of antibiotic resistance expressed were not determined in any of the above studies. In 1984, resistance of several strains of viridans group streptococci were shown to carry *tet*M, and five of these strains contained a Tn*916*-like conjugative element. Subsequently, *tet*O was cloned and characterized from a strain of *S. mutans* (1988), and in 1990, clinical isolates of *S. milleri* were shown to contain the streptomycin resistance determinant *aadE* (7 strains), the kanamycin resistance gene *aph3A* (8 strains), and *ermB*, *tet*M, and *tet*O (11, 14, and 3 strains, respectively).

Currently, numerous tetracycline resistance determinants have been identified in a variety of oral bacterial species: *tet*B in isolates of

A. *actinomycetemcomintans* and *T. denticola*; *tet*L, normally considered a gram-positive bacterial gene, in *E. corrodens*, *Neisseria sicca*, *F. nucleatum*, and *Veillonella parvula*; *tet*Q in *Prevotella* species, *V. parvula*, and *Capnocytophaga* species; and *tet*M in a variety of gram-positive and gram-negative species. More recently, the relatively new determinant, *tet*W, was detected in isolates of oral species belonging to the genera *Streptomyces*, *Lactobacillus*, *Actinomyces*, *Veillonella*, *Streptococcus*, *Neisseria*, and *Prevotella*.

Since the late 1980s, a number of oral bacterial species, both gram-positive and gram-negative, have been shown to produce β-lactamases. The presence on plasmids of genes encoding β-lactamase activity has been demonstrated in isolates of *E. corrodens* and *Neisseria sicca*, but the location of β-lactamase-encoding genes in such oral microorganisms as *F. nucleatum*, *Prevotella* species, *Tannerella forsythia*, *Porphyromonas* species, and *Veillonella* species has not been established. In addition, as mentioned earlier, PBP-mediated resistance to β-lactam antibiotics has been disseminated among the viridans group streptococci, as well as *S. pneumoniae,* by transformation among strains able to achieve a state of natural competence.

It seems obvious at this time that at least some species of oral bacteria have either developed or acquired resistance to virtually all clinically useful antibiotics, as is true of species normally occupying other niches. Although the vast majority of these oral species are considered commensals and are not generally associated with infectious diseases, they clearly can and often do serve as reservoirs of antibiotic resistance, ready to transfer their traits by one or more genetic mechanisms, to pathogenic species that share or pass through the oral environment.

ANTIBIOTIC RESISTANCE IN THE 21ST CENTURY

Genetic Elements in Resistance Spread

We have seen that bacterial pathogens have evolved and/or acquired numerous mechanisms by which they may resist the lethal or inhibitory effects of antibiotics. Strains of virtually every species of bacteria that inhabit humans or animals, pathogenic or commensal, have been shown to express resistance to one or more, and often several, different antibiotics and antibiotic classes. New resistance traits and new species expressing older traits have been and continue to be selected by our appropriate and inappropriate use of antibiotics following their dissemination on a variety of genetic elements that may be transferred via several mechanisms. The types of genetic elements associated with antibiotic resistance, and the mechanisms by which they may be disseminated, of which we are currently aware, are summarized in Table 9. Genes encoding antibiotic resistance may be carried on conjugative or nonconjugative plasmids and transposons, or within integrons. The resistance gene repertoire of a transposon or integron may expand by the insertion of new resistance transposons or the addition of new resistance gene cassettes, respectively. Transposons and integrons may be located on any type of replicon, chromosomal, plasmid, or bacteriophage, and the resistance traits encoded by these replicons may be transferred from bacterial strain to bacterial strain via conjugation, transformation, or transduction. Even

TABLE 9 Characteristics of genetic elements involved in resistance gene dissemination

Genetic element	Characteristics
Transmissible plasmid	Double-stranded, circular, autonomously replicating molecule able to mediate its own transfer from cell to cell involving direct contact, or mobilizing for transfer of other genetic elements
Conjugative transposon	Nonreplicating genetic element of a discrete size able to integrate into bacterial replicons, or to excise from such replicons in the form of a circular transfer intermediate; encodes genes essential for conjugative transfer
Mobilizable plasmid	Circular, double-stranded replicating molecule encoding genes that permit the use of a conjugative plasmid to facilitate its transfer from cell to cell via conjugation
Transposon	Nonreplicating element of a discrete size able to move from one segment of a replicon to another, or from one replicon to another replicon in the same cell
Gene cassette	Circular, nonreplicating segment of DNA encoding an open reading frame without promoters; inserts into integrons
Integron	Integrated segment of DNA encoding an integrase, a promoter, and an insertion site (att) for the integration and expression of gene cassettes
Transducing bacteriophage	Bacterial virus able to package non-phage-encoded DNA, which may be transferred to cells of the same or very closely related species by transduction
Bacterial chromosome	Major replicon of bacterial cells that may encode resistance to antibiotics and which may subsequently be transferred by transformation to species able to achieve a state of natural competence

resistance traits that have evolved by one or more mutational events within a gene may be disseminated by one of these transfer mechanisms, especially by the transformation of those species of bacteria able to achieve a natural state of competence.

The Many Mechanisms of Antibiotic Resistance

Historically, resistance to penicillin began with the plasmid-mediated synthesis, by strains of *S. aureus*, of an enzyme, penicillinase, that cleaved the β-lactam ring of penicillin, rendering it ineffective as an antimicrobial. Subsequently, a large variety of β-lactam antibiotics were developed and introduced into clinical practice, many so as to increase the spectrum of antibacterial activity, but also to provide newer varieties, such as the cephalosporins, carbapenems, and monobactams, that would be resistant to the existing β-lactamases. However, the introduction of each new type of β-lactam antibiotic was soon followed by the emergence of newer β-lactamases that not only could destroy the newer β-lactams, but in many instances, their predecessors as well.

At least two types of mechanisms by which the newer β-lactamases have evolved have been elucidated. First, mutations in plasmid-mediated β-lactamase-encoding genes have resulted in enzymes with increased affinity for some of the newer β-lactams. Second, an inducible chromosomal gene, *ampC*, common among many gram-negative bacterial species, has very high intrinsic affinity for later generation cephalosporins but is not induced in their presence. However, mutations have occurred in the regulatory genes that control their expression, resulting in derepressed (constitutive) production of higher levels of the enzyme, and consequent resistance to those newer cephalosporins.

Regardless of the mechanism by which they have evolved, more than 200 different β-lactamases have been identified in gram-positive and gram-negative bacteria. In addition, *S. aureus* also found a way to overcome the activity of the β-lactam, methicillin, via the acquisition of a gene, *mecA*, encoding a new PBP with a low affinity for β-lactam antibiotics, including methicillin. Several species of streptococci apparently accumulated, over a period of greater than 50 years since the introduction of penicillin into clinical practice, a sufficient number of mutations in the gene encoding the penicillin-binding protein PBP2a to reduce its affinity to penicillins sufficiently so as to render strains producing it resistant to all β-lactams. These mutated genes were subsequently broadly disseminated among a variety of streptococcal species that are naturally transformable, thus speeding up the process of evolution. Other bacterial species, such as *P. aeruginosa*, have found a way to avoid the lethal activity of these antibiotics by keeping them out of the cell via efflux pumps.

Resistance to the tetracyclines is probably the most common antibiotic resistance phenotype known, and representatives of virtually every bacterial species examined have been shown to be resistant to this class of antibiotics. The most common mechanism of tetracycline resistance involves the transport of the antibiotic out of the cell at such a rate that the ribosomes, although sensitive to tetracyclines, never come into contact with them. Several genes encoding these tetracycline-specific efflux pumps have been identified in gram-negative (*tet*A and *tet*B being the most common) and gram-positive (*tet*K and *tet*L) bacteria. Another mechanism of tetracycline resistance involves the production of a protein that protects the ribosome from the antibiotics. Several genes, such as *tet*M, *tet*O, *tet*Q, and *tet*S, have been detected in gram-positive and gram-negative species, as well as such cell wall-free bacteria as *Mycoplasma* species. Bacterial strains expressing one of these genes are also resistant to minocycline.

Resistance of most bacterial species to the fluoroquinolones generally involves an accumulation of one or more mutations in the QRDR of *gyrA* and/or *parC*, with, in some instances, an occasional mutation in *gyrB* or *parE*. Overexpression of the chromosomally encoded efflux pump genes, *norA* or *pmrA*, by *S. aureus* or *S. pneumoniae*, respectively, may also lead to low-level fluoroquinolone resistance. The intrinsic resistance of *P. aeruginosa* to fluoroquinolones can be attributed to the activity of at least four RND efflux pumps, especially the MexAB-OprM system. Quinolone resistance mediated by a transmissible plasmid was described for the first time in 1998. Since then, strains of members of the *Enterobacteriaceae* that harbor a plasmid carrying the quinolone resistance gene, *qnr*, which encodes a protein that protects DNA gyrase from inhibition by fluoroquinolones, have been isolated.

For every antibiotic in clinical practice, there are bacterial species that produce one or more efflux pumps providing resistance to that antibiotic. Most such pumps, with the exception of the Tet, Mef, and Cml proteins, which mediate resistance to tetracycline, macrolides, and chloramphenicol, respectively, are not antibiotic specific but rather mediate resistance to several antibiotics or antibiotic classes, as well as other types of compounds that are toxic to them. On the other hand, most antibiotics to which resistance is provided by efflux pumps have, like the β-lactams, also selected for other mechanisms of resistance. These mechanisms include enzymes that catalyze the acetylation of aminoglycosides and chloramphenicol; the adenylylation or phosphorylation of aminoglycosides; the methylation of a specific adenine residue in 23S rRNA resulting in the MLS resistance phenotype; the synthesis of an intermediate step in the synthesis of tetrahydrofolic acid, such as dihydropteroate synthetase (sulfonamide resistance) or dihydrofolate reductase (trimethoprim resistance); or the replacement of D-Ala with D-Lac as the terminal residue in the murein pentapeptide precursors of gram-positive bacterial cell walls, resulting in resistance to glycopeptides such as vancomycin. And, of course, there are the single mutations, or accumulation of mutations, that continue to result in resistance of bacterial species to members of whole classes of antibiotics, such as the fluoroquinolones.

■ KEY POINTS

The modern antibiotic era is generally considered to have begun in 1941, when sufficient quantities of the β-lactam antibiotic, penicillin, became available to help prevent and successfully treat what would often have been, up to that time, fatal bacterial infections among Allied troops. Numerous derivatives of penicillin, four generations of cephalosporins, and the newer β-lactams, the carbapenems and monobactams, soon followed, each new version extending the spectrum of susceptible pathogens covered by the previous members of the class or overcoming resistance to some or all of the earlier agents. At the same time, new classes of antibiotics, inhibiting different bacterial targets, such as the aminoglycosides, tetracyclines, macrolides, fluoroquinolones, and most recently, the oxazolidinone linezolid, were being added to the antibacterial armamentarium.

Despite the large number of antibiotics available, they actually target a very limited number of essential bacterial functions, i.e., the synthesis of cell walls; the macromolecular biosynthetic processes, such as replication, transcription, or translation; or steps in intermediary metabolism, such as the folic acid pathway. An occasional agent targets a function other than those mentioned above, such as the cell membrane disrupters, e.g., the polymyxins, or DNA itself, as does activated metronidazole.

Each new antibiotic introduced into clinical practice has been followed, often very rapidly, by the emergence of bacterial pathogens, as well as commensals, that are resistant to it. Such resistance may involve the acquisition of a gene that encodes an enzyme able to destroy or inactivate the antibiotic, or one that allows the cell to bypass the normal target of the antibiotic, e.g., PBPs with lower affinity for β-lactams, or dihydrofolate reductases with decreased affinity for trimethoprim; mutations in a gene encoding, or regulating the expression of, an antibiotic target; or acquisition or activation of a chromosomally determined efflux pump that excretes the antibiotic from the cell and away from the antibiotic target. Thus, for every antibiotic available there is at least one and usually two to three mechanisms available to bacteria by which they may overcome its inhibitory or lethal activity. Because genes mediating antibiotic resistance may be located within transposons or integrons, they may be present on plasmids, the host chromosome, or even bacteriophage DNA. Antibiotic resistance traits may be transferred from strain to

strain of a given species, and even between different species and genera of bacteria by plasmid- or transposon-mediated conjugation, conjugative mobilization, transformation, and occasionally transduction.

Once resistance to any antibiotic emerges, a strain carrying it will be selected, or its transfer to new strains and species may be facilitated and subsequent newly resistant strains selected, by the appropriate and inappropriate use of that antibiotic in human and animal medicine, as a growth promoter in animal feeds, or for the protection of crops and marine forms from infection by plant and fish pathogens, respectively. Because many bacterial species have become resistant to multiple antibiotics, the use of any one of them to which it is resistant will select for its entire resistance phenotype. The presence of so many antibiotics, and so much of each, in the environment has produced strains of enterococci and staphylococci that are resistant to all available antibiotics, and *S. pneumoniae* strains resistant to most clinically useful antibiotics. New untreatable pathogens are sure to arise in the future.

With regard to the discovery and/or development of new antibiotics or classes of antibiotic, it is generally assumed that the low hanging fruit have all been picked. Discovery of chemical compounds that are inhibitory to bacterial cells without an accompanying toxicity to humans has become more difficult with time, and considerably more expensive. Many pharmaceutical companies have abandoned the search for new antibiotics because the monetary rewards do not seem sufficient to warrant the expense of their development. With regard to those companies that have remained in the hunt, all of the available modern technologies, such as high throughput screens to test millions of compounds in short periods (weeks to no more than months) of time; the availability of the genome sequences of numerous pathogenic species to identify and validate the essentiality of potentially new antimicrobial targets, and the advanced genetic and molecular tools by which to do so; microarray, proteomic, and metabolomic technologies to aid in identifying the functions of genes of unknown function; crystallography to elucidate the structures and mechanisms of action of potential new targets, and to aid in the design of chemical entities that

(continues)

KEY POINTS

(Continued from previous page)
will inhibit them; and the latest methods of chemical synthesis, such as combinatorial chemistry, by which many forms of a primary structure can be made, are all being applied to the discovery and development of new antibiotics. We must keep in mind, however, that the introduction of every new antibiotic or antibiotic class into clinical use has been followed by the emergence of bacterial pathogens that are resistant to it. It can also be stated with some degree of certainty that every new antimicrobial agent, no matter how novel the agent or its target, introduced in the future will also be followed by the appearance of resistant strains of at least some pathogenic species. For, as remarked by Nobel laureate Paul Berg, "Mother Nature always bats last."

FURTHER READING

Axelsen, P. H. 2002. *Essentials of Antimicrobial Pharmacology: a Guide to Fundamentals for Practice*. Humana Press, Totowa, N.J.

Dajani, A. S., K. A. Taubert, W. Wilson, A. F. Bolger, P. Ferriery, M. H. Gewitz, S. T. Shulman, S. Nouri, J. W. Newburger, C. Hutto, T. J. Pallasch, T. W. Gage, M. E. Levison, G. Peter, and G. Zuccaro, Jr. 1997. Prevention of bacterial endocarditis. Recommendations by the American Heart Association. *JAMA* **277:** 1794–1801.

Levy, S. B. 2001. *The Antibiotic Paradox*, 2nd ed. Perseus Publishing, Cambridge, Mass.

Walsh, C. 2003. *Antibiotics: Actions, Origins, Resistance*. ASM Press, Washington, D.C.

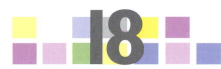

Infection Control in Dentistry

J. Christopher Fenno, Wilson A. Coulter, and
Dennis E. Lopatin

INTRODUCTION

Dental professionals are exposed to a wide variety of microorganisms in the blood and saliva of patients. These microorganisms may cause infectious diseases such as the common cold, pneumonia, tuberculosis, herpes, hepatitis B, and acquired immune deficiency syndrome. The use of effective infection control procedures and universal precautions in the dental office and the dental laboratory prevents cross-contamination that could put dentists, dental office staff, dental technicians, and patients at risk for infection.

Infection control in dentistry, as in other health professions, involves application of a risk management decision-making process, including risk identification, assessment, or analysis, and implementation of design and procedures for risk control. "Cross-infection" is typically defined as the transmission of infectious agents among patients and staff within the clinical environment. Recent research findings suggesting that oral microorganisms cause systemic infections and contribute to the development of chronic diseases such as coronary artery disease highlight the need to place more emphasis on controlling the risks of cross-infection. Moreover, the consequences of dealing with lapse of infection control after the fact are dire, both economically and in public relations terms.
Infection control is an important component of the overall risk management process that should be in place in dental operatories and clinics of all sizes. For this purpose, the concept of "risk" has several possible definitions, each of which has relevance to the practice of dentistry:

- Chance of loss or injury; hazard; danger; peril
- The possibility of suffering harm or loss
- A factor, element, or course involving uncertain danger or hazard
- The danger or probability of loss to an insurer

The primary goal of all infection control measures is to minimize the risk to dental patients and staff of infection caused by exposure to infectious material in the course of dental treatment. At-risk populations include patients, dental professionals, and support staff, all of whom include individuals with different levels of susceptibility to infection. The challenge to the dental professional is to implement infection control procedures and practices that best protect everyone involved without compromising the quality of care.

In medicine, especially as practiced in hospitals, increasing attention is being paid to the problem of infections of nosocomial (hospital-acquired) and iatrogenic (therapy-related) origins, especially those involving antibiotic-resistant bacterial strains. Respiratory and mucosal infections due to hospital-acquired bacterial and viral pathogens are a significant cause of mortality, especially in immunocompromised patients. Many of these infections are extremely difficult to treat due to the high incidence of multiple antibiotic resistance. The most frequently isolated bacterial agents in these infections include *Enterococcus* spp., *Staphylococcus aureus*, and *Pseudomonas aeruginosa*. For example, many nosocomial *S. aureus* infections involve strains resistant to the class of antibiotics most frequently used to treat staphylococcal infections. These strains, designated methicillin-resistant *S. aureus* (MRSA), are typically resistant to all useful antibiotics with the exception of vancomycin. The prevalence of MRSA strains in nosocomial *S. aureus* infections is currently greater than 50%, up from approximately 30% 10 years ago. Transmissible vancomycin resistance is common among enterococci, and MRSA strains with high-level vancomycin resistance have been isolated in at least two U.S. hospitals within the past 2 years. Although the prevalence of antibiotic-resistant bacterial strains is likely lower in the community than in hospital settings, the trend toward prevalence of pathogens resistant to multiple antibiotics is an especially serious public health issue that is likely to have increasing implications for the dental profession, especially in designing appropriate treatment for patients with a higher susceptibility to infection.

For several reasons, infection control in hospitals is a much more complex process than is infection control in the typical dental practice setting. Patient care in the hospital setting, including dental care, usually involves large numbers of staff with differing levels of training and understanding of infection control. Hospitalized patients are much more likely to be susceptible to infection. Moreover, like hospitalized patients, dental patients receiving treatment in a hospital setting are at higher risk for exposure to antibiotic-resistant bacterial pathogens than dental patients treated in the private practice setting. Despite these differences, the principles on which infection control practices are based are essentially identical in both situations.

The goal of this chapter is to identify risks for the transmission of infection in dental treatment settings, define strategies for managing of these risks based on scientific evidence, and provide protocols for risk management. It is crucial for dental practitioners to realize that in addition to dealing with real risks of cross-infection during dental treatment they must also address risk perception. Perception of risk has played a significant and not always positive role in shaping public health policy and has at times dramatically affected the relationship between the health professions and the public. As new potential risks are identified, policy makers, patients, and health care practitioners are prone to either under- or overreact based on fear. Universal precautions (see below) have been developed to address this issue. As scientific evidence becomes available on the actual risk of infection from newly identified threats, it is important that risk management strategies be revised and that health professionals and the public be educated. Perception of risk is currently playing a role in the dialogue surrounding risk management for development of biofilms in dental waterlines, human immunodeficiency virus (HIV) transmission, bovine spongiform encephalopathies, and severe acute respiratory syndrome (SARS).

Many of the most current discussions and procedures for infection control are found on websites of professional organizations and governmental agencies, in particular the American Dental Association (ADA) and the Centers for Disease Control and Prevention (CDC). These sources are updated regularly as new information in the field is assessed and procedures for minimizing the risk of iatrogenic infections in dentistry evolve.

INTRODUCTION TO RISK CONTROL

Quality Assurance Is the Promise of Performance

The commitment to act for the benefit of the patient and the public is the cornerstone of virtually all professional codes of ethics, including the ADA's Principles of Ethics and Code of Professional Conduct. Practice of appropriate infection control procedures is an important part of overall assurance of quality care. Outcomes data from quality assurance assessments provide the evidence that the dentist is meeting his or her ethical and legal obligations to patients and society.

Cross-Infection Control Is Essentially a Set of Management Strategies for Risk Control

Risk control in dentistry uses a single-tier approach in which all patients are treated as though they are a potential source of infectious pathogens. This single-tier approach is known as "universal precautions." It applies the concept of risk to the procedure, not the patient. Whereas all patients are treated equally in terms of the quality assurance mechanisms that comprise infection control, the importance of medical history for determining best patient care must not be overlooked. However, this is not a substitute for proper infection control. The universal precautions system of infectious disease control assumes that all body fluids are infectious and requires every employee exposed to direct contact with body fluids to be protected as though such body fluids were hepatitis B virus (HBV) or HIV infected. Universal precautions are intended to prevent parenteral mucous membrane and nonintact skin exposures of health care workers to bloodborne pathogens. Specifically, dental health care workers should consider blood, saliva, and gingival fluid from all patients to be infectious.

What Is Risk Management?

For the purposes of dental practice, cross-infection control equals risk management. The control of cross-infection involves a particular application of a risk management decision-making process, with risk identification, assessment, or analysis, and implementation of risk control procedures. Although quantitative data on the actual risks associated with many specific procedures are somewhat limited, the design of infection control protocols takes into account several important factors, including the following:

- Known risks and hazards of specific dental procedures (for example, dental surgery in patients with implanted medical devices)
- Known risks and hazards of other procedures (for example, injections)
- Regulatory requirements of governments and professional societies
- Perception of risk in the community served
- Perception of risk within the dental profession

Several concepts in this list require further explanation. The distinction between "hazard" and "risk" is important. Hazard is the potential harm (including number of people exposed and severity of consequences) that may be suffered due to some particular incident or procedure. Risk is the quantification of a hazard in terms of probability of the occurrence of harm. Risk assessment also considers the likelihood of transmission of the infectious agent and the severity of the outcome of being infected. Perceptions of risk are influenced by many factors other than scientifically determined risk. These determinants of perceived risk tend to involve beliefs and feelings that are most easily understood from a sociological or psychological perspective. A common example of perceived risk is that riding in an automobile is safer than flying in an airplane. The statistics on passenger injury or death in airplane and automobile crashes do not support this perception, but it is nevertheless widespread. Any profession that deals with the public must address both real risks and the public's perception of risks associated with the profession.

In designing effective risk management strategies for infection control in dentistry, it is necessary to address actual hazards and risks, as well as to acknowledge the importance of perceived risks to the community and its confidence in the profession. A good example of this has been the public perception of a risk of HIV transmission via dental procedures. Indeed, even the dental profession perceived the risk of treating HIV patients as high and was initially resistant to the treatment of these patients until the facts became clear that there appears to be an extremely low risk of HIV transmission by this route, especially compared with the much higher risk of transmission of HBV or hepatitis C virus (HCV) by the same procedures.

CROSS-INFECTION RISKS IN DENTISTRY

Possible sources of infection in the dental care setting include the following:

- Patients with infectious disease (e.g., influenza, measles, or tuberculosis)
- Patients in the prodromal or convalescent stage of infection (e.g., herpes simplex virus)
- Healthy (or asymptomatic) carriers of disease-causing organisms (e.g., *Streptococcus pyogenes*, *Neisseria meningitidis*, and *Haemophilus influenzae*)
- Environmental sources: airborne organisms or biofilms in waterlines or on equipment or instruments

Routes of Spread of Infection

There are several possible routes of transmission of infectious agents. Certain types of infectious agents are more likely to be transmitted by one route than another, so it is important to understand the significance and possible consequences of a failure of infection control procedures in any of the following transmission routes. The major potential risks include contamination of wounds during surgery and contamination of sterilized instruments during storage.

EXAMPLES OF AIRBORNE ROUTES OF CROSS-INFECTION

Examples of dust-borne routes

- *S. aureus* from skin scales
- *Clostridium tetani* from environmental dust
- These and other organisms released from solid surfaces
- Source: skin scales, wound dressings, solid surfaces
- Risk: contamination of wounds during surgery; contamination of sterilized instruments during storage

Examples of aerosol routes

- Large droplets >100 μm fall to ground within 2 m of source and contribute to surface contamination and dust spread.
- Droplet nuclei <100 μm, usually 5 to 10 μm, remain in air for hours and can be inhaled into lungs. This was an important factor that made the recent incidents involving release of weaponized anthrax spores so highly infectious and difficult to remove from contaminated locations.
- Sources: speaking, sneezing, all intraoral procedures. Massive increase when using ultrasonic scaling, air-rotor, air/water syringe.

MICROORGANISMS SPREAD BY AEROSOL

Viruses: HBV, Epstein-Barr virus, varicella-zoster virus, rubella virus, measles virus, and respiratory viruses (e.g., influenza virus, rhinovirus, and adenovirus)

Bacteria: *Mycobacterium tuberculosis* (tuberculosis), *Bordetella pertussis* (whooping cough), *Legionella pneumophila* (Legionnaires' disease), *N. meningitidis* (bacterial meningitis), *Streptococcus pneumoniae* (bacterial pneumonia), and *S. pyogenes* (strep throat, etc.)

PREVENTION OF AEROSOL TRANSMISSION

Aerosol transmission may be prevented in the following ways:

1. Elimination or limitation of organisms at source:
   - Postpone elective treatment during infective period.
   - Use preoperative antiseptic mouthwash.
2. Interruption of transmission:
   - Use rubber dam and high-speed suction.
   - Use hand instruments when possible.
   - Flush ultrasonic scalers and air/water syringes 30 s between patients.

- Have adequate ventilation in surgery. Typical standards for adequate ventilation are in the range of 5 to 8 liters/s/occupant, or approximately 6 air changes per hour.
- Use vacuum cleaner during surgery environmental cleaning.
3. Protection of the potential recipient:
   - Use masks and protective eyewear.
   - Vaccinate when possible, e.g., HBV, BCG, rubella, and influenza (during epidemics).

EXAMPLES OF CONTACT ROUTES OF CROSS-INFECTION

Person to person

- Person: direct spread from person to person by hands and clothes or fomites (towels, etc.)
- Risk: viruses, e.g., HBV, HCV, herpes simplex virus, respiratory syncytial virus, SARS, gram-negative bacilli, and *S. aureus*
- Prevention: handwashing, gloves, and protective clothing

Equipment

- Dental instruments, chairs and units, and impression materials
- Risk: bacterial and viral infectious agents
- Prevention:
  1. Sterilization of instruments (see below)
  2. Use of disposables. The use of presterilized disposable instruments continues to increase. These are suitable for many applications in dental practice. The relatively high cost of disposables is balanced by the assurance of sterility and reduced costs of autoclave operation
  3. Disinfection of dental materials in contact with patients (impressions, for example)
  4. Environmental hygiene
  5. Defining zones in the dental operatory (contaminated areas and clean areas)
  6. Disposal of infected waste (Table 1)

Fluids

- Dental water supplies, disinfectants, and detergents
- Risk: HBV, HCV, gram-negative bacilli including *Pseudomonas* and *Acinetobacter*
- Prevention: flushing water supply lines and using sterile water and biocide in water.

EXAMPLES OF PARENTERAL SPREAD OF CROSS-INFECTION

- Source of inoculation: blood, saliva, and secretions. Inoculation injury may be via eye, breach in intact skin, mucous membranes, or other sharps injury. The level of inoculation and infective dose of the particular organism determine the actual risk to operator. For example, a needlestick injury with a hollow needle injecting a

TABLE 1 Electronic resources for infection control information

Organization	Publication	Last update	Web address or contact
American Dental Association	Topical Index: Infection Control (see full listing)	Updated regularly	http://www.ada.org/prof/resources/topics/icontrol/index.asp
American Dental Association	Infection Control Recommendations	2003	http://www.ada.org/prof/resources/topics/icontrol/icontrol_rec.asp
American Dental Association	DUWL page	2003	http://www.ada.org/prof/resources/topics/waterlines/index.asp
American Dental Association	SARS page	2003	http://www.ada.org/prof/resources/topics/sars.asp
Centers for Disease Control and Prevention	Recommended Infection-Control Practices for Dentistry	Morb. Mortal. Wkly. Rep. **35**: 237–242, 1986, updated 2001	http://www.cdc.gov/mmwr/preview/mmwrhtml/00033634.htm
Centers for Disease Control and Prevention	Centers for Disease Control and Prevention Oral Health Resources Index	2003	http://www.cdc.gov/OralHealth/infection_control/index.htm
Centers for Disease Control and Prevention	Recommended Infection-Control Practices for Dentistry, 1993	Morb. Mortal. Wkly. Rep. **42**(RR-8), 1993, updated 2001	http://www.cdc.gov/mmwr/preview/mmwrhtml/00021095.htm
Centers for Disease Control and Prevention	Guideline for Hand Hygiene in Health-Care Settings	Morb. Mortal. Wkly. Rep. **51**(RR-16):1–44, 2002	http://www.cdc.gov/mmwr/preview/mmwrhtml/rr5116a1.htm
Centers for Disease Control and Prevention	Bloodborne Pathogens in Dental Settings	2002	http://www.cdc.gov/ncidod/hip/BLOOD/dental.htm
Centers for Disease Control and Prevention	Infection Control: Bloodborne Disease Transmission	2002	http://www.cdc.gov/OralHealth/infection_control/fact_sheet/bloodborne.htm
AIDS Education Training Center	National HIV/AIDS Clinicians' Consultation Center	Updated regularly	http://www.ucsf.edu/hivcntr/
AIDS Education Training Center	National HIV/AIDS Clinicians' Consultation Center	Telephone consultation	HIV Consultation Service (Monday–Friday, 9 am–8 pm eastern standard time): 1-800-933-3413 Clinicians' Post-exposure Prophylaxis Hotline (24 h, 7 days/wk): 1-800-448-4911
United Kingdom Department of Health	Risk Assessment for vCJD and Dentistry	July 2003	http://www.doh.gov.uk/cjd/dentistryrisk/index.htm
United Kingdom Department of Health	Revised TSE Guidelines	June 2003	http://www.doh.gov.uk/cjd/tseguidance/tseguidancepart4.pdf
Centers for Disease Control and Prevention	Sterilization & Disinfection	Updated regularly	http://www.cdc.gov/ncidod/hip/Sterile/sterile.htm
U.S. Food and Drug Administration	Sterilants and High Level Disinfectants	March 2003	http://www.fda.gov/cdrh/ode/germlab.html

significant volume of blood with a high titer of HBV is a high risk.

- Risk: viral infections including HBV, HCV, and HIV. Relative risk following inoculation injury: HBV (30%), HCV (10%), and HIV (0.3%).
- Prevention: adequate training and effective sharps policy including safe disposal of sharps, safe cleaning and sterilization of sharps, safe resheathing of needles; hepatitis B vaccination; wearing gloves and dressing wounds.

Management of Recently Identified Infection Control Risks

EMERGING INFECTIOUS DISEASES

Within the past 2 decades, several new or newly recognized human infectious diseases have emerged and, in some cases, become extremely serious public health concerns. These include HIV, SARS, and transmissible spongiform encephalopathies (TSEs) ("mad cow disease" and related conditions). These are life-threatening diseases with limited or no effective treatment options, and most have a high mortality rate. These factors, combined with uncertainty surrounding epidemiology and relative infectivity, have contributed to the public's concern that they may be at risk of infection during dental treatment. With all of these diseases, there has been emphasis both on identifying potentially infected persons within the population and designing specific infection control methodologies to minimize the risks of transmission.

The AIDS epidemic, in particular, has resulted in revisions of accepted infection control practices, especially with regard to practices that help minimize exposure to blood. Prior to this, the use of gloves and special care with instruments were suggested during treatment of known carriers of hepatitis B. The subsequent acceptance of universal precautions and increased attention to infection control in medicine and dentistry were a direct result of recognition of the infectious nature of HIV during its latent, asymptomatic phase. The mandated use of gloves and other protective equipment, the increased emphasis on proper use of sharps, and increased management of potentially infected waste have served to greatly limit the likelihood of HIV transmission in dental practice. The only documented case of dentally related HIV transmission appears to have been intentional. Available evidence indicates a low occupational risk for HIV infection among dental health care workers. In fact, the increased use of barrier controls and related procedures has most likely resulted in reduced risk for transmission of other pathogens that are much more infectious than HIV.

It is important to note that there is very limited evidence available to date to suggest that dental procedures conducted with rigorous attention to infection control standards present a risk to the public or to the practitioner. There are of course issues of understanding of and compliance with proper infection control procedures, but numerous studies indicate that, with respect to changes mandated since the discovery of HIV, infection control in dentistry has improved markedly in recent years. Even so, infection control standards are constantly evolving in response to new information on specific infectious agents and newly available technologies.

Regularly updated training and education of dental personnel in infection control theory and procedure are especially necessary in regard to diseases such as HIV/AIDS for which new knowledge and information regularly become available. One useful resource for clinicians is the National HIV/AIDS Clinicians' Consultation Center in San Francisco, Calif. (Table 1; also see http://www.ucsf.edu/hivcntr/). This service provides open access to extensive and up-to-date training and educational materials. In addition, the service offers health care providers HIV clinical and drug information through individualized telephone consultation, as well as a telephone hotline for managing occupational exposure to HIV, HBV, and HCV (Table 1).

Two other recently identified emerging infectious diseases have been in the public eye. The acute respiratory disease SARS, which may have originated from civet cats in China, appears to have been at least temporarily contained after significant outbreaks in Asia and Canada. In those cases, isolation and quarantine of infected individuals and their contacts have effectively limited the spread of this highly contagious viral disease, which appears to resolve within a few weeks. Infection control measures concentrated on isolation of potentially infective foci and barrier protection of health care workers. To date, there are no published reports of implications of SARS for the practice of dentistry. Standard practice already suggests postponing dental treatment for contagious individuals, whatever the disease.

The keys to SARS prevention in health care settings (and in the community) are early detection of cases, containment of infection, protection of personnel, and hand hygiene. The dental office should implement infection protocols and administrative strategies to protect personnel and patients from SARS. Those strategies should include education of dental personnel about SARS. Since new information is likely to become available, periodic checks of the websites of the CDC (http://www.cdc.gov/ncidod/sars/index.htm), the World Health Organization (http://www.who.int/csr/sars/en/), and local or state health departments for the latest news about SARS epidemiological information in the community are recommended. Detailed information on appropriate modifications to patient medical history questionnaires is available on the ADA SARS website (Table 1).

The TSE diseases (commonly referred to as mad cow disease) present quite a different scenario and are having a serious impact on the practice of dentistry in Europe. A human TSE with specific neuropathologic and molecular characteristics that distinguish it from the sporadic form of Creutzfeldt-Jakob disease (CJD) has been associated with eating cattle products infected with a prion (transmissible variant protein) that causes the bovine form of TSE. The bovine disease is apparently due to ingestion of infected animal tissue present in certain types of animal feed products, and the human form, designated vCJD, presumably results from ingestion of infected animal tissue.

Although human TSE cases of bovine origin have not been identified in North America at the time of writing, the recent identification of bovine TSE in a Canadian beef herd suggests that there is little reason for a complacent attitude with regard to this disease. Most beef produced in

Canada is exported to the United States, and neither country has instituted the level of inspection at the herd or slaughterhouse level that has become standard in Europe. In addition, significant numbers of game animals (elk and deer) in several states are known to suffer from a "chronic wasting disease" that is closely related to the bovine TSE. This condition was first detected in confined herds east of the Rocky Mountains and has recently spread as far east as Wisconsin. A recent case report documented investigation of the deaths of three men from neurological illnesses that may have been related to the ingestion of wild game. While this and other reports have shown no clear connection between human degenerative neurological disease and bovine or game animal TSEs in North America, continued surveillance remains important to assess the possible risks.

To date, there have been no significant changes in infection control measures in North America in response to the possible threat posed by prion-associated diseases. In this context, the response of the European dental community may prove instructive. A major outbreak of bovine TSE began in the 1980s, vCJD in humans was first observed in 1996 and was found to be associated with the consumption of infected bovine tissue. The disease has primarily affected young adults. There have not been large numbers of deaths to date, but it is expected that the numbers will continue to rise due to the long incubation period of TSEs.

The following definitions have been suggested in Britain for screening patients who may be at risk and would require special attention in dental care. One obvious problem in trying to define such groups is the extended incubation period and slow onset of symptoms characteristic of vCJD.

- Patients diagnosed as having vCJD
- Patients suspected as having above
- Receipt of pituitary gland hormone (before August 1992 in the United Kingdom)
- Receipt of dura mater grafts (before August 1992 in the United Kingdom)
- Family history of vCJD, i.e., close blood line relatives

The following general protocols are suggested for treating at-risk patients:

- When a "risk-prone" procedure is carried out on a patient in the at-risk category, instruments and equipment involved must be incinerated.
- When the procedure is not considered to be risk prone, and it is not practicable to dispose of the instruments and equipment used, then these instruments should be thoroughly cleaned and decontaminated to remove as much organic debris as possible and then dispatched to a CSSD for sterilization in a porous load (high-vacuum) steam sterilizer, according to recommendations.
- Single-use instruments should be used when possible.
- In instances when single-use instruments cannot be used, they must be processed at the most stringent levels after use.

One of the more serious issues in dealing with TSEs is that infective prion particles can survive standard sterilization and disinfection techniques. This is the reason single-use instruments are recommended for certain patient groups. In instances when decontamination is necessary, extremely high levels of disinfection are required. Recommended for vCJD decontamination is use of a vacuum steam sterilizer (134 to 137°C for 18 min), followed by six successive cycles of 3 min each at 134 to 137°C. The recommended chemical disinfectant is 20,000 ppm of chlorine for 1 h, 2 M sodium hydroxide for 1 h or (for histological samples) 96% formic acid. It is suggested that all confirmed and suspected vCJD patients receive dental treatment in a hospital setting. Procedures involving neural tissue for at-risk patients should also be done in a hospital setting. In cases of suspected vCJD (including patients defined as at risk), dental instruments should be quarantined until disease status is known and incinerated if vCJD is confirmed. In confirmed cases, all instruments should be single use and incinerated after use.

In summary, the risk to public health posed by dental transmission of vCJD appears small compared to that for hospital surgery in similar scenarios. In all surgical procedures, the key consideration in minimizing any risk of transmission is ensuring the efficacy of instrument decontamination, with emphasis on cleaning the instruments, even though current methods cannot remove such risks completely.

Following consultation with the Spongiform Encephalopathy Advisory Committee and the Health and Safety Executive and risk assessment analysis, the Department of Health, United Kingdom, has concluded that the risks of transmission of infection from dental instruments are very low provided optimal standards of infection control and decontamination are maintained. There is no reason why patients at risk for or showing symptoms of vCJD or CJD should be refused routine dental treatment (http://www.doh.gov.uk/cjd/tseguidance/tseguidancepart4.pdf). The debate hinged on the fact that the oral tissue has not been shown to pose a risk of transmission of vCJD with the exception of the tonsillar tissue, which dentists are unlikely to abrade.

BIOFILMS IN DENTAL WATER LINES

Biofilms in dental unit water lines (DUWLs) and the potential of biofilm-derived organisms to cause nosocomial infections in dental patients and dental staff have been the subject of continuing study and considerable controversy in recent years. The unique feature of DUWLs is the capacity for rapid development of a biofilm on the dental water supply lines combined with the generation of potentially contaminated aerosols to which patients and dental staff are regularly exposed. Dental equipment such as retracting shut-off valves, antiretracting valves that tend to fail, or water-lines that are inaccessible contribute to a situation in which virtually every standard dental unit contains water with higher numbers of bacteria than the source water for the system. Typical DUWL biofilms are composed primarily of environmental bacteria and other microorganisms derived from the source system, either tap or bottled water. The majority of the organisms in the DUWL biofilm are harmless environmental species, but some dental units may harbor opportunistic respiratory pathogens, such as *P. aeruginosa*, *Mycobacterium* spp., and *Legionella* spp. The presence of organisms apparently derived from the oral cavity has been reported (Table 2). This is assumed to be due to backflow from dental apparatus.

TABLE 2 Microbes that may be present in dental unit water lines[a]

Microbe	Most likely source
Bacteria	
Achromotobacter	Water
Acinetobacter	Water
Actinomyces	Oral
Alcaligenes	Water
Bacillus	Water
Bacteroides	Oral
Flavobacterium	Water
Fusobacterium	Oral
Klebsiella	Water
Lactobacillus	Oral
Legionella	Water
Micrococcus	Water
Mycobacterium	Water
Nocardia	Oral
Ochromobacterium	Water
Pasteurella	Water
Peptostreptococcus	Oral
Pseudomonas	Water
Serratia	Water
Sphingomonas	Water
Staphylococcus	Oral
Streptococcus	Oral
Xanthomonas	Water
Fungi	
Penicillium	Water
Cladosporium	Water
Alternaria	Water
Scopulariopsis	
Protozoa	
Acanthamoeba	Water

[a]Compiled from various studies, not quantified.

Risk assessment analysis suggests a generally low level of hazard from biofilm organisms contaminating DUWLs on the respiratory health of both the dental team and patients. However, definitive case-controlled clinical studies to quantitate these risks have not been done. Nevertheless, to be in general compliance with public health standards for drinking water, the ADA suggests (and many jurisdictions mandate) that water from DUWLs contain fewer than 200 CFU/ml. This standard is relatively easily maintained in the reservoirs of DUWL systems by periodic disinfection and flushing. Higher levels of DUWL organisms are typically found upon initial flushing of lines following a period of inactivity (e.g., early morning).

Several studies have suggested that exposure to *Legionella* spp. from DUWL may pose a health risk to dental personnel due to the opportunistic nature of this organism, its apparent ability to thrive in the DUWL environment, and the chronic exposure of these workers to DUWL aerosols. In recent studies *Legionella* species were detected in over half of DUWL samples although *L. pneumophila* was present in less than 10%. Furthermore, over a third of dental personnel have been found to possess serum antibodies to *L. pneumophila*. Together, these studies suggest that chronic exposure to elevated levels of *Legionella* spp. may be a potential health risk for dental personnel and immune compromised patients.

Current recommendations by the ADA and CDA are summarized below, and are regularly updated on the websites listed in Table 1. At present, commercially available options for improving dental unit water quality are rather limited. They include the use of the following strategies:

- Independent DUWL water reservoirs
- Chemical treatment regimens for DUWL
- Daily draining and air purging regimens
- Point-of-use filters upstream of instruments

Procedural strategies for maintaining DUWL quality and minimizing risk of infection include the following:

- After each patient, discharge water and air for a minimum of 20 to 30 s from any dental device connected to the dental water system that enters a patient's mouth (e.g., handpieces, ultrasonic scalers, or air/water syringes).
- Consult with dental water line manufacturers to (i) determine suitable methods and equipment to obtain the recommended water quality and (ii) determine appropriate methods for monitoring the water to ensure quality is maintained.
- Consult with the dental unit manufacturer regarding the need for periodic maintenance of antiretraction mechanisms.

In summary, the quality of DUWLs is of considerable importance since patients and dental staff are regularly exposed to water and aerosols generated from this system. The significance of such exposure to patients and the dental staff is not well understood, and there is presently no convincing evidence of a public health problem from exposure to dental unit water. However, the goal of infection control is to minimize the risk from exposure to potential pathogens and to create a safe working environment in which to treat patients, and it is relatively simple to minimize the bacterial load in DUWLs. Several infection control methods and prevention strategies designed to reduce the impact of the biofilm on dental water contamination are currently available and suitable for use in general practice. These include in-line filtration systems, periodic flushing and disinfection regimens, and isolated sterile water reservoirs. Bacterial load in dental unit water can be kept at or below recommended guidelines for drinking water (fewer than 200 CFU/ml) by using a combination of readily available measures and strict adherence to maintenance protocols.

PRACTICAL APPLICATION OF INFECTION CONTROL MEASURES IN GENERAL DENTISTRY

Definitions of Terms

Sterilization is the process by which all living cells, viable spores, viruses, and viroids are either destroyed or removed from an object or habitat. A sterile object is totally free of viable microorganisms, spores, and other infectious agents. When sterilization is achieved by a chemical agent, the chemical is called a sterilant.

Disinfection is the killing, inhibition, or removal of microorganisms that may cause disease. Disinfecting agents, usually chemical, can be used on inanimate objects or on skin and mucosal membrane prior to medical intervention. A disinfectant does not necessarily sterilize an object because viable spores and a few microorganisms may remain.

Sanitization is closely related to disinfection. In sanitization, the microbial population is reduced to levels that are considered safe by public health standards. The inanimate object is usually cleaned as well as partially disinfected. For example, sanitizers are used to clean eating utensils in restaurants.

Problems Posed for Prevention of Cross-Infection in General Dental Practice

There are several characteristics of dental technique and the dental operatory itself that contribute to the overall risk of transmission of infection during the course of standard dental procedures. Even the smaller dental practices treat high numbers of patients, resulting in rapid turnover of patients. It is not uncommon for a single practitioner to schedule more than 25 patients per day. A wide variety and number of instruments are typically used, including high-speed instruments that generate aerosols. Many invasive minor surgical procedures result in breaches of epithelial tissue with associated bleeding. Depending on the oral health of the patient, dental hygiene treatment can also result in varying degrees of bleeding.

The practical (as well as the financial) burden of preventing transmission of infection rests with the practitioner. Overall success in minimizing risk to both dental practitioners and patients relies on the design and rigorous implementation of infection control policies and procedures that must be a seamless part of normal daily procedures involving all members of the staff. These procedures can be divided into categories as listed below:

   A. Personal protection for staff

   B. Physical design and written infection control policies, etc.

   C. Rigorous implementation of infection control policies

   D. Interactions with patients during treatment: importance of medical histories

Note that the risk to be assessed is associated with the dental procedure, not the patient; i.e., the procedure on a given patient may constitute a high or low risk of cross-infection (see "Universal Precautions" below).

   A. Personal protection for dental staff:
- Vaccinations as required, including HBV
- Glasses (for both operative and patient) and masks changed regularly
- Routine use of gloves and suitable protective clothing
- Training of staff and regular review of procedures
- Recording of accidents and incidents

   B. Physical design and written infection control policies, etc.:
- Design the operatory to allow zoning and ease of handwashing and disinfection of surfaces
- Choose equipment that is easily cleaned and disinfected
- Protect water lines

   C. Rigorous implementation of infection control policies:
- Sanitization (cleaning) of instruments
- Sterilization of instruments
- Disinfection of impressions
- Use of disposables
- Disinfection of surfaces
- Adequate aspiration and ventilation
- Safe disposal of waste

   D. Interactions with patients during treatment: importance of medical histories. While maintaining universal precautions such that infection control is driven by the dental procedures, it is necessary to take individual patient health issues into account when designing treatment. This is to ensure that patients at higher risk for nosocomial infections due to dental procedures are protected at a level that is appropriate for their situation. For instance, antibiotic prophylaxis to reduce the risk of endocarditis or bacteremia may be indicated for certain classes of patients, including those with implanted medical devices and those with a history of cardiac valvular diseases or disorders.

CONCLUSION

The threat posed by cross-infection in dentistry can be minimized by the application of good clinical dental practices; involving the whole dental team in safe practices; working in a safe, efficient environment; an assessment of the risk involved in the operative procedure on a given patient; and continuous reappraisal of the measures necessary to prevent cross-infection.

Universal Precautions

The following paragraphs provide an example of the specific procedures and behaviors required to implement universal precautions in the dental care setting. Similar procedures should be followed in smaller clinics and practices, with appropriate adaptation for the likely lack of the large centralized sterilization and dispensing facilities of an academic dental clinic.

HANDWASHING

Because health care workers can easily pick up and transmit organisms from patients as well as other contaminated environmental surfaces, handwashing is an essential first step in the practice of universal precautions. Most resident microorganisms found in the superficial layers of the skin are not highly virulent but may be responsible for some skin infections. Ordinary handwashing will remove organisms from skin; however, it may not remove them from around rings and under long fingernails. Make sure handwashing is effective by keeping nails cut short and well manicured. Rings, watches, bracelets, fingernail polish, or false fingernails may not be worn while treating patients. Handwashing or decontamination should take place before putting on gloves and at the intervals listed below:

1. After glove removal
2. Whenever hands or other skin surfaces are contaminated with blood or body fluids containing visible evidence of blood
3. Whenever hands or other skin surfaces inadvertently come in contact with contaminated surfaces or objects

Gloves should be changed between patients and before leaving the operatory.

Ordinary handwashing techniques

Ordinary handwashing should take place before examinations, restorative procedures, or suture removal. No special soap is required.

1. Lather hands well with soap and water; rub vigorously together for at least 10 s so that all surfaces are scrubbed. If hands are visibly soiled, rub the lather over them for longer than 10 s or wash and rinse hands two or three times.
2. Rinse hands thoroughly under a stream of cool or tepid water.
3. Blot hands dry with disposal paper towels.
4. Shut off the faucet using a clean paper towel to avoid contaminating hands with the faucet handle. (When exiting the restroom use a clean paper towel to grab onto the door handle and open the door.)
5. Apply hand lotion periodically throughout the day as needed.

Surgical scrub

A special antimicrobial product is needed anytime a surgical scrub is required.

1. Scrub hands and arms to the elbows with an antimicrobial liquid product for several minutes.
2. Rinse thoroughly to remove soap.
3. Dry hands on sterile towel.

Waterless hand products

In addition to handwashing, hand care is very important. Constant handwashing removes moisture from the skin. Depending on local regulations and practice, waterless hand rinse products may not be acceptable for use in the dental care setting. Alcohol-based rinse products are not a replacement for soap and water, but an acceptable alternative for hands visibly clean. These alcohol gel solutions can effectively destroy transient skin microbes, and they have the advantages of leaving the hands dry for gloving and containing emollients for skin care. Use emollient hand cream or lotion between washings. Avoid using products that contain petroleum or other oil emollients. These formulations weaken the latex barrier of the glove. In addition, moisturizing products should be applied sparingly between glovings to avoid excessive buildup of moisture under the gloves.

PROTECTIVE BARRIERS

Gloves

Wearing gloves protects health care workers by providing an extra barrier against the entry of microorganisms through any breaks in the skin. Gloves also protect patients from becoming infected with microorganisms that may be present on the hands of the health care worker. Wearing gloves, however, is no substitute for handwashing. Wearing gloves and handwashing may not provide enough protection if weeping dermatitis or open sores are present. Health care workers with these conditions must refrain from direct patient contact and handling patient care equipment until the condition has cleared up or should place a waterproof dressing over minor cuts and abrasions before donning gloves.

Gloves must be worn whenever hands are put into a patient's mouth or if a health care worker touches instruments, equipment, or surfaces that may be contaminated. A new pair of gloves should be used for every patient contact. A new pair of gloves should be worn during all cleaning and decontaminating procedures. Gloves used before, during, or after contact should not be worn outside the treatment areas.

The selection of gloves should be consistent with the procedure being performed. Three types of gloves are available:

1. Disposable examination gloves are used for procedures involving contact with the oral mucous membrane. These gloves are made of either vinyl or latex. There are no reported differences in the effectiveness of intact latex and intact vinyl when used as a barrier against contact with blood.
2. General purpose utility gloves are used when cleaning instruments, equipment, and contaminated surfaces. Rubber household gloves are suitable and can be decontaminated with iodophor and reused.
3. Sterile disposable gloves are used when sterility is necessary during either restorative or surgical procedures.

Neither sterile surgical nor examination gloves are designed for reuse. Washing these gloves may damage the gloves and actually cause "wicking," increasing the flow of liquid through undetectable holes in the gloves. General purpose utility gloves may be decontaminated and reused if intact. If a glove is torn, punctured, or becomes compromised, remove it immediately and dispose of it properly. Health care workers who are regularly exposed to latex products are at increased risk for latex hypersensitivity. Latex-free gloves are available as an alternative. Chemicals used in latex glove manufacturing include mercaptobenzothiazoles, thiurams, carbamates, guanidines, amine compounds, and phenolic compounds. Individuals vary in the type and degree of sensitivity to these materials. The following represent the types of reactions commonly experienced by individuals who are hypersensitive to latex:

Irritant contact dermatitis. This is the most prevalent dermal problem noted on the hands of health care workers. Contact dermatitis typically results from direct contact with chemical irritants. Frequent handwashing and improper drying technique of the hands may also contribute to the condition. Irritant contact dermatitis will usually appear as red, chapped, or dry skin. Occasionally fissures and vesicles will develop.

Delayed (type IV) hypersensitivity. This condition is an allergic contact dermatitis typically resulting from residue of the chemicals used in glove manufacturing as well as chemicals from handwashing products. The condition will usually appear as a red rash that forms on the back of the hand. Fissures and fluid-filled vesicles may also develop as part of the condition. The rash will continue to develop for up to 48 h after initial contact with the allergen.

Immediate (type I) hypersensitivity. This condition is typically the most serious dermal reaction. Type I hypersensitivity is an immunoglobulin E-mediated response that, when triggered by contact with latex gloves or other products containing latex, will begin affecting an exposed sensitive individual in 30 min or less. Symptoms can include redness, itching and swelling, asthma, conjunctivitis, and rhinitis. In extreme cases anaphylaxis may occur shortly after the initial exposure, leading to respiratory distress, low blood pressure, and potentially death.

Masks and glasses

There can be extensive spatter of blood and saliva during many dental procedures. Spattered material may enter the practitioner's eyes, nose, and mouth, where mucous membranes can provide easy entrance for microorganisms. Health care workers must wear a mask with protective glasses with side shields or a face shield. These protective barriers must be used for facial protection whenever blood or fluids contaminated by blood may be spattered (i.e., during all patient treatments, while cleaning instruments, while disposing of contaminated fluids). The face mask should be handled by touching the periphery (outside edges) only and should not contact the mouth while being worn.

A new face mask must be used for every patient. Always replace a face mask when it becomes wet during a single treatment. A wet mask may tend to collapse against the face and may not provide a barrier to microorganisms. In addition, face masks should not be pulled down around the chin or neck when not covering the mouth.

Protective glasses and side shields or a face shield must be worn during all dental procedures. Protective eyewear must be decontaminated with detergent and water between patients. If glasses need to be put down before they have been decontaminated, they should be placed on a disposable towel out of the way. Glasses should not be handled with unprotected hands until they have been decontaminated. Nondisposable eye-protective equipment should be washed with soap and water between patients and disinfected with a tuberculocidal "hospital disinfectant" that is registered with the U.S. Environmental Protection Agency (EPA).

Gowns

Impermeable gowns that cover clothing should be worn at all times during patient care and disposed of properly.

USE AND DISPOSAL OF NEEDLES AND OTHER SHARP INSTRUMENTS

Many dental instruments or items are sharp and can easily pierce or cut skin. These instruments include needles, scalpels, explorers, scalers, rotating burs, endodontic files, orthodontic wires, rotating pumice, and stone wheels. Contaminated sharp objects should be disposed in a puncture-resistant leakproof sharps container. Sharps should not be disposed in the regular trash. Disposable needles should not be recapped by hand, and needles should not be bent, broken, or otherwise manipulated by hand.

Important: One exception to the rule against recapping is aspirating syringes, which are not fully disposable and are regularly used in the dental practice setting. If the disposable needle is removed from the syringe without recapping it, injury can occur. Aspirating syringes should be recapped using the one-handed "scoop" technique or a resheathing device. A syringe should not be recapped by using both hands or by any other technique that involves moving the point of a used needle toward the body.

Infection Control Checklist

Before patient treatment:

- Ensure equipment is sterilized or disinfected.
- Put disposable cover in place.
- Place instruments on bracket table.
- Set out materials and mixing instruments.

During patient treatment:

- Treat all patients as potentially infectious.
- Wear new gloves for each patient and discard punctured gloves, wash hands.
- Wear masks and protective eyewear and clothing.
- Use rubber dam when appropriate and high-speed aspiration, ensure good ventilation.
- Only sheath needles using a device.

After patient treatment:

- Dispose sharps and segregate clinical waste.
- Clean and sterilize all instruments.
- Clean and disinfect all contaminated areas.
- Clean and disinfect impressions and dental appliances before sending them to the laboratory.
- Prepare the surgery for the next patient.

At the end of each session:

- Dispose all clinical waste.
- Clean and disinfect all work surfaces.
- Disinfect the aspirator, tubing, and spittoon.
- Clean the chair and the unit.

Sterilization of Instruments

The aim of sterilization of instruments and subsequent storage for use is to deliver sterile instruments to the chairside, thereby preventing the risk of cross-infection from patient to patient and between dental health care workers and patient by contaminated instruments. Several methods are available for sterilization of dental instruments, including the steam autoclave, the

TABLE 3 Advantages and disadvantages of sterilization methods

Method	Advantages	Disadvantages
Steam	Is quick and easy Allows sterile packaging Is very reliable Penetrates fabric- and paper-wrapped packs	May leave instruments wet, causing them to rust Requires packaging Damages plastics May dull certain sharp items
Chemical vapor	Is quick Can be used with packaged items Penetrates paper-wrapped packs Is very reliable Does not rust instruments Leaves instruments dry	Requires good ventilation Cannot handle large loads Does not penetrate fabric-wrapped packs Damages certain plastics Replacing special solution increases cost
Dry heat	Is cheap and easy Is very reliable Leaves instruments dry Does not rust instruments Requires little maintenance	Is slow, requires longer processing time Requires careful loading Damages plastics Melts or destroys some metal or solder joints Chars fabric
Chemical disinfectant/sterilant	Is cheap initially Can sterilize items that would be damaged by heat	Has a limited life Cannot be checked for effectiveness Protective clothing required during use Toxic fumes require special ventilation Cannot be used with packaged items Must be rinsed off with sterile water May corrode instruments

chemical vapor sterilizer ("chemiclave"), and the dry-heat oven. Of these, the autoclave has become the professional standard because of its reliability and relatively rapid cycling time, and its use is mandated in many states. Recommended operating conditions for the steam autoclave for heat-sensitive instruments are 121 to 124°C at 1.1 to 1.25 bar pressure for a minimum of 15 min, or 134 to 137°C at 2.1 to 2.3 bar pressure for a minimum of 3 min (ADA, 1996). These recommended parameters vary slightly, depending on the particular manufacturer's instructions.

Soiled instruments should be cleaned before sterilization, since the presence of blood and other debris can adversely affect steam penetration and thereby prevent the sterilization temperature from being reached on all surfaces. Appropriate hand- and eye-protective equipment should be used when handling contaminated instruments. It is generally recommended to use a two-stage presterilization procedure including soaking in a detergent solution followed by thorough cleaning. Appropriate steam-permeable wrapping material should be used to maintain sterility of instruments until use.

Quality assurance of the sterilization process is an absolute necessity in dentistry. In the case of the autoclave, regular monitoring is necessary to ensure that the instrument is operating at a temperature and pressure that will kill all microbes. While these instruments typically have pressure- and temperature-monitoring equipment, these numerical recordings are potentially subject to mechanical malfunction. Similarly, chemical indicators such as autoclave tape that changes color upon reaching a

TABLE 4 Surface disinfectants

Category	Advantages	Disadvantages
Synthetic phenolics (<3% [vol/vol], approx 1 h)	EPA registered Broad-spectrum activity Tuberculocidal Can be used on metal, glass, rubber and plastic Not readily neutralized by organic matter	Prepare fresh daily May degrade plastic and etch glass with prolonged exposure Difficult to rinse off certain materials
Quaternary ammonium compounds (concn and effective time vary with product and manufacturer)	EPA registered Bactericidal against gram-positive bacteria Low tissue toxicity	Not a tuberculocidal or virucidal (hydrophilic viruses) Inactivated by organic matter, soaps, and hard water Variable activity against gram-negative bacteria
Quaternary ammonium compounds/alcohol (concn and effective time vary with product and manufacturer)	EPA registered Broad-spectrum activity Tuberculocidal Pleasant odor Low tissue toxicity	Inactivated by organic matter, soaps, and hard water Film accumulation
Iodophors (450 ppm, 10 min on precleaned surface; otherwise up to several hours)	EPA registered Broad-spectrum activity Tuberculocidal	Prepare fresh daily May discolor some surfaces Inactivated by hard water
Hypochlorites (600–6,000 ppm [1:10–1:100 diluted bleach]); bacteria: minutes; fungi: up to 1 h	EPA registered Broad-spectrum activity Tuberculocidal Economical	Prepare fresh daily for most May degrade plastic and rubber Corrosive to metal Reduces activity by organic matter Skin and eye irritant
Alcohols (70% ethyl or 70% isopropyl; 20 min required for *Cryptosporidium*, much less for other organisms)	EPA registered Rapidly bactericidal Tuberculocidal Only slightly irritating Economical	May degrade some plastics, rubber, and metal Reduces activity by organic matter Rapid evaporating Not recommended for environmental surface cleaning

certain temperature are suitable for routine use but do not directly demonstrate autoclave performance.

Since it is impractical to test sterility by direct culturing of all instruments, a standardized direct method of functional performance testing using biological indicators has been developed. Biological indicators, generally spores of *Bacillus stearothermophilus* or *Bacillus subtilis*, depending on the type of sterilizer, provide the best assurance of sterility by challenging the sterilizer with quantifiable, highly resistant spores. Many states now mandate the use of these spore tests, which are available in several forms. Paper spore strips impregnated with 10^4 to 10^5 bacterial spores per strip are designed to be incubated in culture medium following sterilization treatment. This type of spore strip system is typically managed by a commercial or institutional sterilization monitoring service. A simpler method of spore testing is the spore test ampule such as ATTEST (3M Healthcare, St. Paul, Minn.), which is designed to be placed in the center of an autoclave load and incubated on removal. The ampule contains a glass vial of culture medium with a color indicator. After sterilization, the vial is "crushed" to join the growth media with the processed spore strip. The ampule is incubated for 48 h for a visual change readout. A color change to yellow indicates surviving spores and a positive result. This system, combined with a mini-incubator, can be

TABLE 5 Disposal of infected waste[a]

Waste	In the office	Out of the office
Needles Scalpels Broken glass Disposable syringes Intravenous tubing with needle attached	"Sharps" container	Dispose every 90 days at an approved landfill or via a commercial medical waste hauler
Orthodontic wire	"Sharps" container	Dispose with other office waste at any time
Liquid blood	Flush into sewer system	
Items dripping with blood or saliva	Options: (i) flush into sewer system or (ii) incinerate	
Blood- or saliva-soaked items	Regulated waste container	Dispose every 90 days (same as sharps)
Pathological waste, unfixed tissue	Autoclave	Label as "Decontaminated Medical Waste" and dispose with other office waste
Teeth	Options: (i) Return to patient (ii) Incinerate (iii) Regulated waste container (iv) Autoclave	 Dispose every 90 days (same as sharps) Label as "Decontaminated Medical Waste" and dispose with other office waste
Items stained with blood Items moist with saliva Gloves, masks, etc. Patient disposable items not soaked or caked with blood or saliva	Office waste container	Dispose with other office waste in the dumpster or garbage can

[a]This table summarizes the handling, discarding, and disposal of medical waste from the dental office in compliance with the Medical Waste Regulatory Act and the Bloodborne Pathogens Standard.

TABLE 6 Hepatitis B virus postexposure management

Status of exposed worker[a]	Treatment when source is found to be:		
	HBsAg positive	**HBsAg negative**	**Unknown or not tested**
Unvaccinated	1. Initiate HBV series. 2. Worker should receive a single dose of hepatitis B immune globulin (HBIG) as soon as possible and within 24 h, if possible.	Initiate HBV series	Initiate HBV series
Previously vaccinated[b]			
Known responder	Test exposed worker for anti-HBs: 1. If adequate,[c] no treatment 2. If inadequate, HBV booster dose	No treatment	No treatment
Known nonresponder	1. Worker should receive two doses of HBIG; second dose is administered 1 mo after the first. or 2. Worker should receive one dose HBIG plus one dose hepatitis B vaccine.	No treatment	If known high-risk source, may treat worker as if source were HBsAg positive
Response unknown	Test exposed worker for anti-HBs: 1. If inadequate, one dose of HBIG plus HBV booster dose 2. If adequate, no treatment	No treatment	Test exposed worker for anti-HBs: 1. If inadequate, HBV booster dose 2. If adequate, no treatment

[a]Once an exposure has occurred, the blood of the individual from whom exposure occurred should be tested for hepatitis B surface antigen (HBsAg) and antibody to human immunodeficiency virus (HIV antibody). The information given in this table is based on recommendations from Centers for Disease Control and Prevention, Updated U.S. Public Health Service guidelines for the management of occupational exposures to HBV, HCV, and HIV and recommendations for postexposure prophylaxis, *Morb. Mortal. Wkly. Rep.* **45**:1–42, 2001.

[b]Exposed worker has already been vaccinated against hepatitis B.

[c]Adequate anti-HBs is >10 mIU.

used in an individual practice. A drawback to all spore test systems is the delay of 12 to 48 h before test results can be read, and longer if an off-site monitoring service is used. However, the spore test system remains the current standard of practice for quality assurance of sterilization.

The information listed above can provide a guide for implementation of a standardized sterilization protocol for the individual dental practice. Specific written protocols should be in place as an integral part of a standardized and documented infection control program. The protocol should include written procedures on how to operate the instrument; how to carry out a daily test; what information must be recorded; and what to do if there is a failed sterilization cycle. The responsible user or administrator must ensure that all operators are fully trained; daily tests are carried out correctly; all faults are recorded; the autoclave/sterilizer is properly maintained; and adequate sterilization records are kept.

The advantages and drawbacks of sterilization procedures available to the dental community are given in Table 3. In the autoclave steam is heated above the boiling point of water by applying pressure. Steam then denatures proteins, ultimately leading to cell death. Autoclaves have a large capacity; however, items damaged by water or that will rust or corrode should not be sterilized by this method. Dry-heat ovens also kill by protein denaturation; however, in the absence of water, this process is less efficient. Hence killing by hot air requires at least 160°C for over an hour. The chemclave uses a mixture of chemicals, often primarily formalde-

TABLE 7 Public Health Service recommendations for chemoprophylaxis after occupational exposure to HIV, by type of exposure and source material[a]

Type of exposure	Source material[b]	Antiretroviral prophylaxis[c]	Antiretroviral regimen[d]
Percutaneous	Blood[e]		
	Highest risk	Recommend	ZDV plus 3TC plus IDV
	Increased risk	Recommend	ZDV plus 3TC, plus IDV[f]
	No increased risk	Offer	
	Fluid containing visible blood or other potentially infectious fluid,[g] or tissue	Offer	ZDV plus 3TC
	Other body fluid (e.g., urine)	Not offer	ZDV plus 3TC
Mucous membrane	Blood	Offer	ZDV plus 3TC, plus IDV[f]
	Fluid containing visible blood or other potentially infectious fluid,[g] or tissue	Offer	ZDV, plus 3TC
	Other body fluid (e.g., urine)	Not offer	
Skin increased risk[h]	Blood	Offer	ZDV plus 3TC, plus IDV[e]
	Fluid containing visible blood or other potentially infectious fluid,[g] or tissue	Offer	ZDV plus 3TC
	Other body fluid (e.g., urine)	Not offer	

[a]The information given in this table is based on recommendations from Centers for Disease Control and Prevention, Updated U.S. Public Health Service guidelines for the management of occupational exposures to HBV, HCV, and HIV and recommendations for postexposure prophylaxis, *Morb. Mortal. Wkly. Rep.* **45:**1–42, 2001.

[b]Any exposure to concentrated HIV (e.g., in a research laboratory or production facility) is treated as percutaneous exposure to blood at the highest risk.

[c]Recommend: postexposure prophylaxis (PEP) should be recommended to the exposed worker with counseling. Offer: PEP should be offered to the exposed worker with counseling. Not offer: PEP should not be offered because these are not occupational exposures to HIV.

[d]Regimens: zidovudine (ZDV), 200 mg three times a day; lamivudine (3TC), 150 mg two times a day; indinavir (IDV), 800 mg three times a day (if IDV is not available, saquinavir may be used, 600 mg three times a day). Prophylaxis is given for 4 weeks.

[e]Highest risk: both larger volume of blood (e.g., deep injury with large-diameter hollow needle previously in source patient's vein or artery, especially involving an injection of source patient's blood) and blood containing a high titer of HIV (e.g., source with acute retroviral illness or end-stage of AIDS; viral load measurement may be considered, but its use in relation to PEP has not been evaluated). Increased risk: either exposure to larger volume of blood or blood with a high titer of HIV (e.g., solid suture needle injury from source patient with asymptomatic HIV infection).

[f]Possible toxicity of additional drug may not be warranted.

[g]Includes semen, vaginal secretions, and cerebrospinal, synovial, pleural, peritoneal, and amniotic fluids.

[h]For skin, risk is increased for exposures involving a high titer of HIV, prolonged contact, an extensive area, or an area in which the skin integrity is visibly compromised. For skin exposures without increased risk, the risk for drug toxicity outweighs the benefit of PEP.

hyde, that are volatilized by heating. The unit operates under pressures of 20 to 25 psi, which produces a temperature of 130°C and allows sterilization in 20 to 30 min. Chemical sterilants are generally alkylating agents that can denture proteins without the presence of water. Chemicals such as ethylene oxide, formaldehyde, and β-propiolactone can all be used for sterilization; however, they are very toxic to humans.

Disinfecting agents (Table 4) are useful when sterilization is not practicable or cannot be achieved, such as large areas of floor or benches, or large pieces of equipment. It is also useful for skin and mucosal surfaces. Disinfectants can be protein denaturants (e.g., alcohols and phenolics), oxidizing agents (e.g., halogens), or active against lipid bilayer membranes (e.g., quaternary ammonium compounds). UV light can also be used to disinfect bench tops.

Methods for the correct disposal of biohazardous waste are given in Table 5. In the event that infection control procedures break down and exposure to HBV- or HIV-infected material is suspected, postexposure management is outlined in Tables 6 and 7.

KEY POINTS

Dental professionals are exposed to a wide variety of microorganisms in the blood and saliva of patients. These microorganisms may cause infectious diseases such as the common cold, influenza, pneumonia, tuberculosis, herpes, hepatitis, transmissible spongiform encephalopathy, and acquired immune deficiency syndrome. The use of effective infection control procedures and universal precautions in the dental office and the dental laboratory will prevent cross-contamination that could put dentists, dental office staff, dental technicians, and patients at risk for infection.

Infection control in dentistry, as in other health professions, involves application of a risk management decision-making process, including risk identification, assessment, or analysis, and implementation of design and procedures for risk control. Cross-infection is typically defined as the transmission of infectious agents among patients and staff within the clinical environment.

Risk control in dentistry uses a single-tier approach in which all patients are treated as though they are a potential source of infectious pathogens. This single-tier approach is known as universal precautions. It applies the concept of risk to the procedure, not the patient. Emphasis should be placed on consistent adherence to recommended infection control strategies, including hand hygiene, the use of protective barriers, appropriate methods of sterilization or disinfection, and vaccination when possible.

Possible sources of infection in the dental care setting include patients with infectious disease (e.g., influenza, measles, or tuberculosis); patients in the prodromal or convalescent stage of infection (e.g., herpes simplex virus); healthy (or asymptomatic) carriers of disease-causing organisms (e.g., *S. pyogenes, N. meningitidis,* and

H. influenzae); and environmental sources such as airborne organisms or biofilms in waterlines or on equipment or instruments.

Routes of spread include airborne such as through dust or aerosols; contact including person to person or with contaminated equipment or fluids; and parenteral through accidental puncture with needles, and so forth.

Sterilization is the process by which all living cells, viable spores, viruses, and viroids are either destroyed or removed from an object or habitat. A sterile object is totally free of viable microorganisms, spores, and other infectious agents.

Sterilization can be achieved by physical or chemical means. Physical methods include the steam autoclave, the hot-air oven, and the chemiclave. Chemical sterilants include ethylene oxide and formaldehyde.

Disinfection is the killing, inhibition, or removal of microorganisms that may cause disease. Disinfecting agents, usually chemical, can be used on inanimate objects or on skin and mucosal membrane prior to medical intervention. A disinfectant does not necessarily sterilize an object because viable spores and a few microorganisms may remain.

Sanitization is closely related to disinfection. In sanitization, the microbial population is reduced to levels that are considered safe by public health standards. The inanimate object is usually cleaned as well as partially disinfected. For example, sanitizers are used to clean eating utensils in restaurants.

ACKNOWLEDGMENTS

We thank Dennis Turner, Assistant Dean for Patient Services, University of Michigan School of Dentistry, for helpful discussions on infection control practices and issues.

FURTHER READING

Cottone, J. A., G. T. Terezhalmy, and J. A. Molinari. 1996. *Practical Infection Control in Dentistry.* Williams & Wilkins, Media, Pa.

Index

mediators of, 28
Porphyromonas gingivalis and, 266–267
Prevotella intermedia and, 278–279
and systemic disease, 372–375
Influenza A virus, 296–297
Innate immunity. *See* Immune system, innate immunity
Insertional mutagenesis, 163–166, 176–178
Insertion-duplication mutagenesis, 176
Instrument sterilization, 441–445
Integration vectors, 159–163
Integrons, in antibiotic resistance, 411–412, 418–419
Interferon, 27, 42, 330–331
Interleukin (IL)
induction of acute-phase proteins by, 27
in mucosal defenses, 367
in periodontitis, 225, 284–285, 287, 293
Intracellular defenses against viruses, 322
Intraoral devices, for caries research, 241
Intravenous drug users, hepatitis B infection in, 316
Isogenic mutants, 139, 145–146
Iteron-regulated replicons, 147
Itraconazole, 345
IVET (in vivo expression technology), 180
IVIAT (in vivo induced antigen technology), 180–182

J

Jenner, Edward, 326
Juvenile periodontitis. *See* Localized aggressive periodontitis

K

Ketoconazole, 345
Knockout of genes, 145–146, 159–160

L

Lactobacillus spp., in cariogenesis, 21, 233, 239, 252
Lactoferrin, 70, 212–213
Lactoferrin-binding proteins, 274
LAP. *See* Localized aggressive periodontitis
Latex hypersensitivity, 439
Lead exposure, and enamel formation, 238
Legionella spp., 434
Leukotoxin, 198, 268, 273, 283, 293
Lincosamide antibiotics, 387
Linezolid, 386, 413–414
Linnaeus, Carl, 4
Lipopolysaccharide (LPS)
of *Actinobacillus actinomycetemcomitans*, 269

of *Eikenella corrodens*, 276
pathogenetic effects of, 9–10, 293, 372
of *Porphyromonas gingivalis*, 9, 263
recognition of, by host cells, 367
Lipoteichoic acids, 10–12
Lithium, antibiotic interactions with, 404
Localized aggressive periodontitis (LAP)
Actinobacillus actinomycetemcomitans and, 193, 198–199, 255, 256, 260
antibody response in, 255, 285
neutrophil function in, 281–282
plaque microbiota in, 58
Localized juvenile periodontitis. *See* Localized aggressive periodontitis
LPS. *See* Lipopolysaccharide
Lymph nodes, 29–31
Lymphocytes. *See also* B lymphocytes; T lymphocytes
antigen recognition by, 37–39
function of, 28–29, 44
in initiation of adaptive immune response, 39, 41–42
intraepithelial, 213–214, 217
mucosal, 213–214, 216–217
recirculation of, 31, 32
types of, 29
Lymphoid system, 28–31
Lysis of bacteria, for DNA recovery, 76–77
Lysozyme, salivary, 69, 211–212

M

Macrolide antibiotics, 388, 397, 399, 404
Macrophage chemoattractant protein, 367
Macrophages
in cell-mediated immunity, 43
in initiation of adaptive immune response, 39, 42, 43
in innate immunity, 23, 25, 322
Mad cow disease. *See* Transmissible spongiform encephalopathies
Major histocompatibility complex, 38, 292, 322–324. *See also* Human leukocyte antigens
Malodor, oral, 117
Masks, 439–440
Mast cells, in innate immunity, 24, 25
Materia alba, 54
MBC (minimal bacteriocidal concentration), 392, 393
Mechanical forces, and plaque formation, 52
Membranes, bacterial. *See* Cytoplasmic membrane
Metronidazole
adverse effects of, 397, 404

resistance to, 401, 413
spectrum of, 390–391, 397, 399
MIC (minimal inhibitory concentration), 392, 393
Micafungin, 340
Mice
caries research in, 220, 241–242
periodontal disease research in, 288–289
Miconazole, 345
Microaerophilic bacteria, 19, 84
Microarrays, for DNA analysis, 80–81, 183–185, 251–252
Microbial physiology, 107–124
acid tolerance, 52, 109–114, 250
acid-base cycling in oral cavity, 108–109, 114
alkali production and tolerance, 109–110, 114–115
in biofilms, 121–123
oxygen levels and oxidation-reduction potentials in plaque, 116–117
oxygen metabolism and oxidative damage, 117–121
oxygen sources, 115
Microscopy of bacteria, 83–84
Minimal bacteriocidal concentration (MBC), 392, 393
Minimal inhibitory concentration (MIC), 392, 393
Molds, 334
Molecular analysis techniques, 76–83, 138–141. *See also* Polymerase chain reaction; Recombinant DNA technology
and bacterial classification, 74–75, 83
DNA hybridization assays, 80–81, 173, 183–185
DNA recovery from samples, 76–77
ribosomal 16S gene cloning and sequence analysis, 74–75, 81–83
Molecular biology, 169–186. *See also* Genetic transfer
gene expression studies, 169–175
gene function studies, 138–141, 175–178
gene regulation studies, 178–182
genomics, 126, 182–183
proteomics, 185–186
transcriptomics, 183–185
Molecular techniques in cariogenesis research, 247–252
Molecular techniques in population genetics research, 195–197
Monobactam antibiotics, 383, 384
Mosaic genes, 127, 129
Motility, in virulence of *Treponema denticola*, 274
Mucins
and bacterial clearance, 66–67
complexes formed by, 65
as host defense, 206–207
in saliva, 209–210